Ultrasound in Cardiology

Ultrasound in Cardiology

EDITED BY

Kurt J. G. Schmailzl

Medical Director
Department of Cardiology and Pulmonology
Ruppiner Hospital, Neuruppin, Germany

AND

Oliver Ormerod

Consultant Cardiologist,
John Radcliffe Hospital, Oxford, UK

ENGLISH TRANSLATION BY
Suzyon O'Neal Wandrey

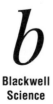

Blackwell Science

© 1994 by Blackwell Science
Editorial Offices:
238 Main Street, Cambridge, Massachusetts 02142, USA
Osney Mead, Oxford OX2 0EL
25 John Street, London WC1N 2BL
23 Ainslie Place, Edinburgh EH3 6AJ
54 University Street, Carlton, Victoria 3053, Australia

Other Editorial Offices

Arnette Blackwell SA
1, rue de Lille
75007 Paris
France

Blackwell Wissenschafts-Verlag GmbH
Kurfürstendamm 57
10707 Berlin
Germany

Blackwell MZV
Feldgasse 13
1238 Wien
Austria

First published in English 1994

First published in German 1994 by
Blackwell Wissenschafts-Verlag, Berlin

Printed in Germany

DISTRIBUTORS

Marston Book Services Ltd
PO Box 87
Oxford OX2 0DT
(*Orders*: Tel: 0865 791155
Fax: 0865 791927
Telex: 837515)

USA
Blackwell Science, Inc.
238 Main Street
Cambridge, MA 02142
(*Orders*: Tel: 800 759-6102
617 876-7000)

Canada
Times Mirror Professional Publishing, Ltd
130 Flaska Drive
Markham, Ontario L6G 1B8
(*Orders*: Tel: 800 268-4178
416 470-6739)

Australia
Blackwell Science Pty Ltd
54 University Street
Carlton, Victoria 3053
(Orders: Tel: 03 347-5552)

A catalogue record for this title is available from the
British Library

ISBN 0-86542-802-6

No one can learn echocardiography from books alone, just as no adequate practical training can be conveyed by courses in which seven or more trainees must share one echocardiograph. Nonetheless, a multitude of monographs on cardiac ultrasound imaging exist, some of them good ones and some less good. Apart from the fact that each author chooses different focal points, the less good ones economize on pictorial material, trying to make up for this with mere verbal descriptions. They also tend to abstain from explanatory schematic diagrams, provide only surrogate physiological discourses instead of explanations of an echocardiographic phenomenon, and replace the systematology by which a syndrome can be described echocardiographically by patchwork of individual findings scattered throughout the book. The sheer multitude of "echo" books already indicates the deficiency. With the knowledge that, in order to obtain a standard imaging view, the transducer must be positioned in the fourth intercostal space in the left parasternal region of the ideal patient, the only experience to be gained is that the ideal patient is seldom found on the examination table.

In addition to relating facts, a book should above all convey a critical sense of the potentials and limitations of a given method. This implies the necessity to examine emerging problems from more than one perspective. We therefore arrive at different solutions that may not always be in agreement. A book dealing with an imaging technique such as echocardiography must explain typical features of disease and show them in various stages of development and from different imaging views. This, exactly, is the endeavor of the present volume.

This book is designed as a manual and atlas for most applications of ultrasound in cardiovascular medicine. I felt that a multidisciplinary approach would be the most suitable way to realize this goal. In contrast to other volumes, this manual includes the practical demands of surgery, intensive care medicine, interventional cardiology and radiology using ultrasound techniques. Each major chapter comprises sections addressing the answers the user wishes to find and the consequences of those answers. In this respect, the present volume is not just another how-to-do-it. Sources of error and pitfalls are systematically discussed and each chapter discussed lists both the advantages and the disadvantages of the ultrasound-based techniques available today.

Any suitable approach promises to be an exchange of paradigms in search of an intelligent noninvasive or minimally invasive method of quantifying cardiovascular diseases. The technological developments that have led to the convergence of seven branches of echocardiography (3D, ultrasound-based tissue characterization and acoustic microscopy, stress echocardiography, transesophageal echocardiography, intravascular sonography, and intracoronary Doppler) in the acquisition of heretofore inaccessible morphological and functional information illustrate the new role of cardiac ultrasound imaging. Although findings seldom point unequivocally to a given diagnosis this is not necessarily bad news for the physician; echocardiography is of use in almost all cardiological diagnoses. Echocardiographic findings have led to new descriptive terms, such as "asymmetric septal hypertrophy" – terms that are now synonymous with the disease itself. New echocardiographic techniques have opened doors to a quantitative cardiology which had been closed for a long time and have made it possible to study and modify individual factors involved in the development and course of disease in the difficult search for the causality in medicine.

The first section on methodology describes the fundamental principles, examination procedures, and basic measurement and assessment tasks of conventional echocardiography and Doppler. It also describes new computer-assisted techniques for cardiac ultrasound diagnosis and interventional echocardiography, the role of cardiac ultrasound imaging in intensive care and emergency medicine, and the perspectives of cardiac ultrasound treatment.

The second section on nosology describes the use of cardiac ultrasound imaging techniques in the diagnosis and quantitation of cardiovascular disease, and discusses related sources of error and follow-up and treatment considerations. Major chapters contain a section that critically assesses the results of echocardiography, then compares the results to those of complementary diagnostic techniques. These chapters also contain a customized quick reference program with a schematic diagram (flow chart) of the diagnostic therapeutic decision-making process.

Main emphases ensued on the one hand from the principal conviction that the method criticism and decision-making should be essential elements of the learning process. On the other hand, common problems came to the fore; problems that often arise in the assessment of valvular heart diseases and ischaemic syndromes were also a main focal point. Even though it is impossible to achieve completeness, no important areas of application should be omitted. With this in mind, a major chapter on pediatric echocardiography was integrated into the book. Even though echocardiography is rapidly advancing, we have made the utmost effort to report and evaluate the latest research findings.

Beside the information that cardiac ultrasound imaging can provide, this book will help the reader to understand something of the revolution that "echo" has brought to cardiology. It has now become established as a supplementary tool to the eyes and ears of the physician.

Kurt J.G. Schmailzl, M.D., Ph.D.

It is not a mere obligation, but a pleasure, for me to express my appreciation to all the people who have helped to make this book possible. I would first like to thank my wife Kirsten, and also Helmut Holtermann, who untiringly processed my thousands of suggestions for improvement of and changes in the graphic illustrations; Dr. Antje Jaensch, D.V.M., and Manuela Klein, M.A., without whose editorial assistance many discrepancies and typographical errors would have remained undetected; and Rainer Kusche, whose infallible eye oversaw the production of every page in each step of the printing process.

Last but not least I would like to mention the enthusiasm of Drs. Karin Förster, D.V.M., and Jürgen Neumann, M.D., from the Schering Corporation, Dr. Jürgen Warnecke, M.D., from G. Pohl-Boskamp GmbH & Co., and Markus Miniböck, formerly of Toshiba Medical Systems, whose assistance went above and beyond superficial commercial interests.

Those familiar with the medical publishing business have undoubtedly heard of the spiritus rector, Dr. Axel Bedürftig, M.D., and know of his loyalty, great sensitivity, and tenacity.

Kurt J.G. Schmailzl, M.D., Ph.D.

Prof. Amer Al-Zarka, M.D.
University of California, Irvine
Cardiology Division
101 City Drive South
Orange, CA 92668
USA

Prof. Naoki Asada
Okayama University
Dept. of Information Technology
1-1, Tsushima Naka 3-Chome
Okayama 700
Japan

Maria Ayuso
Istituto di Malattie
Dell´ Apparato Cardiovascolare
Piazza Guilio Cesare
70124 Bari
Italy

PD Dr. Rudolf Blasini
I. Medizinische Klinik und
Poliklinik der TU München
Klinikum rechts der Isar
Ismaninger Straße 22
81675 München
Germany

PD Dr. rer. nat. Rüdiger Brennecke
Johannes-Gutenberg-Universität Mainz
II. Medizinische Klinik und Poliklinik
Langenbeckstraße 1
55131 Mainz
Germany

P. Anthony N. Chandraratna, M.D.
University of Southern California
School of Medicine
Division of Cardiology
2025 Zonal Avenue, GH Room 7621
Los Angeles, CA 90033
USA

Prof. Denton A. Cooley, M.D.
Surgeon-in-Chief
Texas Heart Institute
Department of Adult Cardiology
P.O. Box 20345
Houston, Texas 77225-0345
USA

Dr. med. Karl-Matthias Deppermann
Universitätsklinikum Benjamin Franklin
Medizinische Klinik und Poliklinik
Abt. für Innere Medizin mit Schwerpunkt
Kardiologie und Pneumologie
Hindenburgdamm 30
12203 Berlin
Germany

Dr. med. Christian Detter
Ludwig-Maximilian-Universität München
Klinikum Großhadern
Herzchirurgische Klinik
Marchioninistraße 15
81377 München
Germany

Prof. Shigeru Eiho
Kyoto University
Dept. of Engineering
Division of Applied Systems Science
Yoshida Honcho, Sakyo-Ku
Kyoto 606-01
Japan

Prof. Dr. med. Raimund Erbel
Abt. Medizinische Kardiologie
Universitätsklinikum Essen
Hufelandstraße 55
45147 Essen
Germany

Dipl.-Phys. Bernd Gaßmann
Krankenhausbetrieb von Berlin-Pankow
Akademisches Lehrkrankenhaus
Institut für Klinische Ultraschalldiagnostik
Hobrechtsfelder Chaussee 96
13122 Berlin
Germany

Prof. Dr. med. Gerd Hausdorf
Charité
Kinderkardiologie
Schumannstraße 20 – 21
10098 Berlin
Germany

Dr. Sabino Iliceto
Istituto di Malattie
Dell´ Apparato Cardiovascolare
Piazza Guilio Cesare
70124 Bari
Italy

Prof. Dr. med. Reiner Körfer
Direktor der Klinik für
Thorax- und Kardiovaskularchirurgie
Herz- und Diabeteszentrum NRW
Universitätsklinikum der
Ruhr-Universität Bochum
Georgstraße 11
32545 Bad Oeynhausen
Germany

Dr. med. Heinrich Körtke
Klinik für Thorax- und Kardiovaskularchirurgie
Herz- und Diabeteszentrum NRW
Universitätsklinikum der
Ruhr-Universität Bochum
Georgstraße 11
32545 Bad Oeynhausen
Germany

Kirsten van Kooten
Immenhof 1
21217 Seevetal
Germany

Dr. med. Irmtraut Kruck
Asperger Straße 48
71634 Ludwigsburg
Germany

Prof. Michiyoshi Kuwahara
Osaka Sangyo University
3-1-1, Nakagaito, Daito-shi
Osaka 574
Japan

Cataldo Memmola
Istituto di Malattie
Dell´ Apparato Cardiovascolare
Universita Degli Studi Di Bari
Piazza Guilio Cesare
70124 Bari
Italy

PD Dr. med. Susanne Mohr-Kahaly
Johannes-Gutenberg-Universität Mainz
II. Medizinische Klinik und Poliklinik
Langenbeckstraße 1
55131 Mainz
Germany

Venanzio F. Napoli
Istituto di Malattie
Dell´ Apparato Cardiovascolare
Universita Degli Studi Di Bari
Piazza Guilio Cesare
70124 Bari
Italy

Prof. Dr. med. Bruno Reichart
Direktor der Herzchirurgischen Klinik
Ludwig-Maximilian-Universität München
Klinikum Großhadern
Marchioninistraße 15
81377 München
Germany

Prof. Paolo Rizzon
Direttore
Istituto di Malattie
Dell´ Apparato Cardiovascolare
Universita Degli Studi Di Bari
Piazza Guilio Cesare
70124 Bari
Italy

Dr. Dr. med. Kurt J.G. Schmailzl
Chefarzt der Medizinischen Klinik A
Schwerpunkt Kardiologie/Pneumologie
Ruppiner Klinikum GmbH
16816 Neuruppin
Germany

Jonathan M. Tobis, M.D.
University of California, Irvine
Cardiology Division
101 City Drive South
Orange, CA 92668
USA

Kostantinus Valsamis
Istituto di Malattie
Dell´ Apparato Cardiovascolare
Universita Degli Studi Di Bari
Piazza Guilio Cesare
70124 Bari
Italy

James Wallis, M.D.
University of California, Irvine
Cardiology Division
101 City Drive South
Orange, CA 92668
USA

Prof. Susan Wilansky, M.D.
Texas Heart Institute
Department of Adult Cardiology
P.O. Box 20345
Houston, Texas 77225-0345
USA

Dr. med. Ursula Wilkenshoff
Universitätsklinikum Benjamin Franklin
Abt. Kardiologie/Station 006
Hindenburgdamm 30
12203 Berlin
Germany

Robert F. Wilson, M.D.
University of Minnesota
Dept. of Medicine
Box 508 UMHC
420 Delaware St. SE
Minneapolis, MN 55455
USA

Part One

FUNDAMENTAL PRINCIPLES
OF CARDIAC ULTRASOUND DIAGNOSIS

In addition to the classical methods of diagnosis, imaging techniques such as ultrasound are gaining increasing influence in medical diagnosis. In contrast with other imaging techniques such as x-ray, computed tomography, and magnetic resonance imaging, ultrasound does not fall under the domain of radiology. Instead, due to its unique capabilities, ultrasound has gained a secure position in each respective medical department.

The outstanding features of ultrasound are its noninvasive nature and repeatability. Static ultrasound recordings permit assessment of the morphology and the topographic anatomy at a given moment in time. *Real-time* imaging technology has now made it possible to assess dynamic processes. Doppler echocardiography, based on the principle of Doppler effect, permits assessment of blood flow characteristics.

In contrast with other medical imaging techniques, ultrasound is an extremely interactive technique. The operator must adjust numerous instrument controls to fit the individual examination conditions. There are no "standard control settings" that ensure optimal image quality.

For optimal imaging in a variety of individual examination conditions, the echocardiograph must have adjustable controls. The operator must interact dynamically with both the machine and the patient during the examination. In order to properly identify artifacts and errors in imaging, the physician must have good background knowledge of the physical principles of ultrasound.

Any book on ultrasound diagnosis must therefore provide at least a brief description of the physical principles of ultrasound. In this section, we will examine the physical and technical aspects of echocardiography. The purpose is not to derive theoretical formulas, but to explain important principles of ultrasound wave transmission, signal processing, and standardization of echocardiographic techniques.

Semiquantitative assessments can be derived from originally qualitative ultrasound diagnostic data by using a combination of hydrodynamic techniques and two-dimensional echocardiographic measurements. One must understand how these models function in order to properly appreciate the results.

A good understanding of the physical principles of ultrasound is the essential basis for maintaining quality results and for developing future techniques.

1. **Fundamentals of Echocardiography**
1.1 **Physical Principles of Conventional Echocardiography**

Conventional echocardiographs have integrated capabilities for two-dimensional and *M-mode* echocardiography. The specifics of ultrasound wave propagation, methods of data acquisition, the physical limitations of ultrasound waves, and their impact on conventional techniques of cardiac ultrasound diagnosis will be discussed. Lastly, the most prominent sources of error in interpretation of ultrasound images will be presented and discussed.

M-mode was the first ultrasound technique to find application in cardiology. In 1949 Edler and Hertz became the first investigators to ultrasonically describe the human mitral valve.

Ultrasound

Sound is a mechanical wave that is propagated through elastic media such as solids, liquids, and gases. The propagated wave has a characteristic volume, called the *sonic field.*

Sound waves are physically described in terms of wavelength λ (lambda), frequency f, and the propagation velocity c at which they travel through the respective medium. The relation of these three variables is described by the following formula:

$c = \lambda \times f.$

Energy is transported with each wave. Various sonic field parameters can be used to describe this energy transport.

Since the ultrasound frequency range is within the acoustic spectrum, the physics of ultrasound falls under the field of acoustics. The total acoustic frequency range is subdivided into different frequency bands relative to the human hearing range.

Acoustic Designation	Frequency Range	Example
Infrasound	$0\ \text{Hz} < f < 16\ \text{Hz}$	Seismic waves
Audible sound	$16\ \text{Hz} < f < 20\ \text{kHz}$	Orchestral sounds
Ultrasound	$20\ \text{kHz} < f < 10\ \text{GHz}$	**Dolphins and bats analyze ultrasound signals for spatial orientation**
Hypersound	$10\ \text{GHz} < f < 1\ \text{THz}$	Technical applications Acoustic microscopy

The Production of Ultrasound

For diagnostic purposes, ultrasound is conventionally produced using the inverse piezoelectric effect. Other techniques used in extradiagnostic areas such as therapy and surgery will not be discussed here.

The *piezoelectric effect*, upon which ultrasound wave reception is based, can be explained as follows: Mechanical deformations of the surface of some natural crystals such as quartz and tourmaline, and of some ceramic materials such as barium titanate and barium zirconate create small electrical charges. These charges are proportional to the size and shape of the respective mechanical deformations. When an ultrasound wave strikes a piezoelectric substance, compression and rarefaction of the substance occurs in rhythm with the wave. This, in turn, produces electrical impulses which can be converted by electrodes to signals suitable for electronic processing.

Diagnostic ultrasound waves are generated using the *inverse piezoelectric effect*. Alternating electrical current applied via electrodes the surface of a piezoelectric substance generates an alternating electrical field. The electrical field causes the piezoelectric substance to produce depth oscillations (compressions and rarefactions), which occur in rhythm with the electric field.

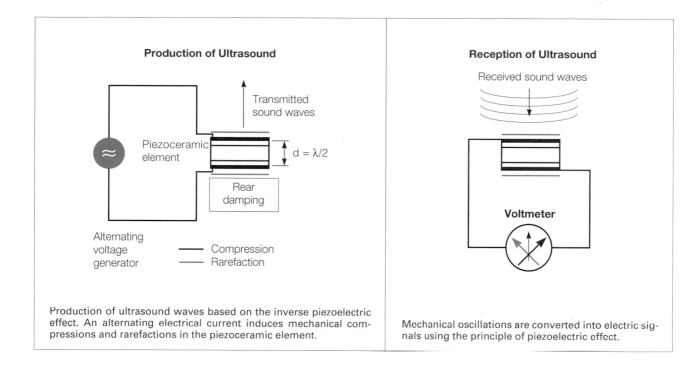

Production of ultrasound waves based on the inverse piezoelectric effect. An alternating electrical current induces mechanical compressions and rarefactions in the piezoceramic element.

Mechanical oscillations are converted into electric signals using the principle of piezoelectric effect.

The system is in a state of resonance when the thickness of the piezoceramic plate equals to one-half the wavelength of the excitation oscillations. Since piezoceramic elements transform mechanical energy into electrical energy and vice versa, they are called piezotransformers or *transducers*. Since oscillations occur in a preferred direction, transducers are also known as *depth-mode oscillators*.

Wave propagation takes place when the oscillations spread through a medium in contact with the piezoelectric crystal. There are primarily two types of waves that play a role in sound wave propagation:

1. *Longitudinal waves*	Atoms and molecules in the wave field move parallel to the direction of propagation of the sound wave (normal wave direction). Regions of particle compression and rarefaction (density fluctuation) occur in the medium.
2. *Shear waves*	Atoms and molecules in the wave field move perpendicular to the direction of wave propagation. No particle compression and rarefaction occurs (*e.g.* water waves).

Since the principle sound waves produced in biological tissue are longitudinal waves, they therefore play a major role in ultrasound diagnosis. Shear waves, which occur primarily in solids, play only a minor role in echocardiography.

The Sonic Field

The volume of the medium through which ultrasound waves are propagated is involved in energy exchange and interactive processes. This volume, called the sonic field, can be described using various physical parameters.

The most important are listed below.

λ	Wavelength	Distance travelled by the wave during one complete oscillation (Units: m, cm, or mm).
T	Period	Time in which the particle completes one complete cycle (Unit: s).
f	Frequency	Reciprocal of the total period ($f = 1/T$) (Units: Hz, kHz, MHz). Once a wave has been generated, it is propagated at a constant frequency regardless of the type of medium.
c	Propagation velocity	Medium-dependent variable that is defined by the equation: $c = \lambda \times f$ (Unit: m/s). It follows that when a wave is transmitted from one medium to another with a different propagation velocity, the wavelength must change, since frequency remains constant.
A	Amplitude	Extent of excursion of particles traversed by a wave from the resting position (Units: m, mm).
V_{max}	Particle velocity	Amplitude of the velocity at which excursion occur: $V_{max} = 2\pi \times f \times A$ (Unit: m/s).
P	Sound pressure	(Also called alternating sound pressure). Describes the deviation of instantaneous pressure from static pressure in longitudinal waves (Unit: Pa).
Z	Impedance	(Also called acoustic impedance or wave impedance). Describes the behavior of waves at the interfaces of two media: $Z = \rho \times c$. Acoustic impedance is the product of the propagation velocity c and density ρ of the respective medium.
I	Intensity	Describes the energy content of a wave (Unit: W/m^2). Intensity is conventionally used to evaluate potential biologic effects of ultrasound. However, it has only limited suitability for assessing the degree of biological effect.

Ultrasound waves are not homogeneously distributed throughout the tranducer's sonic field. The physical laws of wave propagation state that interference will occur near the face of the transducer. Therefore, full visualization is possible only in more distal areas. Sound pressure distribution in the near and far fields can be computed using different mathematical formulas. The distribution of sound pressure in the near field must be expressed numerically, whereas sound pressures in the far field can be described by analytical formulas.

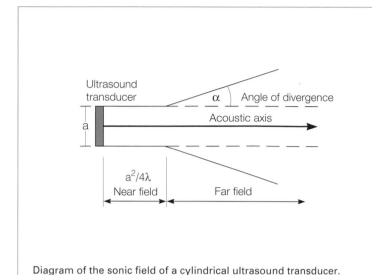

Ultrasound transducer

α　Angle of divergence

Acoustic axis

a

$a^2/4\lambda$

Near field　　　Far field

Diagram of the sonic field of a cylindrical ultrasound transducer.

Geometry of the sonic field under ideal conditions with a cylindrical ultrasound transducer. The amplitude of motion across the entire surface perpendicular to the acoustic axis is uniform. The sonic field can be divided into a near field and a far field. The length of the near field and the magnitude of the angle of divergence are determined by the transducer dimensions and by the wavelength of transmitted ultrasound. The pressure distribution in the near field must be expressed numerically, whereas the far field can be described by various analytical formulas. The acoustic axis extends in a vertical line from the transducer (normal surface).

Wave cancellation or *interference* in the near field limits the imaging capabilities in the near field. The axial length of the near field is proportional to the square of the transducer dimensions and is indirectly proportional to the wavelength. Structures in this area cannot be clearly delineated. Therefore, additional technology for cardiac ultrasound diagnosis had to be developed to enable evaluation of the cardiac apex from an apical transducer position.

Intensity in the far field is inversely proportional to the square of the distance from the transducer. The far field can therefore be described as a spheric wave. The angle of divergence α represents the magnitude of divergence of the ultrasound wave in the far field. Splitting of the far field into *side lobes* in addition to the main beam is an undesirable effect. The main beam lies on the acoustic axis, and side lobes represent peak intensities lateral to the acoustic axis. New technology has been developed to suppress side lobes, which play a major role in the development of artifacts. The geometry of the sonic field has a decisive influence on the instrument's resolving power.

Propagation Phenomena

Transducers used in medical ultrasound diagnosis function according to the *pulse-echo technique*. The transducer emits brief ultrasonic pulses (bursts) and waits for reflected echoes to return. These signals are then processed for imaging. The intensity (amplitude) of returning echoes and the signal transit time between transmission and reception are then measured. The difference between the emitted and returning signal amplitudes is used to generate an image of the reflecting object.

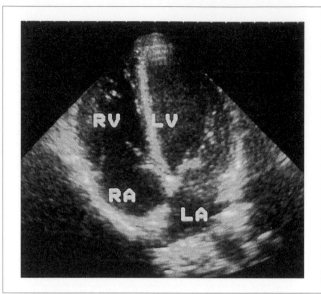

Echocardiographic images interpret wave propagation phenomena differently from those of interdisciplinary ultrasound diagnosis. This image illustrates the hard contour setting that is characteristic of echocardiographic images.

Cardiac ultrasound images are optimized with respect to strong specular reflections and scattered echoes.

As compared with interdisciplinary ultrasound, the frequencies used in echocardiography allow relatively limited tissue characterization.

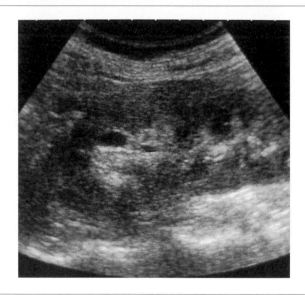

Interdisciplinary ultrasound diagnostic images use much softer contour settings. In order to generate ultrasound images of abdomen, low amplitude scattered echoes must be measured as well as specular reflections. Scattered echoes play a major role in ultrasonic tissue characterization. „Soft" instrument settings permit differential tissue characterization. As compared with the hard contours seen in echocardiography, ultrasound images from other disciplines often seem to be covered by a gray veil.

When an ultrasound wave traverses media of different acoustic impedances, the wave is partially reflected and partially refracted by the interfaces of the media. The proportions of reflection and refraction are angle dependent. The following table describes the behavior of ultrasound waves at interfaces.

Reflection at Planar Surfaces	Refraction at Planar Surfaces
The *reflection* of waves at planar interfaces plays a major role in ultrasound image generation. When a wave front strikes an interface, part of the wave is reflected and part is refracted. For reflection to occur, the interface must be large compared to the wavelength. An interface is thereby defined as the surface separating two media of different acoustic impedances. The angle of reflectance corresponds with the angle of incidence. The reflection coefficient determines the intensity of reflection. When the acoustic impedance of Medium 1 is negligible compared with that of Medium 2 (or vice versa), the wave is completely reflected at the interface (*e.g.* muscle-air interface), as is illustrated in the formula below. When the interface is perpendicular to the angle of incidence of the ultrasound wave: $\alpha_E = \alpha_R$.	When *refraction* occurs, a second part of the wave passes through the interface and is thereby attenuated. The transmission coefficient defines the proportion of energy transmitted through the interface. The direction of propagation of the wave changes when it passes through an interface. According to *Snell's law of reflection and refraction:* $\sin \alpha_E / c_1 = \sin \alpha_R / c_1 = \sin \beta / c_2$. α_E Angle of incidence α_R Angle of reflection β Angle of refraction c_1 Velocity of propagation in Medium 1 c_2 Velocity of propagation in Medium 2 Since the maximal angle of refraction is 90°, the angle of total reflection is calculated as: $\alpha_{Interface} = \arcsin c_1 / c_2$. Note: A different formula is used to calculate total reflection in media with greatly different impedances (*e.g.* muscle and bone, see reflection from planar surfaces). When the angle of incidence of the wave front is perpendicular to the interface: $\alpha_E = \beta = 0°$.
Impedance of Medium 1: $Z_1 = \rho_1 \times c_1$	Impedance of Medium 2: $Z_2 = \rho \times c_2$
Reflection coefficient: $R = \{(Z_2 - Z_1) / (Z_2 + Z_1)\}^2$	*Transmission coefficient:* $T = 4 \times Z_2 \times Z_1 / (Z_2 + Z_1)^2$

The following relation applies:

The sum of intensity of the reflected (I_R) and refracted (transmitted) waves (I_T) is equal to the intensity of the incident ultrasound wave:
$I_0 = I_R + I_T$ and $R + T = 1$.

Reflection and refraction occur under the following conditions:

- When the interface is larger than the wavelength.
- When the propagated wave is characterized as a normal wave traveling perpendicular to the wave fronts. The normal wave corresponds to the direction of propagation.

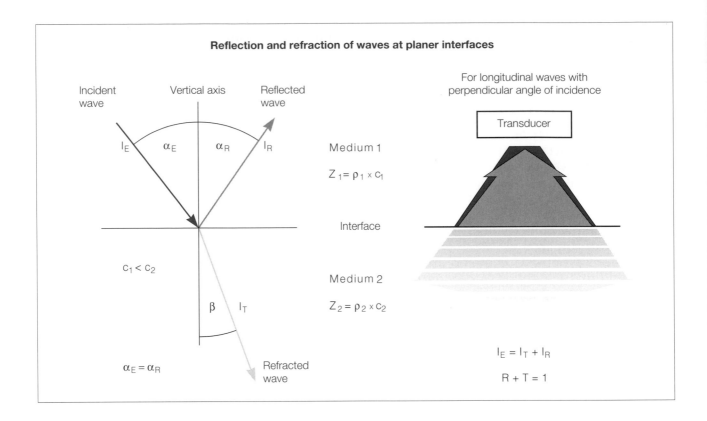

- The interfaces must be planar as compared with the wavelength.
- The reflection coefficient is used to calculate the amplitude of reflection.
- The transmission coefficient is used to calculate the amplitude of the refracted, transmitted beam.
- Reflection and transmission play a fundamental role in diagnostic ultrasound.
- The reflected wave normally does not return to the transmitter unless the angle of incidence of the initially transmitted wave is perpendicular to the interface.

Scatter

Reflection and refraction of ultrasound waves in biological tissue is determined by physical conditions. Large scanning targets such as organ borders create strong specular echoes, whereas targets that are smaller than or equal to the wavelength create weaker *scattered echoes*. Diagnostic ultrasound focuses primarily on structures that range from a few millimeters to one-tenth of a millimeter in size.

Huygens' principle states that when ultrasound strikes small targets containing local inhomogeneities in physical properties, new wave fronts (elementary waves) are generated. Wave fronts generated by adjacent inhomogeneous targets interfere with one another and create a new wave field – the *stray field*. Since scattered energy is not uniformly distributed throughout the stray field, the angle of scatter is not dependent on the angle of the incident ultrasound beam. Some of the new wave fronts return to the transducer, resulting in *backscatter*. The intensity of backscatter is lower than that of echoes reflected from interfaces. Still, scatter plays a major role in the assessment of ultrasound images. The analysis of scatter provides important information on cellular detail. Different investigators have used various methods of textural analysis in an effort to describe the distribution of scatterers within the investigated tissue.

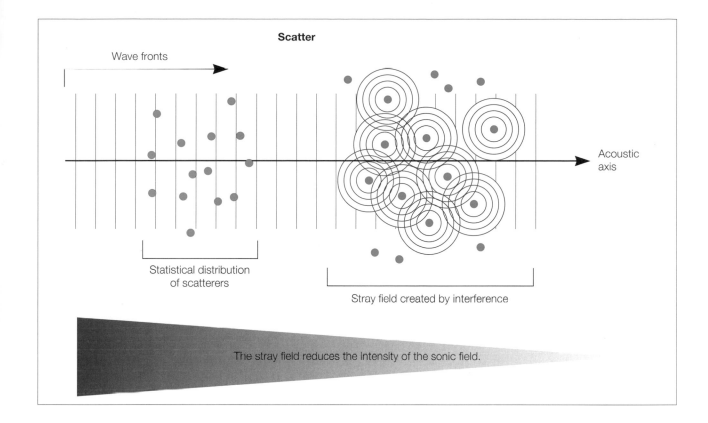

Terms such as echo intensity, echogeneity, echo density, and homogeneity are used in acoustic tissue characterization of parenchymal organs.

Interactions between ultrasound and objects that are very small compared with the wavelength can be described using *Lord Raleigh's theory*. According to this theory, it is not the arrangement of inhomogeneities in tissue, but rather the statistical density of distribution of these inhomogeneities that plays the major role in the development of scatter. The intensity of Rayleigh scatter is proportional to the fourth power of the frequency of the incident wave. The higher the frequency of the incident wave, the greater the degree of scatter. *Rayleigh scatter* is one of the phenomena that impedes signal processing in attempts to use higher frequencies at deeper depths of penetration.

Red blood cells, which are approximately 10 μm in size, are around 100 times smaller than the wavelength of diagnostic ultrasound. In conventional echocardiograpy, blood-filled cavities are visualized as echo-free spaces. Rayleigh scatter is caused by the statistical fluctuation in red blood cell population density. Because the red blood cells themselves are in motion (blood flow), the frequency of Rayleigh scatter deviates from that of the incident wave. This deviation can be measured to obtain the *Doppler frequency* (Doppler shift). Rayleigh scatter of red blood cells therefore provides a physical basis for detecting Doppler shifts.

Sound Attenuation and Absorption

When sound waves travel through biological tissue, the wave intensity (energy per unit area and time) is attenuated in proportion to the distance traveled by the wave.

The various factors involved in sound wave attenuation are listed below:

- **Geometry of the sonic field**
  The sonic field of ultrasound transducers diverges in the far field. The sonic energy is therefore spread out over a larger area in the far field, and the wave intensity decreases.

- **Reflection and Refraction**
  At planar interfaces, part of the incident wave is diverted from its initial direction of propagation due to the effects of reflection and refraction.

- **Scatter**
  Scatter mechanisms lead to attenuation due to "undirected reflectance".

- **Absorption**
  Due to atomic and molecular processes, part of the wave's energy is converted to other energy forms (primarily heat). This energy loss is directly proportional to the distance traveled by the wave. Absorption increases exponentially as the depth of penetration of the wave in biological tissue increases. The damping variable D is used to describe the decrease in amplitude (in decibels) per unit of distance traveled by the wave. The damping variable D is medium- and frequency-dependent, as is described by the following formula:

  $$D = a \times f.$$

  The proportionality factor a describes the distance and frequency dependency of damping.

These factors have a direct impact on image generation.

1. Organ borders proximal and distal to the transducer should be identified as like interfaces. Therefore, they should be represented with the same intensity on the generated image. However, because attenuation and absorption increase with distance, the signal amplitudes received from the far organ borders are lower than those from the near borders.

2. In order to neutralize these effects and in order to obtain comparable signals from like interfaces at different depths of penetration, the attenuated distant echoes must be enhanced by means of depth-selective *time-gain compensation* (TGC). Since the attenuation conditions of tissue are not known, the operator must estimate how much time-gain compensation is required and check the results by inspecting the display image.

3. Every amplifier and every transducer has an inherent noise level. Only those returning signals that exceed the noise level contribute information for the generated image. The maximum depth from which usable signals return to the transducer is defined as the *maximum depth of penetration*. The penetration depth can be increased by increasing the transmission frequency. However, in order to prevent undesirable biological effects, restrictions are placed on the allowable transmitter power.

Resolution

How well does the image approximate the true conditions? An important parameter of image quality is *resolution* or *resolving power*.

Ultrasound resolution is defined as the minimum distance at which two adjacent reflecting objects can be distinguished or identified. Theoretically, the resolving power in the direction of propagation of the wave, or *axial resolution*, must be at least equal to one wavelength. Mathematical analyses of echocardiographic frequencies (2 to 5 MHz) predicts axial resolution that is clearly less than 1 mm. However, the maximum resolution obtained in clinical practice is only around 2 mm.

As mentioned before, phenomena associated with sound wave propagation and sonic field geometry cause blurring that reduces the resolving power from the theoretical norm.

Resolution can be improved by using higher frequencies. However, higher frequencies require excessive damping, which has undesirable effects. Lower frequency transducers (2 to 3.5 MHz) must be used to visualize higher penetration depths. Experience has shown that the penetration depth is reduced by one-half when then the transmission frequency is doubled. The operator has no choice but to compromise between the necessary penetration depth and the highest possible resolution.

When using the pulse-echo technique, axial resolution is also dependent on the pulse duration, which is controlled by the ultrasound machine and the transducer. These parameters can be used to test the system quality.

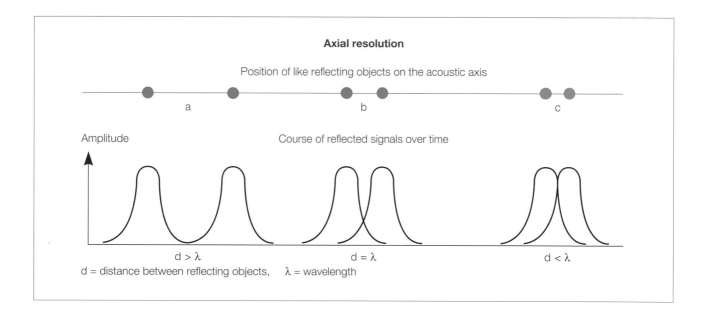

Axial resolution

Position of like reflecting objects on the acoustic axis

a   b   c

Amplitude   Course of reflected signals over time

$d > \lambda$ $d = \lambda$ $d < \lambda$

d = distance between reflecting objects,   λ = wavelength

In contrast with axial resolution, where one assumes that reflecting objects are located one behind the other in the direction of propagation, *lateral resolution* is defined as the smallest distance at which two adjacent reflecting objects lying perpendicular to the direction of propagation can still be distinguished from one another.

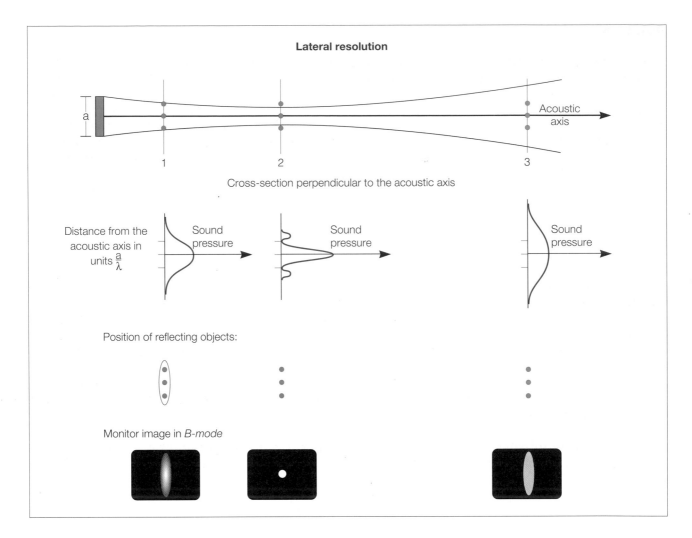

Lateral resolution depends largely on the geometry of the sonic field, particularly the distribution of intensity perpendicular to the acoustic axis. As a rule of thumb, lateral resolution will be two to three times poorer than axial resolution at certain transmission frequencies. The geometry of the sonic field can be adjusted to improve the lateral resolution. This is done by varying the aperture and focus.

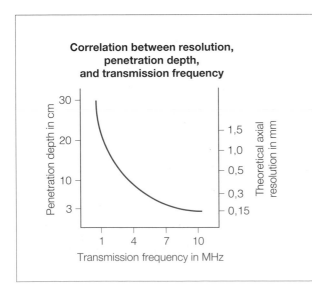

The graph highlights the technical compromises that must be made in diagnostic ultrasound.

Sound conduction in biological tissue is poorer in older patients than in adolescents. However, since the maximum transmission frequency is restricted by regulations, a lower frequency must be selected to achieve the necessary depth of penetration. This, however, results in relatively crude axial resolution. The operator should keep this in mind during the examination.

When structures of interest lying proximal to the transducer are interrogated at higher frequencies, the axial resolution is significantly improved. The transmission frequency determines the amount of accuracy and detail with which a tissue structure can be visualized.

Aperture

The surface area of the transducer or transducer elements through which ultrasound travels is called the *aperture*. In circular transducers, the aperture is equal to the diameter of the transducer. The length of the near field can be varied by changing the aperture and the wavelength, however, imaging of structures in the near field is limited because of interference. The size of the aperture also influences the angle of divergence in the far field. A large aperture can be used to reduce the degree of divergence in the far field, at the price of elongation of the near field. In electronically steered systems, the aperture can be dynamically adjusted in accordance with the desired depth of penetration.

Focus

The axial and lateral resolution of normal transducers is usually best at the near and far field transition zone, where the highest concentration of the sonic field *(focus)* is located. When the sonic field is further narrowed, the site of greatest beam concentration is called the *focal point*. An acoustic lens with a geometrically fixed focus can be fitted onto the face of the transducer to improve resolution. This works similar to an optical lens. In electronically steered scanners, the time of element activation for proximal targets is delayed with respect to element activation for distant targets. By variably manipulating the timing of element activation, the focal point can be variably positioned. This technique is known as *dynamic focussing*. Dynamic focussing of both transmission and reception is achieved by additionally delaying the reception of returning signals.

All modern echographs have integrated capabilities for both dynamic focussing and aperture adjustment. In transducer arrays, the aperture may also be equipped with an additional *sensitivity control* for suppressing side lobes (apodization), thereby further improving resolution.

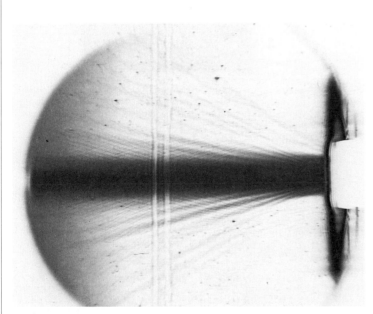

Schlieren photograph of a sonic field.

This photograph shows the sound pressure distribution in front of the transducer. Dark areas in the photograph correspond to high-density zones; light areas represent low-density zones. Density in the medium through which a wave is propagated is directly proportional to the alternating sound pressure.
The refraction index of light is density-dependent. In schlieren optics, the refraction index is used to make optical observations of alternating sound pressure distribution.

The region of interference in the near field directly in front of the transducer and the region of lateral divergence in the far field are clearly visible. The concentration of sonic energy around the acoustic axis (main beam) and the presence of pressure maxima lateral to the acoustic axis (side lobes) are also clearly visible.

The axial position of the focal point greatly influences the quality of axial and lateral resolution. This can be studied in phantom studies and in comparison studies.

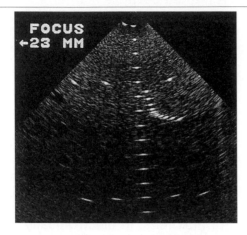

Image of a tissue-like phantom. Horizontal and vertical wires are used to test image quality. Precise visualization of the arc-shaped wires requires excellent resolving power. The focus is set at a depth of 23 mm.

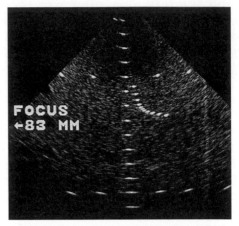

Same phantom as in left panel. The focus is now set at a depth of 83 mm. The arc-shaped wires now are much more sharply delineated than before (improved axial and lateral resolution).

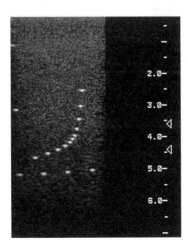

Image of a tissue-like phantom. Two focal points (triangles on the depth scale) have been set near the arc-shaped group of wires.

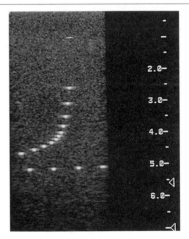

Image of a tissue-like phantom. Two focal points (triangles on the depth scale) have been set beneath the arc-shaped wires. The resolution in the vicinity of the wires is clearly worse than in the image on the left.

The Transducer

The desired result of scanning is to obtain a cross-sectional view of the structure of interest. In ultrasound, the transducer is used to carefully interrogate or "raster" the investigated region. The ultrasonic beam is swept incrementally across the structure. The transducer's electric pulses are converted into mechanical oscillations, which are propagated through the medium lying directly in contact with the transducer. After it has transmitted the initial pulse, the transducer waits for the sound waves that have been reflected and scattered by the medium to return. All returning signals are assigned positions relative to the acoustic axis in accordance with their spatial orientation. This produces a line of information for image generation. When echoes from the furthest part of the interrogated region have returned, thereby completing one transmission-reception step (pulse-echo technique, see "Image Generation"), the ultrasonic beam is shifted by a small angle or linear increment, and another pulse is emitted.

The simplest scanners use parallel or linear array transducers, in which the individual scan lines are located parallel to one another. Since these scanners require a relatively large sonic window, they are unsuitable for the echocardiographic window, which is limited by the size of the intercostal spaces. Optimal transducers for echocardiography should therefore be punctiform in shape.

Sector scanning transducers meet these requirements. They create ultrasound beams using sector elements with a variable sector angle.

Basically, two types of transducers are used in sector scanning:

1. Electronically steered or *phased array transducers* consist of multiple small piezoceramic elements arranged side by side to form an array. By electronically controlling the sequence of firing of the individual elements, the acoustic axis of the transducer can be moved laterally out of the original orthogonal plane. All elements of the array contribute information for image generation. The sonic fields of the individual elements are superpositioned to create the acoustic axis of the transducer. The controlled firing sequence makes it possible to scan the region of interest from one stationary central point. The number of piezoelectric elements in modern phased array transducers ranges from 64 to 128.

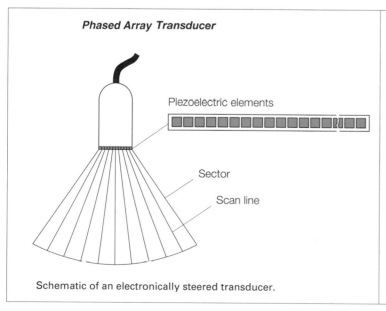

Phased Array Transducer

Piezoelectric elements

Sector

Scan line

Schematic of an electronically steered transducer.

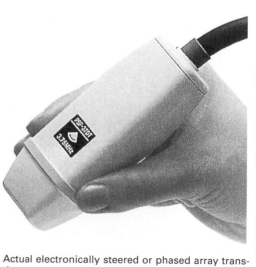

Actual electronically steered or phased array transducer.

2. Almost all *mechanically steered transducers* available now are wobbler systems. In contrast with rotating scanners, almost all mechanical sector scanners for echocardiography are designed with a rotating disc construction that sweeps the transducer element along the axis to create the desired sector angle. The ultrasonic beam is thus steered both electronically and by means of a linear motor. Electronically steered scanners always have a planar transducer surface, whereas mechanically steered transducers have a hemispher-ical, dome-like application surface. *Annular array transducers* were designed to provide mechanical transducers with electronic focussing capabilities. Annular array transducers contain concentrically arranged circular rings of equal area. The rings are steered in a manner similar to that of phased array scanners. The position of the focal point can there-fore be adjusted to improve axial and lateral resolution.

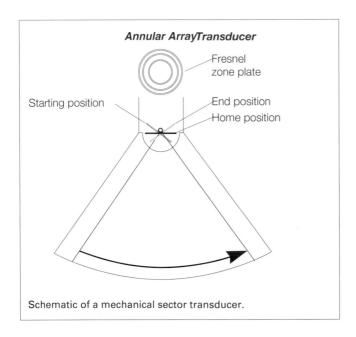

Schematic of a mechanical sector transducer.

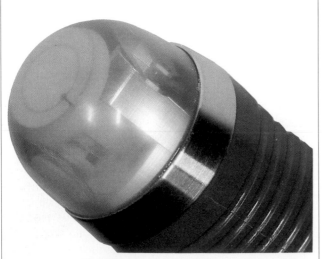

Close-up view of an annular array transducer. The axially suspended, concentrically arranged, circular piezoelectric ring elements are clearly visible.

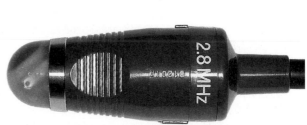

Photograph of a mechanical sector transducer with a transmission frequency of 2.8 MHz. The circular piezoelectric disc is in the sector edge position. Sweeping is steered by a servomotor. Because the disc rotates around an axis, all mechanical sector scanners for ultrasound have a hemispherical, dome-shaped tip.

Image Generation

To be acceptable for ultrasound diagnosis in general and cardiac ultrasound in particular, the imaging technique must be easy to use and reproducible. By applying the physical laws of transmission and reflection, the piezoelectric transducer can be used as both transmitter and receiver. The transducer sends very brief ultrasonic pulses into the biological tissue medium, then waits for reflected and scattered echoes to return and converts them into electrical impulses *(pulse-echo technique)*. By measuring the signal transit time and the amplitude of returning echoes, the spatial orientation of the reflecting object can be derived. In order to calculate the distances involved, the mean velocity of sound in biological tissue (1540 m/s) is assumed to be constant. All relevant signals received by the transducer (those greater than the noise level) are assigned to their respective scan line, regardless of their site of origin. This, however, is a major cause of artifacts and other image deficiencies.

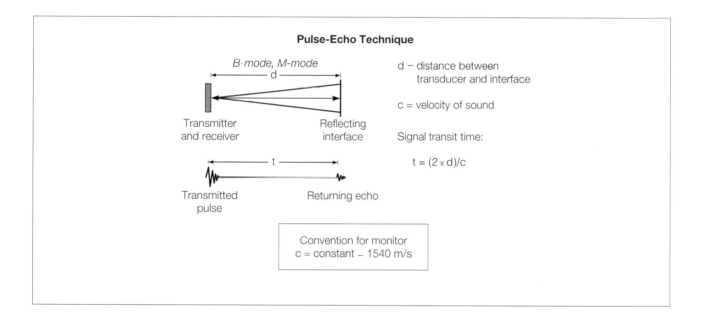

Pulse-Echo Technique

B-mode, M-mode

d — distance between transducer and interface

Transmitter and receiver — Reflecting interface

c = velocity of sound

Signal transit time:

$$t = (2 \times d)/c$$

Transmitted pulse — Returning echo

Convention for monitor
c = constant – 1540 m/s

The returning echoes are in the same frequency range as the transmitted pulse. By electronic manipulation, the returning signal can be broken down to derive a simplified signal containing only amplitude information. This simplified signal can be used to derive the spatial orientation of impedance shifts on the acoustic axis.

There are several ways to process the signal to obtain a representation of the investigated structure on a monitor. The principle of amplitude modulation was the first to be used. Further developments in electronics soon made it possible to apply this one-dimensional amplitude modulation technique to rapidly moving cardiac structures such as mitral leaflets. With the further development of technology, it was possible to obtain two-dimensional images of a very thin layer of tissue by converting amplitude into units of brightness.

Although the term "ultrasound image" is frequently used, the present book makes an effort to describe the operational mode of the echocardiograph by using the terms B-mode and M-mode instead of B-scan and M-scan. Echocardiographic signal acquisition is a dynamic process. The image, however, represents a static moment in time. Naturally, a B-scan is made up a given number of B-mode lines of information (scan lines). Thus, B-mode and M-mode signal processing is a one-dimensional process, whereas the image represented on the monitor is two-dimensional.

A-Mode

The *A-mode format* (A = amplitude) can precisely measure the distance of reflecting objects from each other and from the transducer. Using a cathode ray tube, the amplitude (intensity) of a returning echo is recorded as a deflection perpendicular to the distance axis. More distant echoes are recorded at the appropriate distance further down on the axis. The distance between the two spikes represents the distance between the two reflecting objects, assuming the echograph has been calibrated for the mean velocity of sound in the medium (1540 m/s). The signal transit time is converted to distance using the equation: $c = 2s/t$ (c = velocity of sound, s = depth of penetration, t = signal transit time). The factor of 2 is used because the signal transit time represents the round-trip time from the transducer to the reflecting object and back.

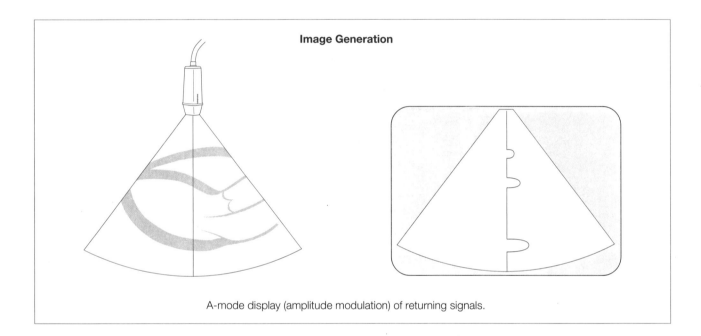

Image Generation

A-mode display (amplitude modulation) of returning signals.

B-Mode

The *B-mode* format (B = brightness) is a modified version of A-mode: A-mode amplitude deflections are converted to a B-mode brightness dots. The intensity (amplitude) of returning signals is expressed numerically on a gray scale of 0 to 16, 32, 64, or 256 shades of gray. The lowest intensity signal is usually assigned the value 0 (black), and the highest intensity signal is assigned the highest value on the scale (white). However, the human eye is capable of distinguishing only around 20 different shades of gray in a given image.

In B-mode, the two-dimensional A-mode scan line is reduced to a brightness-modulated line of information. This makes it possible to juxtapose several adjacent B-mode scan lines on the monitor. For this purpose, an image memory *(scan converter)* is used to store individual B-mode scan lines, then display them adjacent to one another to create a complete cross-sectional image of the investigated structure. The monitor image is therefore a composite of sequential B-mode scan lines that have been created by sweeping the axis of the transducer across the region of interest.

It takes 0.2 ms to generate one B-mode scan line at a penetration depth of 15 cm. In modern instruments, this procedure is electronically steered at speeds which the eye can no longer follow. This enables virtually instantaneous or *real-time imaging* of processes in the region of interest.

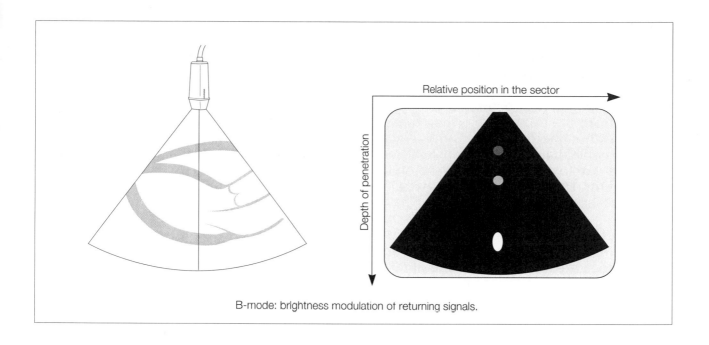

B-mode: brightness modulation of returning signals.

The term B-mode does not describe the generation of the monitor image, but rather the format of signal processing. The terms *B-mode* and *B-scan* are not identical. The B-scan is a composite of multiple individual B-mode scan lines. We have emphasized this difference by preferentially using the term *B-mode* instead of *B-scan*.

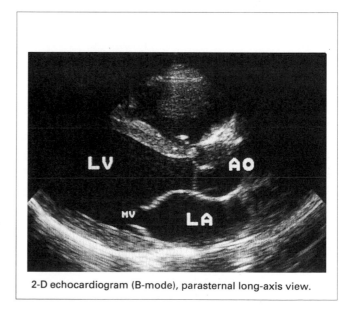

2-D echocardiogram (B-mode), parasternal long-axis view.

M-Mode

The term *M-mode* is derived from the word motion. Although two-dimensional (B-mode) echocardiography utilizes a relatively fast frame repetition rate, it is still too slow to efficiently record high-frequency fluttering. In B-mode the acoustic axis is kept constant with respect to the investigated structure, and each reflecting object is recorded at the appropriate distance from the transducer. When these objects move, their position on the distance axis changes. When the individual B-mode scan lines are displayed on a vertical axis relative to distance (while maintaining a constant beam position), a one-dimensional display of moving structures with excellent temporal resolution can be generated by assembling the scan lines on a monitor. M-mode scans have excellent temporal resolution and are therefore ideal for use in cardiac valve assessment.

In contrast with 2-D echocardiography, M-mode does not generate a cross-sectional image, but lines of information that record the motion of reflecting objects over time. M-mode therefore provides the maximum degree of temporal resolution.

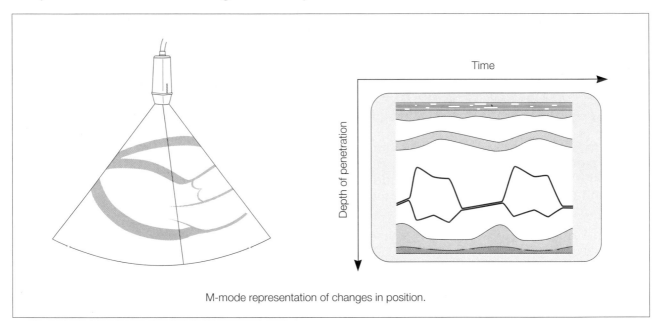

M-mode representation of changes in position.

Combined Two-Dimensional and M-Mode Display

In echocardiography, comparison studies that require standardization of the transducer position must be performed. The transducer position can be targeted and studied using combined two-dimensional and M-mode echocardiographic techniques. This not only increases accuracy, but also saves time. M-mode tracings are made after the beam has been targeted by means of two-dimensional guidance.

Artifacts

Wave propagation phenomena such as reflection, refraction, scatter, absorption, interference, etc. sometimes are not completely accounted for in signal processing. This results in artifactual or deficient images.

Speckle is one of the major artifacts. Speckle, which is generated by interference from the stray field, is distributed randomly throughout the ultrasound image.

In speckle, the receiver detects reflected amplitudes which have no morphological equivalent. Efforts are being made to reduce speckle by means of statistically based filtration.

Some artifacts can be imitated using phantoms. Phantom studies have shown that the higher the resolution, the better the phantom can be visualized.

The following images show common examples of B-mode artifacts.

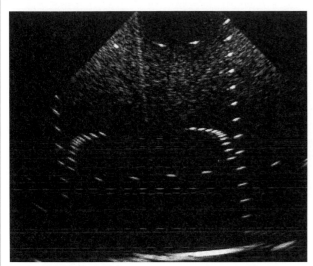 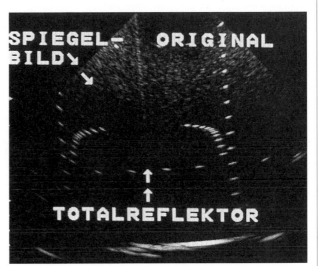

Two-dimensional echocardiogram of a group of wires in a tissue-like phantom.

Explanation of specular artifact on the wall of the phantom. Phantom-air interface.

In the above photographs, the phantom-air interface functions as a perfect reflector, thereby producing mirror images of structures within the phantom. The intensity of the specular artifacts is lower than that of the original structure. Additionally, the combination of several artifacts makes it difficult to properly interpret the image. For correct interpretation, these structures must therefore be interrogated from multiple imaging planes.

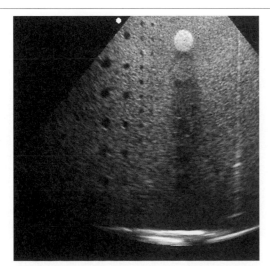 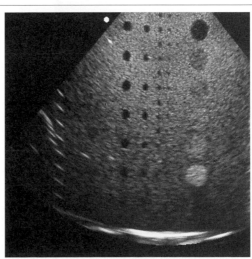

Two-dimensional echocardiogram of a group of cylinders in a tissue-like phantom. The distal structures behind the first cylinder are only vaguely recognizable (shadowing artifact).

If the highly echo reflective structure is located at a great depth of penetration, all proximal structures can be adequately assessed.

This vertically arranged group of cylinders of unequal acoustic impedances is interrogated from diametrical 2-D echocardiographic planes. The relatively high acoustic impedance of the first cylinder in the left panel permits only limited assessment of deeper structures. This effect is called *acoustic shadowing*. The transmitted portion of energy is clearly less than that lateral to the structure. Changing the transducer position made it possible to properly assess the structures.

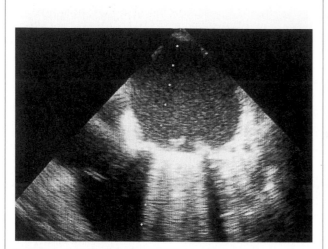

Prosthetic mitral valve. A comet-like artifact appears due to great differences in impedance.

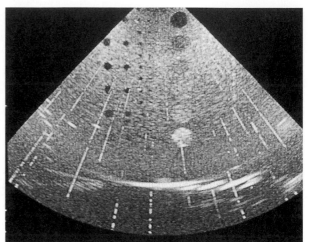

The transducer may register high-frequency artifact-producing signals from surrounding structures.

In clinical practice, it is necessary to echocardiographically assess prosthetic valve function. The impedance of materials used in these valves differs greatly from that of human tissue. Valvular prostheses reflect sound at a high velocity, thereby causing multiple reflections that resemble the tail of a comet. This comet-like structure is delimited by echo-free zones caused by absorption of sonic energy by the valve ring.

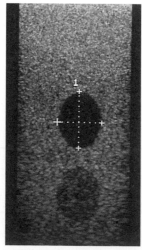

Two-dimensional echocardiogram of a circular cylinder within a phantom. Different sound velocities result in dimensional distortion.

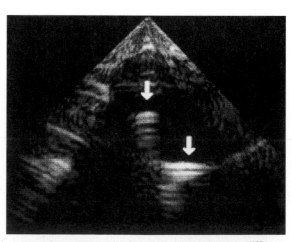

Here, a wire courses horizontally through two different media. Discontinuity of the two-dimensional image results because a constant velocity of sound was assumed.

From a technical point of view, diagnostic ultrasound is a form of high-frequency technology. It is necessary to screen out frequencies from the surroundings, because the echograph is not capable of identifying the origin of received signals. In other words, the transducer functions as an antenna for foreign signals.

The basic measurement parameter for depth of penetration is the signal propagation time. For display purposes, the velocity of ultrasound is assumed to be constant (1540 m/s). Any variation from this sound velocity will result in dimensional distortion.

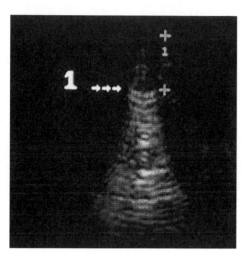

Two-dimensional echocardiogram of a wire in the near field of the transducer. The geometry of the sonic field causes distortion of the wire.

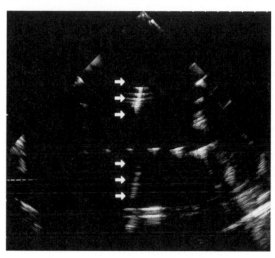

Multiple reflections arise when there are large changes in impedance between the transducer and the structure. This is visualized as repeated echoes.

The geometry of the sonic field, particularly that of the near field, is characterized by interference. Returning signals may originate from highly echo reflective objects that lie outside the acoustic axis of the respective B-mode scan line. This is due to divergence of the sonic field which, in turn, results in image distortion.

Reflected echoes from the imaged structure as well as from the medium-transducer interface cause repeated echoes of the structure to appear at a depth two times deeper than that of the actual structure. The intensity of the repeated echoes is significantly lower than that of the original echoes. Repeated echoes can be reduced or emphasized by adjusting the appropriate instrument setting.

| 1. | Fundamentals of Echocardiography |
| 1.2 | Physical Principles of Conventional and Doppler Color Flow Imaging |

Echocardiography can no longer be described as a purely morphological technique. It is now possible to assess blood flow velocity by means of *duplex sonography, i.e.,* the combined use of two-dimensional echocardiography and Doppler echocardiography.

Doppler has greatly expanded the potentials for assessment of local and global cardiac function. The clinical significance of the Doppler effect, which enables measurement of blood flow velocity, still is not completely understood. Due to ongoing methodological and technical advances, the range of application of Doppler technology in medicine is constantly expanding.

The physical principles underlying the Doppler technique were first described in 1842 by Christian Doppler.

Doppler Effect

A characteristic change in the frequency of ultrasound waves is changed is caused by solid particles moving in the bloodstream (*i.e.* red blood cells). This characteristic change in frequency (frequency shift) is called the *Doppler effect.* The frequency shift provides information as to the velocity and direction of blood flow.

Red blood cells function as scatter centers in the bloodstream. Their diameter is clearly smaller than the wavelength in conventional diagnostic ultrasound. The red blood cell-related Doppler effect is thus attributable to Rayleigh scatter. The intensity of Rayleigh scatter is around 1000 times smaller than that of reflections measured in conventional two-dimensional echocardiography.

Therefore, quality of Doppler instruments is determined primarily by their amplification and signal analysis capabilities.

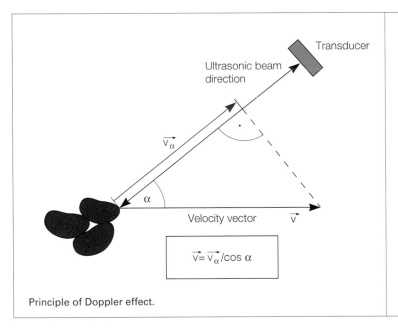

Principle of Doppler effect.

$$\vec{v} = \vec{v}_\alpha / \cos \alpha$$

An ultrasound beam emitted by the transducer is deflected by moving red blood cells. The change in frequency of the ultrasound wave is proportional to the velocity to the red blood cells. When the signal returns to the transducer, the difference between the transmitted and returning frequency is measured. This difference frequency is called the Doppler frequency shift.

The magnitude of the Doppler frequency shift is dependent on the size of the angle formed between the ultrasound beam and the red cell velocity vector. Only the site where the velocity vector intersects the ultrasound beam is assessed. This must be taken into account when performing quantitative assessments.

Doppler Equation

The Doppler equation mathematically defines the Doppler effect. This makes it possible to convert the Doppler frequency shift to blood flow velocity.

$$\Delta f = |f_{TM} - f_{RC}| = f_{TM} \times \{(2 \times v \times \cos\alpha)/c\}$$

Δf	*Doppler frequency shift*
f_{TM}	*Transmission frequency*
v	*Blood flow velocity*
c	*Velocity of sound through tissue (assumed to be a constant 1540 m/s)*
α	*Angle between velocity vector and acoustic axis of the transducer*

The effects of angle size become clear when the equation is solved to obtain blood flow velocity:

$$v = (\Delta f \times c) / (2 \times f_{TM} \times \cos\alpha)$$

Due to the cosine function in the denominator, only angles of up to 20° can be considered tolerable. Larger angles will lead to underestimation of velocity.

Cardiac ultrasound transducers transmit at frequencies of 2 to 10 MHz. The Doppler frequency shift caused by the interaction of cardiac ultrasound with human blood flow is in the audible range (20 Hz to 20 kHz). Doppler studies can therefore be tracked acoustically.

The following diagrams demonstrate the Doppler effect. A blood vessel containing a single stationary red blood cell is shown in the first diagram. The red blood cell deflects the transmitted ultrasound waves, and a small portion of reflected energy returns to the transducer (left). When plotted over time, the wave-forms of transmitted and received signals are shown to be in phase (equidistant). The loudspeakers on the transmitter and receiver emphasize the fact the Doppler frequency shift is an audible phenomenon. The frequency is measured after a wave crest has been transmitted or received.

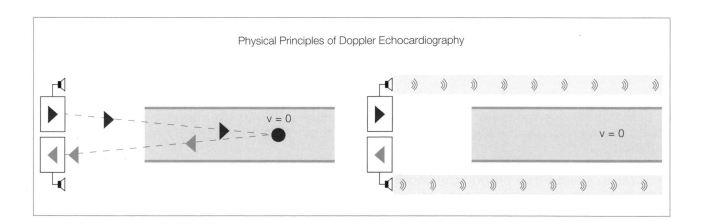

Physical Principles of Doppler Echocardiography

In the following diagram, a red blood cell is moving *towards* the transducer at a velocity other than zero. The moving red blood cell compresses the reflected waves. The number of waves registered on the receiving end is greater than the number emitted by the transmitter. The frequency of returning waves is higher than the transmitted frequency. The signals are no longer in phase. By convention, an increase in frequency is defined as positive velocity. Blood flowing towards the transducer is represented as positive blood flow velocity.

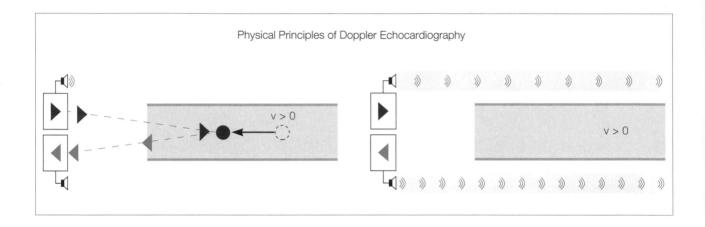

In the next diagram, the red blood cell is moving *away from* the transducer at a velocity other than zero. The number of waves scattered by the red blood cells per unit time decreases. The waves are now "pulled apart". The receiver registers a significantly lower number of waves per unit time than was transmitted. The frequency of the received signal is lower than that of the transmitted signal. The motion of blood away from the transducer is represented as negative blood flow velocity.

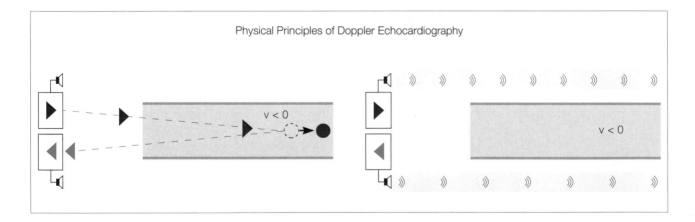

Doppler spectral analysis is conventionally used in echocardiography. Spectral analysis permits simultaneous measurement of different velocities. In real situations, not one red blood cell, but several, are investigated. Furthermore, they do not necessarily move at the same velocity.

In order to assess true blood flow conditions, the received signal must be broken down into individual components by means of **spectral analysis**. The spectral display is not charted as amplitude versus time, but as amplitude versus frequency.

The mathematical procedure used in spectral analysis is the *Fast Fourier Transform* (FFT). The FFT makes it possible to break down a signal composed of several different frequencies into its individual frequency components (spectral analysis).

In addition to the frequency components, one also assesses the amplitude of the received signal, *i.e.*, the contribution of each individual component to the total signal. The measured spectral shift can be represented as the Doppler frequency shift, or it can be used to calculate the blood flow velocity.

The spectral display is conventionally displayed as a velocity versus time diagram. Similar to the procedure in B-mode, the amplitude of each individual spectral component is modulated in terms of brightness. Frequently occurring velocities are encoded on the spectral display as bright dots, and velocities that contribute little to the total signal are encoded as dark dots.

Two different techniques for measuring the Doppler effect have been developed. Since their areas of application in cardiac ultrasound vary, the underlying principle of these techniques should first be explained.

Continuous-Wave Doppler

Continuous-wave Doppler (CW Doppler) is performed using a transducer containing two adjacent piezoelectric crystals. One crystal functions as the transmitter, while the second functions as the receiver. As the name implies, this enables the transducer to continuously transmit and receive ultrasound signals.

In CW Doppler all blood flow velocities detected on the axis of the transducer are summed (see figure below).

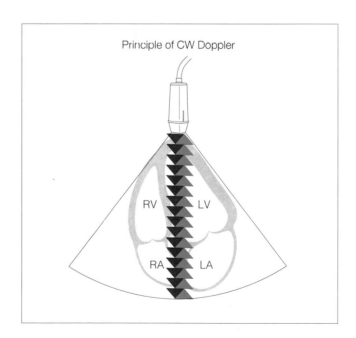

Principle of CW Doppler

The CW Doppler beam appears as a line on the 2-D echocardiogram. The CW Doppler line of interrogation can be positioned freely within the 2-D sector.

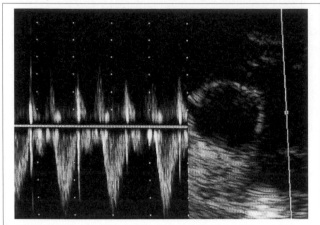 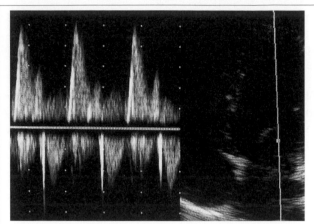

| CW Doppler recording through the pulmonary artery demonstrating systolic flow directed away from the transducer (v < 0), and corresponding 2-D echocardiogram. | CW Doppler spectral display of the mitral valve, demonstrating diastolic flow directed towards the transducer (v > 0), and corresponding apical four-chamber 2-D echocardiogram. |

Pulsed-Wave Doppler

In contrast with CW Doppler, *pulsed-wave Doppler (PW Doppler)* uses a single transducer to generate a spectral display by alternately transmitting and receiving ultrasound pulses over a selected period of time in order to evaluate only the frequency of echoes returning from a chosen depth.

A region of interest (ROI) is positioned on the two-dimensional echocardiogram before activating the PW Doppler beam. Only signals returning from the depth of the ROI are included in the spectral analysis. The size and position of the ROI can be defined anywhere on the two-dimensional image. The acquired information is obtained from a definable volume, because the sonic field also occupies a volume at the region of interest. Therefore, this region of interest is called the *sample volume or range gate.*

Local, selective flow measurement is possible with PW Doppler.

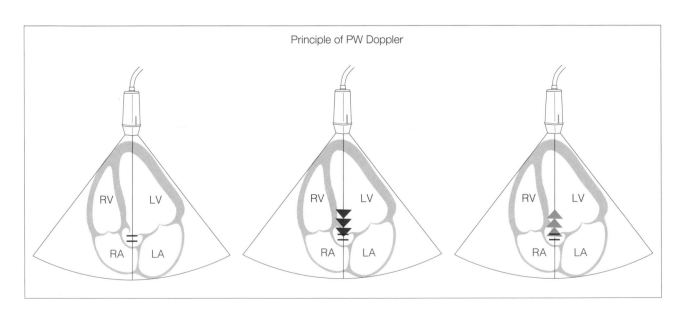

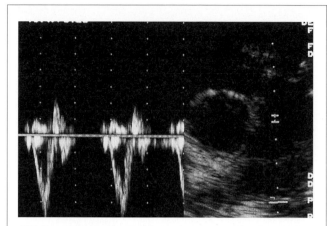

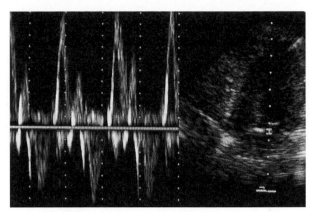

PW Doppler recording of the pulmonary artery demonstrating systolic flow directed away from the transducer (v < 0); corresponding parasternal short-axis 2-D echocardiogram.

PW Doppler spectral display of the mitral valve, demonstrating diastolic flow directed towards the transducer (v > 0, and corresponding apical four-chamber 2-D echocardiogram.

Pulse Repetition Frequency (PRF)

The PW Doppler technique uses a pulsed operating mode. After a pulse is emitted, the transducer functions as a receiver until the signal has returned from the specified depth of penetration. Only then can the next signal be transmitted. The transit time of the PW Doppler signal determines the sampling rate of the transmitted pulse, or *pulse repetition frequency* (PRF). The PRF is indirectly proportional to the depth of penetration. The higher the PRF, the lower the depth of the range gate, and vice versa.

The depths of penetration required for echocardiographic purposes (up to ca. 20 cm) require a PRF of 3.8 kHz, which is in the same range as the Doppler frequency shift.

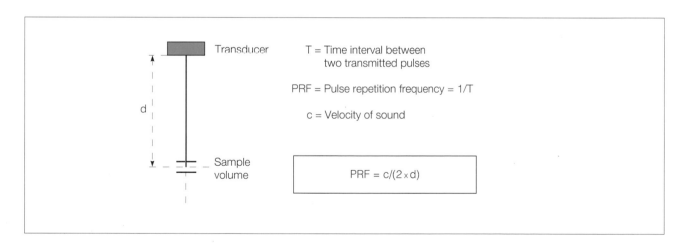

Transducer

T = Time interval between
    two transmitted pulses

PRF = Pulse repetition frequency = 1/T

c = Velocity of sound

Sample
volume

$$PRF = c/(2 \times d)$$

The fact that PW Doppler permits only intermittent (pulsed) measurement of Doppler frequency shift comprises a mathematical and technical problem. Only when the frequency shift is equal to less than half the PRF can the velocity be properly assessed. When the Doppler frequency shift exceeds one-half the sampling rate (PRF/2), the direction of flow is depicted as being opposite to the true direction.

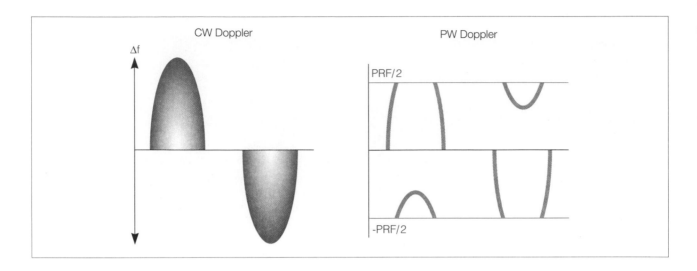

The PW Doppler spectrum usually has only a narrow frequency band (small Doppler gate), whereas the CW Doppler spectrum sums all velocities detected along the CW beam, thereby creating an appearance of fullness.

For any given transmission frequency, a curve of maximum measurable blood flow velocities at the selected depth of the Doppler gate can be derived.

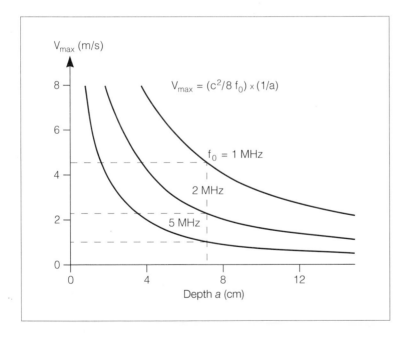

Doppler Color Flow Imaging

By placing multiple gates along the sector of the 2-D echocardiogram, and by separately assessing the Doppler frequency shifts for each of these gates, a two-dimensional distribution of Doppler frequency shifts can be obtained. Because moving tissue also causes a Doppler effect, a *tissue filter* is used to differentiate between blood flow and tissue to ensure that only blood flow signals are encoded in color.

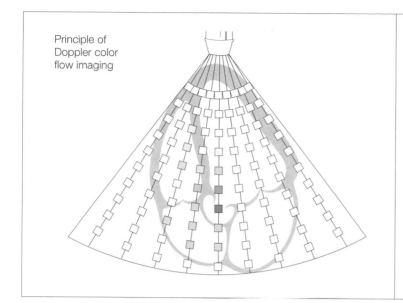

Principle of Doppler color flow imaging

Multiple range gates are placed within the defined region of the 2-D echocardiogram. Signals from each gate are evaluated separately by Doppler spectral analysis. A tissue filter is used to differentiate between tissue and flowing blood particles. This ensures that only blood flow signals are encoded in color. There are no binding rules for color assignment. Conventionally, flow towards the transducer is encoded in red, and flow away from the transducer is encoded in blue. The color-encoded image is superimposed on the two-dimensional image, and both are displayed simultaneously on the monitor.

Doppler frequency shift, amplitude of Doppler frequency shift, and spectral broadening in each individual gate is analyzed. This data is then used to assess the mean flow velocity, direction of flow, and degree of turbulence in each gate.

Various conventions exist for expressing these values on a color scale. Only the signals from gates containing blood flow information are encoded in color and superimposed on the two-dimensional image.

Because of the enormous amount of information that has to be processed for each individual gate, the temporal resolution of Doppler color flow imaging is significantly lower than that of conventional pulsed and continuous-wave Doppler. In order to obtain color flow images synchronous with cardiac phases, a small scanning sector must be selected, or the color Doppler M-mode format must be used instead. Combined use of color-encoded 2-D/M-mode and conventional PW and CW Doppler echocardiography is possible.

When conventional Doppler techniques are combined with color Doppler 2-D or M-mode echocardiograms, it is important to remember that the images are not produced simultaneously, but in rapid sequence by different methods of signal processing. However, the naked eye cannot recognize the difference.

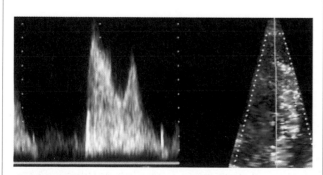

CW Doppler recording of the mitral valve and corresponding color Doppler four-chamber 2-D echocardiogram.

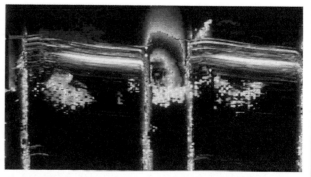

Color Doppler M-mode echocardiogram demonstrating a mitral valve prosthesis.

Because only one color can be assigned to a gate at a given point in time, the color assignment is based on the mean *blood flow velocity* within the gate.

When quantitative assessments are needed, pulsed or continuous-wave Doppler measurements must therefore be used.

Although Doppler color flow imaging is helpful and time-saving, it should be used only as an auxiliary technique in conjunction with PW and CW Doppler examinations.

Aliasing

The way that pulse repetition frequency (PRF) limits the ability of the ultrasound machine to accurately measure blood flow velocity was mentioned under the principles of PW Doppler.

These limitations also apply for Doppler color flow imaging, which is merely a modified version of conventional PW Doppler.

Aliasing is a phenomenon inherent to all pulsed measurement techniques.

Aliasing occurs when the Doppler frequency shift exceeds the *Nyquist limit,* which is defined as half the pulse repetition frequency (PRF/2).

In conventional PW Doppler, the top of the velocity curve is cut off and displayed in the opposite channel.

In Doppler color flow imaging, signals are *wrapped around or folded over* the time axis of the velocity spectrum, thereby resulting in color reversal, *i.e.* a reversal of color from red to blue, or vice versa. In other words, aliasing simulates a reversal in blood flow direction.

Although it is possible to determine the spatial orientation of a particular flow velocity in PW Doppler, it is not possible to individually assess all Doppler frequency shifts within the sample volume.

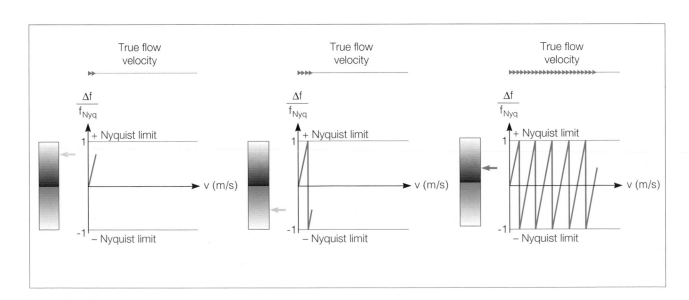

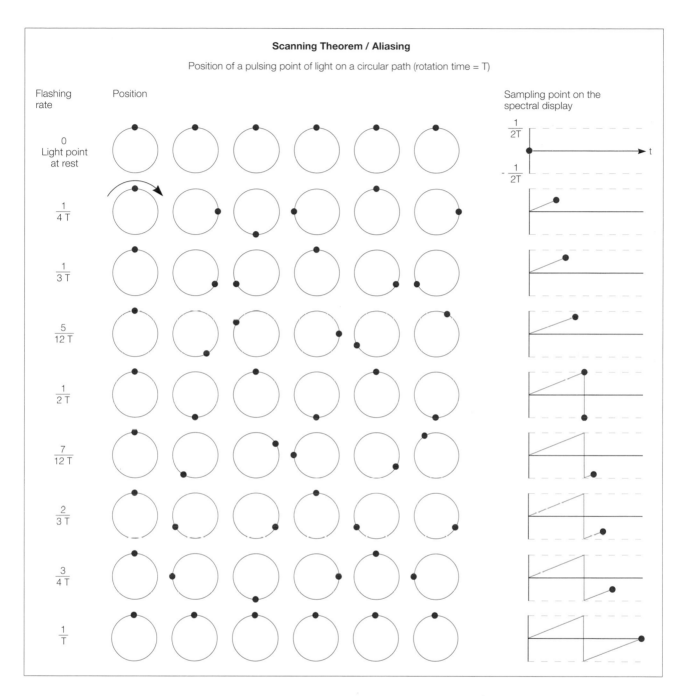

Scanning Theorem / Aliasing

Position of a pulsing point of light on a circular path (rotation time = T)

In the above diagram, a point of light travels in a circular path. The light travels at a constant velocity and pulses with different intensities (frequencies) of brightness. The frequency is measured and charted over time. At first it is easy to determine which direction the point of light is traveling in. The direction of rotation and the blinking rate can be determined by observing the point of light as it rotates (rows 1-4).

However, when the blinking rate is equal to one-half the rotation velocity (row 5), the point of light appears to be in two different places. Now it is no longer clear whether the point of light is traveling to the left or the right. The blinking rate has reached the Nyquist limit and aliasing occurs. When the blinking rate increases again (rows 6-8), the rotation velocity appears to have slowed down. In the last row of the diagram, the blinking rate has reached the rotation velocity. Although motion clearly is taking place, the point of light appears to rest in position (measured value = 0). These phenomena occur in any imaging system based on intermittent, pulsed measurement of motion.

Intra- and interobserver variability of findings in cardiac ultrasound is largely to blame for the lack of technical standardization. Fundamental variables such as the transducer frequency, angle of incidence, gain setting, and signal processing for imaging must be evaluated and set by the user on the basis of his or her level of skill and experience, and with the goal of the examination in mind. A second user has a different level of skill and experience, and he may prioritize the goal of the examination differently, or decide to select another examination technique instead. There are no binding rules for deciding which transducer frequency to use, nor can the transducer be continuously adjusted to maintain the desired level of compromise between resolution and depth of penetration. There is no truly reliable way to determine whether the most favorable angle of incidence has been found, and angle correction techniques tend to increase this uncertainty. There are as many "ideal" gain settings for an individual case as there are echocardiographers. When using filters, one cannot determine whether important details have also been filtered out, or whether noise has been included in the interpretation. The processing of signal data to obtain amplitude, brightness, and motion-modulated images (A, B, and M-mode) is on the one hand industrial standard and on the other hand a well kept secret.

As long as echocardiographic documents are compared with the naked eye alone instead of by means of mechanical methods with clearly defined rules, the lack of standardization will persist, and the standardization of implemented algorithms will only play a silent role in sales talks. In addition to price, number of technical features, and ergonometric design, the decision to buy an echocardiograph is usually based on its "superior imaging capabilities". Manufacturers sometimes attempt to explain why their transducer is superior to others, or why other transducers are inferior, by comparing construction features, the number of transducer elements, etc. However, it is impossible to make a truly quantitative comparison of raw and processed echocardiographic data obtained from different ultrasound systems. The same is true of color flow imaging, in which case all problems concerning the linearity of the color scale and the translation of the color scale into primary and secondary colors have been solved in practice, but not in theory.

The year-long standardization efforts have been focused on the problems of digital information technology and, thus, on the conditions for later processing, storage, and transfer of echocardiographic images.

It is still impossible to tell when and whether justifiable standardization techniques of signal production and signal processing for the generation of echocardiographic images will be established. In addition to the wide range of differences in transducer frequency, angle of incidence, gain settings, and signal processing for image generation, usable information is also lost due to arbitrary, conventional or unavoidable - at any rate non-standardized - choices made using the available alternatives.

Over the decades, the users of cardiac ultrasound technology have gained experience and expertise, which can be described as "rules of the trade". Some institutions have published recommendations, rules, and tips on how to obtain the quality echocardiographic images in clinical practice which, however, are sometimes arbitrary. One such institution is the *American Society of Echocardiography* [1-9].

The experience gained in designing and constructing echocardiographic systems and in interpreting the ultrasound signals has produces some rules of operation and technical standardizations. As a result, some systems are now compatible, and qualitative differences are more readily identifiable.

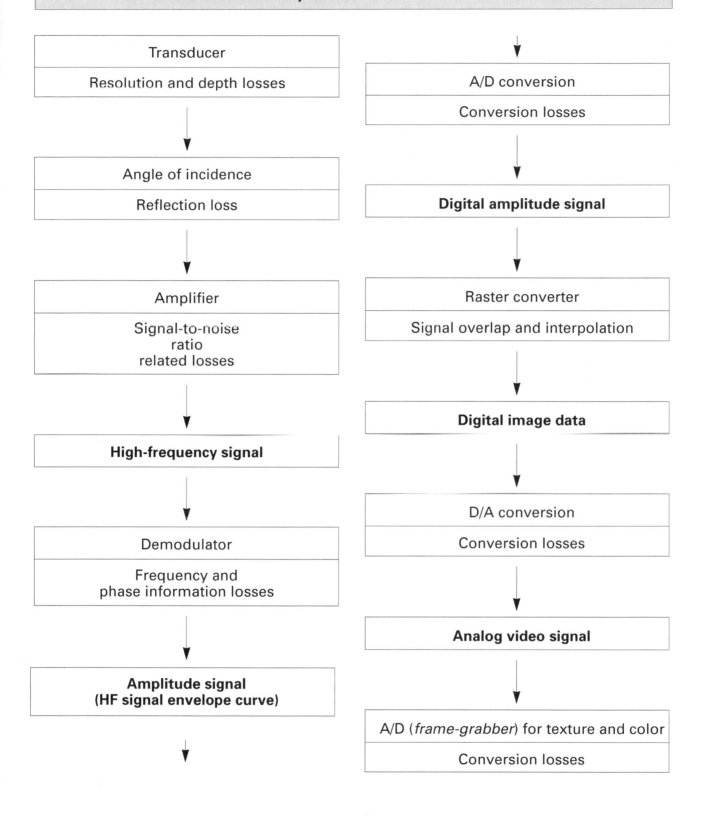

1.3   **Instrumentation and Technical Standardization**   **38**
of Cardiac Ultrasound Systems
1.3.1   **Instrumentation**

Modern echocardiographic instruments must have M-mode and two-dimensional echocardiographic capabilities as well as pulsed and continuous-wave Doppler capabilities. Doppler color flow imaging is becoming a standard procedure. The trend towards reduced prices in the microelectronic industry is helping to spread this technology.

Overview of Echocardiographic Instrumentation	
Basic unit	The basic unit is comprised of the power supply unit and the electronics needed to steer the ultrasound transducer in the different operating modes. It serves as a carrier for documentation technology, the monitor and peripheral equipment.
Transducer	The standard equipment of any echocardiographic system should include an ultrasound transducer with a transmission frequency of around 2.5 to 3.5 MHz (M-mode and 2-D echocardiography, PW and CW Doppler).
	Higher frequency transducers are also available. Optional: Transducer probes for single plane, biplane, or multiplane transesophageal echocardiography.
	A pencil transducer with a transmission frequency of 2.0 MHz should also be a part of the standard equipment.
Monitor	The monitor is used to display ultrasound images generated by the various operating modes. All assessment and measurement tasks are performed using the monitor. For better imaging quality, a black-and-white monitor should be used instead of a color monitor in systems that do not employ Doppler color flow imaging. On the other side, a color monitor should be used in systems employing Doppler color flow imaging. Some manufacturers offer instruments with two integrated monitors, one for black-and-white and a second for color display. Monitors now operate on internationally standardized video standards (Europe = standard PAL; USA = NTSC).
Documentation	In order to record dynamic processes, a video recorder must be installed. Color and black-and-white video printers for single-frame documentation are optional, but useful. A 35 mm camera can be installed to make slides for training purposes. Alternatively, a multiformat camera can be used with planar x-ray film.
	Computer assisted documentation techniques are gaining increasing application in echocardiography. However, interfaces have not yet been standardized.
ECG	An ECG should always be recorded simultaneously with the electrocardiogram. ECG triggering is helpful, but not mandatory, since the image storage device (cine loop) is large enough in the majority of ultrasound machines. Ports are provided for connecting a phonocardiograph and other external signals.
Software	Should include fundamental cardiologic measurement programs.

With an adequate knowledge of the most important physical principles, the physician should view the echocardiographic examination as an interaction between the machine, the patient, and the operator. In other words, the operator must properly manipulate the instrument settings to achieve optimal results. Every physician-trainee should be properly trained in the use of the echocardiographic control panel.

The echocardiographic control panel is often organized in functional groups of mostly instrument-independent control elements. The most important elements for instrument operation should be explained.

Nomenclature

The monitor of the ultrasound machine displays images that have been synthesized using various echocardiographic modes of operation (M-mode and 2-D echocardiography, PW and CW Doppler, Doppler color flow imaging). In this volume, B-mode has sometimes been used to denote two-dimensional echocardiography, which is generated using multiple individual B-mode scan lines. M-mode and TM-mode may also be used synonymously. Unless otherwise stated, Doppler color flow imaging, or color Doppler, refers to the combination of two-dimensional echocardiography and color-encoded Doppler.

**1.3   Instrumentation and Technical Standardization
         of Cardiac Ultrasound Systems**
1.3.2   Technical Standardization of Cardiac Ultrasound Systems

Pulsed and continuous-wave Doppler techniques provide spectral displays (velocity versus time) that document the functional correlation between blood flow velocity and cardiac phase. However, Doppler signals are processed very different from two-dimensional (B-mode) and M-mode echocardiographic signals.

Instrument Operation and Settings

It is important to differentiate between settings used when the transducer is activated (pre-processing), and those used simply for cosmetic image improvement (post-processing).

The following list is not complete. It describes settings that can be found on every echocardiograph.

Pre-Processing

M-Mode and 2-D Echocardiography (B-Mode)

- **Total gain**
  This control adjusts the gain setting for all received signals. Noise is amplified along with the signal.

- **Depth-selective gain or time-gain compensation (TGC)**
  Signals reflected from like interfaces located at different depths of penetration should be displayed with the same gray level intensity. However, because signals from greater depths are attenuated and refracted, their amplitude is significantly lower than that of returning echoes from tissues structures located proximal to the transducer.

Time gain compensation utilizes depth-selective amplification of signals to make up for the intensity lost due to longer transit times.

- **Depth of penetration**
  Signals from the desired depth of penetration can be obtained by activating the receiving mode of the transducer at the appropriate time. Since signals from deeper depths require longer transit times, they are not recorded. The depth of penetration is set at the level of the structure of interest.

- **Sector angle (2-D echocardiography only)**
  The size of the sector angle and the depth of penetration are decisive determiners of the refresh rate (number of frames per second). The temporal resolution is good when the depth is small and the sector is narrow (30°), but assessment of the total cardiac structure is limited. The sector can be rotated within certain limits.

- **Sweep rate (only in M-mode)**
  This function spreads or compresses the time axis on the M-mode display. It can be used to vary the number of heart actions displayed on the monitor.

Pulsed and Continuous-Wave Doppler

- **Total gain**
  This control adjusts the gain setting for all received signals. Noise is amplified along with the signal.

- **Wall motion filter**
  Regardless of whether they are comprised of blood particles or tissue, all moving scatterers and reflecting objects in the path of the CW Doppler beam or within the Doppler gate create a Doppler effect. A wall motion filter can be used to filter out strong signals from tissue, such as those caused by motion of the walls of the heart.

- **Baseline shift**
  Usually the spectral display begins with a symmetrical velocity scale (equal measurement range for positive and negative velocity directions). By shifting the baseline in a positive or negative direction, one measurement range is expanded while the other is reduced. The total measurement range remains constant. Flow velocities that result in aliasing on PW Doppler recordings can sometimes be displayed adequately when the baseline is shifted. Baseline shift is included as a post-processing function on some systems.

- **Position of the CW Doppler beam, placement of the PW Doppler sample volume**
  The position from which velocity distribution is to be measured is displayed on the 2-D echocardiogram. It can be freely defined within the 2-D sector. The depth of the PW Doppler sample volume is defined in the same manner.

- **Size of the PW Doppler sample volume**
  The size of the sample volume ranges from ca. 2 to 20 mm, and can be increased or decreased in small increments. Signal intensity is proportional to sample volume size. Local, sharply delimited flow phenomena should be interrogated using a small sample volume.

1.3   **Instrumentation and Technical Standardization**   41
           of Cardiac Ultrasound Systems
1.3.2   **Technical Standardization of Cardiac Ultrasound Systems**

- **Sweep Rate**
  This function spreads or compresses the time axis on the Doppler spectral display. It can be used to vary the number of heart actions displayed on the monitor.

- **Pulse Repetition Frequency (only for PW Doppler)**
  The size of the PW Doppler measurement range is dependent on the depth of the sample volume. The pulse repetition frequency (PRF) therefore determines the maximum velocity that can be measured without causing aliasing. The PRF should always be adjusted in accordance with the depth of penetration in order to properly display the entire velocity spectrum. Conventionally, the PRF can be adjusted in steps of 0.5 or 1 kHz within a range of ca. 3 to 12 kHz.

Doppler Color Flow Imaging

- **Total gain**
  This control adjusts the gain setting for all received signals; noise is amplified along with the signal.

- **Wall motion filter**
  All moving and reflecting objects within the color-encoded region create a Doppler effect. The motion of the heart walls generates a Doppler signal that sometimes is superimposed upon the structure of interest in the two-dimensional echocardiogram. By manipulating the wall filter, it is possible to maintain the integrity of cardiac structures in 2-D echocardiograms. The velocities that the wall filter fades out are not included in the computations for color-encoding.

- **Size of the color-encoded sector**
  Conventionally, the area to be color-encoded is defined as a sector (or portion of a sector) on sector transducers. The position of the color sector can be freely defined on the two-dimensional echocardiogram. The angle of the color sector can also be variably defined on the 2-D echocardiogram. Because Doppler color flow imaging is a very time-consuming process (compared with PW or CW Doppler), temporal resolution is dependent on the size of the color sector.

- **Baseline shift**
  Usually color flow imaging begins with a symmetrical spectral velocity scale (equal measurement range for positive and negative velocity directions). By shifting the baseline in a positive or negative direction, one measurement range is expanded while the other is reduced. The total measurement range remains constant. Flow phenomena that result in aliasing in Doppler color flow imaging can sometimes be displayed en bloc by employing baseline shift. Baseline shift is included as a post-processing function on some systems.

- **Pulse Repetition Frequency (PRF)**
  The size of the PW Doppler measurement range is dependent on the depth of the color sector. The PRF at a fixed depth of penetration determines the Nyquist limit. Aliasing occurs when velocities within the color-encoded area exceed the Nyquist limit, *i.e.*, there is color reversal from red to blue, or vice versa. Conventionally, the PRF can be adjusted in steps of 0.5 or 1 kHz within a range of ca. 3 to 12 kHz.

All of the above-mentioned parameters can be stored as *presettings*. When the ultrasound machine is started up, the personally preferred settings are displayed and are utilized in the various modes of operation.

Post-Processing

M-mode and Two-Dimensional Echocardiography (B-Mode)

- **Gray scale display**

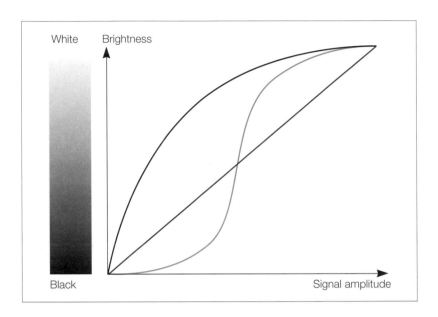

The M-mode and 2-D (B-mode) echocardiographic data stored in the image memory can be converted (scan converter) by means of various functions to a gray scale display. Each function manipulates the display differently. The red-encoded function utilizes linear transmission. In the blue curve, the signal was spread in the mid-range of the gray scale. This can be used to sharply delineate contours or to boost the system's contrast resolution.

Doppler Color Flow Imaging

- **Color assignment**
  Color flow imaging is based on a color scale. The number of shades on the color scale may vary. Similar to the gray scale used in two-dimensional imaging, the velocities measured at each Doppler gate are assigned a corresponding shade of color. The scale can be manipulated to optimize high or low velocity display, or to emphasize variance, which is represented as the degree of flow turbulence in Doppler color flow images.

All Operating Modes

- **Noise Filter**
  A noise filter can be used in all operating modes. The filter level can be adjusted. Part of the signal is also filtered out at higher levels of filtration.

Reproducibility

Image documents generated by cardiac ultrasound exist as monitor images, video printouts, slides, and video tapes. Documents generated on systems produced by different manufactures will be comparable as long as the same display standards have been used.

For all displays, the depth of penetration is determined as a function of transit time. In order to convert the transit time to depth, a constant velocity of sound (1540 m/s) is assumed.

Additional conventions to ensure the reproducibility of documents are summarized below.

Compatibility

The compatibility of image documents is basically a question of recording standards. All manufactures offer standardized signal outlets that can be used to document single frames and to record sequences in the appropriate video standard (VHS and S-VHS in Europe, and NTSC in the USA).

Images can easily be recorded on videotape. Internal measurement software for digitization of single frame documents obtained from videotape functions only in compatible systems.

| 1.3.2 | Technical Standardization of Cardiac Ultrasound Systems |
| 1.3.2.2 | Standardization of Algorithms Used in M-Mode and Two-Dimensional Echocardiography, Doppler Spectral Displays, and Color Flow Imaging |

The most important conventions for each individual operating mode are listed below.

Two-Dimensional Echocardiography

The horizontal and vertical axes of the monitor represent dimensions. The depth of penetration of ultrasound in the body is shown on the vertical axis, and the lateral dimension of the sector arc extending at a right angle to the ultrasound beam is shown on the horizontal axis. Both dimensions are given in centimeters.

1.3.2   **Technical Standardization of Cardiac Ultrasound Systems**   **44**
1.3.2.2   **Standardization of Algorithms Used in M-Mode and Two-Dimensional**
                Echocardiography, Doppler Spectral Displays, and Color Flow Imaging

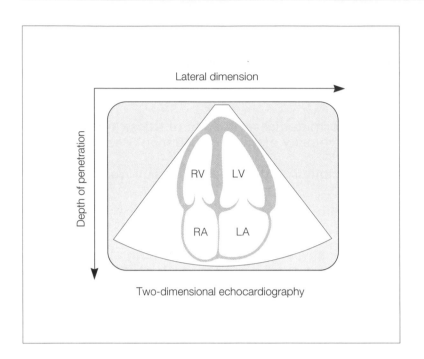

M-Mode Echocardiography

The depth of beam penetration into the body (cm) is represented on the vertical axis, and time is shown on the horizontal axis (units: s and ms).

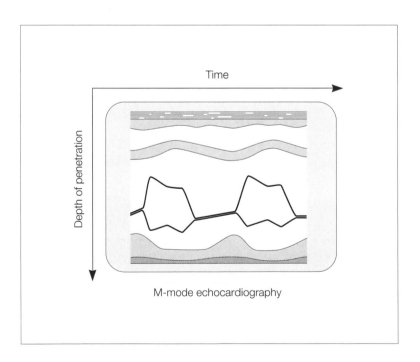

PW Doppler, CW Doppler, Doppler Color Flow Imaging

Frequencies and the relationship of frequencies to one another are key elements in Doppler signal analysis. Doppler frequency shifts can be analyzed to determine the direction of blood flow, the contribution of different components lying on the acoustic axis, the frequency of occurrence of a particular velocity, and temporal changes in distribution of velocities in diastole and in systole. Another key aspect is *spectral broadening,* which occurs when there is turbulent flow.

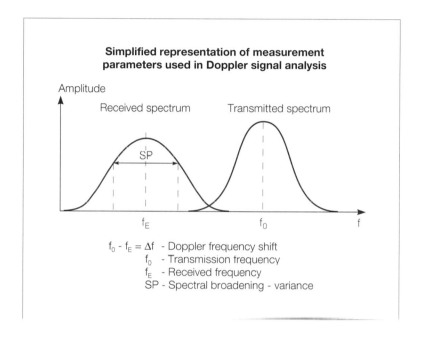

PW Doppler and CW Doppler spectral displays show the course of blood flow velocity over time. Velocity (m/s or cm/s) is displayed on the vertical axis, and time is represented on the horizontal axis. The time axis can be scaled up or down, similar to the method used in M-mode.

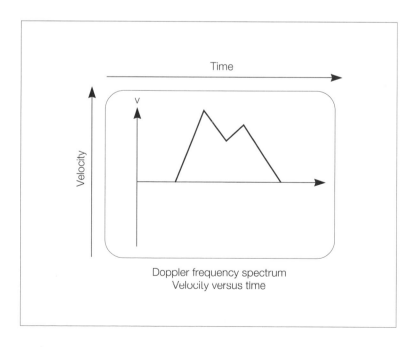

Doppler Color Flow Imaging

The *direction of flow* is described using the colors red and blue, as described below:

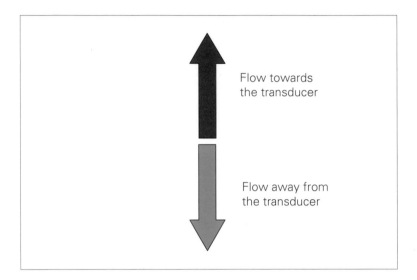

Flow towards the transducer

Flow away from the transducer

The *velocity of flow* is described using different shades of red and blue. The number of shades used on the color scale may vary from one system to another.

The *quality of flow* can also be described. Turbulence, which is characterized by spectral broadening in pulsed and continuous-wave Doppler, is indicated by the color green. Laminar flow, on the other hand, is indicated by the primary colors red and blue.

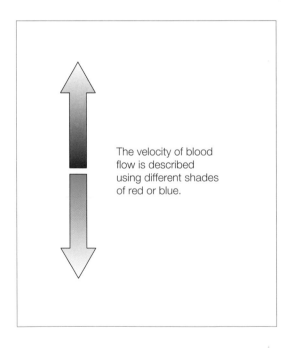

The velocity of blood flow is described using different shades of red or blue.

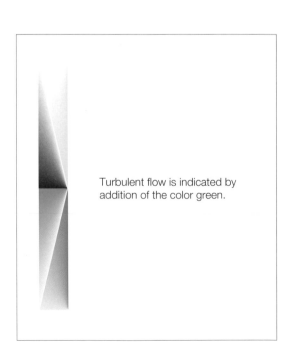

Turbulent flow is indicated by addition of the color green.

The following guidelines apply to all cardiac ultrasound systems.

By storing the instrument settings in the memory, one can be sure that the same settings can be reproduced for later examinations. When more than one operator must use the same machine, each operator should store his or her personalized presettings.

Furthermore, the pertinent technical data should always be recorded both on the monitor and the image document to ensure reproducibility and comparability.

Echocardiographic examinations must be performed with simultaneous ECG recording. Without the ECG recording, it would be impossible to properly determine the timing of cardiac events over the course of the cardiac ultrasound examination.

References

---

1. American Society of Echocardiography Committee on Standards, Subcommittee on Quantitation of Two-dimensional Echocardiograms. Recommendations for quantitation of left ventricle by two-dimensional echocardiography. J Am Soc Echo 1989; 2: 358-367.
2. American Society of Echocardiography Committee on Doppler Standards and Nomenclature. Recommendations for terminology and display for Doppler echocardiography.
3. Pearlman AS, Gardin JM, Randolph MP, Parisi AF, Popp RL, Quinones MA, Stevenson JG. Guidelines for optimal physician training in echocardiography. Recommendations of the American Society of Echocardiography Committee for physician training in echocardiography. Am J Cardiol 1987; 60: 158-163.
4. Pearlman AS, Gardin JM, Randolph MP, Parisi AF, Popp RL, Quinones MA, Stevenson JG, Schiller NB, Seward JB, Stewart WJ. Guidelines for physician training in transesophageal echocardiography: Recommendations of the American Society of Echocardiography Committee for physician training in echocardiography. J Am Soc Echo 1992; 5: 187-194.
5. Report of the American Society of Echocardiography Committee on Nomenclature and Standards in Two-dimensional Echocardiography.
6. Report of the American Society of Echocardiography Committee on Nomenclature and Standards: Identification of myocardial wall segments.
7. Report of the American Society of Echocardiography: Contrast echocardiography.
8. Schiller NB, Maurer G, Ritter SB, Armstrong WF, Crawford M, Spotnitz H, Cahalan M, Quinones M, Meltzer R, Feinstein S, Konstadt S, Seward J. Transesophageal echocardiography. J Am Soc Echo 1989; 2: 354-357.
9. Society of Pediatric Echocardiography Committee in Nomenclature. Suggested nomenclature of cardiac septa. Addendum to: Report of the American Society of Echocardiography Committee on Nomenclature and Standards: Identification of myocardial wall segments.

2. Conventional Echocardiography: Examination Procedure, Fundamental Measurement and Assessment Tasks
(Kurt J.G. Schmailzl)

49

The plethora of terms describing echocardiography (A, B and M-modes, 1, 2, 3, and 4-dimensional echocardiography, pulsed and continuous-wave Doppler, and Doppler color flow imaging) reflects the diverse technical development and history of echocardiography. However, the nomenclature itself tends to become historical as soon as its components are popularized in general diagnosis-oriented "echo".

Any diagnostic approach that is oriented with respect to the chronological sequence of scientific and technical developments of echocardiography is similarly antiquated and hardly practical.

Over the years, echocardiographic examinations have become less routine, and they must provide much more than basic measurements and assessments. To go beyond the routine, the echocardiographer must have a high level of personal skill and technical experience, and a good knowledge of all available diagnostic techniques. These vital aspects will be discussed in this chapter.

In diagnostic screening, the echocardiographer must investigate the questions posed by the referring physician. He must do this by combining all echocardiographic techniques at his disposal.

2. Conventional Echocardiography: Examination Procedure, Fundamental Measurement and Assessment Tasks
2.1 Diagnostic Screening

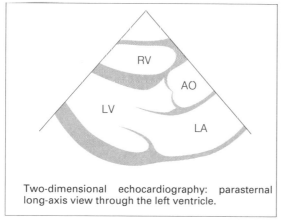

Two-dimensional echocardiography: parasternal long-axis view through the left ventricle.

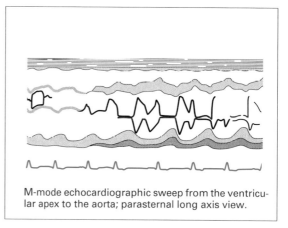

M-mode echocardiographic sweep from the ventricular apex to the aorta; parasternal long axis view.

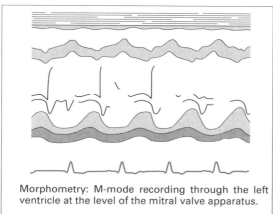

Morphometry: M-mode recording through the left ventricle at the level of the mitral valve apparatus.

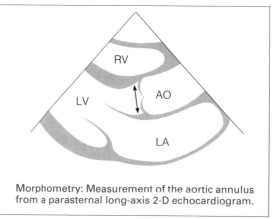

Morphometry: Measurement of the aortic annulus from a parasternal long-axis 2-D echocardiogram.

2.   **Conventional Echocardiography: Examination Procedure,**   50
               Fundamental Measurement and Assessment Tasks
2.1   **Diagnostic Screening**

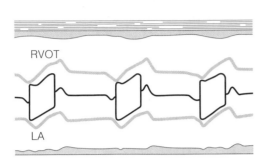

Morphometry: M-mode echocardiogram through the right ventricular outflow tract (RVOT), aorta (AO), and left atrium (LA).

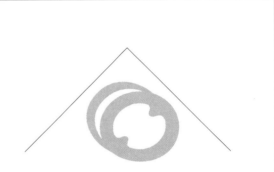

Doppler color flow map of parasternal long-axis 2-D echocardiogram through the left ventricle.

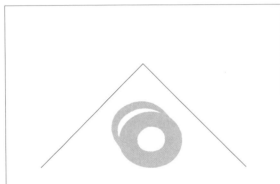

Parasternal short-axis view through the ventricle at apex level (2-D echo).

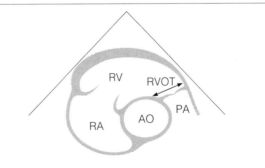

Parasternal short-axis view through the ventricle at papillary muscle level (2-D echo).

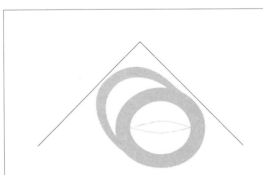

Parasternal short-axis view through the ventricle at mitral valve level (2-D echo).

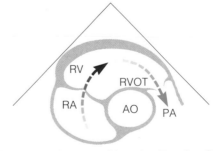

Parasternal cross-sectional view of the aortic root and longitudinal view of the right heart cavities and main pulmonary trunk (2-D echo), used for morphometry of the pulmonary annulus.

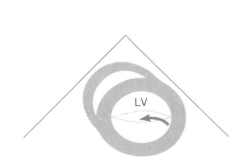

2-D echocardiogram with color Doppler flow mapping; parasternal short-axis view through the ventricle at mitral valve level.

2-D echocardiogram with color Doppler flow mapping; parasternal short-axis view of the aortic root and long-axis view of the right heart cavities and main pulmonary trunk.

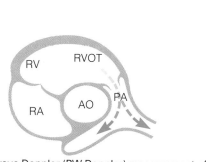

Pulsed-wave Doppler (PW Doppler) measurement of transpulmonary flow velocity obtained from 2-D long-axis scan through the main pulmonary trunk.

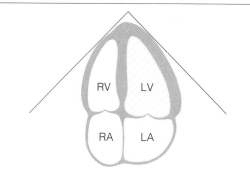

Wall motion analysis and planimetry using an apical four-chamber 2-D echocardiogram.

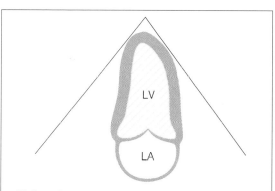

Wall motion analysis and planimetry of the left ventricle using an apical two-chamber 2-D echocardiogram.

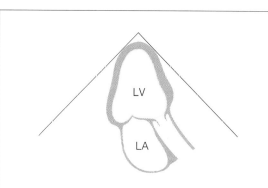

Wall motion analysis using an apical long-axis 2-D scan through the ventricle (RAO view).

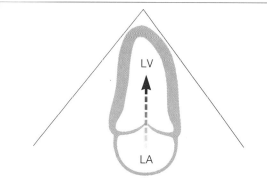

Apical two-chamber 2-D echocardiogram with color Doppler flow mapping.

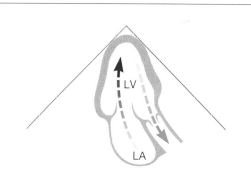

2-D echocardiogram with color Doppler flow mapping; apical long-axis view through the left ventricle (RAO view).

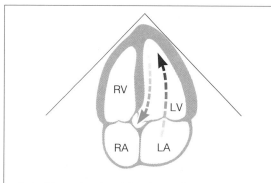

Apical four-chamber 2-D echocardiogram with color Doppler flow mapping.

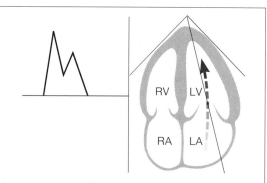

Apical four-chamber 2-D echocardiogram using color-guided CW Doppler to assess transmitral flow.

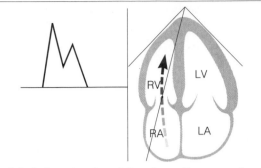

Apical four-chamber 2-D echocardiogram using color-guided CW Doppler to assess transtricuspid flow.

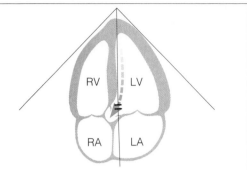

Apical four-chamber 2-D echocardiogram using color-guided PW Doppler to measure flow velocity in the outflow tract.

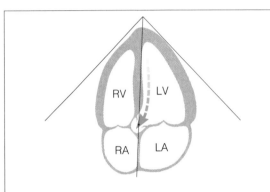

Apical four-chamber 2-D echocardiogram using color-guided CW Doppler to assess transaortic flow.

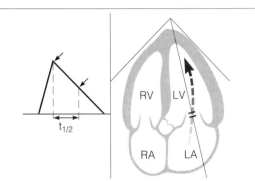

Apical four-chamber 2-D echocardiogram using color-guided PW Doppler to assess the mitral valve area (MVA).

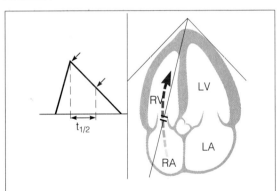

Apical four-chamber 2-D echocardiogram using color-guided PW Doppler to assess tricuspid valve area (TVA).

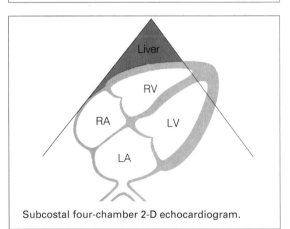

Subcostal four-chamber 2-D echocardiogram.

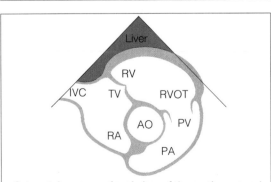

Subcostal cross-sectional view of the aortic root and long-axis view of right heart cavities and main pulmonary trunk.

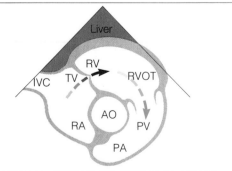

Subcostal cross-sectional view of the aortic root and long-axis view of the right heart cavities and main pulmonary trunk; with Doppler color flow imaging.

2.   **Conventional Echocardiography: Examination Procedure,**
        Fundamental Measurement and Assessment Tasks   **53**
2.1   **Diagnostic Screening**

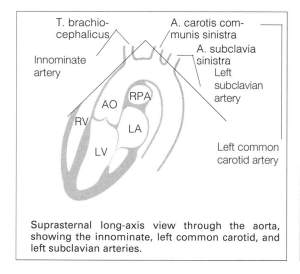

Suprasternal long-axis view through the aorta, showing the innominate, left common carotid, and left subclavian arteries.

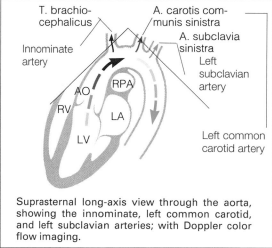

Suprasternal long-axis view through the aorta, showing the innominate, left common carotid, and left subclavian arteries; with Doppler color flow imaging.

2.   **Conventional Echocardiography: Examination Procedure,**
        Fundamental Measurement and Assessment Tasks
2.2   **Transducer Locations and Imaging Planes**

In echocardiography, the imaging planes used to visualize the heart are defined according to three orthogonal planes, namely: the *long-axis plane,* the *short-axis plane,* and the *four-chamber plane.* These planes are not based strictly on the traditional morphological coordinate system (sagittal, transverse, coronal), but on the manner in which they transsect the heart.

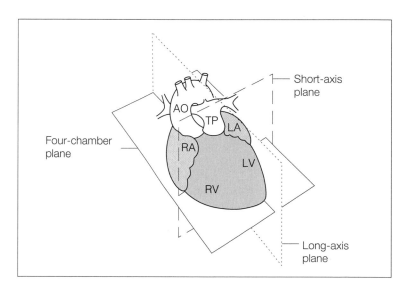

Two-dimensional echocardiograms are classified with respect to the transducer location and the echotomographic plane. All two-dimensional imaging transducers should have an *index mark* indicating the edge of the imaging plane, *i.e.,* the direction of the ultrasound beam.

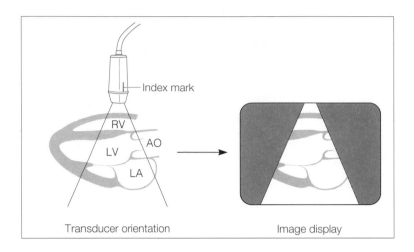

The index mark indicates the part of the image plane that should appear on the right side of the image display. If, for example, the index mark is pointing towards the aorta from a parasternal long-axis view, the aorta will appear on the right-hand side of the image display. As a rule of thumb, the mark should always point either towards the head or towards the left-hand side of the patient.

The conventional but arbitrary orientation of the *apical four-chamber* view is contrary to morphological relationships. On the image display, the ventricle is located on top, the atria on the bottom, the right heart cavities on the left, and the left heart cavities on the right. In the *subcostal four-chamber* view the right heart cavities appear on the top, the atria appear on the left, the left heart cavities appear on the bottom, and the ventricles appear on the right of the image display.

Long-axis views (LAX) of the heart can be obtained from parasternal, apical and suprasternal transducer locations.

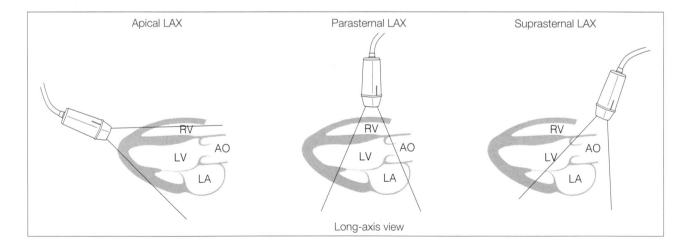

There are recommendations that specify exactly where to place the transducer (parasternal location = 3rd to 4th intercostal space; apical location = site of apex beat; subcostal location = epigastric region; suprasternal location = jugular fossa), and that describe exactly how to rotate the transducer along the spatial axis to achieve a standard view. However, this type of recommendation disregards the inter-individual differences in topography. As a rule, the transducer should be positioned in such a way that the closest possible approximation of the standard echocardiographic view is obtained.

2.   **Conventional Echocardiography: Examination Procedure,**
                 Fundamental Measurement and Assessment Tasks
2.2   **Transducer Locations and Imaging Planes**

55

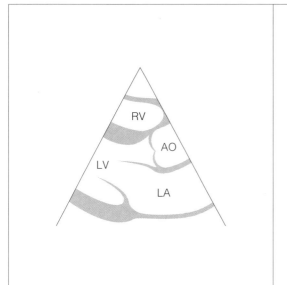

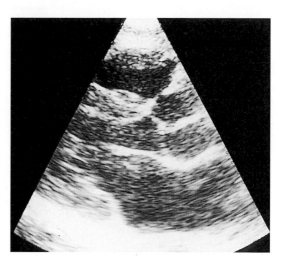

Left parasternal long-axis 2-D echocardiogram.

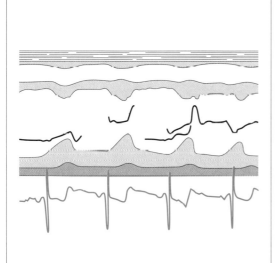

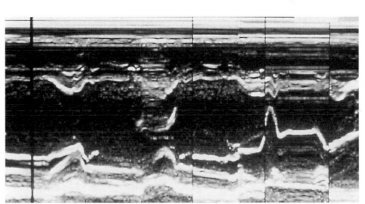

M-mode recording obtained from a left parasternal long-axis 2-D scan at the level of the mitral valve apparatus.

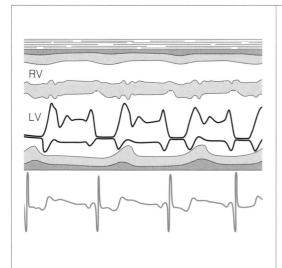

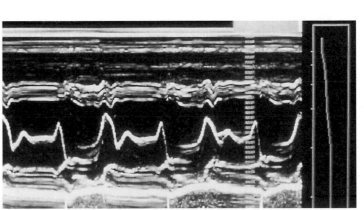

M-mode recording obtained from the left parasternal long-axis view at mitral valve level.

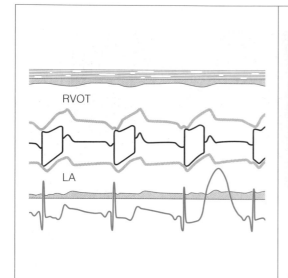

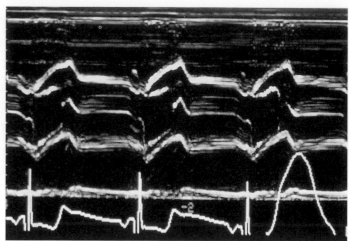

M-mode recording obtained from the left parasternal long-axis view at the level of the right ventricular outflow tract, aortic root, and left atrium.

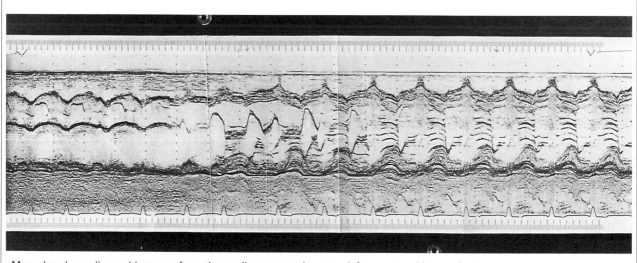

M-mode echocardiographic sweep from the cardiac apex to the aorta, left parasternal long-axis view.

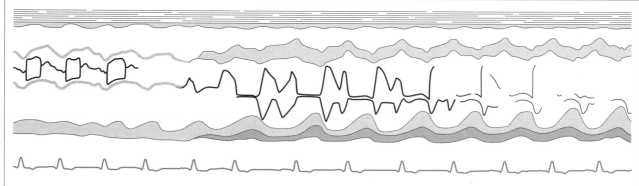

M-mode echocardiographic sweep from the cardiac apex to the aorta, obtained from the left parasternal long-axis view.

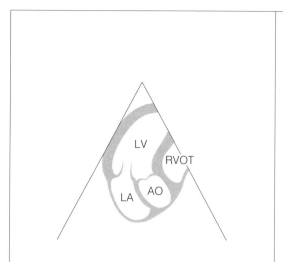

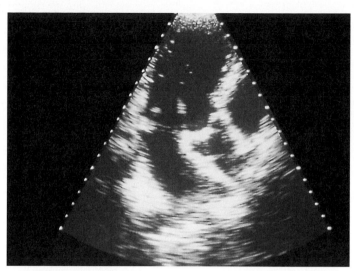

Apical long-axis view through the left ventricle (RAO equivalent view).

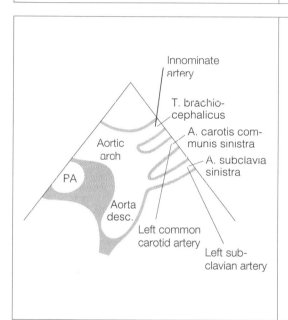

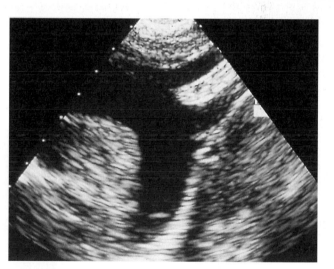

Suprasternal long-axis view through the aorta and its larger branches, right pulmonary artery, and left atrium.

Short-axis views (SAX) of the heart are normally obtained from parasternal and subcostal transducer positions. Additional images can be obtained from the suprasternal position, if necessary.

2.   **Conventional Echocardiography: Examination Procedure,**   **58**
             Fundamental Measurement and Assessment Tasks
2.2   **Transducer Locations and Imaging Planes**

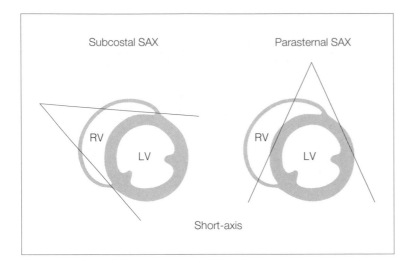

The left *parasternal short-axis view* is obtained by rotating the transducer 90° clockwise along the long axis. By variably rotating and angulating the transducer about the longitudinal axis of the left ventricle, short-axis images can be obtained at the following levels: cardiac apex; papillary muscles; mitral valve; aorta and right cardiac outflow tract from the inferior vena cava across the right atrium, right ventricle and right ventricular outflow tract to the pulmonary valve, the main pulmonary trunk and its primary bifurcation into the pulmonary arteries; the coronary sinus, and the left atrium.

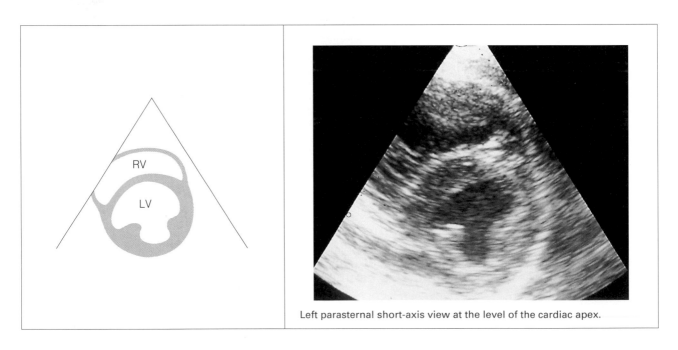

Left parasternal short-axis view at the level of the cardiac apex.

2. **Conventional Echocardiography: Examination Procedure,**
Fundamental Measurement and Assessment Tasks
2.2 **Transducer Locations and Imaging Planes**

59

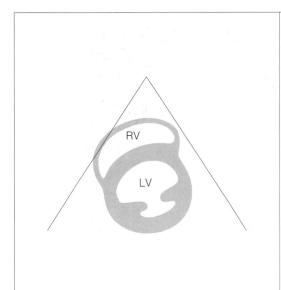

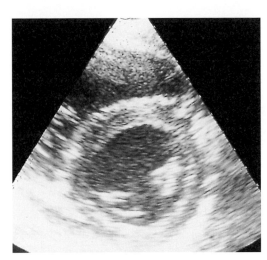

Left parasternal short-axis view at papillary muscle level.

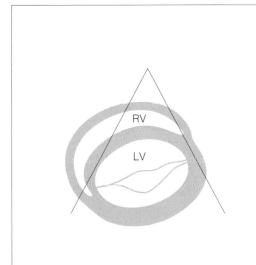

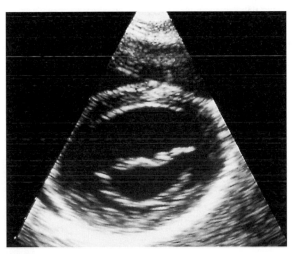

Left parasternal short-axis view at mitral valve level.

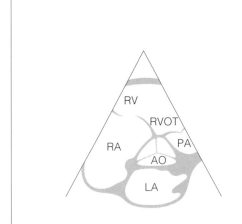

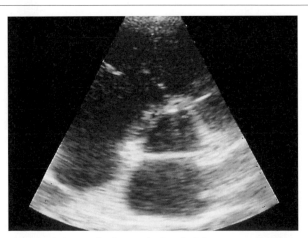

Left parasternal short-axis view at the level of the aorta and right cardiac outflow tract from the inferior vena cava, showing the right atrium, right ventricle and right ventricular outflow tract, pulmonary valve, and main pulmonary trunk.

2.　　**Conventional Echocardiography: Examination Procedure,**
　　　　Fundamental Measurement and Assessment Tasks　　　**60**

2.2　　**Transducer Locations and Imaging Planes**

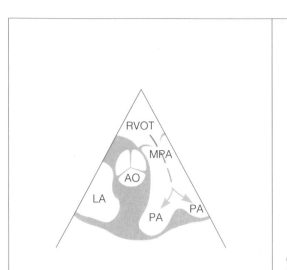

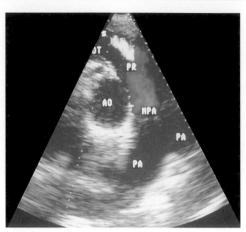

Color flow map of the left parasternal short-axis view at the level of the aorta, showing the right cardiac outflow tract from the IVC across the right atrium, right ventricle and RVOT to the pulmonary valve, the main pulmonary trunk and its primary bifurcation into the pulmonary arteries, the coronary sinus and the left atrium.

The *subcostal short-axis view* is obtained by rotating the transducer 90° counter-clockwise along the four-chamber axis. Depending on which structure was visualized in the four-chamber view, a short-axis view through either the left ventricle or the aorta will be obtained. This view corresponds to the long-axis view through the right ventricle and its inflow and outflow tract, including the right atrium and the bifurcation of the pulmonary arteries.

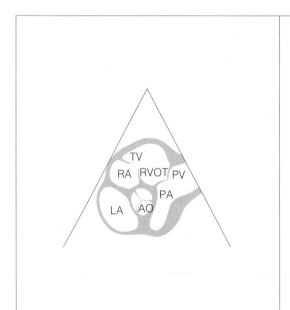

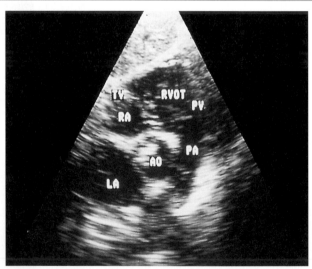

Subcostal short axis 2-D echocardiogram, showing cross-sectional view of the aorta and longitudinal view of the heart cavities.

Four and five-chamber views of the four heart cavities and, in the case of the five-chamber view, the aorta are obtained from apical and subcostal portals.

2.   **Conventional Echocardiography: Examination Procedure,**   **61**
          Fundamental Measurement and Assessment Tasks
2.2   **Transducer Locations and Imaging Planes**

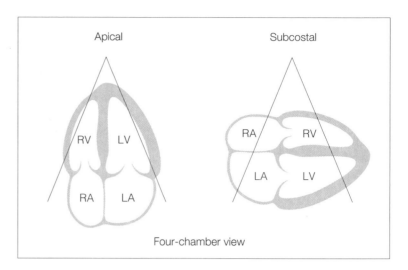

The *apical five-chamber view* of the four heart cavities and the aorta is obtained by superiorly angulating the transducer from the apical four-chamber view towards the sternum. The *subcostal five-chamber view* is obtained by angulating the transducer towards the stomach while slightly rotating it clockwise. This provides visualization of the left ventricular outflow tract, including sub- and supravalvular regions of the aortic valves and, in some cases, the ascending aorta and the aortic arch including the origins of the main branches.

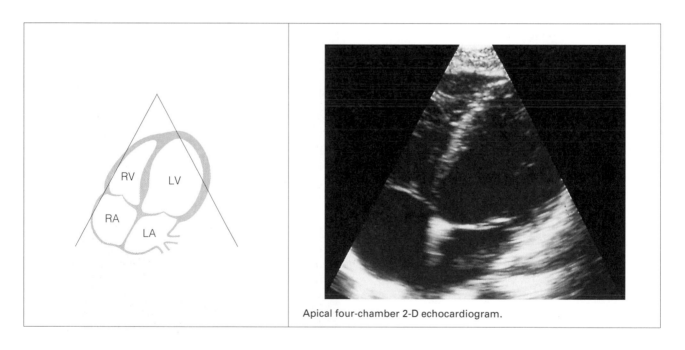

Apical four-chamber 2-D echocardiogram.

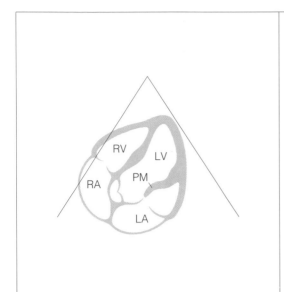

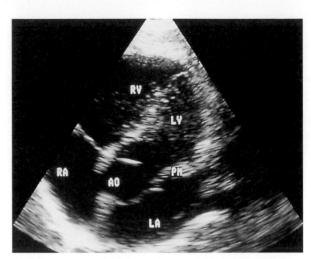

Apical five-chamber 2-D echocardiogram.

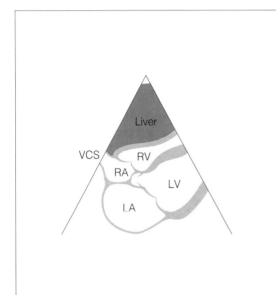

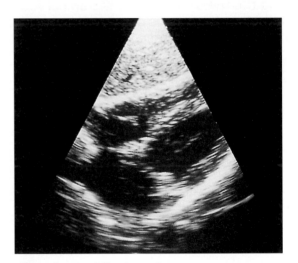

Subcostal four-chamber 2-D echocardiogram.

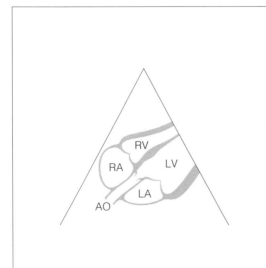

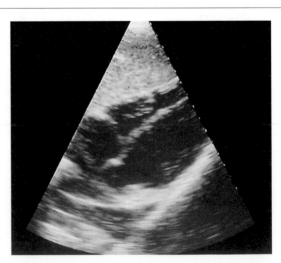

Subcostal five-chamber 2-D echocardiogram, demonstrating the left ventricular outflow tract.

2.   **Conventional Echocardiography: Examination Procedure,**   **63**
            Fundamental Measurement and Assessment Tasks

2.3   **Morphometry**

Echocardiography distinguishes itself from competing and complementary diagnostic techniques by virtue of two seemingly contradictory features. The first is its high precision of measurement. Echocardiographic left ventricular morphometry has made the roentgenographically derived cardio-thoracic ratio for determination of cardiac hypertrophy a seemingly medieval technique. On the other hand, echocardiographic images often are sometimes practically worthless due to limitations of the echocardiographic window, lack of technical expertise of the physician, and noncritical acceptance of findings.

The range of error in one-dimensional measurements should not exceed 5%. It this is not possible, one should either use semiquantitative assessments or dispense altogether with units of size, velocity, etc.

Measurement error must be kept within an acceptable and calculable range. Routine quality control is therefore essential for both new and experienced echocardiographers. If, for example, a left ventricular end-diastolic dimension of 50 mm is measured today, and a dimension of 55 mm is measured 6 months later, two possible explanations exist: 1. disease-related enlargement, or 2. measurement error. The physician must then decide whether to take further diagnostic action or whether to declare the measurement findings invalid. This is particularly important with respect to measurements of interventricular septum thickness, posterior left ventricular wall thickness, left ventricular dimension, aortic diameter, left atrial diameter, and diameter of the pulmonary and aortic valve rings.

Two basic rules of M-mode echocardiography are:
- The plane of section should be perfectly perpendicular to heart and vessel walls.
- This should be visually confirmed, *i.e.*, endocardial lines should be visible and easily distinguishable, and no double contour lines should appear. M-mode echocardiograms should be two dimensionally guided to ensure accurate placement of the beam.

Each echocardiography laboratory should maintain good quality standards by allowing physician-trainees adequate training time and by assessing inter- and intra-observer measurement variability for all echocardiographers at regular intervals.

Each laboratory should have a standardized examination procedure that routinely starts with the patient in the left lateral position, and with echocardiograms acquired at end-expiration. Electrocardiograms should always be recorded simultaneously with echocardiography. Failure to do so constitutes malpractice.

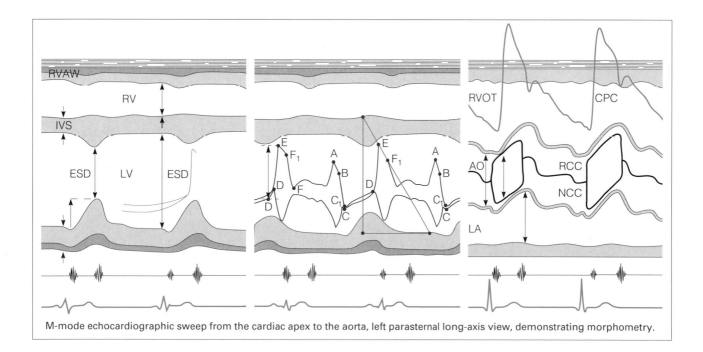

M-mode echocardiographic sweep from the cardiac apex to the aorta, left parasternal long-axis view, demonstrating morphometry.

Measurements are made using *leading edge methodology, i.e.,* from the leading edge of the first echo boundary to the leading edge of the second echo boundary [11]. For example, one measures from the outer surface of the anterior endocardial boundary to the anterior surface of the posterior endocardial boundary of the interventricular septum, or from the adventitia of the anterior aortic wall to the endocardium of the posterior aortic wall. *Exception:* Inner edge methodology is then used when measuring ventricular outflow tract diameter at the level of the semilunar valve insertions (used for computation of the subvalvular cross-sectional area).

End-diastolic measurements are timed with the point of the Q wave on the simultaneously recorded ECG [11]. Particularly in pediatric patients, significant variation may occur if the point of the R wave is used instead. End-systolic measurements are timed to occur with the minimal diameter in cardiac cycle. End-systolic measurements may alternatively be made at the time of maximal interventricular septum thickness or as maximal thickness of the posterior left ventricular wall, defined as the end of T wave on the simultaneously recorded ECG or immediately prior to the second heart sound (S_2) on the phonocardiogram (PCG). The peak downwards excursion of the posterior wall of the interventricular septum occurs before peak upwards excursion of the posterior left ventricular wall. The former corresponds better with hemodynamic criteria for end systole. Only in patients with abnormal or paradoxical septal motion must the maximal thickness of the posterior wall of the left ventricle be used to determine the end-systolic dimension of the left ventricle.

M-mode echocardiograms for left ventricular measurement are conventionally recorded between the mitral valve and papillary muscles at the level of the mitral valve apparatus; the chordae tendineae are also visible. Due to individual differences in the shape of the ventricle, it is sometimes better to direct the beam further towards the mitral valve in patients with small heart sizes and in pediatric patients.

It is neither prudent nor reliable to extrapolate volumes from the M-mode-derived left ventricular diameter. Only the volume of a sphere can be calculated using a single diameter. Volumetric equations magnify exponentially any error in diameter measurement.

The same limitation applies for attempts to calculate left ventricular mass by subtracting the "inner" volume from the "outer" volume derived from epicardial measurements.

Due to its more unfavorable angle and more complex geometry, right ventricular dimensions cannot be measured with the same accuracy and precision as left ventricular dimensions using M-mode echocardiograms obtained from parasternal long-axis 2-D echocardiograms. Low-frequency transducers often provide only unsatisfactory images of the right ventricle. To properly measure right ventricular anterior wall thickness, one should either use a 5 MHz transducer or obtain measurements from the subcostal position. Since the right ventricle resembles a pyramid with tapered ends, diameter measurements are highly dependent on the site of measurement. Furthermore, the reference range of measurements obtained from the left lateral position are significantly higher than those obtained from the supine position.

The aortic root, left atrium, and aortic annulus at the level of the insertions of the aortic cusps are measured in the imaging plane that visualizes the right ventricular outflow tract, aorta, and left atrium. Two-dimensional (aortic annulus) and M-mode echocardiography are used for this purpose. The aortic valve ring is measured at mid or end systole, the aortic root at end diastole, and the left atrium at end systole or at the time of maximum diameter. Multiple indistinct echoes corresponding to artifacts are located in front of the posterior left atrial wall. The wall can usually be found behind these echoes. In cases where the left atrial geometry deviates greatly from the spherical model, M-mode measurements should be made from the suprasternal position.

2.   **Conventional Echocardiography: Examination Procedure,**   **65**
           Fundamental Measurement and Assessment Tasks
2.4   **Valve Morphology**

One and two-dimensional echocardiography, *i.e.* M and B-mode, permit assessment of the morphology and dynamics of the four cardiac valves. Quantitation of valvular defects is usually impossible or very limited.

2.4   Valve Morphology
2.4.1   Tricuspid Valve

The tricuspid valve has three leaflets, namely, the anterior (ATL), posterior (PTL), and septal (STL) tricuspid leaflets. The leaflets are tensed by an anterior papillary muscle, a short posterior papillary muscle, and two septal papillary muscles. The septal tricuspid leaflet with its chordae tendineae may also originate directly at the interventricular septum. Echoes resembling those of the anterior and posterior mitral leaflet are registered primarily from the septal and anterior tricuspid leaflets only.

Two-dimensional echocardiography, which provides information on the leaflet insertions and leaflet dynamics, is particularly helpful in diagnosing Ebstein's anomaly, whereas M-mode echocardiography is helpful in clarifying suspected tricuspid valve endocarditis. One and two-dimensional echocardiograms should preferably be obtained from parasternal short-axis and apical four-chamber views. In patients with right ventricular enlargement due to overload, the tricuspid valve can often be visualized in parasternal long-axis 2-D echocardiograms.

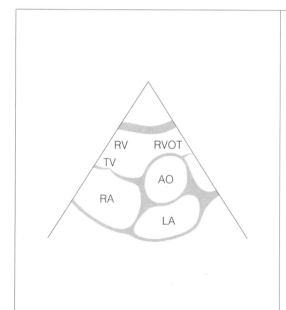 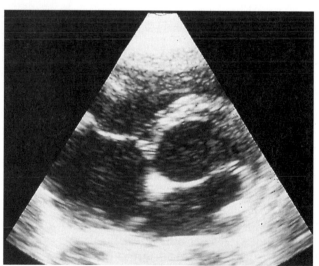

Parasternal short-axis 2-D echocardiogram demonstrating the tricuspid valve.

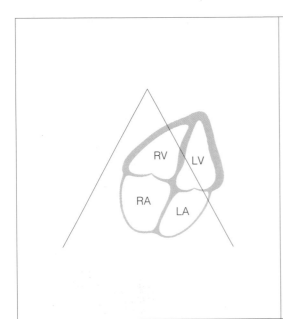

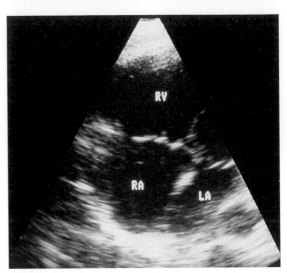

Apical four-chamber 2-D echocardiogram at tricuspid valve level.

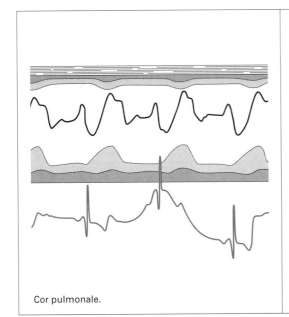

Cor pulmonale.

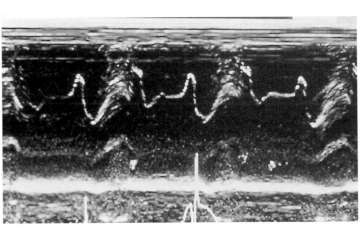

M-mode recording through the tricuspid valve.

Neither accelerated opening nor slow early diastolic closure of the tricuspid valve is specific of structural lesions, which are influenced not only by the valve itself, but also by compliance from the venous bed, impedance from the right ventricle and pulmonary artery tree, and the transvalvular stroke volume. Because of the normally low pressure level, these factors have a stronger influence on the tricuspid valve than the mitral valve.

The pulmonary valve is formed by three semilunar valve cusps, namely, the anterior (APC), right (RPC), and left (LPC) pulmonary cusps.

Two-dimensional echocardiograms of the pulmonary valve, obtained from the parasternal short axis view, are not necessarily diagnostic, even in severe pulmonary stenosis. The M-mode criteria for pulmonary valve defects or for pulmonary hypertension are nonspecific, but helpful, clues as to the diagnosis. The key parameters for echocardiographic diagnosis of pulmonary valve disease and for assessment of the inflow and outflow tracts are: right atrial diameter, diameter of the right ventricular inflow and outflow tracts, dimensions of the pulmonary trunk and its bifurcation, and Doppler-derived pressure gradients and regurgitant jets.

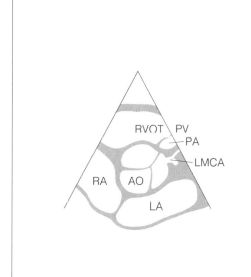

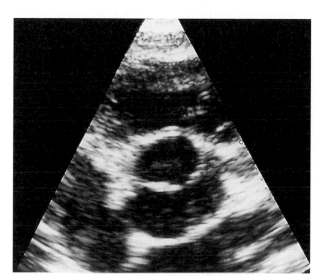

Parasternal short-axis 2-D echocardiogram: pulmonary valve.

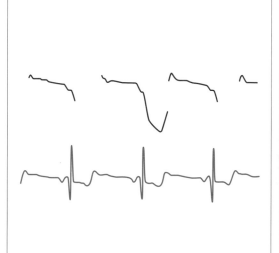

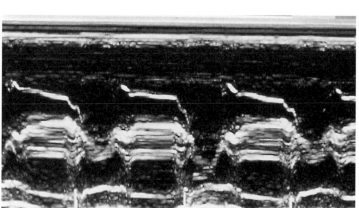

M-mode echocardiogram through the pulmonary valve.

The mitral valve consists of a large anterior leaflet and a smaller posterior leaflet, both of which are tensed by single or multiple-headed anterior (anterolateral) and posterior (posteromedial) papillary muscles and chordae tendineae. Due to its saddle-shaped configuration, the mitral valve is a complex echotomographic target, despite its characteristic appearance.

The mitral valve apparatus, consisting of papillary muscles and chordae, is neither a morphological nor a functional part of the individual leaflets. Each papillary muscle has chordae tendineae that extend to the adjacent sections of the leaflets. The commissural chordae, which originate at the free leaflet edges, as well as the strut chordae have great functional significance. A strut chordae rupture renders surgical correction difficult to impossible.

The anterior leaflet of the opened mitral valve has an M-shaped motion pattern that is described using the points D-E-F-A-B-C. The posterior leaflet has a W-shaped motion pattern that is described using the points D-E'-F'-A'-C.

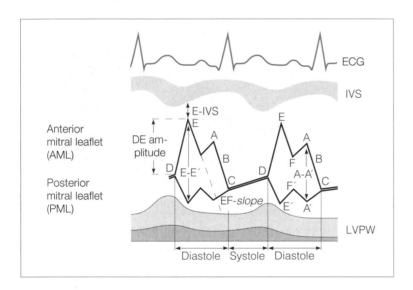

Since the mid-sixties repeated attempts have been made to subdivide mitral valve motion into individual phases [5]. This problem became more complex after a later redefinition of the individual phases of diastole was made [3].

To ensure the quality of mitral valve images, both leaflets should be visualized simultaneously, and double contours should not appear. The gain should be set in such a way that the fine lines of the tips of the mitral leaflets are only discretely visible.

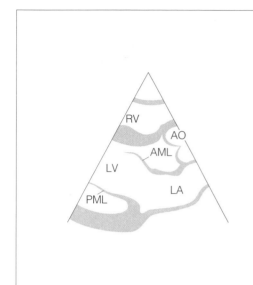

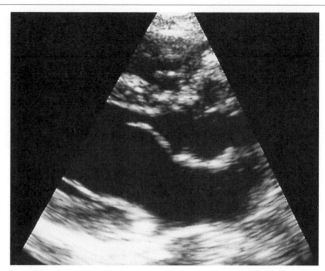

Parasternal long-axis 2-D echocardiogram at mitral valve level in diastole.

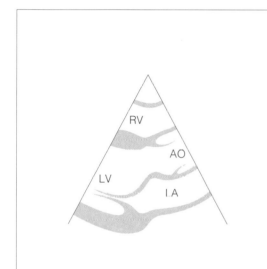

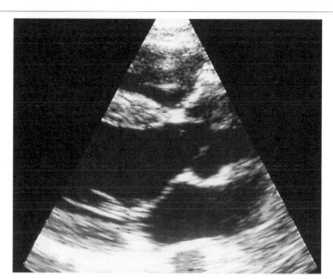

Parasternal long-axis 2-D echocardiogram at mitral valve level in systole.

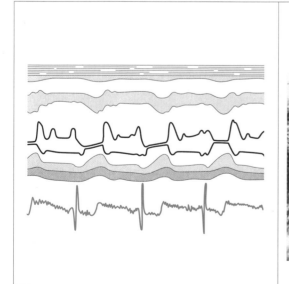

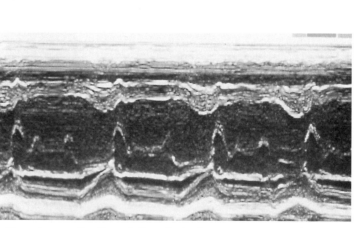

M-mode recording through the mitral valve.

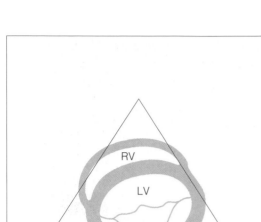

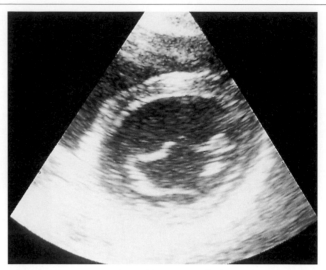

Parasternal short-axis 2-D echocardiogram at mitral valve level, in diastole.

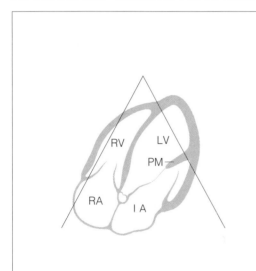

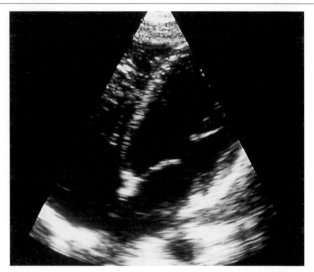

Apical four-chamber 2-D echocardiogram at mitral valve level, in diastole.

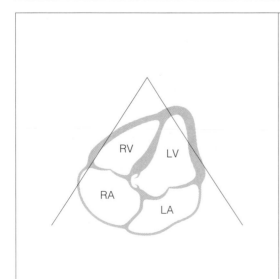

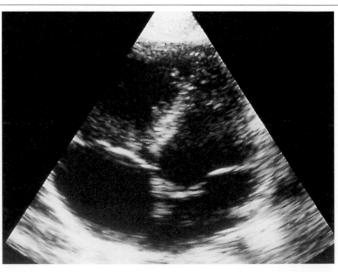

Apical four-chamber 2-D echocardiogram at mitral valve level, in systole.

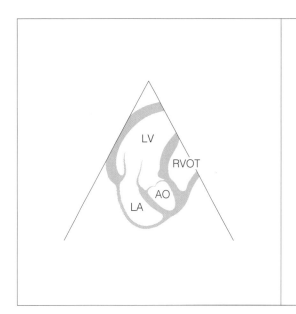

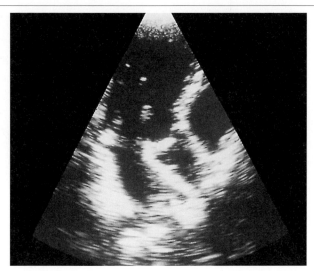

Apical two-chamber 2-D echocardiogram at mitral valve level, in diastole.

2.4   **Valve Morphology**
2.4.4   **Aortic Valve**

The aortic valve consists of three cusps: the right coronary (RCC), noncoronary (NCC), and left coronary (LCC) cusps. Only the RCC and NCC are visible in the parasternal long-axis view. All three aortic cusps are visible in the short-axis view.

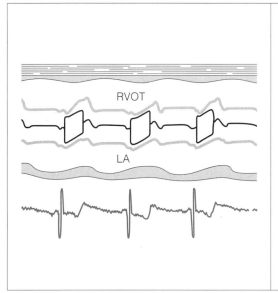

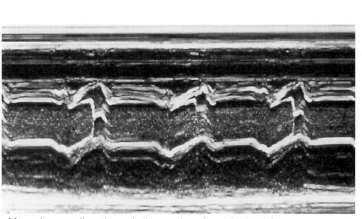

M-mode recording through the aortic valve, obtained from parasternal long-axis 2-D echocardiogram.

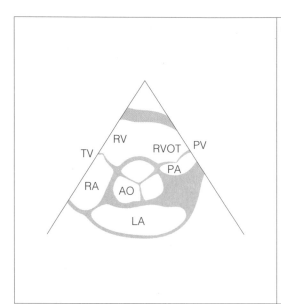

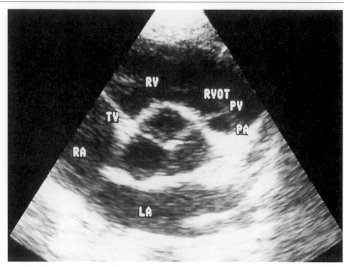

Aortic valve: parasternal short-axis 2-D echocardiogram.

The *eccentricity index,* a measure of the distance of the diastolic closure line relative to mid-line of the aorta, permits diagnosis of normal, tricuspid or bicuspid aortic valve. However, aortic valve abnormalities are now preferentially diagnosed by direct visualization of two or three leaflets (bicuspid or tricuspid) in parasternal short-axis echocardiograms. Aortic valves with more than three leaflets and with sub- or supravalvular membranes are rare.

| 2. | Conventional Echocardiography: Examination Procedure, Fundamental Measurement and Assessment Tasks |
| 2.5 | Echocardiographically Derived Hemodynamic Information |

Hemodynamic information can be derived from parameters such as the thickness, size, motion and topography of cardiac and vascular walls, and valvular morphology and dynamics.

Many of these hemodynamic parameters have lost their former significance since the advent of Doppler echocardiography. One of these is *tricuspid valve motion.* Since the tricuspid valve frequently lies at an acute angle to the ultrasonic beam, recordings were often highly unreliable. A reduced DE slope was thought to be due to reduced early diastolic right ventricular filling. Separation of the septal and anterior tricuspid leaflets and an increased amplitude of motion of the anterior tricuspid leaflet were thought to be indicators of transtricuspid flow.

The *mitral valve* is a more favorable scanning target.

The early diastolic opening velocity of the mitral valve *d(DE)/dt* is prolonged in low flow states. It is accelerated in the presence of elevated left ventricular end-diastolic pressure, during a brief portion of atrial systole in left ventricular filling, in low cardiac output, and in pulmonary hypertension.

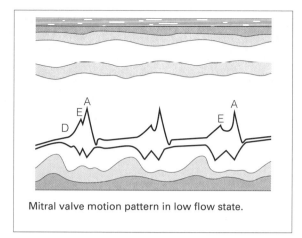

Mitral valve motion pattern in low flow state.

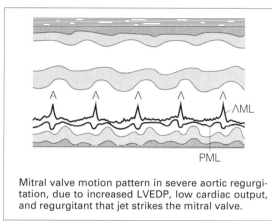

Mitral valve motion pattern in severe aortic regurgitation, due to increased LVEDP, low cardiac output, and regurgitant that jet strikes the mitral valve.

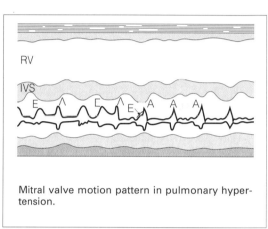

Mitral valve motion pattern in pulmonary hypertension.

Factors that influence the early diastolic opening amplitude DE include structural changes in the valve, preload and afterload conditions, and transmitral stroke volumes. *E point septal separation, i.e.* the distance between the anterior mitral leaflet and the interventricular septum, is considered specific of low cardiac output, even before direct proof is obtained by morphometry of the left ventricle and Doppler measurement of stroke volume and cardiac output. *Mitral cusp separation* or EE' separation, which was formerly used to calculate stroke volume, is now only of historical interest.

The *early diastolic EF slope* may be reduced due to mitral stenosis. However, it may also be reduced due to slow early diastolic filling due to reduced left ventricular compliance and, in some cases, pulmonary hypertension.

Aortic valve motion pattern directly reflects the connection between contraction and perfusion. *Aortic cusp separation* has been used to calculate transaortic stroke volume. However, like mitral cusp separation, it is now only of historical interest.

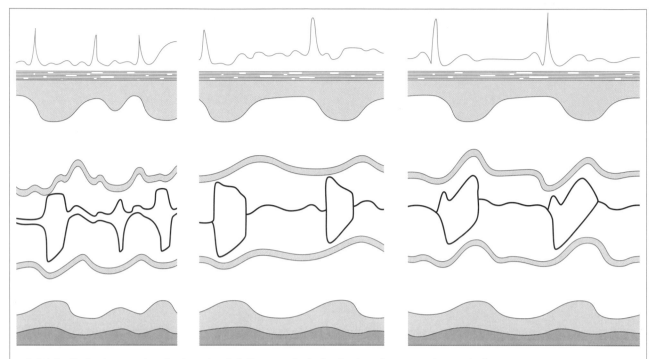

1. Brief mitral valve opening due to pulse deficit or paradoxical pulse in pulmonary artery embolism.
2. Gradual systolic closure corresponding to flow reduction in reduced left ventricular function and mitral regurgitation.
3. Mid-systolic closure due to sudden early systolic flow reduction in hypertrophic obstructive cardiomyopathy, mitral regurgitation, ventricular septum defect, or aortic root ectasia.

The *left atrial emptying index* is also outdated. This index was established by studying the amplitude of motion of the posterior aortic wall, which lies adjacent to the left atrial anterior wall. The amplitude of motion in the first third of diastole is normally greater than 40% of the total amplitude.

Echo contrast agent dilution methods for determination of cardiac output, which are similar to dye dilution and thermodilution methods, are still being discussed.

With some reservations, valve motion patterns and other measurement and calculation data can provide indications of such intracardiac and intravascular pressure relationships as:

- increased left ventricular systolic pressure (LVSP),
- increased left ventricular end-diastolic pressure (LVEDP),
- increased right ventricular systolic pressure (RVSP), and
- increased right ventricular end-diastolic pressure (LVEDP).

The *mass index* or the ratio of end-diastolic thicknesses of the interventricular septum and the posterior left ventricular wall has been shown to correlate with left ventricular systolic pressure. Premature closure of the mitral valve and prolongation of the A to C interval indicate a of pathological elevation in left ventricular diastolic pressure.

Prolongation of the A to C interval is also observed in the presence of diminished left ventricular compliance due to hypertrophy, ischemia or scarring. A point occurs prematurely, and a "notch" or B *bump* is observed between A and C. The B bump, in particular, indicates that the left ventricular end-diastolic pressure is in excess of 20 mmHg.

2.   **Conventional Echocardiography: Examination Procedure,**   **75**
           Fundamental Measurement and Assessment Tasks
2.5   **Echocardiographically Derived Hemodynamic Information**

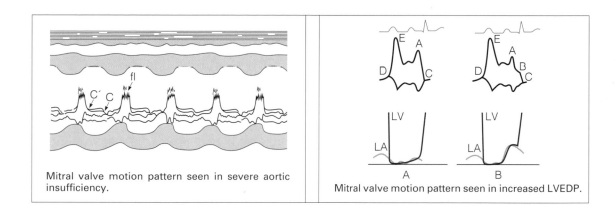

Mitral valve motion pattern seen in severe aortic insufficiency.

Mitral valve motion pattern seen in increased LVEDP.

Increased RV systolic pressure due to right ventricular hypertrophy, obstruction of the right ventricular outflow tract or increased pulmonary artery pressure is sometimes reflected in pulmonary valve motion.

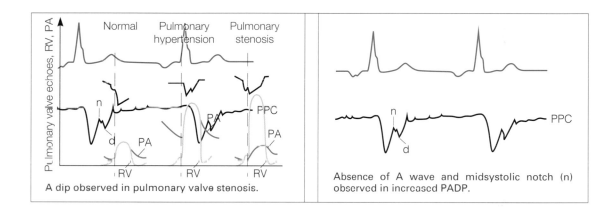

A dip observed in pulmonary valve stenosis.

Absence of A wave and midsystolic notch (n) observed in increased PADP.

The *PEP/RVET ratio* and Doppler-derived data are probably the most reliable techniques to determine the presence or absence of pulmonary hypertension.

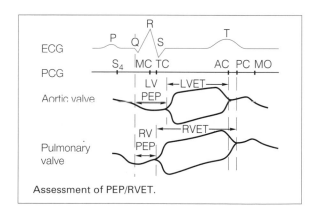

Assessment of PEP/RVET.

Delayed tricuspid valve closure and premature pulmonary valve opening are insensitive and nonspecific in the presence of increased right ventricular end-diastolic pressure. Except in severe cases, inferior vena cava dilation and hepatic vein dilation are also insensitive and nonspecific qualitative assessment criteria.

The routine M-mode and two-dimensional echocardiographic indices of ventricular function are as follows.

Left Ventricular Systolic Function

Global systolic function
  LVFS
  Mean Vcf
  LVEF (Teichholz method)
  LVEF (area-length method or Simpson's single plane method)
  LVEF (Simpson's biplane method)
Regional systolic function
  Wall motion analysis

Left Ventricular Diastolic Function

Global diastolic function
  DE slope
  EF slope
  E/A ratio
  AC notch (B bump)
  Peak rate of change of dimension and wall thickness
    - $d(LVEDD)/dt_{max}$ in early diastole
    - $d(LVEDD_{PW})/dt_{max}$ in early diastole
  IRP: AVC-MVO or LVD_{min}-MVO
Regional LV diastolic function?

Right Ventricular Systolic Function

Global systolic function
  RVEF
  3-D Reconstruction
Regional systolic function
  Wall motion analysis
  3-D reconstruction

Right Ventricular Diastolic Function?

Fractional shortening and the mean *velocity of circumferential fiber shortening* are the simplest and most reliable indices of left ventricular systolic function. Fractional shortening represents the transverse diameter fractional shortening of the left ventricle at the level of the mitral valve apparatus, and the mean velocity of circumferential fiber shortening is the mean velocity of circumferential fiber shortening of the left ventricle at the level of the mitral valve apparatus.

LVFS	= (LVEDD - LVESD) / LVEDD
Mean Vcf	= (π LVEDD - π LVESD) / (π LVEDD x LVET) = (LVEDD - LVESD) / (LVEDD x LVET) = LVFS/LVET

The mean velocity of circumferential fiber shortening therefore corresponds to the fractional shortening divided by the left ventricular ejection time, which is obtained from M-mode aortic valve motion analysis.

The greatest limitation of these indices is that they reflect only the regional contractile behavior in the basal to middle segment of the interventricular septum and the basal to middle segment of the posterolateral wall, and apply only in healthy individuals or in those with heart diseases that uniformly involve the entire left ventricle. Only when these conditions are met can the data be used to extrapolate global systolic function. This obviously is not the case in coronary artery disease, the leading cause of left ventricular dysfunction. Fractional shortening may be normal in the presence of large areas of scarring in inferior and apicoseptal wall segments, or in significant reduction in overall pump function. Conversely, fractional shortening may be pathologically reduced in localized myocardial infarction of the basal or middle septum with normal overall pump function.

In volume and/or pressure overload, the use of fractional shortening and mean velocity of circumferential fiber shortening may become problematic, because these indices are preload and afterload-dependent. Due to the effects of remodelling, the left ventricle becomes more globular in shape, whereas the short axis increases out of proportion with the long axis. This leads to overestimation of the overall pump function in patients with large hearts. Also, the mean velocity of circumferential fiber shortening is directly proportional to the heart rate. However, neither of these parameters correlates linearly with systolic left ventricular function across the entire range of measurement. In other words, an fractional shortening of 0.40 is not necessarily one-third higher than an fractional shortening of 0.30. Practical problems may arise in accentuated triaxial rotation of the heart. Because ultrasonic beam then intersects the septum or anterior wall segment diagonally, the short axis measured in diastole or systole will then be falsely large. These limitations and problems related to the use of fractional shortening and mean velocity of circumferential fiber shortening are outweighed by their advantages: they are relatively easy to use, and their limitations are readily definable and comprehensible. This cannot be said of competing parameters.

M-mode derived ejection fraction is included in the standard reports of most echocardiographic systems. Furthermore, the overwhelming majority of users of echocardiographic findings are accustomed in using it in angiography and nuclear cardiology, whereas they still are not appreciative of the echocardiographic fractional shortening. That is why left ventricular ejection fraction has become the established parameter for the overall pump function. In the most frequent and the most incorrect application together, ejection fraction simply is given as an M-mode derived parameter. The computation of ejection fraction from M-mode data is based on two assumptions: 1. that the imaged M-mode section correctly reflects the left ventricular short axis and 2. that the geometry of the left ventricle corresponds to a *prolate ellipse*, the volume of which can be calculated as follows:

$$V = \pi/6 \times L \times D1 \times D2$$

L	Long axis
D1, D2	Short axis of the prolate ellipsoid

If, for simplification, one also assumes that both short axes D1 and D2 are of equal length and that they equal one-half the length of the long axis (L = 2 x D1; D1 = D2), the equation can be simplified as follows:

$$v = \pi/6 \times D^2 = \pi/3 \times D^3,$$

and with the final simplification:

$$\pi/3 = 1.$$

LVEDV = LVEDD^3, or
LVESV = LVESD^3, and

LVEF   = LVSF/LVEDV
          = (LVEDV - LVESV)/LVEDV
          = (LVEDD^3 - LVESD^3)/LVEDD^3

The problem with this simplified equation is that, in addition to the limitations and problems associated with the use of fractional shortening, any error in measurement of the LVEDD and LVESD are multiplied to the third power. Therefore, left ventricular ejection fractions calculated by this method have a wide range of error. If, for example, the measured LVEDD and LVESD are off by 5 percent each, the stroke volume will be miscalculated by more than 30 percent [1]. For this reason, one should obstain from using M-mode-derived stroke volumes and ejection fractions with this equation.

Of all methods for calculation of the ejection fraction using M-mode derived data, the *Teichholz formula method* seems to correlate best with angiographic data [8, 12]. This method was established performing comparison studies with angiographic volumetric data and by making necessary adjustments.

$$V = AL/2 + 2/3 \, (AL/2) = 5/6 \, AL$$

A	*Cross-sectional area perpendicular to the long axis at mitral valve level*
L	*Long axis*

$$V = [7/(2.4 + D)] \times D^3$$

D	*Short axis*

LVEF = {[7 / (2.4 +LVEDD)][LVEDD^3] - [7 / (2.4 LVESD)][LVESD^3]} / {[7 / (2.4 LVEDD)][LVEDD^3]

Diameter miscalculation is also a major source of error in calculations based on the Teichholz formula. This greatly restricts its applicability in routine clinical practice. It should not be used when endocardial boundaries are poorly delineated or when the heart is enlarged.

The basic problem in using M-mode derived data to calculate left ventricular function is that it lacks multidimensional information. Two-dimensional echocardiography has overcome this obstacle. Since it permits qualitative and quantitative assessment of global and regional left ventricular function, 2-D echocardiographic parameters have replaced the systolic time interval.

Using integrated planimetry functions and commercially available software, 2-D echocardiography provides relatively reliable methods of volumetry which can be applied, for example, to calculate the ejection fraction. The primary methods are:

> ▸ the single plane area-length method and
> ▸ the single plane and biplane modified Simpson's rule method
>   (slice summation method)

Single plane measurements are usually obtained from the apical four-chamber view. Using the biplane Simpson's rule technique, measurements are obtained from apical two and four-chamber views.

Single Plane Area-Length Method

$V = \pi/6\ D^2L = 8/3\ \pi\ (A^2/L)$

D	*Short axis*
L	*Long axis*
A	*Cross-sectional area perpendicular to the long axis*

Biplane Modified Simpson's Rule Method

$$V = \pi/3\ h\ \left(\sum_{o=1}^{n-1} D_{o1}D_{o2} + 1/2 \sum_{e=2}^{n} D_{e1}D_{e2} \right)$$

D_i	*Slice diameter in both axes*
n	*Number of slices*
h	*Thickness of slices*
o	*Odd-numbered slices*
e	*Even-numbered slices*

The modified Simpson's rule is superior to other methods, because no geometric assumptions must be made. Therefore, the modified Simpson's rule can also be used even when the shape of the left ventricle is distorted.

Volumes computed by echocardiography are usually smaller than those measured at angiography. There are two reasons for this:

1. Although the radiocontrastography agent penetrates into the trabeculae, current echocardiographic systems do not visualize these interstices. They therefore blend in with endocardial contours.
2. Echocardiographic error in measuring the true long axis is greater than in cardangiography.

Regional left ventricular function is described by visual qualitative assessment or by computerized quantification of wall motion in the different wall segments (for wall motion analysis, see Section 14.1: Identification of Ischemic Myocardial Regions, and Section 5.2: Stress Echocardiography).

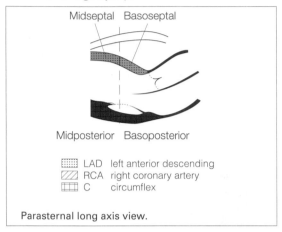

Midseptal   Basoseptal

Midposterior   Basoposterior

LAD   left anterior descending
RCA   right coronary artery
C   circumflex

Parasternal long axis view.

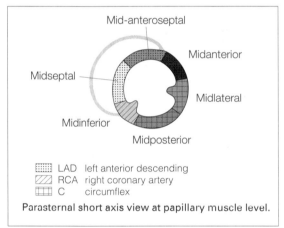

Mid-anteroseptal

Midseptal

Midanterior

Midlateral

Midinferior

Midposterior

LAD   left anterior descending
RCA   right coronary artery
C   circumflex

Parasternal short axis view at papillary muscle level.

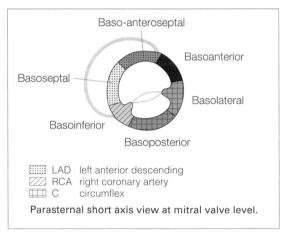

Baso-anteroseptal

Basoseptal

Basoanterior

Basolateral

Basoinferior

Basoposterior

LAD   left anterior descending
RCA   right coronary artery
C   circumflex

Parasternal short axis view at mitral valve level.

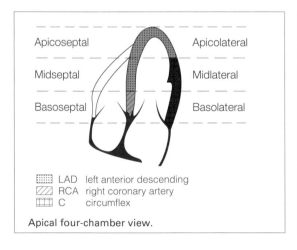

Apicoseptal   Apicolateral

Midseptal   Midlateral

Basoseptal   Basolateral

LAD   left anterior descending
RCA   right coronary artery
C   circumflex

Apical four-chamber view.

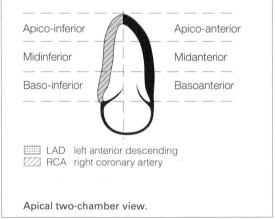

Apico-inferior   Apico-anterior

Midinferior   Midanterior

Baso-inferior   Basoanterior

LAD   left anterior descending
RCA   right coronary artery

Apical two-chamber view.

The left ventricular wall can be divided into basal, middle, and apical segments, which can further be described as septal, posterior, anterior, inferior, and lateral. With certain limitations, they may be further classified with respect to the corresponding supply areas of the three main coronary arteries. In visual qualitative assessment, wall motion is conventionally described as hyperkinetic, normokinetic, hypokinetic, akinetic or dyskinetic. These motion patterns can be assigned values on a numerical scale in order to establish a semiquantitative wall motion score.

Physiological, invasive and noninvasive descriptions of left ventricular diastolic function vary. Therefore, although dozens of conventional and Doppler echocardiographic parameters of left ventricular diastolic function have been tested, most studies have concluded, at best, that none of these parameters is suitable for all applications, and that none can reliably differentiate between compliance and relaxation.

The new physiological model of the heart as an *integrated muscle and pump system* has reformulated the classical hydrodynamic and clinical cardiologic definitions of systole and diastole. The new model subdivides the cardiac cycle into three phases (contractility, relaxation, and compliance). Load dependence is defined as a characteristic of the relaxation phase, which incorporates the second part of the ejection period (EP), the isovolumic relaxation period (IRP), and the rapid filling phase (RFP) [2].

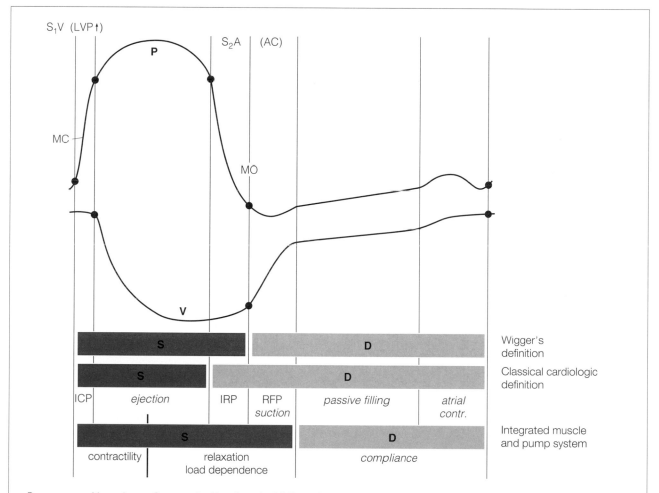

P = pressure; V = volume; S = systole; D = diastole; MVC = mitral valve closure; S$_1$V = 1st heart sound with reshaping of the left ventricle and increase in LV pressure; S$_2$A = 2nd heart sound with aortic valve closure; MVO = mitral valve opening; ICP = isovolumic contraction phase; EP = auxotone ejection phase; IRP = isovolumic relaxation phase; RFP = Rapid filling phase; PFP = passive filling phase; AC = atrial contraction.

Therefore, current parameters of left ventricular diastolic function based on the clinical cardiologic definition are inevitably influenced by energy-consuming myocardial processes, passive ventricular filling capacities, and overall compliance. These factors, in turn, are affected by different load conditions and heart diseases. The multitude of schematic overviews on the influence of relaxation and compliance on different parameters documents the deficiency of current practical methodology.

The mitral valve motion pattern and peak rates of change in left ventricular diameter and wall thickness are popular indices of left ventricular diastolic function.

A *diminished DE slope* is seen in reduced early diastolic filling due to elevated left ventricular end-diastolic pressure and correspondingly depressed LA-LV filling pressure. Any disease that causes either a reduction in cardiac output or severe aortic insufficiency may be the underlying cause.

A *diminished EF slope* is characteristic of mitral stenosis, but may also occur in any condition causing reduced compliance.

The *E/A ratio* (ratio of E wave to A wave velocity) often becomes inverted in the presence of disturbed compliance, *e.g.,* left ventricular hypertrophy. Unfortunately, the E/A ratio is an unspecific indicator that has been shown to vary in the same heart in consecutive beats.

A connection between the *B notch* (bump between A and C) and diminished LV compliance has also been reported. The B notch is frequently observed when the left ventricular end-diastolic pressure exceeds 20 mmHg.

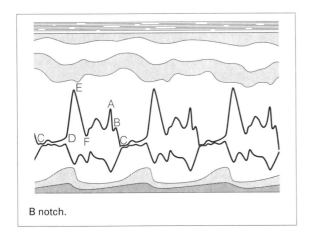

B notch.

The *peak filling rate* (PFR; peak early diastolic rate of change in left ventricular end-diastolic diameter) and *anterior wall thickness* are dependent on preload, afterload, heart rate, and left ventricular systolic function [4].

The *isovolumetric relaxation period* (IRP) is dependent on relaxation velocity, afterload, atrium-chamber interactions, and myocardial capacities [6].

The parameters of regional left ventricular diastolic function are still not available for echocardiography.

The geometry of the right ventricle is very complex. When the right ventricle is dilated, remodelling occurs, making it difficult to assess right ventricular systolic function - even with 2-D echocardiography [9]. Conventional echocardiographic assessment of right ventricular dimensions and global systolic function has been limited to qualitative visual assessments. Efforts have been made to approximate the right ventricular ejection fraction using single plane or biplane echocardiographic techniques. Some investigators performed contrast echocardiographic studies of the endocardial boundaries using specific right-heart echocontrastography agents. However, the reproducibility of these results is still unsatisfactory.

Regional functional disturbances can be more easily assessed. This is done by performing wall motion analyses using echocardiograms obtained from parasternal, apical, and subcostal views, similar to the procedure for the left ventricle. New developments in three-dimensional reconstruction seem to hold promising potentials for improving global and regional functional assessment of the right ventricle.

At the present time, there are no practical parameters for assessing right ventricular diastolic function.

| 2. | Conventional Echocardiography: Examination Procedure, Fundamental Measurement and Assessment Tasks |
| 2.7 | Basic Measurement Program and Reference Ranges - Quick Reference |

Conventional echocardiographic and transthoracic color Doppler echocardiographic examinations are now extensively combined in clinical practice, except where billing is concerned. The referral sheet used by our hospital does not list these items separately, whereas special semi-invasive examination and/or other examinations that explicitly require informed consent are listed as options.

CARDIAC ULTRASOUND DIAGNOSTICS (ADULT)

Height: _____
Weight: _____
Current blood pressure (Riva-Rocci): _____

REQUESTED EXAMINATION(S)

Doppler color flow imaging
▸ **Transthoracic echocardiography**
▸ **Transesophageal echocardiography**
▸ **Stress echocardiography**
   Stressor: _____
▸ **Contrast echocardiography**
   Contrast medium: _____

▸ **Percutaneous transluminal sonography**
   Site: _____
▸ **Tissue characterization**
   Site: _____
▸ **3-D reconstruction**

1. Primary cardiovascular diagnosis: _____
2. Pertinent secondary diagnoses: _____
3. Questions posed by referring physician: _____

4. Previous findings from __/__/___ exist and can be found: enclosed / in the patient records.
Pertinent data:

_____

5. Sites of healed myocardial infarctions:

_____

6. Patient transport required?   yes/no

7. Referring department / Phone: .... / ....
Date / Signature of referring physician: .... / ....

SUMMARY OF FINDINGS AND THERAPY CONSIDERATIONS

Video: S-VHS

_____

_____

_____

Image quality: good / limited quality for calculations / unsatisfactory

Date / Signature:

In any thorough conventional measurement program (M-mode, 2-D), wall thicknesses, diameters, ventricular function, morphologic features and dynamics of the valves must be measured and assessed. In justified individual cases, supplementary measurements can be made for calculation and assessment of ventricular mass and volumes, stroke volumes, and ejection fraction.

Morphometry and Ventricular Function

Wall thickness, mass

RV-AW-EDD	_____	($\leq$ 5 mm)
IVS-EDD	_____	(6-11 mm)
LV-PW-EDD	_____	(6-11 mm)
LV-MI	_____	($\leq$ 134/$\leq$ 109)

Systolic Function

LVFS	_____	($\geq$ 0.25)
mVcf	_____	(1.0-1.9 circ/s)

Global Systolic Function
Method: _Teichholz_

LVEF	_____	_____

Diameter

RVEDD	_____	(9-26 mm)
RVOT-MSD	_____	(19-29 mm)
LVEDD	_____	(37-56 mm)
LVESD	_____	(27-37 mm)
LAD-maxD	_____	(28-45 mm)
ARD-maxD	_____	(20-37 mm)
LVOT-MSD	_____	(17-26 mm)
RV-LAX-ED	_____	(36-48 mm/m²)
RV-LAX-ES	_____	(25-35 mm/m²)
RV-SAX-ED	_____	(13-22 mm/m²)
RV-SAX-ES	_____	(9-17 mm/m²)
RVFS	_____	($\geq$ 0.21)

RA-LAX-ED	_____	(11-20 mm/m²)
RA-LAX-ES	_____	(19-29 mm/m²)
RA-SAX-ED	_____	(11-19 mm/m²)
RA-SAX-ES	_____	(14-23 mm/m²)

Regional Systolic Function
(Wall motion analysis)

RV _____

LV				
Septal	_____ /	_____ /	_____	
Ant.	_____ /	_____ /	_____	
Lateral	_____ /	_____ /	_____	
Post.	_____ /	_____ /	_____	
Infer.	_____ /	_____ /	_____	
Apical	_____ /		_____	

LA-LAX-ED	_____	(11-23 mm/m²)
LA-LAX-ES	_____	(17-30 mm/m²)
LA-SAX-ED	_____	(0.8-16 mm/m²)
LA-SAX-ES	_____	(14-23 mm/m²)

Volumes, Volume Indices
Method: _____

RVEDV	_____	_____
RVESV	_____	_____
RVEF	_____	_____
	_____	

Method: _____
RA volume _____ _____ _____

Method: _Simpson's Biplane_

LVEDVI	_____	(52-82/37-85 ml/m²)
LVESVI	_____	(18-36/12-40 ml/m²)
LVSVI	_____	(28-52/22-48 ml/m²)
LVEF	_____	(0.49-0.70/0.46-0.71)
CI	_____	(2.36±0.37 l/min m²)

Method: _____
LA volume _____ (12-51 ml/m²)

Valves

Valve Morphology and Dynamics

_____

_____

Like the echocardiography laboratory itself, other specialized laboratories such as the cardiovascular laboratory, the electrophysiology laboratory, the nuclear cardiography laboratory, and the catheterization laboratory are able to perform complementary diagnostic techniques to help clarify special diagnostic questions posed by the referring physician or special clinical problems.

ANAMNESIS / SYMPTOMATOLOGY / PHYSICAL EXAMINATION FINDINGS

| Resting ECG | Exercise ECG | Chest x-ray in 2 planes | Doppler color flow imaging |

CARDIOVASCULAR LABORATORY

LUNG FUNCTION LABORATORY

ELECTROPHYSIOLOGY LABORATORY

NUCLEAR CARDIOLOGY LABORATORY

ECHOCARDIOGRAPHY LABORATORY

CATHETERIZATION LABORATORY

The following tables and graphs were **printed with permission from:** Geigy Scientific Tables, Vol. 5, Heart and Circulation, 8th Ed., C. Lentner (ed.), Basel, Ciba-Geigy Ltd., 1990.

Table 1. Angiocardiography and 2-D echocardiography: methods for the calculation of left ventricular volumes.

Method	Application	Formula	Remarks
Area length method [1] (ellipsoidal model; $A = [\pi\,D\,L]/4$)	Angiocardiography and echocardiography	Single plane: $V = \dfrac{\pi}{6} D^2 L = \dfrac{8}{3\pi} \dfrac{A^2}{L}$ Biplane: $V = \dfrac{\pi}{6} D_1 D_2 L = \dfrac{8}{3\pi} \dfrac{A_1 A_2}{L}$ or $V = \dfrac{8}{3\pi} \dfrac{A_1 A_2}{L}$	D = minor axes in the respective planes A = area perpendicular to the major axes in the respective planes L = major axis, or the longer of the major axes in the two planes
Modified ellipsoidal model [2] (Teichholz)	Echocardiography	$V = \left(\dfrac{7.0}{2.4 + D}\right) D^3$	D = left ventricular internal dimension, determined by echocardiography
Hemicylinder hemi-ellipsoidal method [3]	Echocardiography	$V = A\dfrac{L}{2} + \dfrac{2}{3} A \dfrac{L}{2} = \dfrac{5}{6} AL$	A = area perpendicular to the major axis at the level of the mitral valve L = major axis
Disc-summation method [4] (Simpson's rule)	Angiocardiography and echocardiography	Single plane: $V = \dfrac{\pi}{4} h \sum\limits_{i=1}^{n} D_i^2$ Biplane: $V = \dfrac{\pi}{4} h \sum\limits_{i=1}^{n} D_{i1} D_{i2}$ $V = \dfrac{\pi}{3} h \left(\sum\limits_{o=1}^{n-1} D_{o1} D_{o2} + \dfrac{1}{2} \sum\limits_{e=2}^{n} D_{e1} D_{e2} \right)$	D_i = disc diameter in the respective plane n = number of discs h = height of disc o = odd-numbered discs e = even-numbered discs
Modified disc-summation method (right ventricle)			

References
1. Dodge et al., Am Heart J, 60, 762 (1960).
2. Teichholz et al., Am J Cardiol, 37, 7 (1976).
3. Folland et al., Circulation, 60, 760 (1979).
4. Gentzler et al., Circulation, 50, 324 (1974); Redington et al., Brit Heart J, 59, 23 (1988).

Table 2. Angiocardiography: ventricular and atrial volumes, left ventricular free wall thickness and left ventricular mass in children and adults (volumes and mass related to body surface area).

	Unit	Mean	s	Range	Method	Ref.
Right ventricular volume						
End-diastolic:						
— 7 infants and children, < 1 year	ml/m²	39	8	30–49	Biplane (AP and LAT projections) disc-summation method, area-length method and 2-chamber method	1
— 9 children, > 1 year	ml/m²	70	13	48–93		
— 14 adults, 32–69 years	ml/m²	97	19	75–127	Biplane (RAO and LAO projections) disc-summation method*	2
— 10 adults, 29–47 years	ml/m²	64	13	–		3
— 9 adults	ml/m²	81	13	63–101	Biplane (AP and LAT projections) disc-summation method*	4
End-systolic:						
— 9 adults	ml/m²	39	9	24–53		
— 14 adults, 32–69 years	ml/m²	41	13	23–64	Biplane (RAO and LAO projections) disc-summation method*	2
Left ventricular volume						
End-diastolic:						
— 19 infants and children, < 2 years	ml/m²	42	10	–	Biplane (AP and LAT projections) area-length method*	5
— 37 children, > 2 years	ml/m²	73	11	–		
— 10 adults	ml/m²	77	7	–	Single-plane (RAO projection) area-length method*	6
— 13 adults, 19–48 years	ml/m²	81	15	53–98		7
— 17 adults, 34–59 years	ml/m²	72	15	46–92	Biplane (RAO and LAO projections) area-length method*	8
— 50 adults	ml/m²	71	16	–		9
— 22 adults, 31–59 years	ml/m²	59	17	34–85	Biplane (AP and LAT projections) area-length method*	10
— 8 adults, 24–64 years	ml/m²	76	11	60–94		11
— 17 adults, 28–59 years	ml/m²	93	18	–	Single-plane (RAO projection) disc-summation method	12
— 18 men, 20–67 years	ml/m²	95	15	–	Biplane (RAO and LAO projections) area length method	13
	ml/m²	99	15	–	Single-plane (RAO projection) area-length method	
— 7 women, 20–67 years	ml/m²	73	12	–	Biplane (RAO and LAO projections) area length method	
	ml/m²	78	14	–	Single-plane (RAO projection) area-length method	
End-systolic:						
— 17 adults, 34–59 years	ml/m²	20	8	8–33	Biplane (RAO and LAO projections) area-length method*	8
— 50 adults	ml/m²	26	8	–	Biplane (AP and LAT projections) area-length method*	9
— 8 adults, 24–64 years	ml/m²	21	8	12–34		11
— 17 adults, 28–59 years	ml/m²	27	9	–	Single-plane (RAO projection) disc-summation method	12
— 18 men, 20–67 years	ml/m²	35	6	–	Biplane (RAO and LAO projections) area length method	13
	ml/m²	33	6	–	Single-plane (RAO projection) area length method	
— 7 women, 20–67 years	ml/m²	26	7	–	Biplane (RAO and LAO projections) area length method	
	ml/m²	24	8	–	Single-plane (RAO projection) area length method	

Table 2. Angiocardiography: ventricular and atrial volumes, left ventricular free wall thickness and left ventricular mass in children and adults (volumes and mass related to body surface area) (continued).

	Unit	Mean	s	Range	Method	Ref.
Left atrial volume						
Maximum:						
– 16 infants and children, < 2 years	ml/m²	26	5	–		5
– 25 children, > 2 years	ml/m²	38	8	–	Biplane (AP and LAT projections) area-length method*	
– 8 adults, 24–64 years	ml/m²	41	7	32–51		
Minimum:						11
– 8 adults, 24–64 years	ml/m²	16	5	12–24		
Left ventricular anterior free wall thickness						
End-diastolic:						
– 8 adults	cm	0.83	0.12	0.64–1.00	RAO projection	14
– 13 adults, 19–48 years	cm	0.78	0.11	0.59–0.97	AP or RAO projection	7
– 6 adults	cm	0.85	0.13	–	AP projection	15
– 18 men, 20–67 years	cm	0.87	0.13	–	RAO projection	
	cm	0.83	0.11	–	LAO projection	13
– 7 women, 20–67 years	cm	0.83	0.10	–	RAO projection	
	cm	0.75	0.12	–	LAO projection	
Maximum systolic:						
– 6 adults	cm	1.68	2.9	–	AP projection	15
Left ventricular mass						
– 11 infants and children, < 2 years	g/m²	96	11	–		5
– 34 children, > 2 years	g/m²	86	11	–	Rackley et al., Circulation, 29, 666 (1964):	
– 10 adults	g/m²	73	15	–		6
– 13 adults, 19–48 years	g/m²	81	18	57–117	$\text{LVM} = 1.05 \frac{\pi}{6} \{[(D_{AP}+2h)$	7
– 50 adults	g/m²	93	18	–		9
– 17 adults, 28–59 years	g/m²	93	27	–	$(D_{LAT}+2h)\,(L+2h)]-D_{AP}D_{LAT}L\}$	12
– 18 men, 20–67 years	g/m²	96◇	16	–	[LVM in g; all dimensions in cm	
	g/m²	98†	19	–	(h: average ventricular wall thickness)]	13
– 7 women, 20–67 years	g/m²	80◇	15	–		
	g/m²	84†	17	–		

* Calculated volumes are corrected for "true volume" with a regression equation computed from cast volumes versus volumes determined by angiocardiography.
◇ Calculated from biplane measurements.
† Calculated from single-plane measurements.

References
1. Graham et al., Circulation, 47, 144 (1973).
2. Unterberg et al., Z Kardiol, 77, 120 (1988).
3. Redington et al., Brit Heart J, 59, 23 (1988).
4. Gentzler et al., Circulation, 50, 324 (1974).
5. Graham et al., Circulation, 43, 895 (1971).
6. Schwarz et al., Circulation, 60, 48 (1979).
7. Huber et al., Circulation, 64, 126 (1981).
8. Wynne et al., Am J Cardiol, 41, 726 (1978).
9. Kennedy et al., Am Heart J, 97, 592 (1979).
10. Peterson et al., Circulation, 49, 1088 (1974).
11. Toma et al., Cardiovasc Res, 21, 255 (1987).
12. Rousseau et al., Am J Cardiol, 50, 1028 (1982).
13. Thüring et al., Fortschr Röntgenstr, 150, 562 (1989).
14. Fester and Samet, Circulation, 50, 609 (1974).
15. Hood et al., Am J Cardiol, 22, 550 (1968).

Table 3. *M-mode* echocardiography: cardiac dimensions, fractional shortening and left ventricular mass in adults.

	Unit	Mean	s	95% interval (range in parentheses)	Reference
Right ventricular internal dimension (RVD) End-diastolic RVD:					
– Adults	cm	1.9	0.4	0.9–2.6	1
– 83 adults	cm	1.7	0.4	0.9–2.6	2
– 40 adults, 19–68 years	cm	1.7	0.4	≤2.5	3
– Men	cm	2.2	0.5	≤3.1	4
– Women	cm	1.9	0.5	≤2.8	4
– 52 women, 20–63 years	cm	1.7	0.4	–	5
End-systolic RVD:					
– 40 adults, 19–68 years	cm	1.6	0.4	≤2.4	3
Left ventricular internal dimension (LVD) End-diastolic LVD:					
– Adults	cm	4.7	0.56	3.7–5.6	1
– 82 adults	cm	4.7	–	3.7–5.6	2
– 40 adults, 19–68 years	cm	5.0	0.4	–	3
– Men	cm	4.9	0.5	≤5.8	4
– Women	cm	4.4	0.5	≤5.3	4
– 52 women, 20–63 years	cm	4.7	0.4	–	5
– 166 active men, 31–55 years	cm	5.5	0.5	(4.4–7.0)	6
– Related to body surface area:					
166 active men, 31–55 years	cm/m^2	3.0	0.3	(2.2–3.4)	6
End-systolic LVD:					
– Adults	cm	3.5	0.6	2.7–3.7	1
– 40 adults, 19–68 years	cm	3.0	0.3	–	3
– Men	cm	3.1	0.5	≤4.1	4
– Women	cm	2.7	0.5	≤3.7	4
– 52 women, 20–63 years	cm	2.6	0.3	–	5
Maximum aortic root dimension (AO)					
Adults	cm	2.7	0.7	2.1–4.4	1
121 adults	cm	2.7	–	2.0–3.7	2
Men	cm	3.2	0.5	≤4.1	4
Women	cm	2.7	0.4	≤3.5	4
52 women, 20–63 years	cm	2.7	0.3	–	5
Left atrial dimension (LA)					
133 adults	cm	2.9	–	1.9–4.0	2
Men	cm	3.3	0.5	≤4.2	4
Women	cm	3.2	0.4	≤3.9	4
52 women, 20–63 years	cm	3.1	0.4	–	5
Related to body surface area:					
– 50 adolescents, 14–16 years	cm/m^2	1.66	0.28	–	7
Left ventr. posterior free wall thickness (PWT) End-diastolic PWT:					
– 137 adults	cm	0.9	–	0.6–1.1	2
– 22 adults, 22–61 years	cm	0.83	0.18	–	8
– 20 adults, 19–63 years	cm	0.9	0.2	–	9
– 106 men	cm	0.9	0.1	≤1.2	10
– 119 women	cm	0.8	0.2	≤1.1	10
– 52 women, 20–63 years	cm	0.8	0.1	–	5
– 166 active men, 31–55 years	cm	0.9	0.1	(0.6–1.3)	6
– Related to body surface area:					
50 adolescents, 14–16 years	cm/m^2	0.39	0.06	–	7
166 active men, 31–55 years	cm/m^2	0.50	0.05	(0.3–0.6)	6
End-systolic PWT:					
– 20 adults, 19–63 years	cm	1.5	0.3	–	9

Table 3. *M-mode* echocardiography: cardiac dimensions, fractional shortening and left ventricular mass in adults (continued).

	Unit	Mean	*s*	95 % interval (range in parentheses)	Reference
Ventricular septal thickness (ST) End-diastolic ST:					
– Adults	cm	0.9	0.2	0.6–1.2	1
– 137 adults	cm	0.9	–	0.6–1.1	2
– 22 adults, 22–61 years	cm	0.92	0.18	–	8
– 20 adults, 19–63 years	cm	0.7	0.2	–	9
– 106 men	cm	1.0	0.2	≤1.3	10
– 119 women	cm	0.9	0.2	≤1.2	10
– 52 women, 20–63 years	cm	0.9	0.1	–	5
End-systolic ST:					
– 20 adults, 19–63 years	cm	1.2	0.3	–	9
Fractional shortening (FS)					
22 adults, 22–61 years	–	0.38	0.04	–	8
20 adults, 19–63 years	–	0.40	0.01	–	9
Men	–	0.36	0.06	≥0.25	4
Women	–	0.36	0.06	≥0.25	4
52 women, 20–63 years	–	0.43	0.05	–	5
Left ventricular (LVM)					
106 men*	g	176	45	<266	10
119 women*	g	121	40	≤201	10
166 active men, 31–55 years*	g	197	45	(105–341)	6
Related to body surface area:					
– 50 adolescents, 14–16 years◇	g/m²	72	15	–	7
– 106 men*	g/m²	89	21	≤134	10
– 119 women*	g/m²	69	19	≤109	10
– 166 active men, 31–55 years*	g/m²	98	20	(56–153)	6

* Calculated as "Penn-cube" LVM with formula of Devereux and Reichek (Circulation, 55, 613 (1977))
◇ Calculated as "ASE-cube" LVM with formula of Troy et al. (Circulation, 45, 602 (1972)).

References

1. Biamino and Lange, Echokardiographie, Hoechst Aktiengesellschaft, Frankfurt a. M. (1983) 44.
2. Feigenbaum, H., Echocardiography, 4th ed., Lea & Febiger, Philadelphia (1986) 622.
3. Manyari et al., Am J Cardiol, 57, 1147 (1986).
4. Devereux, R. B., Cardiology, 71, 118 (1984).
5. Michelsen et al., Eur Heart J, 9, 61 (1988).
6. Washburn et al., Am J Cardiol, 58, 1248 (1986).
7. Laird and Fixler, Pediatrics, 67, 255 (1981).
8. Hahn et al., Z Kardiol, 71, 445 (1982).
9. St. John Sutton et al., Circulation, 66, 790 (1982).
10. Devereux et al., J Am Coll Cardiol, 4, 1222 (1984); Devereux, R. B., Hypertension, 9, Suppl. 2, 19 (1987).

Table 4. M-mode echocardiography: cardiac dimensions and fractional shortening in neonates and infants (longitudinal study) [1].

Age	Number	Body mass		Body length		Right ventricular anterior wall thickness (RVAWT)*		Right ventricular internal dimension (end-diastolic) (RVD [ED])*		Right ventricular outflow tract dimension (RVOT)*		Ventricular septal thickness (end-diastolic) (ST [ED])*		Left ventricular internal dimension end-diastolic (LVD [ED])*		end-systolic (LVD [ES])*		Left ventricular posterior free wall thickness (PWT [ED])*		Pulmonary artery root dimension (PA)	
		Mean	s	Mean	s	Mean	s	Mean	s	Mean	s	Mean	s	Mean	s	Mean	s	Mean	s	Mean	s
		kg		cm		mm															
1st hour	32	3.313	0.353	50.1	1.76	2.6	0.2	9.8	1.3	13.6	1.3	3.5	0.4	17.3	1.7	11.5	1.3	3.3	0,3	11.2	0.8
1st day	53	3.283	0.478	49.9	2.0	2.6	0.3	9.8	1.2	14.1	1.1	3.4	0.4	18.1	1.4	12.1	1.1	3.2	0.3	11.4	0.9
3 days	53	3.213	0.481	49.9	2.0	2.7	0.2	9.6	0.9	13.6	1.3	3.5	0.3	17.6	1.3	11.7	1.0	3.3	0.3	11.2	0.7
6 days	53	3.197	0.456	50.1	2.0	2.7	0.2	9.6	1.0	13.7	1.2	3.5	0.3	17.9	1.1	11.9	0.7	3.4	0.3	11.1	0.7
1 month	20	3.714	0.447	–	–	2.9	0.2	9.5	1.3	14.2	1.4	3.7	0.4	19.5	1.8	13.1	1.3	3.7	0.4	11.8	0.9
2 months	42	4.914	0.984	57.9	5.3	2.9	0.2	9.6	0.9	14.4	1.4	4.1	0.5	21.7	2.0	14.5	1.7	4.0	0.4	12.1	1.0
6–11 months ..	13	9.149	1.227	72.4	3.4	3.2	0.2	10.7	2.3	16.3	3.2	5.0	0.6	24.1	2.8	16.8	2.0	4.9	0.6	14.6	1.3
12–14 months .	23	10.162	0.837	76.9	2.6	3.2	0.3	9.7	1.0	16.9	1.8	5.0	0.6	26.8	2.3	17.6	1.4	5.0	0.5	14.3	1.0

Age	Number	Body mass		Body length		Aortic root dimension (AO)*		Maximum aortic valve separation (AOV)		Maximum left atrial dimension (LA)		LA/AO		Tricuspid valve amplitude (TV ampl)		Mitral valve amplitude (MV ampl)		Fractional shortening (FS)	
		Mean	s	Mean	s	Mean	s	Mean	s	Mean	s	Mean	s	Mean	s	Mean	s	Mean	s
		kg		cm		mm						...		mm				...	
1st hour	32	3.313	0.353	50.1	1.76	9.5	0.8	7.6	0.7	11.9	1.4	1.3	0.1	9.5	1.2	8.4	1.1	0.33	0.03
1st day	53	3.283	0.478	49.9	2.0	9.9	0.7	7.7	0.6	12.1	1.2	1.2	0.1	8.9	1.0	8.3	1.2	0.33	0.03
3 days	53	3.213	0.481	49.9	2.0	10.0	0.7	7.8	0.7	11.8	1.0	1.2	0.1	8.8	1.0	8.5	1.2	0.33	0.04
6 days	53	3.197	0.456	50.1	2.0	10.2	0.6	8.0	0.6	11.8	0.8	1.2	0.1	8.7	1.1	8.6	1.1	0.34	0.03
1 month	20	3.714	0.447	–	–	11.2	0.9	8.3	0.7	12.9	1.2	1.1	0.1	9.1	1.3	9.0	1.2	0.33	0.03
2 months	42	4.914	0.984	57.9	5.3	11.7	1.0	9.4	0.7	13.7	1.4	1.2	0.1	9.9	1.2	10.0	1.2	0.33	0.04
6–11 months ..	13	9.149	1.227	72.4	3.4	14.0	1.5	10.8	1.0	16.1	2.1	1.1	0.1	11.2	1.5	11.5	1.9	0.34	0.02
12–14 months .	23	10.162	0.837	76.9	2.6	14.1	1.2	11.9	1.2	15.8	1.6	1.1	0.1	12.6	0.9	12.6	0.9	0.34	0.03

* Dimensions obtained in accordance with standard measurement recommendations of the American Society of Echocardiography (ASE) [2].

References
1. Oberhänsli et al., Helv paediat Acta, 36, 325 (1981).
2. Sahn et al., Circulation, 58, 1072 (1978).

Table 5. M-mode echocardiography: cardiac dimensions in children* (aged 1–15 years).

Body surface area	Right ventricular internal dimension◇ (end-diastolic) (RVD [ED])[†]		Maximum left ventricular internal dimension◇ (end-diastolic) (LVD [ED]$_{max}$)		Maximum left atrial internal dimension◇◇ (LA)		Aortic root dimension[††] (end-diastolic) (AO)		Ventricular septal thickness◇ (end-diastolic) (ST [ED])[†]		Left ventricular posterior free wall thickness◇ (end-diastolic) (PWT [ED])[†]	
	Mean	95% interval	Mean	95% interval	Mean	95% interval	Mean	95% interval	Mean	95% interval	Mean	95% interval
						mm						
0.4 m²	8.7	3.0–14.3	29.0	20.5–37.2	19.0	12.9–25.4	16.7	12.6–20.7	5.8	3.5– 8.0	4.7	2.5– 6.8
0.5 m²	9.4	3.8–15.0	30.4	32.0–38.8	19.9	13.7–26.2	17.6	13.5–21.5	6.0	3.8– 8.3	5.0	2.8– 7.2
0.6 m²	10.0	4.5–15.7	33.3	23.6–40.2	20.8	14.5–26.9	18.5	14.4–22.4	6.3	4.1– 8.6	5.4	3.2– 7.5
0.7 m²	10.8	5.1–16.4	34.8	25.2–41.8	21.6	15.2–27.8	19.3	15.3–23.2	6.6	4.3– 8.8	5.7	3.5– 7.8
0.8 m²	11.6	5.9–17.1	36.1	26.8–42.5	22.3	16.0–28.5	20.0	16.1–24.0	6.9	4.6– 9.1	6.0	3.8– 8.2
0.9 m²	12.3	6.7–17.9	37.8	28.5–45.0	23.1	16.9–29.3	20.9	17.0–24.9	7.2	5.0– 9.4	6.3	4.2– 8.5
1.0 m²	13.0	7.4–18.9	39.5	30.0–46.5	24.0	17.8–30.1	21.8	17.9–25.8	7.5	5.3– 9.7	6.6	4.5– 8.8
1.1 m²	13.7	8.1–19.3	41.0	31.6–48.4	24.8	18.5–30.9	22.7	18.8–26.7	7.8	5.6–10.0	7.0	4.8– 9.2
1.2 m²	14.3	8.8–20.0	42.8	33.2–50.0	25.6	19.3–31.8	23.6	19.6–27.6	8.1	5.8–10.2	7.3	5.2– 9.5
1.3 m²	15.0	9.5–20.7	44.8	34.8–51.5	26.8	20.1–32.7	24.4	20.4–28.4	8.4	6.1–10.5	7.7	5.5– 9.8
1.4 m²	15.7	10.1–21.4	46.5	36.5–53.0	27.0	20.9–33.5	25.2	21.2–29.2	8.7	6.4–10.8	8.0	5.8–10.2
1.5 m²	16.4	10.8–22.1	48.5	38.0–54.8	27.9	21.7–34.3	26.1	22.0–30.1	8.9	6.8–11.1	8.4	6.1–10.5

* 47 males, 33 females (15% from Mediterranean, and 85% from Central European countries).
◇ Measurement at the level of the mitral valve.
◇◇ Measurement at the level of the aortic root.
[†] Measurement at the moment of maximum end-diastolic left ventricular dimension (end of QRS complex).
[††] Measurement at the peak of R wave.

Reference
Lange et al., Herz, 8, 105 (1983).

Table 6. 2-D echocardiography: cardiac chamber dimensions, related to body surface area, and fractional shortening in adults (aged 18–38 years).

	Unit	26 men			25 women		
		Mean	2 s	90 % tolerance interval	Mean	2 s	90 % tolerance interval
Parasternal long-axis view							
Left ventricular anteroposterior dimension:							
– end-diastolic	cm/m²	2.7	0.4	2.3 –3.1	2.7	0.4	2.3 –3.1
– end-systolic	cm/m²	1.8	0.4	1.4 –2.2	1.8	0.4	1.4 –2.2
– fractional shortening	...	0.34	0.08	0.27–0.41	0.35	0.11	0.25–0.45
Left atrial anteroposterior dimension:							
– end-diastolic	cm/m²	1.3	0.3	1.0 –1.6	1.3	0.3	0.9 –1.7
– end-systolic	cm/m²	1.7	0.4	1.3 –2.1	1.8	0.4	1.4 –2.2
Parasternal short-axis view at level of the tips of papillary muscles							
Left ventricular anteroposterior dimension:							
– end-diastolic	cm/m²	2.5	0.3	2.2 –2.8	2.6	0.3	2.3 –2.9
– end-systolic	cm/m²	1.7	0.3	1.4 –2.0	1.8	0.3	1.5 –2.1
– fractional shortening	...	0.34	0.08	0.27–0.41	0.33	0.07	0.27–0.39
Left ventricular mediolateral dimension:							
– end-diastolic	cm/m²	2.6	0.3	2.3 –2.9	2.8	0.4	2.4 –3.2
– end-systolic	cm/m²	1.7	0.4	1.3 –2.1	1.8	0.3	1.5 –2.1
– fractional shortening	...	0.36	0.1	0.27–0.45	0.36	0.1	0.27–0.45
Apical 4-chamber view							
Left ventricle, major axis:							
– end-diastolic	cm/m²	4.5	0.4	4.1 –4.9	4.7	0.5	4.3 –5.1
– end-systolic	cm/m²	3.1	0.4	2.7 –3.5	3.3	0.4	2.9 –3.7
Left ventricle, minor axis:							
– end-diastolic	cm/m²	2.6	0.3	2.3 –2.9	2.8	0.4	2.4 –3.2
– end-systolic	cm/m²	1.7	0.3	1.4 –2.0	1.8	0.4	1.4 –2.2
– fractional shortening	...	0.35	0.07	0.3 –0.42	0.36	0.01	0.27–0.45
Left atrium, major axis:							
– end-diastolic	cm/m²	1.5	0.4	1.1 –1.9	1.8	0.6	1.3 –2.3
– end-systolic	cm/m²	2.1	0.4	1.7 –2.5	2.4	0.7	1.8 –3.0
Left atrium, minor axis:							
– end-diastolic	cm/m²	1.2	0.3	0.9 –1.5	1.2	0.4	0.8 –1.6
– end-systolic	cm/m²	1.8	0.3	1.5 –2.1	1.8	0.5	1.4 –2.3
Right ventricle, major axis:							
– end-diastolic	cm/m²	4.1	0.6	3.6 –4.6	4.3	0.6	3.8 –4.8
– end-systolic	cm/m²	3.0	0.6	2.5 –3.5	3.1	0.5	2.7 –3.5
Right ventricle, minor axis:							
– end-diastolic	cm/m²	1.7	0.4	1.3 –2.1	1.8	0.4	1.4 –2.2
– end-systolic	cm/m²	1.3	0.4	0.9 –1.7	1.3	0.4	0.9 –1.7
– fractional shortening	...	0.3	0.1	0.21–0.39	0.31	0.11	0.21–0.41
Right atrium, major axis:							
– end-diastolic	cm/m²	1.4	0.3	1.1 –1.7	1.5	0.5	1.1 –2.0
– end-systolic	cm/m²	2.3	0.4	1.9 –2.7	2.4	0.6	1.9 –2.9
Right atrium, minor axis:							
– end-diastolic	cm/m²	1.5	0.4	1.1 –1.9	1.6	0.3	1.3 –1.9
– end-systolic	cm/m²	1.8	0.4	1.4 –2.2	1.9	0.4	1.5 –2.3

Reference
Erbel et al., Dtsch. med. Wschr., 110, 123 (1985).

Table 7. 2-D echocardiography*: right ventricular dimensions at enddiastole in 41 adults (aged 19–46 years).

	Absolute measurements			Measurements related to body surface area				Absolute measurements			Measurements related to body surface area		
	Mean	2 s	Range	Mean	2 s	Range		Mean	2 s	Range	Mean	2 s	Range
	cm			cm/m²				cm			cm/m²		
Right ventricular chamber							*Diameter of tricuspid valve annulus*						
Major axis (RVLAX)	7.6	0.5	6.9–8.9	4.4	0.4	3.6–5.4	RVA₁	3.4	0.3	2.5–4.0	2.0	0.2	1.6–2.4
Minor axis (RVSAX)	3.0	0.3	2.4–3.7	1.8	0.2	1.4–2.2	RVA₂	2.4	0.3	1.6–3.1	1.5	0.2	1.1–1.8
Right ventricular inflow tract							*Right ventricular wall thickness*						
RVIT₁	4.5	0.5	3.7–5.4	2.6	0.3	2.0–3.3	T1	0.3	0.07	0.2–0.5	0.2	0.04	0.1–0.3
RVIT₂	3.0	0.3	2.4–3.9	1.7	0.2	1.4–2.0	T2	0.3	0.07	0.2–0.5	0.2	0.05	0.1–0.3
RVIT₃	2.4	0.4	1.5–3.0	1.4	0.2	1.0–1.8	T3	0.3	0.05	0.3–0.5	0.2	0.04	0.1–0.3
RVIT₄	5.1	0.5	4.0–7.0	2.9	0.4	2.3–3.6	T4	0.4	0.07	0.2–0.5	0.2	0.04	0.1–0.3
							T5	0.3	0.08	0.2–0.5	0.2	0.05	0.1–0.3
							T6	0.3	0.06	0.2–0.5	0.2	0.04	0.1–0.3
Right ventricular outflow tract							T7	0.4	0.07	0.3–0.5	0.2	0.05	0.1–0.3
RVOT₁	2.2	0.3	1.8–3.0	1.3	0.2	1.0–1.7	T8	0.4	1.0	0.3–0.6	0.2	0.06	0.1–0.4
RVOT₂	2.3	0.3	1.8–2.9	1.3	0.3	1.0–2.9	T9	0.4	0.07	0.3 0.6	0.2	0.05	0.1–0.3
RVOT₃	2.0	0.3	1.4–2.6	1.1	0.1	0.9–1.4	T10	0.4	1.0	0.3–0.7	0.2	0.06	0.1–0.4
RVOT₄	2.7	0.2	2.0–3.2	1.6	0.2	1.2–2.0							

Reference
Foale et al., Brit Heart J, 56, 33 (1986).

ˣ For sites of measurement, see pages 762–764.

Table 8. 2-D echocardiography: end-diastolic dimensions of aorta
and pulmonary artery according to body mass in neonates, children and adolescents
(regression lines and 905 tolerance intervals).

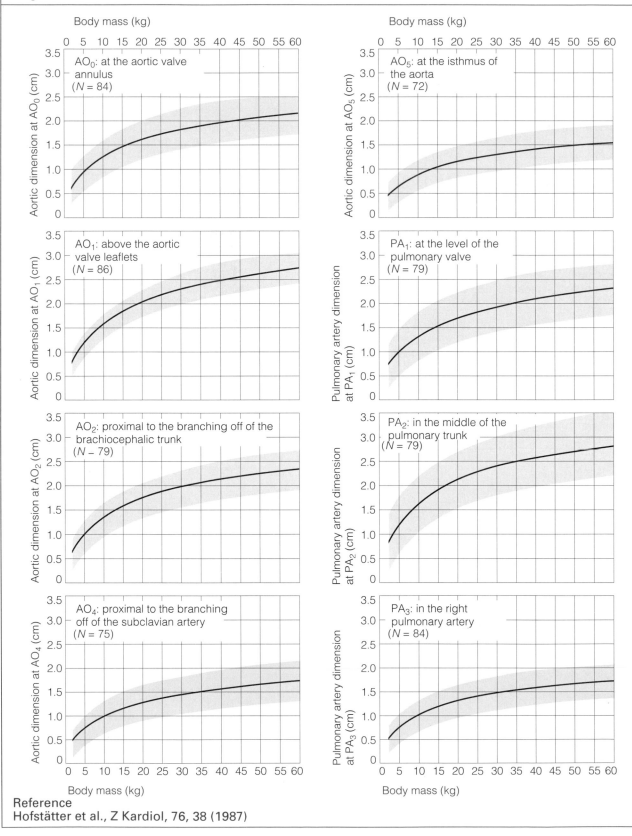

Reference
Hofstätter et al., Z Kardiol, 76, 38 (1987)

Table 9. 2-D echocardiography*: mitral valve dimensions in 35 adults (aged 37 [s 14] years).

	Mean	s
	cm	
Anterior leaflet length◇	2.00	0.31
Posterior leaflet length◇	1.45	0.22
Diameter of mitral valve annulus:		
– end-diastolic	2.68	0.39
– end-systolic	2.91	0.34

* Parasternal long-axis view; computerized analysis.
◇ Just before mitral valve closure.

Reference
Pini et al., Circulation, 80, 915 (1989).

Table 10. 2-D echocardiography*: left ventricular volumes and ejection fraction in adults.

	Unit	35 men◇ (18–40 years) [1]			20 women◇ (22–35 years) [1]			22 adults[†] (22–61) years) [2]	
		Mean	s	90% tolerance interval	Mean	s	90% tolerance interval	Mean	s
Left ventricular volume:									
– end-diastolic	ml	127	18	96–157	98	21	59–138	100	29
– – related to body surface area	ml/m^2	67	9	52– 82	61	13	37– 85	–	–
– end-systolic	ml	50	10	33– 68	42	12	18– 65	35	17
– – related to body surface area	ml/m^2	27	5	18– 36	26	7	12– 40	–	–
Cardiac output	l/min	–	–	–	–	–	–	4.2	1.0
Cardiac index	l min^{-1} m^{-2}	–	–	–	–	–	–	2.36	0.37
Stroke volume	ml	76	13	55– 98	57	11	36– 77	65	17
Stroke volume index	ml/m^2	40	7	28– 52	35	7	22– 48	39	9
Left ventricular ejection fraction	...	0.59	0.06	0.49–0.7	0.58	0.07	0.46–0.71	0.66	0.1

* Apical 4-chamber view and RAO-equivalent view.
◇ Left ventricular volumes calculated by biplane disc-summation method.
[†] Left ventricular volumes calculated by biplane area length method.

References
1. Erbel et al., Dtsch med Wschr, 107, 1872 (1982).
2. Hahn et al., Z Kardiol, 71, 445 (1982).

Table 11. Correlation between left ventricular volumes determined by 2-D echocardiography and X-ray cineangiocardiography* in 35 patients (CAD, valvular disease, constrictive pericarditis).

Method of calculation from 2-D echocardiografic measurements	Correlation for			
	LVEDV		LVESV	
	r	$S_{y,x}$ (ml)	r	$S_{y,x}$ (ml)
Biplane area length method	0.67	49	0.72	44
Single-plane area length method	0.61	52	0.64	48
Modified ellipsoidal model (Teichholz)	0.72	46	0.81	37
Hemicylinder hemiellipsoidal method	0.68	49	0.75	42
Disc-summation method	0.76	43	0.86	32

* Angiocardiographic volumes calculated by single-plane area length method and the regressions of Kennedy et al., Am Heart J, 80, 343 [1979]).

Reference
Folland et al., Circulation, 60, 760 (1979).

Table 12. Calculation of left ventricular wall stress.

Assumption	Formula	Ref.
Spherical model	Spherical wall stress (according to LaPlace): $$S_{spheric} = \frac{PD}{4h}$$	
Ellipsoidal model Model approximating thick-walled geometry	Circumferential wall stress: $$S_1 \frac{PD\,(2L^2 - D^2)}{4h\,(L^2 + Dh)}$$ Meridional wall stress: $$S_2 = \frac{PD^2}{4h\,(D + h)}$$	1.2 1.2
Thin-walled model	Circumferential wall stress: $$S_3 = \frac{PD}{2h}\left[1 - \frac{D^3}{2L^2(D + h)}\right]$$	2.3

P: left ventricular pressure or systolic blood pressure (in kPa or kdyn/cm^2)

References
1. Falsetti et al., Circulation Res, 26, 71 (1970).
2. Krayenbühl, H. P., Eur Heart J, 6, Suppl. C, 33 (1985).
3. Sandler, H., Dodge, H.T., Circulation Res, 13, 91 (1963).

Table 13. Systolic left ventricular wall stress.*

	Subjects	Mean	s	Range	Ref.
		kPa$^\diamond$			
$S_{spherical}$ (spherical wall stress)					
Peak-systolic	22 adults, 22–61 years	28.3	5.9	–	1
S_2 (meridional wall stress)					
End-systolic	14 subjects, 8–32 years	4.7	1.0	3.0–6.2	2
	45 adults, 43 (s 10) years	4.7	1.1	–	3
	87 adults, 19–65 years	6.3	1.9	–	4
	10 men, 20–37 years	6.3	1.6	4.0–9.1	5
	20 men, 49 years.............	4.2	0.8	–	6
	Men	6.3	1.5	–	7
	Women	5.9	0.9	–	7
	160 black and white adults, 44 (s 12.7) years	6.3	2.1	–	8
Peak-systolic	14 subjects, 8–32 years	14.2	2.3	11.6–20.0	2
	45 adults, 43 (s 10) years	12.6	2.5	–	3
	10 men, 20–37 years	13.7	2.8	10.1–19.3	5
	20 men, 49 years	14.5	2.3	–	6
	Men	17.1	2.9	–	7
	Women	16.8	2.4	–	7

* Calculated from systolic blood pressure and echocardiographic left ventricular dimensions.
$\diamond$ 1 kPa = 10 kdyn/cm^2.

References
1. Hahn et al., Z Kardiol, 71, 445 (1982).
2. Colan et al., Am J Cardiol, 52, 1304 (1983).
3. De Simone et al., Am J Cardiol, 60, 1317 (1987).
4. Lutas et al., Hypertension, 7, 979 (1985).
5. Wilson et al., Am J Med, 68, 664 (1980).
6. Hartford et al., Hypertension, 7, 97 (1985).
7. Nakashima et al., Am J Cardiol, 53, 1044 (1984).
8. Hammond et al., J Am Coll Cardiol, 7, 639 (1986).

Left Ventricular Wall Stress

Left ventricular wall stress (S) is an estimate of the force stretching the myocardial fibers (end-diastolic wall stress) or of the force resisting systolic shortening of the myofibrils (systolic wall stress); it is a resultant of left ventricular pressure, internal dimensions and wall thickness. Assuming spherical or ellipsoidal geometry of the left ventricle, wall stress is calculated according to the formulae given in Table 12.
Unit: kPa, kdyn/cm^2 (1 kPa = 10 kdyn/cm^2).

Methods

Left ventricular internal dimensions and wall thickness may be obtained by angiocardiography, as well as by M-mode echocardiography, 2-D echocardiography and magnetic resonance imaging; left ventricular pressures may be determined by left heart catheterization or by measurement of arterial systolic blood pressure (as an approximation of left ventricular peak systolic pressure).

Table 14. Cineangiocardiography, centerline method*: regional wall motion in adults ($\bar{x} \pm s$).

Left ventricle — 30° RAO projection / 60° LAO projection

Right ventricle — 15° RAO projection / 75° LAO projection

* Centerline method developed by Sheehan and Bolson (University of Washington, Seattle, Wash.): the motion is measured along 100 chords drawn perpendicular to a centerline constructed midway between the end-diastolic and nend-systolic contours. The measured motion of the 100 chords in normalized for heart size by dividing by the length of the end-diastolic perimeter.

Reference: Sheehan et al., Circulation, 74, 293 (1986); Sheehan and Bolson, personal communication.

Table 15. M-mode echocardiography: mean velocity of circumferential fiber shortening (Vcf_{mean}) in children and adults.

	Vcf_{mean}			Ref.
	Mean	s	95 % interval	
	circ/s			
32 boys and young men, 2–24 years	1.6	0.34	–	1
10 adults, 20–35 years	1.09	0.13	0.86–1.29	2
22 adults, 22–61 years	1.24	0.22	–	3
38 adults	1.3	–	1.02–1.94	4
20 men, 49 years	1.11	0.18	–	5

References
1. Goldberg et al., Circulation, 62, 1061 (1980).
2. Rankin et al., Circulation, 51, 910 (1975).
3. Hahn et al., Z Kardiol, 71, 445 (1982).
4. Feigenbaum, H., Echocardiography, 4th ed., Lea & Febiger, Philadelphia, 1986, page 622.
5. Hartford et al., Hypertension, 7, 97 (1985).

Table 16. M-mode echocardiography: interventricular septal and left ventricular posterior wall thickness, wall thickening and rate of change of wall thickness in children and adults.

	Unit	31 children (3–12 years) [1]						20 adults (19–63 years) [2]	
		Level of mitral valve cusps		Level of tips of mitral valve cusps		Level of papillary muscles		Level of chordae tendineae of mitral valve	
		Mean	s	Mean	s	Mean	s	Mean	s
Interventricular septum									
End-diastolic thickness	mm	6.3	1.5	6.7	1.0	6.1	1.3	7	2
End-systolic thickness	mm	9.7	1.0	11.0	2.0	11.0	2.0	12	3
Relative systolic thickening	...	0.34	0.13	0.63	0.31	0.66	0.25	0.53	0.13
Peak rate of systolic thickening	mm/s	28	8	31	10	27	7	–	–
Peak rate of diastolic thinning	mm/s	42	10	40	20	32	10	–	–
Normalized peak rate of systolic thickening ..	s^{-1}	–	–	–	–	–	–	3.9	0.8
Normalized peak rate of diastolic thinning .	s^{-1}	–	–	–	–	–	–	3.4	0.9
Left ventricular posterior wall									
End-diastolic thickness	mm	6.4	2.0	6.4	2.0	5.8	2.0	9	2
End-systolic thickness	mm	9.9	2.0	11.0	2.0	11.0	2.0	15	3
Relative systolic thickening	...	0.55	0.27	0.77	0.37	1.06	0.51	0.69	0.23
Peak rate of systolic thickening	mm/s	35	10	36	10	36	8	–	–
Peak rate of diastolic thinning	mm/s	64	30	90	30	100	30	–	–
Normalized peak rate of systolic thickening ..	s^{-1}	–	–	–	–	–	–	4.6	1.4
Normalized peak rate of diastolic thinning .	s^{-1}	–	–	–	–	–	–	9.1	4.3

References
1. Shapiro et al., Brit Heart J, 45, 264 (1981).
2. St. John Sutton et al., Circulation, 66, 790 (1982).

Table 17. Diastolic time intervals and left ventricular lengthening (M-mode echocardiography* and ECG) in 28 adults (aged 17–46 years).

	Time interval		Left ventricular lengthening (ΔD)		Fractional lengthening $\left[\dfrac{\Delta D}{LVD(ED) - LVD(ES)}\right]$	
	Mean	s	Mean	s	Mean	s
	ms		mm		...	
Relaxation time index (from minimal internal dimension to mitral valve opening	13[†]	15	0.6	0.5	–	–
Rapid filling period	111	32	10.7	2.2	0.62	0.1
Diastasis (slow filling period)	264	156	4.1	1.9	0.22	0.09
Filling period during atrial contraction	115	44	2.8	1.8	0.16	0.1

* Parasternal short-axis view; left ventricular internal dimension at the level of the free edges of the mitral valve leaflets.
† Range: –29 to 35 ms

Reference
Hanrath et al., Am J Cardiol, 45, 15 (1980).

Table 18. M-mode echocardiography*: peak rate of posterior wall thinning (*peak*-dh/dt) in adults.

	Age	Condition	*Peak*-dh/dt		Reference
			Mean	s	
			cm/s		
20 untrained adults	17–60 years	Rest	9	2	1
10 athletes◇	16–32 years	Rest	10	1	1
12 adults	34–63 years	Rest	8.2	3.7	2
11 adults	30–64 Jahre	Rest	8.4	2.7	3
		Exercise†	11.8	4.0	3

* Parasternal short-axis view at the level of the mitral valve.
◇ Top-class endurance swimmers.
† Bicycle ergometry in supine position (heart rate: 101 [s 13] min^{-1}).

References
1. Shapiro and McKenna, Brit Heart J, 51, 637 (1984).
2. Bourdillon et al., Circulation, 67, 316 (1983).
3. Mason et al., Circulation, 59, 50 (1979).

1. Biamino G, Lange L. Echokardiographie. Hoechst AG, Frankfurt/Main 1983; 176.
2. Brutsaert DL et al. Circ Res 1980; 47: 637.
3. Brutsaert DL, Rademakers FE, Sys SU, Gillebert TC, Housmans PR. The heart as an integrated muscle and pump system: triple control and subdivision of the cardiac cycle. Acta Cardiologica 1984; 39: 89-95.
4. Colan SD, Borow KM, Neumann A. Effects of loading conditions and contractile state (methoxamine and dobutamine) on LV early diastolic function in normal subjects. Am J Cardiol 1985; 55: 790-796.
5. Edler I. Ultrasound cardiogram in mitral valve disease. Acta Chir Sand 1956; 111: 230.
6. Gamble WH, Shaver JA, Alvares RF, Salerni R, Reddy PS. A critical appraisal of diastolic time intervals as a measure of relaxation in left ventricular hypertrophy. Circulation 1983; 68: 76-87.
7. Geigy Scientific Tables, Vol. 5, Heart and Circulation, 8th Ed., C. Lentner (ed.), Basel, Ciba-Geigy Ltd., 1990.
8. Kronik G, Slany J, Mösslacher H. Comparative value of eight m-mode echocardiographic formulas for determining left ventricular stroke volume. Circulation 1979; 60: 1308-1316.
9. Levine RE, Gibson TC, Aretz T et al. Echocardiographic measurement of right ventricular volume. Circulation 1984; 69: 497-505.
10. Report of the American Society of Echocardiography Committee on Nomenclature and Standards in Two-dimensional Echocardiography.
11. Sahn DJ, DeMaria A, Kisslo J, Weyman A. Recommendations regarding quantitation in m-mode echocardiography: results of a survey of echocardiographic measurements. Circulation 1978; 58: 1072.
12. Teichholz LE et al. Am J Cardiol 1976; 37: 7.

The indications for conventional Doppler echocardiography and Doppler color flow imaging (color Doppler) are:

- Valvular heart disease,
- Prosthetic cardiac valves,
- Intracardiac wall defects,
- Pathological changes in supply and drainage vessels,
- Filling disturbances of the cardiac cavities.

The ultimate motive of the Doppler examination is to quantitate or define the severity of regurgitation or stenosis. Doppler is normally very useful in this regard, although it has limitations.

The standard transducer positions for Doppler echocardiography are shown in the figure below. It is also legitimate to use any other transducer position that successfully images the region of interest when the findings can be properly documented.

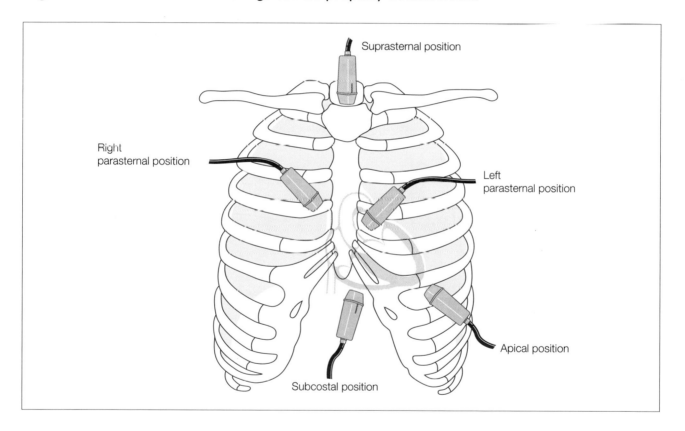

3.   **Conventional Doppler Echocardiography and Doppler Color Flow**   **106**
            Imaging: Examination Procedure and Assessment Tasks
3.1   **Blood Flow Velocities**

Since the introduction of Doppler techniques in clinical practice, numerous studies have been performed to define normal and pathological blood flow velocities in various heart diseases.

A major problem with comparing these studies is the lack of standardization of collectives with respect to age and composition.

Velocity has been used as a fundamental measurement parameter in a number of methods for quantitation of pathological and normal flow phenomena. The following reference diagram shows normal blood flow relationships in the heart of a healthy adult. The length of the arrows is a simplified connotation of local flow velocity in the healthy heart. Measurement of flow velocities in this manner is restricted, because the heart can rarely be imaged in its entirety from conventional transducer positions. Since it is extremely difficult to perform precise angle corrections, these techniques should be used with reservations.

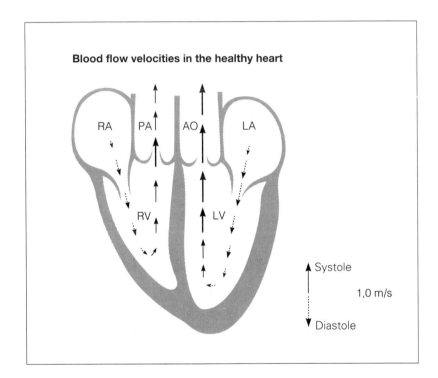

Blood flow velocities in the healthy heart

RA   PA   AO   LA

RV   LV

▲ Systole

1,0 m/s

▼ Diastole

It is impossible to postulate normal blood flow velocities. There is a range of normal and a scope of pathological blood flow velocities for every subgroup of patients. Furthermore, these ranges may overlap.

Blood flow phenomena across the cardiac valves must be assessed according to cardiac phase. It is therefore necessary to perform Doppler echocardiography with simultaneous ECG recording. Two flows that occur in rapid sequence, or even overlap, would be falsely interpreted without an ECG recording. The expected mean flow velocities for normal and pathological blood flow, as synchronized with the ECG recording, are shown in the following illustration.

3.   **Conventional Doppler Echocardiography and Doppler Color Flow**   107
     Imaging: Examination Procedure and Assessment Tasks
3.1   **Blood Flow Velocities**

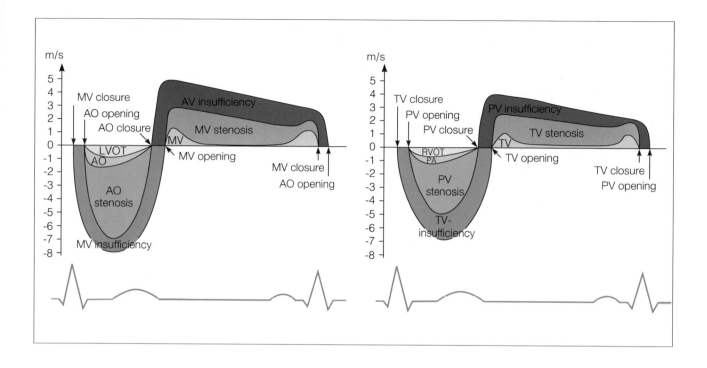

3.   Conventional Doppler Echocardiography and Doppler Color Flow Imaging: Examination Procedure and Assessment Tasks
3.2   Pressure Gradients

In hydrodynamics, one studies the relationships between flow velocity and pressure. Only when a pressure difference exists between two points in a system can liquids flow from the point of higher pressure to the point of lower pressure. The volume of flow (volume per unit time - dV/dt) is proportional to the flow velocity. Flow is maintained only for as long as the pressure difference between the two points continues to exist. This pressure difference is called the *pressure gradient;* its slope is directly proportional to the distance between the two points.

Pulsed-wave (PW) Doppler can be used to measure local flow velocities, which in turn can be used to calculate the pressure gradient across a cardiac valve *(transvalvular pressure gradient)*. The transvalvular pressure gradient plays a major role in the quantitation of valvular stenosis.

The *Bernoulli equation* provides a physical description of flow relationships. A simplified version of the Bernoulli equation can be used in Doppler echocardiography, because the proportion of viscous friction and flow acceleration in long stenoses do not play a role in cardiac diagnosis.

The *simplified Bernoulli equation* is used to calculate the pressure gradient.

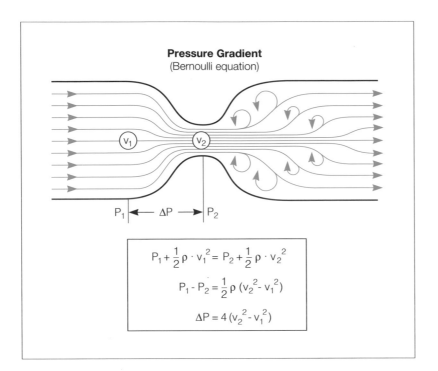

Pressure Gradient
(Bernoulli equation)

$$P_1 + \frac{1}{2}\rho \cdot v_1^2 = P_2 + \frac{1}{2}\rho \cdot v_2^2$$

$$P_1 - P_2 = \frac{1}{2}\rho\,(v_2^2 - v_1^2)$$

$$\Delta P = 4\,(v_2^2 - v_1^2)$$

The *transvalvular pressure gradient* (mmHg) is derived from intrastenotic and prestenotic velocities (m/s). The equation can be further simplified when the prestenotic velocity is small compared with intrastenotic velocity. The standard simplified Bernoulli equation used in Doppler echocardiography for computation of pressure gradients is given below.

$\Delta P = 4 \times v^2$	
ΔP	*Pressure gradient*
v	*Intrastenotic velocity*

The heart functions as a pump. In other words, there is no stationary flow in the heart. All flows occur according to a specific time sequence which is controlled by muscular contractions of the heart and which is mediated by pressure gradients. Cardiac flows are pulsatile in nature. Therefore, the pressure gradient calculated using the Bernoulli equation is representative only of the pressure gradient at that specific moment in time when the velocity was determined.

The *peak pressure gradient* (ΔP_{peak}) is the gradient calculated using the peak velocity measured at a particular point. The *mean pressure gradient* (ΔP_{mean}), on the other hand, is calculated as the arithmetic mean of all individual gradients calculated over the entire duration of flow. The mean pressure gradient is calculated by applying the simplified Bernoulli equation using the mean velocity (v_{mean}).

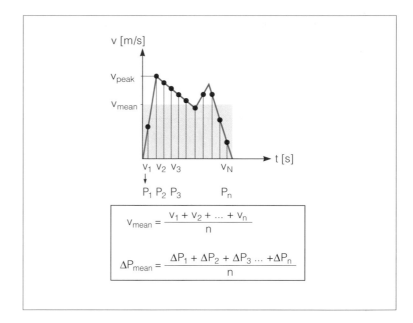

$$v_{mean} = \frac{v_1 + v_2 + \dots + v_n}{n}$$

$$\Delta P_{mean} = \frac{\Delta P_1 + \Delta P_2 + \Delta P_3 \dots + \Delta P_n}{n}$$

3.

Conventional Doppler Echocardiography and Doppler Color Flow Imaging: Examination Procedure and Assessment Tasks

3.3

Assessment of Central and Peripheral Flow

The experienced echocardiographer is able to adjust the transducer position slightly to find the optimum Doppler signal. However, the angle between the velocity vector and the acoustic axis should be kept as small as possible (< 20°).

Mathematical post-scanning angle correction can lead false interpretations, especially when velocities are in the upper limits of normal.

Assessment of Central Flow

The figure below shows the typical M-shaped pattern of the normal diastolic velocity profile of the mitral valve, when obtained from an apical position using PW Doppler. The M-shape correlates with active (E wave) and passive (A wave) filling of the left ventricle.

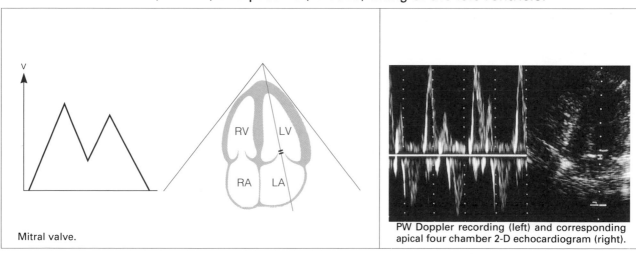

Mitral valve.

PW Doppler recording (left) and corresponding apical four chamber 2-D echocardiogram (right).

Flow across the tricuspid valve is measured similar to flow across the mitral valve.

The same M-shaped spectrum is obtained in diastole. Velocities across the tricuspid valve are normally around 30 to 50 % lower than in the left ventricle. Due to the lower flow velocities, right ventricle often cannot be visualized as well as the left ventricle in Doppler color flow imaging.

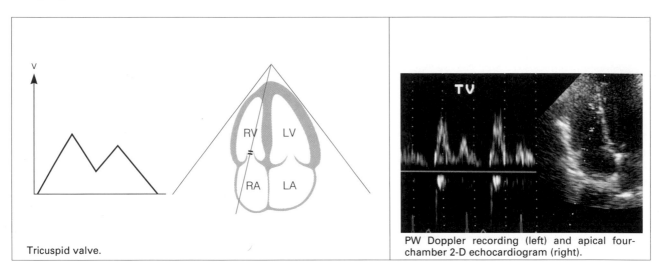

Tricuspid valve.

PW Doppler recording (left) and apical four-chamber 2-D echocardiogram (right).

The systolic flow velocity profile across the aortic valve or in the left ventricular outflow tract (LVOT) is measured using continuous-wave Doppler (CW Doppler). In PW Doppler, such high-velocity flow (ca. 1.50 m/s in normals) would result in aliasing. Since the necessary depth of penetration requires a low PRF, velocities in the LVOT would exceed the Nyquist limit.

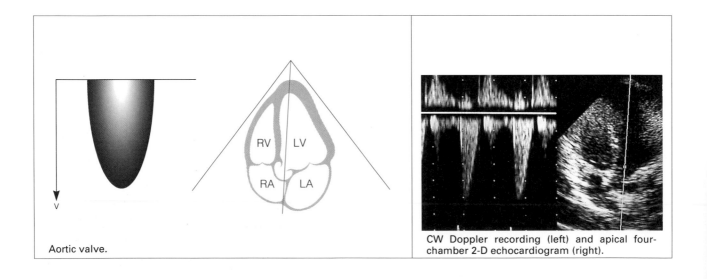

Aortic valve.

CW Doppler recording (left) and apical four-chamber 2-D echocardiogram (right).

Particularly in adolescent patients, the pulmonary artery and valve can be visualized well from the parasternal short-axis view. The PW Doppler sample volume can be positioned exactly in the middle of the pulmonary artery at the level of the valve. PW Doppler can normally be used for flow velocity measurement in this case, because velocities in the lesser circulation are relatively low due to low peripheral resistance of the lungs.

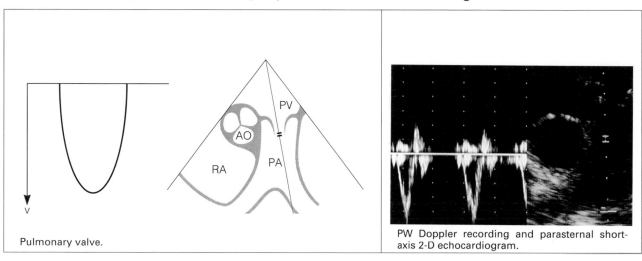

Pulmonary valve.

PW Doppler recording and parasternal short-axis 2-D echocardiogram.

Assessment of Peripheral Flow

Assessment of flow in the peripheral regions of the heart requires much more skill and experience than assessment of central flow. The depth from which Doppler signals are obtained requires high sensitivity of the Doppler technique.

Peripheral flow measurements play a major role in the assessment of cardiac function. Only in the last few years has it become possible to obtain reliable flow measurements from the pulmonary veins at the roof of the left atrium.

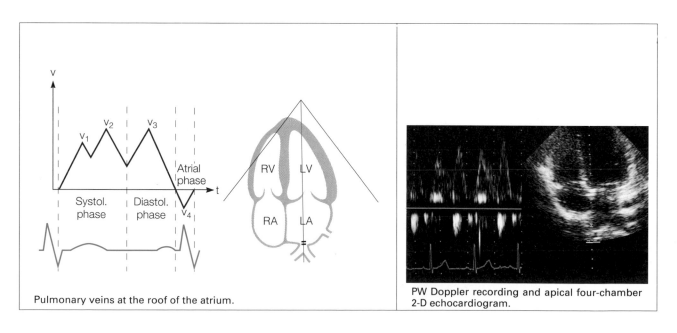

Pulmonary veins at the roof of the atrium.

PW Doppler recording and apical four-chamber 2-D echocardiogram.

The measurement of flow in the pulmonary veins has been the subject of various studies.

The following guidelines values were proposed:

	v_{peak} (m/s)
Early systolic phase	0.50
Late systolic phase	0.60
Diastolic Phase	0.45
Atrial phase	0.20

These guideline values, which demonstrate a large range of variation, have yet to be validated. The diagnostic significance of pathological flow is not yet entirely clear. However, pulmonary venous flow can be used as a parameter for quantification of mitral insufficiency.

The typical flow pattern of right atrial filling is measured in a hepatic vein. The horizontal orientation of the inferior vena cava in 2-D echocardiograms is not suitable for Doppler signal acquisition. Using the hepatic vein instead does not compromise image quality. In patients with pathological right ventricular overload or hemodynamically significant tricuspid insufficiency, dilation of the hepatic veins can be visualized by means of 2-D echocardiography, and systolic flow towards the transducer can be registered using PW Doppler.

Systolic flow from the liver into the inferior vena cava is normally biphasic. The two phases are defined as the *x-trough* and the *y-trough*.

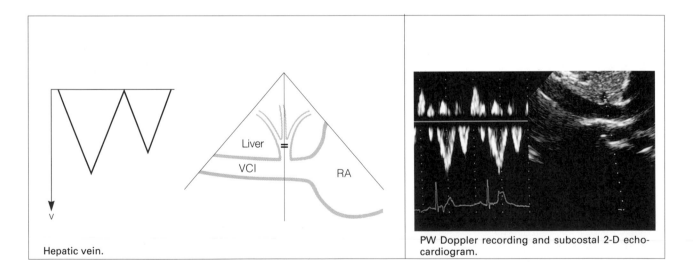

Hepatic vein.

PW Doppler recording and subcostal 2-D echocardiogram.

The aortic arch can be visualized from the suprasternal position. PW Doppler can be used to study the origins of the large head and neck vessels. Flow measurement using CW Doppler is indicated when stenosis of the aortic isthmus is suspected. The following color-encoded image of the aortic arch demonstrates angle-related problems and aliasing.

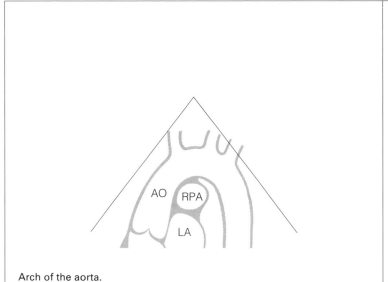

Arch of the aorta.

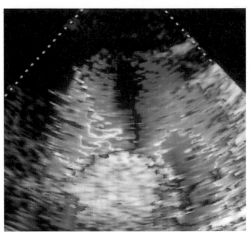

Color flow map of suprasternal short-axis echocardiogram.

3. **Conventional Doppler Echocardiography and Doppler Color Flow**
Imaging: Examination Procedure and Assessment Tasks
3.4 **Doppler Echocardiographic Parameters of Ventricular Function**

Assessment of ventricular performance using Doppler-derived measurements can be problematic, because parameters such as preload and afterload are extremely difficult to integrate into dynamic models. A number of indices of left ventricular (LV) function have been suggested, but only a few have gained significance in clinical practice. The most important of these are listed below.

Deceleration Rate

Left ventricular diastolic performance demonstrates a characteristic M-shaped velocity profile at mitral valve level. Many investigators have attempted to establish reliable indices of diastolic function. These include the *E/A ratio* (ratio of E wave to A wave velocity) and various time intervals. The *deceleration rate* has been found to correlate with LV contractility and, to a limited degree, with LV compliance.

Stroke Volume Across Atrioventricular Valves

Similar to the tricuspid valve measurements, *stroke volume across the mitral valve* is measured in two steps. First the time-velocity integral (TVI) is derived from the Doppler spectrum. The mitral valve orifice area is measured using a two-dimensional image obtained from the parasternal short-axis position.

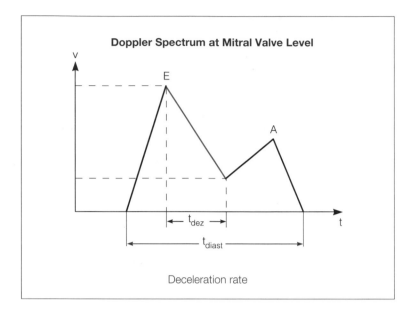

Since the orifice area does not remain constant throughout diastole, the measured area must be corrected. The velocity-time integral and the mitral valve orifice area are multiplied to obtain the transmitral stroke volume. When there is coexistent aortic insufficiency, the difference between aortic and mitral stroke volumes can provide an estimate the volume of aortic regurgitation.

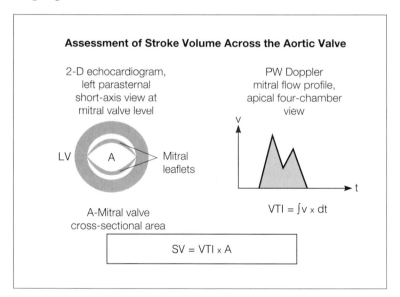

Continuity Equation

The *continuity equation* states that volume rate of flow (dV/dt) in a given system remains constant, regardless of the vessel diameter. When the beam intersects a layer of fluid perpendicular to the direction of flow, the flow stream will traverse a certain length of the vessel in one unit of time. The flow volume in vessel segments of different diameters is maintained by means of the flow velocity.

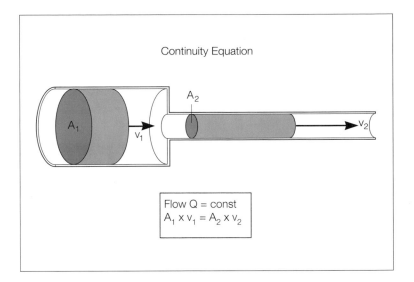

Using relationships in the heart, the continuity equation can be applied to determine the residual orifice area of cardiac valves.

The theoretical model is explained in the following figure. In two-dimensional echocardiography, it is often difficult to measure the residual orifice area of calcified or stenotic valves. The continuity equation provides a solution to this problem.

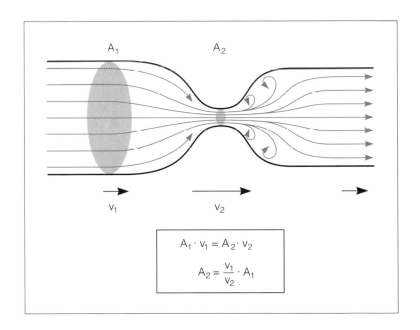

In cardiac applications, the continuity equation is classically used to determine the aortic valve area (AVA). First, the poststenotic cross-sectional area is measured in the left ventricular outflow tract. Next, PW Doppler is used to determine the flow velocity in the LVOT. Finally, CW Doppler is used to determine the intrastenotic velocity.

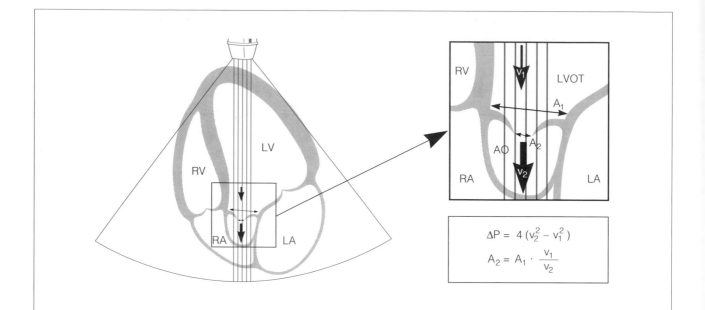

$$\Delta P = 4 \, (v_2^2 - v_1^2)$$

$$A_2 = A_1 \cdot \frac{v_1}{v_2}$$

Calculation of Stroke Volume Using Aortic Flow

The calculation of *stroke volume using aortic flow* is similar to the calculations used with atrioventricular valves. First, the cross-sectional area of the aorta is measured at the level of the valve ring from the 2-D parasternal long-axis. The velocity-time integral (VTI) is then obtained from the Doppler spectrum. The stroke volume is the product of area times the time-velocity integral.

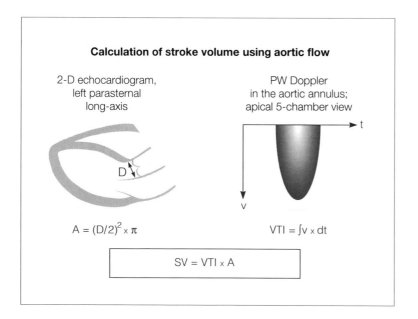

Calculation of stroke volume using aortic flow

2-D echocardiogram, left parasternal long-axis

PW Doppler in the aortic annulus; apical 5-chamber view

$$A = (D/2)^2 \times \pi$$

$$VTI = \int v \times dt$$

$$SV = VTI \times A$$

These functional parameters have inherent sources of error, which will be discussed in the following section.

First of all, blood flow is pulsatile in nature. The above measurements must be made across several cardiac cycles, because flow is not constant from one heart beat to the next.

Secondly, blood flow is not stationary. The blood flow velocity rises and falls. Therefore, sensitivity problems of the transducer or system electronics must be taken into consideration when performing these measurements.

Thirdly, the spatial orientation of the velocity vector is unknown. This gives rise to angle-related problems which may lead to over- or underestimation of blood flow velocity.

For calculation purposes, most theoretical models assume that the flow profile in the vessel cross-section is flat and box-shaped. In reality, however, the flow profile is often parabolic. This can lead to underestimation of flow volume.

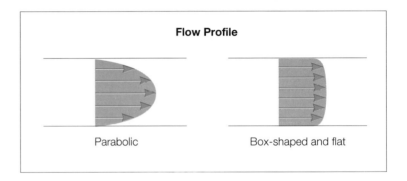

Flow Profile

Parabolic   Box-shaped and flat

Pressure gradients across the aorta derived by means of the Bernoulli equation normally are not comparable with invasively measured pressure gradients.

The invasively determined peak-to-peak gradient (ΔP_{peak}), which is measured at different times in the aorta and in the ventricle, does not occur in the heart. Doppler-derived gradients are instantaneous gradients. They are derived from the flow velocity profile at a specific moment in time.

In cases where a direct comparison of pressure gradients is desired, we recommend that one should compare only the Doppler-derived instantaneous peak pressure gradient with the peak pressure gradient obtained at cardiac catheterization.

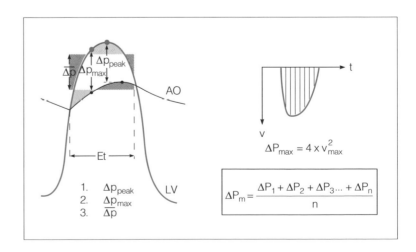

$$\Delta P_{max} = 4 \times v_{max}^2$$

$$\Delta P_m = \frac{\Delta P_1 + \Delta P_2 + \Delta P_3 \ldots + \Delta P_n}{n}$$

1. Δp_{peak}
2. Δp_{max}
3. $\overline{\Delta p}$

There is no physical evidence of a correlation between color jet size and hemodynamic significance.

Echocardiographic measurement data must be presented to the physician in a form that permits diagnosis. Parameters derived from physical calculation methods make it easier to comprehend echocardiographic images and to compare them with those of other diagnostic techniques. These physical methods, which can be applied to a given disease only under certain conditions, are computed using the echocardiograph's central processing unit or on an external computer. Before these methods are applied in the clinical setting, they must be extensively validated by reliable serial measurement studies.

The majority of research work is performed using external computers. Therefore, every echocardiograph should have interfaces that can connect it to the outside world. The monitor, which is the primary output medium for visualization of echocardiographic data, is an analog device. Manufactures have agreed to standardize the analog interface from the echocardiograph to the monitor. The video standard further ensures uncomplicated documentation of ultrasound images. The video standard can be easily converted to the appropriate national television standard. World-wide communication has unlimited potentials. Quality and processing-related limitations of analog technology have compelled physicians to turn to digitization. Monitor images cannot be fed directly into an external computer. They must first be digitized by means of a digitizer (frame-grabber) card. Monitor images generated during echocardiography and Doppler examinations are stored in digital form on the echocardiograph's internal memory unit. A digital interface can be used for direct data transfer to an external computer. The format of digital output data depends how far they were processed by the internal computer before being extracted. Specially developed software in the external computer can be accessed only when the mode of data transfer, *i.e. the data protocol,* is known. This is a decisive problem in computed-assisted ultrasound diagnosis, because almost every manufacturer strives to provide their own brand of specialized software for external computer-assisted cardiac ultrasound diagnosis. There currently is no uniform standard for either the data protocol or the interface.

This situation has created extensive instrumentation and software incompatibility problems. These difficulties are a topic of discussion at several national and international standardization organizations, scientific and medical societies, and manufacturer's organizations. Still, many advances in computer-assisted cardiac ultrasound diagnosis, in addition to the already established methods of image documentation, will have a tremendous impact on the future of echocardiography.

One such development is on-line assessment of ventricular function by automatic boundary detection and ultrasonic backscatter analysis [1, 35]. Two-dimensional *ultrasonic backscatter analysis* (acoustic quantification) permits real-time detection and tracking of blood-tissue interfaces. This may improve the reliability of volumetric calculations. Efforts are being made to utilize these and other methods for ultrasonic tissue characterization.

Automatic boundary detection is another development that is of particular significance in stress echocardiography. The simultaneous assessment of cardiac ultrasound images at rest and under stress and from multiple standardized imaging positions must be analyzed by computer, because the human eye cannot adequately follow this flood of information. The operator interactively controls the computer, which determines whether kinetic disturbances are present in the studied wall regions.

Also, preliminary reports of *3-D reconstruction* of the heart from echocardiographic data are now available. The algorithms are similar to those used in 3-D reconstruction of CT and MRI images. Parallel efforts are being made to simultaneously and automatically generate 3-D data records of echocardiographic images. This would obviate the roundabout way of stacking two-dimensional images to obtain a cubic data record.

When considering computer-assisted cardiac ultrasound diagnosis, one must naturally decide upon how to integrate the technology into the hospital's computer network. If the hospital uses a digital information system, echocardiographic software would be a meaningful addition. The *Picture Archiving and Communicating System* is one such system currently under discussion. With the development of computers that are more powerful yet smaller than ever, the "digital hospital" is gaining increasing significance. The advantages are obvious. Standardization organizations are addressing problems related to the link-up of radiologic and echocardiographic data. The near future will bring adapted systems that can transport patient data and high-quality diagnostic images at high speeds throughout the entire hospital computer network. The increasing dependence on digital data transmission within the hospital has introduced new problems. Problems regarding the protection of data privacy and long-term storage of single frame displays and digital film sequences must be addressed. New legal issues are closely associated with these problems.

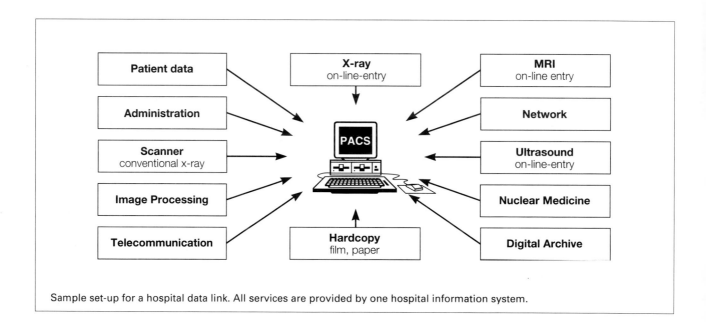

Sample set-up for a hospital data link. All services are provided by one hospital information system.

This, by no means, exhausts the entire potentials of digital technology and its application in echocardiography. This list includes only those developments that are already available or that should soon be available. They will be described and assessed in more detail in the following. The value of computers in medicine is sometimes overrated. Not every echocardiographer needs an external computer for additional data acquisition. A thorough cost-benefit analysis should therefore be made before purchasing any cardiac ultrasound diagnostic system. Furthermore, a computer cannot judge the echocardiographic findings on the basis of the overall clinical picture. The computer should, therefore, be viewed as an aid for improving methodology and as a step from qualitative towards quantitative echocardiographic assessments.

Computer-assisted assessment usually permits off-line evaluation of the echocardiographic findings. On-line assessment is possible only in exceptional cases. Additional data provided by external computer algorithms can support the diagnosis. Once these algorithms have been validated, efforts should be made to integrate them in the echocardiograph.

Historically, computer-assisted cardiac ultrasound diagnosis was first performed using digitized M-mode data. Now all established techniques of M-mode, 2-D, and Doppler echocardiography can be used for this purpose.

The type of signal that is fed into the computer in digital form is of great significance in computer-assisted assessment. It is important to know to what degree signals have been processed by the internal computer on the echocardiograph. Signals transferred to the computer should be unadultered *raw data*. Although raw data are influenced by the transducer and by instrument settings, they are largely independent of post-processing by the echocardiograph and by the operator.

4.1 **Computerized Image Analysis**
4.1.1 **Measuring the Volume of Cardiac Cavities**

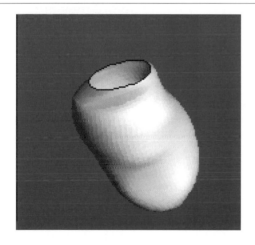

Computer model of the left ventricle, generated from transthoracic two-dimensional echocardiographic data.

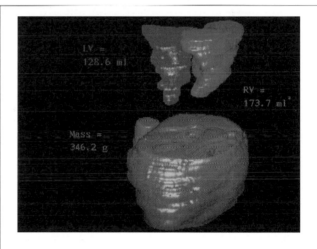

Computer model of the left and right ventricles, generated from MRI images.

All established methods for assessing left ventricular ejection fraction (LVEF) are incorporated in modern echocardiography machines. We will first review the sources of error in conventional echocardiographic determinations of left ventricular systolic and diastolic volumes in order to properly assess the following methods. The Teichholz formula is probably the best known method for M-mode determination of left ventricular volume.

Measurement parameters in M-mode echocardiography	
LVEDD	Left ventricular end-diastolic volume (mm)
LVESD	Left ventricular end-systolic volume (mm)

End-diastolic volume (EDV) and end-systolic volume (ESV) are calculated as follows:

$$EDV = \frac{7}{2.4 + LVEDD} \cdot LVEDD^3 \qquad \text{and} \qquad ESV = \frac{7}{2.4 + LVESD} \cdot LVESD^3$$

One-dimensional parameters (LVEDD, LVESD) are thereby used in a *quasi* empirical formula for volume determination. The relevant derived parameter is *fractional shortening* (FS in %).

$$FS = \frac{LVEDD - LVESD}{LVEDD}$$

The *ejection fraction* (EF) is also derived from the linear and local parameters LVEDD and LVESD. When determining the EF in M-mode echocardiography, local parameters are used to extrapolate global volumes.

$$EF = \frac{LVEDD^3 - LVESD^3}{LVEDD^3}$$

In these equations, one must assume that the theoretical calculation model corresponds with reality. However, this is hardly ever the case in the left ventricle. Therefore, volume calculations based on M-mode images should be reviewed very critically before they are considered in the diagnosis.

LV volumes can also be calculated using 2-D echocardiography. The *area-length method* and the *modified Simpson's rule* are the most widespread. In both methods, measurements (systolic and diastolic) must first be obtained from the apical four-chamber view. However, since the apical region is located in the near field of the transducer, imaging inaccuracy is an inherent problem. Because ventricular length, measured from the apex to the valve level, serves as the basic calculation parameter in both methods, such measurements tend to be imprecise.

In the next step, the inner contours of the left ventricle are defined. Since the acoustic impedances of the endocardium and left ventricular cavity are very similar, these two structures are practically indistinguishable in 2-D echocardiography. This results in overestimation of the cross-sectional area. The contours are almost always marked along the myocardium. Subsequent volume calculations using either the *prolate ellipse model* or the *modified Simpson's rule* based on summation of multiple cylindrical slices are only as accurate as the measurement variables upon which the calculations are based. It should also be noted that only parameters from two dimensions are used in volume calculation. The critical examiner should be aware that deviation from methodology or the measurement of non-normokinetic wall segments affects the reliability of these volume calculations. Aneurysms that remain undetected in the apical four-chamber view can falsify the results, making them useless.

Right ventricular volume cannot be calculated using these methods, because the prolate ellipse model does not apply to right ventricular geometry and contraction behavior.

Some hemodynamically significant stenosis, regurgitation, and septal defects that have a decisive effect on dimensional relationships, kinetics, and stroke volume of the cardiac cavities remain undetected in M-mode and 2-D echocardiography. They therefore remain unaccounted for in the above volume calculation methods. In view of their limitations, the above methods will hardly comprise an advance in echocardiographic quantitation efforts. The continued search for new methods of calculating the volume of cardiac cavities using Doppler echocardiography is therefore of utmost importance.

Newer concepts for volume calculation are based on hemodynamic principles. Cardiologic MRI volume calculation is the current gold standard [8, 30, 34, 35]. Echocardiographically determined regurgitant volumes and stroke volumes should be used as reference values for comparison with MRI measurements.

After the initial euphoric reception of Doppler color flow imaging, it now has a more realistic status. The severity of regurgitation cannot be derived from physical parameters such as the linear extent of the color regurgitant jet. The length, width and area of the color jet are unsuitable parameters for quantitative calculations. The stenotic and regurgitant jets of color flow imaging are so impressive and elegant, that one often forgets the physical laws that govern these phenomena.

4.1 **Computerized Image Analysis**
4.1.2 **Flow Calculation Models**

Physical models can be applied with Doppler flow data to calculate the volume of flow through cardiac valves. In one method, Doppler color flow imaging is used to described flow phenomena proximal to a stenotic or regurgitant orifice. A second method for quantitation of volume is based on the conservation of momentum theory.

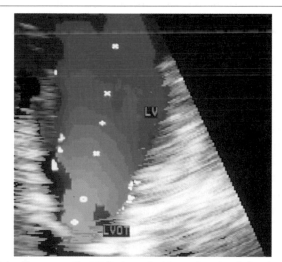

Color flow map of ventricular apical four-chamber 2-D echocardiogram, in systole.

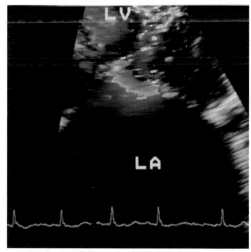

Color flow map of apical four-chamber 2-D echocardiogram, demonstrating mitral regurgitation with proximal flow phenomena.

Proximal Isovelocity Surface Area (PISA)

In the *proximal isovelocity surface area* (PISA) method, the flow convergence region proximal to a stenotic or regurgitant orifice is used to quantify the flow rate from Doppler color flow images. This method assumes that liquids are incompressible and that pressure is a physically isotropic parameter. In the presence of a pressure gradient, pressure increases as blood flows out of a heart cavity towards an orifice. Therefore, the flow rate increases as blood approaches the stenotic or regurgitant orifice. In an ideal situation, the proximal isovelocity surface area (PISA) can be visualized on Doppler color flow images as a semicircular red-blue color aliasing zone. The velocity at this zone equals the Nyquist limit. Viewed three-dimensionally, this semicircular zone is really a hemisphere. The aliasing surface of the hemisphere is the place where all velocity vectors that have reached the Nyquist limit unite when flowing towards the regurgitant or stenotic orifice. The *continuity equation* states that orifice flow must be equal to the flow through the hemispherical proximal isovelocity surface area. The velocity at red-blue color aliasing zone (Nyquist limit) is known, and the radius of the hemisphere can be measured. Taking into account the pulsatile flow cycle, the total stenotic or regurgitant flow volume can be measured.

Color-encoded M-mode echocardiography is used to track temporal changes in the PISA. The regurgitant flow volume can be calculated using the PISA radius (the distance from the orifice to the first color alias in the proximal convergence zone). Computer programs for interactive volume calculation are commercially available. When using the continuity equation, the peak velocity in the stenosis or the leak must be determined in order to calculate the orifice area. This can be determined using CW Doppler [2]. A *frame-grabber* must be used to digitize the images for computer-assisted image analysis. Once the echocardiographic image has been fed into the computer, the red-blue color aliasing zone is detected, and the PISA radius is measured. The Nyquist limit can be read from the calibrated color scale. The computer technology for this method can easily be integrated into the echocardiograph. The criteria for application of this method and the accuracy of the derived flow volumes have not been adequately validated.

Calculation of Regurgitant Flow Volume

First, the red-blue color aliasing zone and the level of the valve are identified using color Doppler M-mode [36]. Color Doppler M-mode can also display the radius between the first color alias and the regurgitant orifice versus time, from the beginning to the end of the PISA phenomenon. The total regurgitant volume can be calculated by integrating the PISA radius R squared over the period of flow. Regurgitant volumes calculated by this method are adjusted to correspond to the body surface are, and are given as index variables [5, 12, 24].

$$V = \int_{onset}^{end} Q \cdot dt = 2 \cdot \pi \cdot v_{Nyq} \int_{onset}^{end} R^2 \cdot dt$$

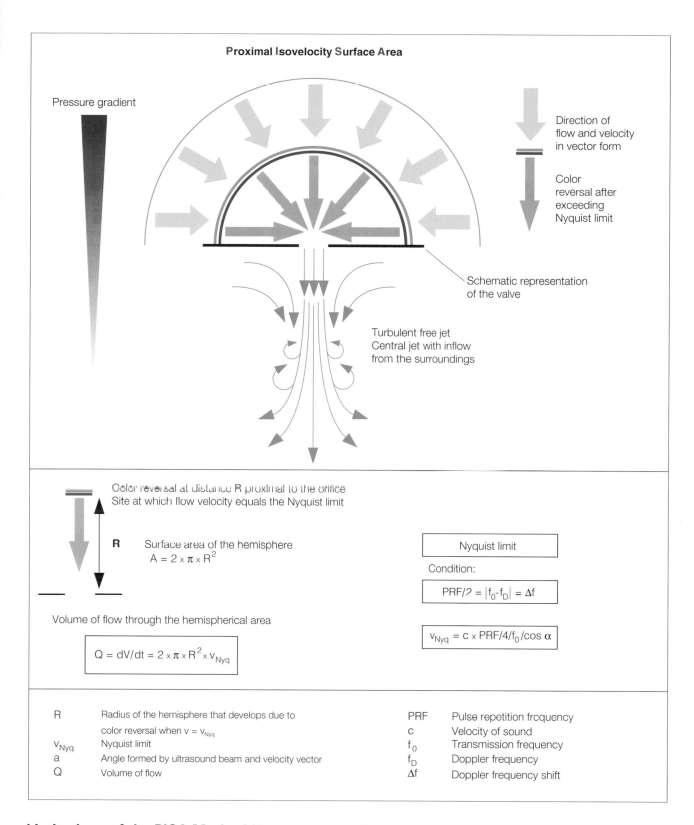

Proximal Isovelocity Surface Area

Pressure gradient

Direction of flow and velocity in vector form

Color reversal after exceeding Nyquist limit

Schematic representation of the valve

Turbulent free jet
Central jet with inflow from the surroundings

Color reversal at distance R proximal to the orifice
Site at which flow velocity equals the Nyquist limit

R   Surface area of the hemisphere
$$A = 2 \times \pi \times R^2$$

Nyquist limit

Condition:

$$PRF/2 = |f_0 - f_D| = \Delta f$$

Volume of flow through the hemispherical area

$$Q = dV/dt = 2 \times \pi \times R^2 \times v_{Nyq}$$

$$v_{Nyq} = c \times PRF/4/f_0/\cos \alpha$$

R	Radius of the hemisphere that develops due to color reversal when $v = v_{Nyq}$	PRF	Pulse repetition frequency
v_{Nyq}	Nyquist limit	c	Velocity of sound
a	Angle formed by ultrasound beam and velocity vector	f_0	Transmission frequency
Q	Volume of flow	f_D	Doppler frequency
		Δf	Doppler frequency shift

Limitations of the PISA Method [2, 4, 9, 16, 20, 32]

- Adjustment of the instrument settings can alter the position of the red-blue color aliasing zone (low flow density)
- The proximal isovelocity surface area is only rarely hemispherical in reality.
- The beam angle at the stenotic or regurgitant orifice may be difficult to determine (funnel-shaped stenoses)
- Angle-related problems: color flow imaging does not correspond to the true conditions.

- Measurement of the radius R is prone to error; this variable is then squared in calculations.
- The midpoint of the hemispherical red-blue zone often is not identical with the morphological site of the stenosis of leak.
- Tracking the temporal change in pulsatile flow requires averaging over several cardiac cycles.
- Reverberations from the morphological structure complicate measurement of the radius R.

The Principle of Conservation of Momentum

Jet volumes still cannot be used for routine clinical quantitation of hemodynamically significant pathologic flow. In this regard, the *principle of conservation of momentum* seems to hold promising potentials for color Doppler assessment of pathologic flow. The principle can be applied to evaluate color jets that do not exceed the Nyquist limit, *i.e.* those ranging up to around 4 m/s. Under these conditions, regurgitant volumes can be reliably quantitated from jet velocities measurable by Doppler color flow imaging [6, 7, 10]. Momentum is transferred when flow occurs in the presence of a pressure gradient. This momentum is subject to the physical laws of the conservation of momentum principle.

Free turbulent jets are well described in the theoretical hemodynamic literature. The conservation of momentum principle can be used to describe cardiac flow if the jet to be studied is a centrally directed free jet, not a wall jet. This method, like the PISA method, permits assessment of jet volume [18, 23, 29]. Before this model can be properly validated, the number of limitations for its use must be minimized. It is important to remember that only the mean velocity of each volume element (range gate) can be measured in Doppler color flow imaging, whereas CW Doppler and PW Doppler measure peak velocities. Momentum is proportional to the product of the volume and velocity of moving fluid. The momentum of the free turbulent jet at the orifice is assumed to be equal to the momentum at any distance x along the jet axis.

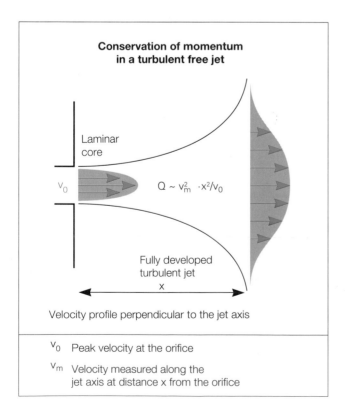

Conservation of momentum in a turbulent free jet

Laminar core

v_0

$Q \sim v_m^2 \cdot x^2/v_0$

Fully developed turbulent jet

x

Velocity profile perpendicular to the jet axis

v_0 Peak velocity at the orifice

v_m Velocity measured along the jet axis at distance x from the orifice

As the free turbulent jet moves outward from the orifice, it interacts with surrounding fluid and increases in fluid mass. The velocity of the jet must therefore decrease over distance, assuming no externally applied gradients come into play. These principles have been used to develop equations for deriving regurgitant flow from velocities measured within the jet. Free jet velocity is characteristic when plotted as a function of axial distance. When the flow rate is normalized to orifice velocity, the total regurgitant volume can be calculated as follows:

$$Q = const \cdot \frac{V_m^2}{V_0} \cdot x^2$$

In free jets created by pulsatile flow, the regurgitant volume is calculated as follows:

$$V = \int Q \cdot dt = Q_{peak} \cdot \frac{\int V_0 \cdot dt}{V_0}$$

The direction of blood flow is sometimes reversed. In other words, blood might not flow from the orifice into the ventricle, but from the ventricle towards the orifice. This occurs when the left ventricle empties into the aorta in systole. In the near future, improved color Doppler systems may enable assessment of LV systolic flow from the cardiac apex to the left ventricular outflow tract without color aliasing. Then, it would be theoretically possible to use a modified version of the above formula to derive the stroke volume. Changes in test conditions require a corresponding adjustment in the proportionality factor. In *in vitro* trials, the results of momentum analyses were comparable to those of laser anomometry [7]. Very little *in vivo* experience with this method has been reported [18, 29].

Left ventricular systolic flow velocities up to 4 m/s do not exceed the Nyquist limit (aliasing).

Example of stroke volume calculation using the conservation of momentum principle:
The flow rate in the LVOT is measured by CW Doppler. The exact location of the sample volume is defined on a color two-dimensional echocardiogram obtained from the apical four-chamber view.
The conservation of momentum principle states that the momentum of a free jet at any distance along the jet axis must be equal to the momentum at the orifice in the absence of externally applied pressure gradients. The regurgitant flow rate (ml/s) is determined by measuring centerline velocities at different distances from the LVOT. The stroke volume is obtained by integrating the temporal changes in velocities measured in the LVOT.

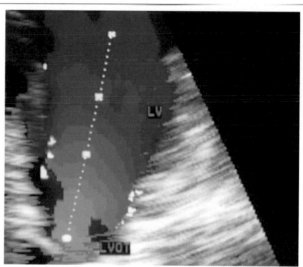

Color flow map of apical four-chamber 2-D echocardiogram (without aliasing).

Limitations of the conservation of momentum method

- The jet must be a turbulence free jet.
- The correction factor must be individually determined.
- The angle at which the beam intersects the jet is unknown.
- Unfavorable imaging conditions limit the use of color flow imaging.
- Results are dependent on instrument settings.
- The method is very time-consuming.
- Lack of reference methods for comparison.

The *in vitro* backscatter behavior of blood and muscle tissue has been extensively investigated. In vivo differentiation is possible when the signal-noise ratio is good. In backscatter analysis, not the received signal, but the frequency content and phase relation of the signal is measured. This method can be used to assess the acoustic characteristics of media located in the sonic field. Backscatter analysis (BA) is performed on line, and is also called *acoustic quantification.* In echocardiographic backscatter analysis, the blood-tissue interface appears as a contour line projected onto the 2-D image. Therefore, this method was first applied for automatic contour detection, particularly in images obtained from parasternal short-axis and apical scanning positions. The result is automatic marking of the endocardial boundaries on 2-D echocardiograms.

The computer performs on-line computation of the area enclosed in the automatically generated endocardial boundaries. The computed area is calculated as a curve synchronized with the ECG recording. This curve is used to obtain the *fractional area change* (FAC), or percent area change [13, 14, 21, 22]. The area rate of change can be calculated in a similar manner. This value is similar to the *mean velocity of circumferential fiber shortening* (Vcf).

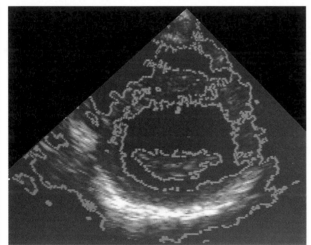

Parasternal short-axis 2-D echocardiogram of the ventricle, with automatic contour detection of the endocardium via backscatter analysis (BA).

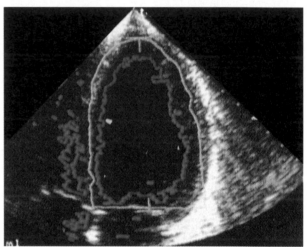

Apical four-chamber 2-D echocardiogram of the left ventricle, with automatic contour detection of the endocardium via backscatter analysis.

LV function can also be assessed on-line [30]. Previous experience has shown that correlation between endocardial contours detected in 2-D echocardiography and backscatter analysis is greatly dependent on both the acoustic suitability of the patient and instrument settings. The transmitter power, depth-selective gain control, and total gain must be maintained at optimal settings.

Noise and speckle in 2-D echocardiograms are sometimes identified as contours. Available study results indicate that automated border detection can be performed in around 60 to 70% of all patients [33]. The intuitive expectations of the operator influence the instrument settings, thereby creating interindividual differences in the method. The use of backscatter analysis in transesophageal echocardiography may make it possible to overcome some of the problems associated with the transthoracic approach.

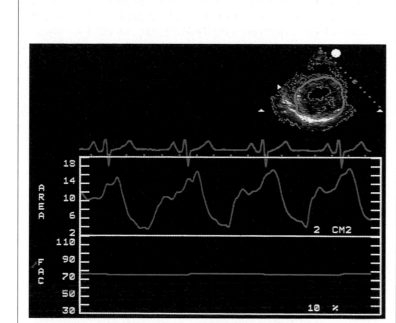

Parasternal short-axis view of the left ventricle with continuous backscatter analysis.

Parasternal short-axis 2-D echocardiogram of the left ventricle, with automatic, continuous contour detection of the endocardium using backscatter analysis. Temporal changes in area and the fractional area change are also shown.

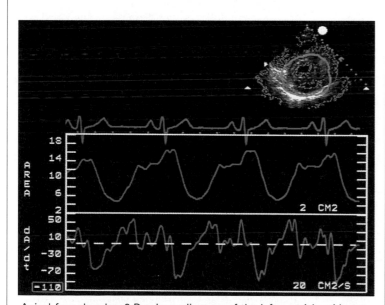

Apical four-chamber 2-D echocardiogram of the left ventricle with continuous backscatter analysis.

Apical four-chamber 2-D echocardiogram of the left ventricle, with automatic, continuous contour detection of the endocardium by means of backscatter analysis and display of temporal changes in LV volume, using Simpson's rule (slice summation method) or the area-length method. The volume rate of change (dV/dt) is also calculated.

Video densitometry has already become a classical method of computerized echo image analysis. The favorable price trends in the computer industry have contributed to the widespread use of this technique. Temporal information on echo contrast agent effects (changes in echo-intensity) permits assessment of global cardiac performance and of pathologic flow phenomena such as regurgitations and intracardiac shunts. After the video images of the contrast study have been entered into an off-line computer, one or more regions of interest (ROI) on the 2-D echocardiogram can be defined and studied. The gray level in the ROI is then calculated sequentially over time. This data is used to generate a curve of the time course of echo contrast agent concentration in the blood [3, 26, 27].

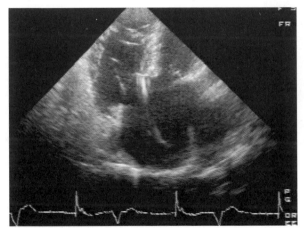

Apical four-chamber 2-D echocardiogram before administration of echo contrast agent.

Contrast echocardiography to quantitate the severity of tricuspid regurgitation.

The transducer is positioned to obtain the apical four-chamber view before the venous injection of echo contrast agent is administered. This view permits assessment of the right ventricle, right atrium, and tricuspid valve. The entire sequence of the contrast study is recorded on video tape.

Note: A pacemaker electrode is visible in the right ventricle.

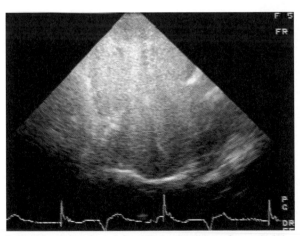

Apical four-chamber 2-D echocardiogram after administration of echo contrast agent.

The echo contrast agent floods the right atrium and the right ventricle. The rate of "wash-out" is determined by right ventricular performance and the degree of severity of tricuspid regurgitation.

The contrast study is digitally analyzed by computer to evaluate the severity of tricuspid regurgitation. Two regions of interest distal and proximal to the tricuspid valve are defined. The mean gray level in these regions is recorded.

In volumetric studies of the heart, the echo contrast agent homogeneously enhances the left ventricle. The echo-intensity of the endocardium is significantly lower than that of the myocardium and of contrast-enhanced blood in the ventricle. Automatic contour detection algorithms can now be used to determine the ventricular cross-sectional area. This area can be integrated into various models for volume calculation [25].

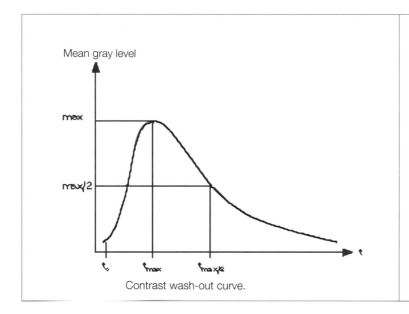

Contrast echocardiography:

Contrast wash-out curves can be used to assess functional indices, the grade of severity of regurgitation, and the hemodynamic significance of septal defects. The use of contrast echocardiography with algorithms for contour detection and 3-D reconstruction to calculate the volume of the individual heart cavities is already under discussion.
All mathematical principles of pharmacokinetics can be utilized to generate wash-out curves. Extracted parameters for quantitation of tricuspid insufficiency are not yet standardized.

Contrast wash-out curve.

These techniques have several advantages, but also have many sources of error. Standardization studies should therefore be performed to ensure the reproducibility and comparability of results [19, 31].

Instrument settings have a great influence on the quality of contrast echocardiograms. In contrast echocardiographic quantitations, it is imperative that the operator be highly skilled and experienced in adjusting the instrument [25].

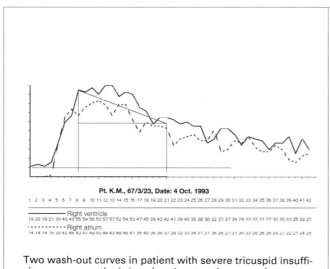

Two wash-out curves in patient with severe tricuspid insufficiency; unsmoothed. (x-axis = heart actions, y-axis = mean gray-scale value in the ROI).

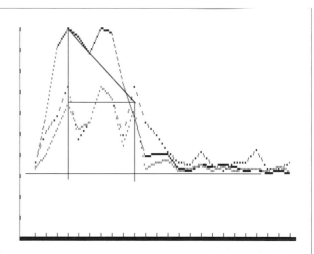

Three wash-out curves in patient with normal right ventricular function; unsmoothed. (x-axis = heart actions, y-axis = mean gray-scale value in the ROI).

Digital subtraction angiography techniques can also be used in contrast echocardiography, *i.e.*, in digital subtraction echocardiography [25]. Subtracted images obtained from multiple planes can be utilized as input data in 3-D reconstruction.

Raw data (raw RF signals) are of particular interest in efforts to devise new techniques of signal analysis that are largely independent of instrument settings. Complicated technology is used to extract the raw analog signal (RF data, RF signal) from the echocardiograph. In contrast with the transmitted signal, the raw analog signal contains all the information describing the biological structure that was examined. The frequency content of this raw signal amounts to around three-times that of the mean transmitted frequency (wide-band transducer). The subsequent process of digitization must be performed with around four to five-times the sample frequency to ensure that harmonic waves and nonlinear effects are also extracted from the signal. After the data has been digitized, its frequency content, phase angle, and a number of other parameters can be assessed. Due to the enormous amount of data collected, the data to be evaluated must be reduced to a region of interest (which is defined on the 2-D echocardiogram). The input signal is extracted from this window only. This technique of signal analysis will be highly useful if it succeeds in defining the local orientation of structural parameters (mean distance between scatterers, attenuation in tissue, etc.), and in providing information for tissue [1].

The audio frequency signal used in Doppler is a quasi raw signal. The expected range of the Doppler frequency shift (in the audible range) poses no great transmission problems. Doppler signals can still be extracted when conditions are poor for extraction of 2-D echocardiographic data. The minimum required Doppler signal amplitude is around 30 dB lower than the amplitude needed for generation of 2-D echocardiograms.

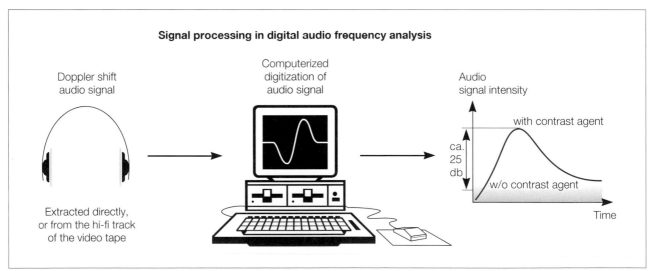

Flow information can be enhanced by echo contrast agents (enlargement of the signal-to-noise ratio). After the analog audio signal has been extracted, it is digitized with ca. 40 kHz. The computer technology needed for analysis of signal amplitude is relatively simple. The result is a temporal curve of the audio signal in digital format, with and without echo contrast agent effects. The amplitude difference between these two curves is used as a measure of echo contrast agent concentration in the selected sample volume. This information can be used as the basis for calculating flow measurements and circulation times. It is feasible to assess flow phenomena in poor-quality of 2-D echocardiograms or when the assessed volumes are very small when this technique is used [28].

Stress echocardiography currently permits computer-assisted wall motion analysis. It is a proven technique for diagnosis of ischemic heart disease.

Conventional Technique

Stress echocardiography is not particularly demanding, as far as the computer technology is concerned. The computer must provide the physician parallel, split-screen images of the echocardiographic resting and exercise sequences. It is relatively easy for the trained echocardiographer to recognize motion (kinetic) abnormalities. Filigree wall motion analysis is, of course, possible, but is very time-consuming and requires interaction with the analytical computer.

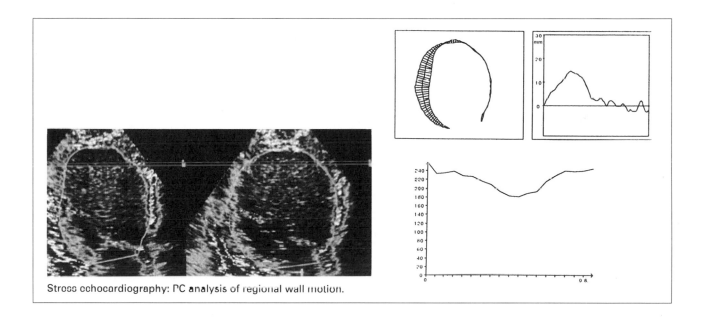

Stress echocardiography: PC analysis of regional wall motion.

Furthermore, *frame-grabbers* usually are also used to digitize the video output signal. The required pixel resolution and digital image processing capabilities are relatively low. A frame-grabber with 8 bit per pixel resolution (256 gray-scale levels) is sufficient for stress echocardiographic analyses.

Motion analysis using Doppler color flow imaging

In order to create a color flow map of cardiac blood flow, a filter is used to mask out low-range frequencies. Because it is in motion, the myocardium itself produces a frequency shift. By changing the filter characteristics for representation of the Doppler color flow signal, blood flow can be completely deleted from the image in order to analyze only the Doppler effect attributable to myocardial motion. The power spectrum of this image and the velocity profile, together with the corresponding 2-D echocardiographic data, make it possible to assess the kinetics of the heart. Pathological areas can be isolated by means of color Doppler analysis. This technique intervenes in the echocardiograph's signal processing process. Reproducibility again is dependent on the uniformity of instrument settings [17].

Color flow mapping of moving structures is not a stress echocardiographic technique *per se*. However, since it permits assessment of motion abnormalities, is can justifiably be included in the category of stress echocardiography.

This technique is closely linked with the development of highly stable, intravenously administered ultrasound contrast agents that also provide acoustic enhancement of the arterial section of the heart. Only a small portion of the echo contrast agent reaches the necessary ranges of reflected signal intensity necessary for imaging the myocardium, because part of the left ventricular blood volume is distributed to the aorta and coronary arteries. Theoretically, the increase in signal amplitude is proportional to the amount of blood flow in the region under study. Residual amounts of contrast agent in the left ventricular cavity have a negative influence on the results. Distal regions of the left ventricle (from the perspective of the transducer) are shadowed over by residual contrast medium in the ventricle. This makes it very difficult to assess the blood flow there. The inclusion of this shadowing effect by means of scatter can be calculated using a computerized model, which can be used for measurement correction [19, 25, 31].

| 4. | Computer-Assisted Cardiac Ultrasound Diagnosis |
| 4.2 | Manual and Computer-Assisted Documentation of Findings |

The *manual documentation* of findings is a standard clinical practice. Manual documentation is cumbersome and create piles of daily paperwork. Since manufacturers have widely standardized interfaces, *computerized documentation* of findings is now wide-spread. Naturally, the images obtained at echocardiography must also be documented. Inexpensive systems usually provide a lower quality of image documentation. However, considering the price of some high-quality systems, it is questionable whether they are really needed for routine clinical practice. Another important document for patients with special heart diseases is their *personal data record* or "passport".

Manual Documentation of Findings

Usually, the echocardiographer uses only those measurement functions that he has learned from experience and training. These measurement data should be included in his or her report of findings. The report should, of course, indicate where image documents are stored. The manually prepared medical report has no limitations as to what is included in it. It should, at any rate, include the basic patient data, the measurement data obtained at echocardiography, and the diagnosis. Since the echocardiographic examination usually proceeds systematically, it is a good idea to catalogue the measurement parameters and summarize them in the report. A comparison of patient data with normal values can also be integrated in the report. One can also design a form sheet where the necessary measurement values, personal data, etc. needs only to be filled in by hand. This also saves time and effort. When echocardiographic findings are abnormal, the images must, of course, be documented in some way. Video printouts of the image should be included in the medical report, or the report should indicate where and on which video tape the patient images can be found. When following the patient, it is rather time-consuming and impractical to search for previously videotaped image sequences.

Computerized Documentation of Findings

The echocardiograph summarizes the measured values in a report that can be transferred directly from the machine to a computer or to a printer. The computer can convert the measurement data and other patient data to a printable format using word processing software or a data bank program. Assuming one has a good knowledge of the computer program, it is easy to design a standard layout for the reports so that the computer can automatically process them.

It is also possible to enter the patient and other data into a mask programmed to correspond with the designed report form. In that case, the printer simply inserts the entered variables in the corresponding spaces on the form. Image documentation is also subject to certain limitations. It is, of course, possible to store echocardiographic images (M-mode, 2-D, CW Doppler, PW-Doppler, color Doppler) using computer technology, and it is possible to include these computer records in the documentation of findings.

Computerized Image Documentation

Since the obtained images are usually assessed off-line, stored images must be used for this purpose. For proper documentation of color Doppler images, either an expensive color video printer or a high-quality color graphics printer must be connected to the computer. The hard-copy printout of 2-D echocardiographic images should be made using a laser printer with at least 32 gray-scale levels (preferably 64) and at least 300 dpi resolution. Practical experiences with laser printers with 600 dpi resolution are very encouraging. The documentation of images on such digital storage media as floppy disks, hard disks, magneto optical disk, etc. requires a large memory unit. However, this is a source of legal problems that will have to be solved in the future. One alternative is to store echocardiographic images and sequences in analog format on video laser disk (that can be written on once or many times). Copies made from video laser disk approximate the quality of the original image. One can make as many copies as desired, including copies for the medical report.

Valve ID Card for Patients With Cardiac Valve Replacements

In addition to the usual patient data, the valve model, size and position, the date of implantation, examination date, and such valve-specific measurement values as effective prosthesis orifice area, mean velocity and, when applicable, pressure half-time are listed on the front of the valve ID card. On the back of the card, there is enough space to document two images (M-mode, 2-D, PW Doppler, CW Doppler, color Doppler). The images are appropriately formatted on a computer, and are printed on the card by means of a color video printer. The valve ID card is the same size as standard credit cards. It is sealed in a watertight plastic cover. The patient should always carry the card along with other personal documents. In case of suspected prosthetic valve malfunction, the obtained images can be compared with the post-operative reference images.

References

1. Angermann CE. Digitale Bildverarbeitung in der Echokardiographie. Internist 1990; 31: 313-320.
2. Barclay SA, Changsheng X, Loyd D, Andersson G, Ask P, Wranne B. The flow convergence region proximal to a regurgitant orifice has a non-hemispherical velocity field. Circulation 1991; 84: II-105.
3. Boyd JS, Paterson C, Dukes J. An ongoing study on the use of albumin microspheres as an echocontrast agent in some domestic animals. Eurodop `92 Conference Proceedings and Abstracts: British Medical Ultrasound Society 1992: 130.
4. Cape EG, Levine RA, Muralidharan E, Heinrich R, Yoganathan AP. Increased heart rate can cause under-estimation of regurgitant flow by proximal isovelocity surface area (PISA).Circulation 1992; 86 : I-804.
5. Cape EG, Yoganathan AP, Rodriguez L, Weyman AE, Levine RA. The proximal flow convergence method can be extended to calculate regurgitant stroke volume; in vitro application of the color Doppler m-mode. J Am Coll Cardiol 1990;15: 109A.
6. Cape EG, Skoufis EG, Weyman AE, Yoganathan AP, Levine RA. A new method for noninvasive quantification of valvular regurgitation based on conservation of momentum. Circulation 1989; 79: 1343-1353.
7. Cape EG, Yoganathan AP, Levine RA. A new theoretical model for noninvasive quantification of mitral regurgitation. J Biomechanics 23: 27-33.
8. Chen C, Koschyk D, Mehl C, Klarhöfer M, Kupper W, Bleifeld W. Comparison of quantifying mitral regurgitation using color Doppler proximal isovelocity surface area and angiography. Circulation 1991; 84: II-637.
9. Chen C, Vandervoort PM, Heik S, Weyman AE, Thomas JD. Is the proximal flow convergence method accurate in the presence of a second outflow? Circulation 1992; 86: I-805.

10. Dousse B, Grossniklaus B, Scheuble C. Two years experience in measuring velocities beyond the Nyquist limit with color flow mapper. Eurodop `92 Conference Proceedings and Abstracts: British Medical Ultrasound Society 1992: 219.

11. Gopal AS, King DL, Keller AM, Rigling R. Superiority of three-dimensional echocardiography in human subjects for ventricular volume computation compared to two-dimensional apical biplane summation of discs method. Circulation 1992; 86: I-270.

12. Grayburn PA, Cigarroa CG, Peters AL, Brickner ME. Color flow assesment of regurgitant flow: superior-ity of proxi-mal isovelocity surface area over momentum analysis in eccentric wall jets. Circulation 1991; 84: II-637.

13. HP Acoustic Quantification waveforms. Hewlett-Packard Company U.S.A. 6/91: 5091-1841E.

14. HP Acoustic Quantification: volumes. Hewlett-Packard Company U.S.A. 9/92: 5091-4627E.

15. Jiang I, Siu SC, Handschumacher MD,. Guerrero JL, de Prada JV, King ME, Picard MH, Weyman AE, Levine RA. Three-dimensional Echocardiography: in vivo validation for right ventricular volume and function. Circulation 1992; 86: I-272.

16. Kang SU, Zhang J, Weintraub R. Effect of frame rate change quantification of color flow imaging: an experimental study. Circulation 1992; 86: I-806.

17. McDicken WN, Sutherland GR, Moran CM, Gordon LN. Colour Doppler velocity imaging of the myo- cardium. Euro-dop `92 Conference Proceedings and Abstracts: British Medical Ultrasound Society 1992: 182-183.

18. Mele D, Guerrero JL, Vandervoort PM, Rivera JM, Cape EG, Yoganathan AP, Vlahakes G, Thomas JD, Weyman AE, Levine RA. Doppler-echocardiographic quantification of tricuspid regurgitation by the momentum method: in vivo validation. Circulation 1992; 86 : I-258.

19. Miszalok V, Fritzsch T, Schartl M. Myocardial perfusion defects in contrast echocardiography: spatial and temporal localisation. Ultrasound i Med & Biol 1986; 12: 581-586.

20. Moises VA, Chao K, Shandas R, Murillo A, Belot JP, Valdez-Cruz L, Sahn DJ. Effects of orifice size and shape on flow rate estimated from flow convergence region imaged by color Doppler flow mapping proximal to restrictive orifices: an in vitro study. J Am Coll Cardiol 1990; 13: 109A.

21. Mügge A, Daniel WG, Niedermeyer J, Grote J, Hausmann D, Lichtlen PR. Akustische Quantifizierung- ein neues On-Line-Verfahren zur automatischen Erfassung von linksventrikulären Flächen und Flächen-änderungen im Echokar-diogramm. Z Kardiol 1992; 81: 681-686

22. Perez JE et al. On-line assesment of ventricular function by automatic boundery detection and ultra-sonic back-scatter imaging. J Am Coll Cardiol 1992; 19: 313-320

23. Reimold SC, Thomas JD, Lee RT. Jet momentum determines color flow Doppler jet area in patients with aortic regurgitation. Circulation 1991; 84 II-637.

24. Rodriguez L, Anconina J, Harrigan P, Levine RA, Monterroso VH, Weyman AE, Thomas JD. Validation of a new method for valve area calculation using the proximal isovelocity surface area in patients with mitral stenosis. J Am Coll Cardiol 1990; 13: 109A.

25. Schlepper M, Berwing K. Kontrast-, Doppler-, Farb-Doppler- und transösophageale Echokardiographie. Stuttgart: Schattauer, 1990.

26. Schlief R, Schürmann R, Niendorf HP. Ultraschallkontrastmittel auf Galaktose-Basis: Grundlegende Eigenschaften und Ergebnisse klinischer Prüfungen. Jahrbuch d Radiologie 1991: 259-265.

27. Schlief R. Echovist: physikalisch-pharmakologische Eigenschaften, Ergebnisse klinischer Prüfungen und Anwen-dungspotential eines neuartigen Ultraschallkontrastmittels. Jahrbuch d Radiologie 1988: 163-170.

28. Schwarz KQ, Bezante GP, Chen X, Schlief R. Volumetric flow measurements by echo contrast. Compar-ison of 3 ultrasonic intensity methods: radio-frequency, videodensity and Doppler. Circulation 1992: 86: I-504.

29. Seifart C. Estimation of cardiac output using high velocity colour Doppler. Eurodop `92 Conference Proceedings and Abstracts: British Medical Ultrasound Society 1992; 78.

30. Stewart W, Gunawardena S, Rodkey S, White R, Luvisi B, Klein A, Salcedo E. Left ventricular volume calculation using integrated backscatter from echocardiography: comparison with MRI and off-line echo analysis. J Am Coll Cardiol 1992; 5: 334.

31. Uhlendorf V, Stein M, Siegert J, Fritzsch T. Erkennbarkeit von Gewebeinhomogenitäten im B-Bild bei Variation des Streukoeffizienten. Wiss Z d Martin-Luther-Univ. Halle-Wittenberg: 1991; 40: 59-68.

32. Utsonomiya T, Quan M, Doshi R, Patel D, Gardin JM. Effect of flow rate, orifice size and aliasing veloc-ity on volume calculation using Doppler color proximal isovelocity surface area method. J Am Coll Cardiol 1990; 15: 89A.

33. Vandenberg B, Cardona H, Miller JG, Skorton GJ, Perez JE. On-line left ventricular volume measurement in patients using automated border detection: comparison with conventional echocardiography (multicenter trial). Circulation 1992; 86: I-262.

34. Weintraub R, Shandas R, Cranney G, Walker P, Yoganathan A, Sahn DJ. Comparison of flow convergence calcu-lations using color Doppler flow mapping and phase velocity encoded MRI: an in vitro study. Circulation 1991; 84: II-636.

35. Wells PNT. Future of Doppler. Eurodop `92 Conference Proceedings and Abstracts: British Medical Ultrasound Society 1992: 232-235.

36. Zhang J, Jones M, Murillo A, Yamada I, Kang SU, Weintraub R, Shandas R, Valdez-Cruz L. Effects of variation of aliasing velocity limit on the accuracy of color m-mode flow convergence methods for assessing mitral regurgi-tation: studies in instrumented sheep yield a new multiple alias method. Circulation 1992; 86: I-805.

4.   **Computer-Assisted Cardiac Ultrasound Diagnosis**   **137**
4.3   **Digital Information Technology for Cardiac Ultrasound Systems**
(Rüdiger Brennecke)

In modern ultrasound systems, most of the image acquisition, storage, and processing is done using digital technologies. All of the ultrasound diagnostic methods introduced in this book can be assumed to be essentially digital techniques. Still, the final documentation and archiving is usually analog, *i.e.*, images are recorded and their results evaluated on video tape or on video hard copy.

The transition to digital methods for everything including information processing outside the ultrasound unit would give us all of the benefits of versatile, programmable computers. The main advantages would be:

- off-line processing of stored echocardiographic images,
- digital image archiving and data communication,
- databases for diagnostic data (images and conventional data).

Initial systems of this kind are already being offered at a commercial level, and are being updated and advanced continuously. In the following I would like to point out some of the common features and risk a final look at the kind of standardization we are hoping for.

4.3   Digital Information Technology for Cardiac Ultrasound Systems
4.3.1   Off-Line Processing of Stored Image Data

In hospital practice, doctors prefer to evaluate findings during the examination (on-line) using the methods and procedures described in the clinical chapters of this book. In just about all ultrasound diagnostic units available on the market, programs are implemented in digital processors for basic functions, such as calculating the volume of the heart from 2-D echocardiograms or evaluating Doppler spectral curves. And yet the physician often wants to utilize the diagnostic data produced by the equipment (text, measurement values) on existing computer systems or evaluate image data off-line.

One of the main motivations for this off-line evaluation of ultrasound images is to try out new examination techniques in practice. They require new algorithms that either have not yet been implemented on existing equipment, or which cannot be installed because of hardware restrictions. This could be observed in the development of stress echocardiography over the past few years. Since stress echocardiography requires storage and manipulation of several sequences of images, it cannot be implemented in existing ultrasound systems without further ado. Even if the necessary technology were implemented, this would not always be a particularly economical approach. Further examples for this kind of off-line processing are tissue characterization and the quantitative evaluation of color Doppler images.

Another reason for developing off-line systems for processing ultrasound images is the considerable time that scientific evaluation of such images can take. In such cases we try to move the evaluation process from the ultrasound unit to an off-line workplace so that the expensive ultrasound unit is not busy with evaluation when it is needed for examination. This category of application includes all examinations on intra- and inter-observer variability which require repeated perusal and processing of image material.

What all of the off-line ultrasound processing applications have in common is the need to transfer images from the ultrasound unit to the computer. By far the most frequent solution to this problem is to digitize video pictures, either during the examination or at a later time from the video tape archive.

The illustration below shows the techniques used today for this kind of video image processing. The simplest approach is to extend the existing computer system to include a video interface. In many cases this simply involves adding a "frame-grabber" card and the appropriate digitizing software. The images stored on the computer and the overlay windows are often displayed on a second monitor connected to the digitizer card. The more modern versions of these cards are not only configured to digitize single images, but can store whole sequences of images in real time. A black-and-white image is usually stored with a resolution of 512 x 512 pixels and 256 gray levels (8 bits deep), but this means the pixels are not square. A true color image requires about three times as much memory (red, green, and blue) for each pixel, so the storage requirement for an ultrasound image is between 256 KB and almost 1 MB.

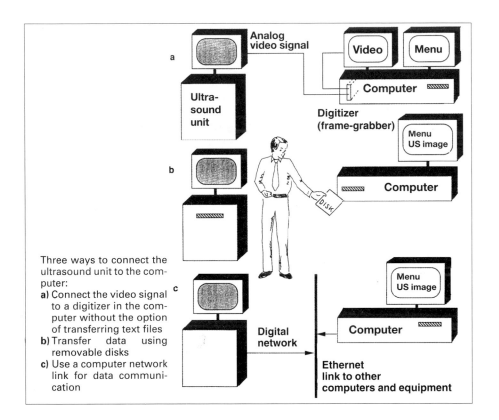

Three ways to connect the ultrasound unit to the computer:
a) Connect the video signal to a digitizer in the computer without the option of transferring text files
b) Transfer data using removable disks
c) Use a computer network link for data communication

This form of storage has a number of drawbacks. For example, the video image at the output of the ultrasound unit has already lost some of the image quality of the original digital information in the ultrasound image. This video image quality is further degraded by the next digitizing step in the connected computer. And all the auxiliary information, such as the patient's name, the measurement data (e.g. ventricle volume), and the ECG, are directly superimposed on the image and cannot always be correctly acquired from the video signal later. This would require a technically complex procedure. For these reasons there is a need for digital transfer of ultrasound data from the ultrasound unit to the external computer system. There are two main solutions to this problem:
- transfer the data on optical disks, or
- transfer the image data through a digital network connection.

In the first method, magneto-optical disks are usually used to transfer the image data. The ultrasound unit is equipped with a drive for reading and writing these disks. Individual images or entire *cineloops* (images of one or more heart cycles) can then be transferred to the disk from the menu of the ultrasound unit.

The advantage of this method of storage is that the diagnostic data can be digitally archived and reproduced in the ultrasound unit.

If the evaluating computer has a suitable disk drive and the appropriate software installed, disks written in the ultrasound unit can be used directly for off-line image evaluation. Today's magneto-optical disks have a storage capacity of 650 MB to 1.3 GB (more than one billion pixels, or 4,000 black-and-white images).

Several thousand images with the above-mentioned resolution can thus be stored on the two surfaces of a single disk. However, the storage speed is nowhere near the real-time capabilities of analog media (video tape recorder). While a full analog image (2 half-frames) can be stored on video tape in about 40 ms (*i.e.* in real time), digital storage of the same image, without resorting to special measures such as data compression, takes one second or more. Accordingly, storing the images of a heart cycle can take anything from 30 to 60 seconds. This makes the storage of digital image sequences too slow by present-day standards, so this method is not generally used in hospital practice.

As an alternative to equipping the ultrasound unit with add-on image data archiving functions using removable magneto-optical disks, the ultrasound unit and computer can be linked by a digital data line. Standard networking technologies are the basis for this connectivity today. The illustration shows a schematic example of this type of link. Under practical conditions, even slower transfer speeds often have to be accepted (about 2 to 5 seconds per image). To manage large numbers of images, it is a good idea to integrate an optical storage drive of the kind mentioned above into the computer.

A comparison of the three illustrated methods of image transfer between ultrasound unit and computer reveals that digital transfer is superior in quality to analog transfer. The digital techniques have the disadvantage of higher costs and lower speed, especially when storing long sequences of images. Finally, another problem with digital image storage is that the type of standards used for analog transfer and storage of the video signal are not available. This problem is discussed in Section 4.3.5 of this summary.

All previously described methods of transferring ultrasound image data to the computer are based on transferring the video raster image in analog or digital form. However, color Doppler images stored on advanced digital systems are not stored as a color image; rather, the 2-D echocardiogram is stored in a special data format digitally separated from the color Doppler data (speed, variance etc.). It is then up to the computer system to unite this data again and synthesize the color Doppler image (with a changed color palette if desired) on the screen.

The three ways of storing image information in television raster format described above are the state-of-the-art at present. We will also discuss two further methods of digital image storage. Until now they have been used only in isolated applications, but are expected to gain significance in the future. To illustrate this technique, let us first return to the internal workings of the ultrasound unit. The following illustration shows a greatly simplified block diagram of the signal route for 2-D echocardiographic representation in ultrasound units. The stages relevant to our discussion are, with reference to the illustration:
- primary signal amplification,
- demodulation (envelope detection) of the high-frequency signal,
- digitizing of this rectified signal by the analog/digital converter (ADC),
- its conversion to raster television picture format, followed by its conversion to a normal video signal by the digital/analog converter (DAC).

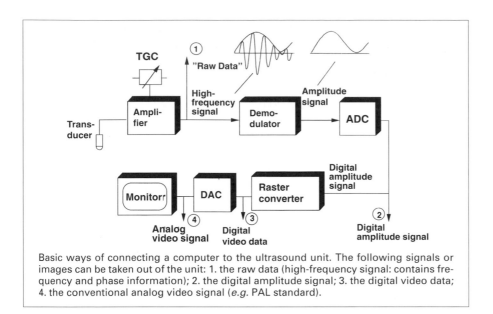

Basic ways of connecting a computer to the ultrasound unit. The following signals or images can be taken out of the unit: 1. the raw data (high-frequency signal: contains frequency and phase information); 2. the digital amplitude signal; 3. the digital video data; 4. the conventional analog video signal (*e.g.* PAL standard).

The primary information delivered by the transducer is modified in each of these steps. During rectification, for example, the frequency and phase information of the high-frequency signal is lost, leaving only the amplitude information. In the second step - the conversion of the ultrasound amplitude signal to the raster television picture - information is lost near the transducer (superimposition of primary acquired data in the narrow part of the sector) and in areas remote from the transducer, information that does not exist as primary data is added by interpolation. The illustration below visualizes this process. The situation has been deliberately exaggerated by using 10 beams instead of the 100-plus beams typically used in the equipment. Even more detrimental than this signal corruption is the disadvantage of the undesired increase in storage space requirements caused by the raster conversion: about 100 ultrasound beam directions are replaced by about 500 television scan lines.

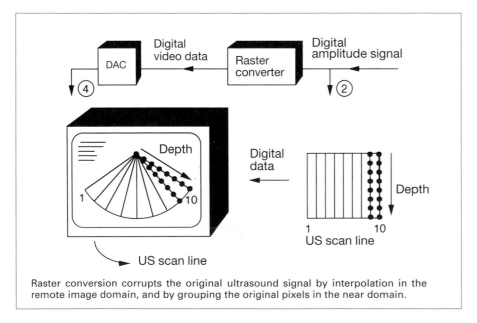

Raster conversion corrupts the original ultrasound signal by interpolation in the remote image domain, and by grouping the original pixels in the near domain.

The above-mentioned advanced approaches to digital image storage try to eliminate these internal signal conversion disadvantages. The methods that play a particularly important in tissue characterization involve digitizing and evaluating the signal, or transferring it to an external computer while it is still high-frequency (before rectification and generation of the envelope signal).

Examples are the analysis of the frequency dependence of ultrasound signal attenuation and acquisition of the *integrated backscatter, i.e.* the integral across the power spectrum of the back-scattered signal parts. This variable is calculated in a simplified way by forming the mean value of the square of the high-frequency echo signal. The much needed standardization is far from being a reality in this highly researched field. One of the minimum requirements here, besides the high-frequency ultrasound signal, is to provide a signal which describes the time gain compensation (TGC). This would allow acquisition of an important part of the influences that depend on the operator.

The high data rate and storage capacity requirements of high-frequency ultrasound signal acquisition are only felt today in basic research projects, however. By contrast, storage of digital data in polar coordinates could be a good solution because of the above advantages (freedom from corruption and low storage space requirements). But the problem here, again, is the need for high-speed raster conversion when storing this data on computers for further processing. This makes the system more complicated and increases the costs of the computer system. For these reasons, both methods are still only employed in research projects.

4.3   Digital Information Technology for Cardiac Ultrasound Systems
4.3.2   Digital Image Archiving

Conventional archives in echocardiography laboratories consist of a large number of video cassettes. For a follow-up examination, for example, it will usually be possible to search through manually kept lists to gather the patient's earlier image material, but it does take a considerably amount of time to find the right cassette and then wind it to the relevant video scene. Furthermore, irreversible data loss is possible due to ageing of the magnetic tape after only a few years.

The ultrasound image storage on magneto-optical disks described in the previous section has some major advantages here. Image quality is much higher than analog video recordings, and the technology of the disk allows fast random access to the data, which is safe for at least ten years by current estimates. The disadvantages are the limited data transfer rate and storage capacity. While many minutes of each examination are typically documented on an analog video tape, the relatively long time taken to transfer digital images form the disk to the image display system will generally force the technician to make do with single images or, at best, a few seconds of moving pictures (cineloops). This reduction in the amount of image data is also known as "clinical data reduction". Image data compression techniques which suppress irrelevant parts of the image and optimize the rest could considerably improve our options for the use of digital storage systems. But they have been adopted reluctantly so far because of the risk of losing medically relevant image information.

For this reason it can be assumed that the conventional analog archive storage method based on video tapes will remain with us for some time to come, and that digital storage of selected image material on removable magneto-optical media will be used as an additional resource. Whether or not it will one day be possible to do without the cumbersome video tape archives will depend not so much on new technical capabilities and developments, as on the experience gained with the time problems and accuracy of this clinical data reduction.

In addition to the image archiving with removable disks described above, we will see more department-wide network integration of ultrasound units and computer systems for image archiving and processing. At this level, image communication and archiving will be more coordinated.

Future cardiology departments will manage image data along with administrative and other text-oriented information (diagnoses, medical reports etc.) at this network level. While it used to be common to have a central computer architecture for this kind of information system, today we are witnessing the emergence of hierarchically organized structures of multiple linked information systems. The hospital information system (HIS) covers the common requirements of the entire hospital. In particular, administrative patient information (central registration etc.) and billing are part of a typical HIS. The individual departments have opti-mized departmental information systems (DIS) for their own specific tasks, with functional units (FUs) connected to them for things like writing medical reports. In other, complex areas, however, global image information systems can be expected. The ultrasound laboratory(and the heart catheter laboratory, for example) produces such an intense flow of internal data that these local work groups (LWG) will often be grouped separately from the departmental information system. But the LWGs communicate with the DISes, and they in turn communi-cate with the HIS.

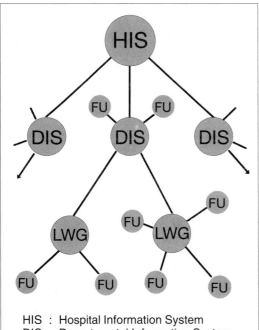

HIS : Hospital Information System
DIS : Departmental Information System
LWG: Local Work Group
FU : Functional Unit

Levels of network communication. Data pro-cessing is based on the local work group (LWG). A system designed for future compatibility must provide for communication with the higher levels of a hospital information system.

The advantage of having clearly structured complex tasks is paid for by the need for a lot of "interfaces" between the individual nodes of the information system hierarchy. Here too, long-term standardization of the data communication and archiving systems will be necess-ary. This is discussed in Section 4.3.4.

If we see the information architecture of the ultrasound laboratory as a local work group, we can understand its structure as a grouping of the typical functional units involved. A large laboratory in the future will have one or more ultrasound units, one or more workstations (personal computers) for image processing and archiving, and several administrative (secretary) workplaces. And this future laboratory will also have a separate image bank, perhaps consisting of an automatic magneto-optical disk changer.

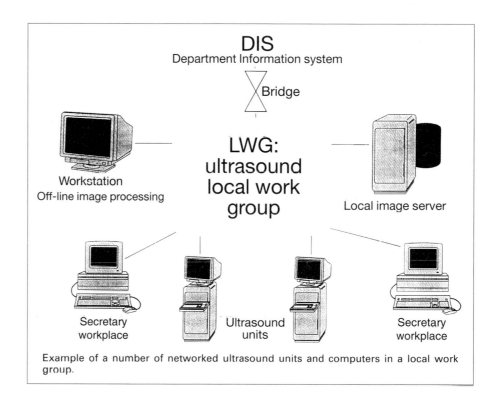

Example of a number of networked ultrasound units and computers in a local work group.

The figure shows the functional units of this type of local work group in the ultrasound laboratory. Again, only the implementation of standards will let equipment from different vendors work together. This local work group will often be connected to the departmental information system by a bridge or gateway to separate the internal and external data flows, and to maintain operations within the work group even if the central system breaks down.

The network connection enables each unit on the network to connect to any other unit, given the appropriate network protocols. This network topology contrasts with the point-to-point connectivity common in the past.

The Ethernet system is often used for the "physical" connection between in-house devices today; the network protocol software running on the personal computers might be Novell NetWare or, on workstations, the Unix TCP/IP protocol. Ethernet usually uses coaxial cables to connect the devices, although twisted pairs are becoming more popular of late. Sometimes a single cable runs through the entire building, with each computer "hooked in" (bus topology). But for reasons of reliability and to increase transfer speed, star networks are becoming increasingly widespread. The maximum signal transmission speed on the Ethernet is 10 MB/s, so a two-dimensional image would take about 1/5 of a second to transfer.

The maximum speed under practical conditions, however, is usually only about 10 to 50% of this maximum speed. As a consequence, Ethernet is only sufficient when demands on image data throughput are low. Image systems of the future are likely to use other network technologies for digital data. The FDDI technique (fiber distributed data interface for fiber optic and copper lines) currently has the best chances of becoming standard for data rates of at least three times what Ethernet can handle (theoretically, ten times).

As planning and administration of the described network systems requires considerable expense and knowledge, and conventional network technologies have not yet been optimized for transferring image data, it is likely that concepts employing archive and removable media such as the magneto-optical disk will catch on faster than the essentially superior network solutions.

4.3   **Digital Information Technology for Cardiac Ultrasound Systems**
4.3.4   **Standardization of Data Archiving and Transfer**

Achieving interoperability between different hardware vendors and functions (*e.g.*, ultrasound unit and computer) is not a simple task even when digital data is used. Certain levels of communication are specified by industry standards, including Ethernet connections and media such as the above-mentioned magneto-optical disk (capacity 650 MB or 1.3 GB), but the problem of correctly interpreting the stored contents and matching the various data formats and the different data structures in the data blocks remains.

In the medical arena there is a fair degree of consensus, as far as data communication is concerned, that we must manage to store not only images but also the data that provides a link to the patient and to the equipment parameters used during the recording. This data is transferred on top of the image information in the form of a "header". Cardiology also requires storage of associated data such as ECG and pressure curves.

Some official committees are currently trying to enforce standards, but progress is slow. A number of industrial consortia are therefore striving to establish de facto standards. The user organizations of radiologists and cardiologists are trying to create a basis for the minimum requirements of their users, for whom generally applicable specifications for the stored contents (headers, image groups etc.) are actually what counts: they are happy to leave storage media and protocol specifications to the companies. What the upshot of these efforts will be is not yet known. The whole situation makes it difficult to plan extensive systems in the hospitals. In the long term it would be good to have a standard for echocardiography and angiocardiography, or even a blanket standard covering medical technology, office communications, and text and image processing in general.

4.   **Computer-Assisted Cardiac Ultrasound Diagnosis**   **145**
4.4   **Three-Dimensional Echocardiography**
(Michiyoshi Kuwahara, Shigeru Eiho, Naoki Asada)

Two-dimensional echocardiography enables us to obtain non-invasive real-time motion images of arbitrary cross-sections of the heart. With 2-D echocardiograms of the left ventricle, the cardiologist can identify abnormal cardiac wall motion by mentally superimposing the 2-D image on the real, three-dimensional heart. Since such subjective 3-D reconstruction is strong-ly dependent on individual experience, this method cannot provide a quantitative assess-ment of cardiac function. Three-dimensional images of the left ventricle reconstructed throughout a cardiac cycle provide not only a spatial display of the form, shape and move-ment of the heart, but also give suitable data for the assessment of regional and global car-diac function. Used in conjunction with computer programs for 3-D left ventricular recon-struction from multiplane 2-D echocardiograms, the ultimate purpose of 3-D echo-cardiography is to enable a quantitative evaluation of left ventricular function.

This section introduces some technical aspects of 3-D echocardiography such as:

1. Projection of multiple 2-D echocardiograms of the left ventricle from different planes to provide spatial and temporal information on the position and orientation of each image. This also gives information about each cardiac phase.

2. Determination of endo- and epicardial boundaries during a given cardiac cycle for each individual cross-section.

3. 3-D reconstruction of the left ventricle by mapping the detected boundaries on a cor-responding 3-D coordinate system, using the spatial and temporal information obtained at image acquisition.

4. Evaluation of cardiac functions based on the 3-D reconstruction of the left ventricle, and demonstration of the results by mapping the functional information to obtain a 3-D display of the left ventricle.

4.4   **Three-Dimensional Echocardiography**
4.4.1   **Acquisition of Multiplane 2-D Echocardiograms**

Theoretically, the more 2-dimensional planes scanned, the more precise the 3-D reconstruc-tion of the left ventricle will be. Two basic strategies for acquiring multiplane 2-D echocardio-graphic images via the restricted acoustic window to avoid the lung and ribs involve:

1. Translation of cross-sectional planes along the chest wall;

2. Rotation of cross-sectional planes along the fixed axis of the transducer.

The first technique is usually applied for short-axis views from the parasternal position [6, 8], and the second is used for long-axis views from the apex [3, 10].

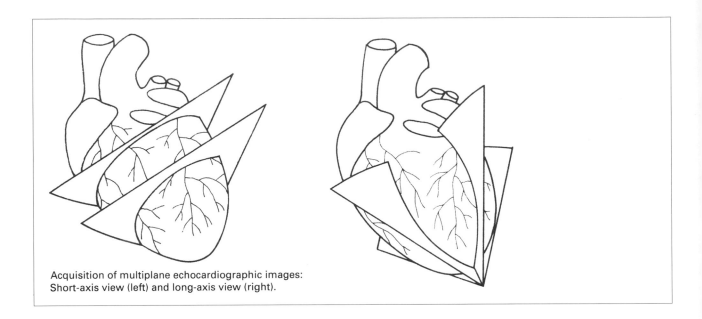

Acquisition of multiplane echocardiographic images:
Short-axis view (left) and long-axis view (right).

The apical approach requires a simple holding attachment for the transducer. This makes it possible to maintain a fixed axis of rotation and to reproducibly locate the proper angle of the cross-sectional planes.

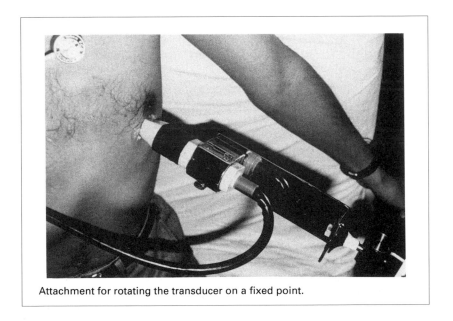

Attachment for rotating the transducer on a fixed point.

The following figure shows a series of six different apical views during the end-diastolic phase. They were obtained by rotating the echo plane at increments of 30° along the transducer axis. An advantage of the apical approach is that it provides total visibility of the left ventricle at every rotating angle of the cross-section. However, there is also a disadvantage in that myocardial borders lying parallel to the ultrasound beam may remain unclear.

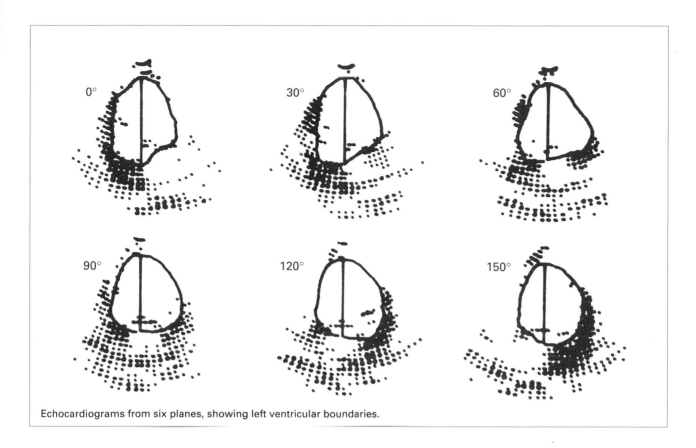

Echocardiograms from six planes, showing left ventricular boundaries.

Long- and short-axis views can be acquired from the parasternal position. On these images, the endocardium and epicardium are usually clearly visible, whereas the apical region is hardly seen. The transducer must be stabilized by a rather complex holding attachment in order to properly register the position and orientation of the cross-sections for 3-D reconstruction. The use of both apical and parasternal views yields the most precise results of 3-D reconstruction.

The acquisition of images for 3-D reconstruction during the cardiac cycle provides a huge number of echo data on several cross-sections. When six different planes are used, for example, approximately 180 frames are digitized and stored in the computer. This amounts to over 11 MB (megabytes) for an image consisting of 256 by 256 sampling points when each point is quantized into 8 bits, *i.e.*, 256 grey levels (8 bits = 1 byte = 256 points)*.

Normally, such a large number of images are recorded on video tape and then digitized for off-line processing. However, since digital memory devices such as IC and hard disks are getting larger in capacity and cheaper in price, it may soon be possible to digitize all images needed for 3-D reconstruction during the cardiac examination, then transfer them directly to an on-line computer. The most recent conventional echocardiography devices are equipped with a scan converter which transforms the image format from sector to raster scan for conventional video systems. This makes it easy to digitize echo images with commercially available image digitizers. However, one must be aware that the true echo signal exists only on the sector scanning lines. Images on raster format have some distortion due to transform processes such as *resampling, smoothing*, etc. A system for direct acquisition of 3-D data was recently proposed [11].

---

* A byte consists of 8 bits and can be assigned a value of 0 to 255. This means that a total of 256 different grey levels can be represented by one byte. At this gray level depth, each image point can be represented by one byte. This computes to 65,536 bytes per frame for an image with 256 x 256 sampling points, and 11,796,480 bytes for 180 frame. This figure divided by 1,024 equals 11,520 kilobytes which, again divided by 1,024 yields a sum of 11.25 megabytes.

For 3-D reconstruction of the left ventricular myocardium, one must first locate the endo- and epicardial boundaries on 2-D echocardiograms. The manual tracing method is sometimes used for conventional processing of 2-D echocardiograms. One usually evaluates two specific frames (end-diastolic and end-systolic) for a quantitative assessment of cardiac function. However, automated methods of boundary detection are desirable to obtain objective and reproducible results.

Many researchers have developed computer-assisted methods with or without operator interaction to detect boundaries from 2-D echocardiograms by using image processing techniques such as enhancement and edge detection [1, 2, 4, 12]. Three-dimensional echocardiography, which deals with several times more images than 2-D echocardiography, requires such sophisticated techniques for boundary detection.

Some of the suggested methods are designed for fully automated boundary detection [5, 7]. However, it is difficult to extract the boundaries of the left ventricle as smooth and connected curves, irrespective of image quality. Two reasons for this are that echo images are generally noisy and that the border of the myocardium is often unclear. Thus, cooperation between the computer and the operator is required to yield stable and reliable results. In a semiautomated procedure, the operator first enters the initial contour data into the computer, then uses the computer to detect the contours of the heart during the desired cardiac phase based on data from a series of consecutive frames [4]. A good knowledge of the shape and motion of the left ventricle is the key to reliable computerized boundary detection, because the contours of the heart remains very similar throughout the cardiac cycle, and only gradual changes can be seen in the successive frames.

One practical procedure for the detection of endo- and epicardial boundaries is summarized below [4]. First, the operator maps several points of the endocardial boundary onto the end-diastolic echocardiogram. The initial contours are then determined by generating a smooth curve across the manually entered points.

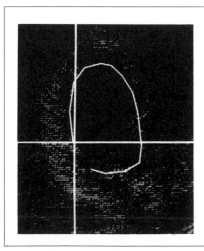

Initial edge points for boundary search.

All frames are subsequently rescanned radially from the center of gravity of the initial contour so that the boundary points can be sought one-dimensionally on the radial lines. A threshold method is used for detection of endocardial boundary points. Once the boundary has been detected on one frame, the same procedure is applied sequentially, frame by frame, in forward and backward order, assuming the regularity (periodic property) of boundary motion. The subsequent frame uses as a reference the boundary determined from the prior frame, which provides the searching range of interest on the radial line.

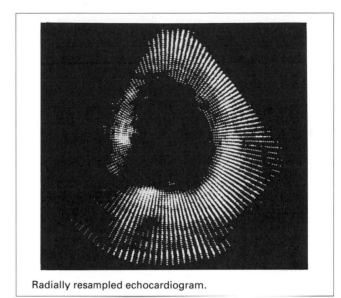

Radially resampled echocardiogram.

By applying a maximum value detection method on each radial line, the epicardial boundary can be determined by referring to the endocardial boundary point already detected on the same frame.

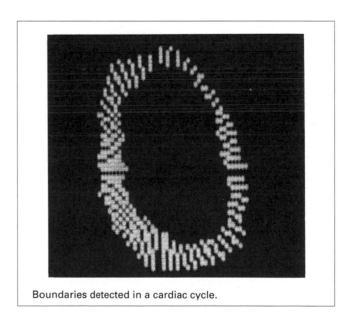

Boundaries detected in a cardiac cycle.

The boundary detection method for single plane echocardiography is applied to each cross-sectional echocardiogram. Thus, all endo- and epicardial boundaries required for 3-D reconstruction can be obtained.

3-D reconstruction of the left ventricle is performed by transferring the endo- and epicardial boundaries determined from multiple cross-sections onto the registered plane in the corresponding 3-D coordinate system, based on whether the apical, parasternal, or both views were used. First, the multiplane echocardiograms are synchronized with the help of an ECG signal. The multiple boundaries of the same cardiac phase are placed on the planes that spatially correspond to those in the planes of image acquisition. Subsequently, the data is interpolated by connecting the individual data points that were entered into the coordinate system.

In the case of the six planes from the apical long-axis view, taken at every 30° rotation, six endocardial boundaries from the same cardiac phase are rearranged in such a way that the rotating axis of each plane should coincide.

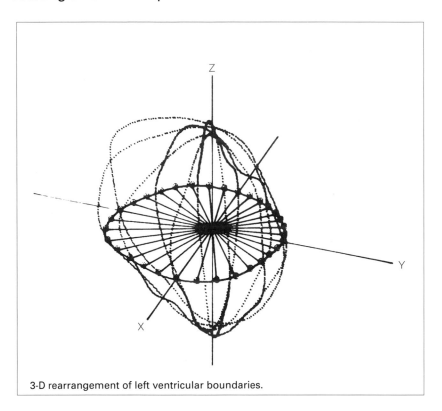

3-D rearrangement of left ventricular boundaries.

Then, the six boundaries are then interpolated with a spline curve by connecting the 12 points of the boundaries of each of the 16 planes perpendicular to the axis of rotation. A three-dimensional reconstruction of the myocardium is produced by applying this procedure to the boundaries of each cardiac phase [9].

As a result of 3-D reconstruction, three-dimensional representation of the left ventricle is obtained as a data set of coordinates *(x, y, z)*. By using the 3-D data sets of consecutive cardiac phases, any cross sectional view of the myocardium at every cardiac phase can be displayed. The 3-D display of the ventricle is realized by means of the wire-frame or shading methods. The wire-frame method is performed by connecting the surface points of the 3-D object and eliminating the hidden, *i.e.* invisible, line from the view angle. The following figure shows the wire-frame display of the endocardium at end-diastolic and end-systolic phases.

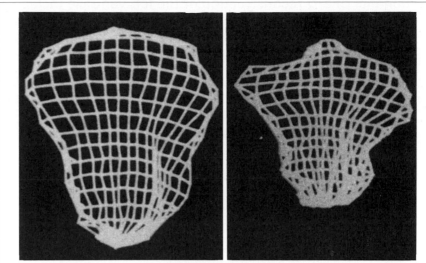

3-D endocardium of the left ventricle at end-diastolic (left) and end-systolic (right).

The shaded display, which provides a more realistic impression of the three-dimensional object, is performed by putting the reflected brightness on the object surface. The following figure shows the shaded representation of the 3-D myocardium throughout a cardiac cycle.

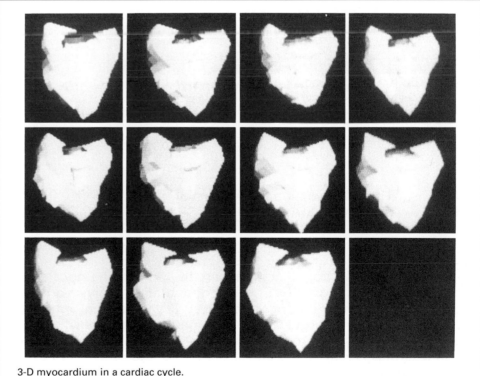

3-D myocardium in a cardiac cycle.

In addition to the static image, the dynamic image, *i.e.* the pulsating left ventricle, also is displayed by showing repeatedly the consecutive 3-D images along the cardiac phase within a given cardiac cycle.

The benefits of 3-D reconstruction of the left ventricle include global information on cardiac function (*e.g.* chamber volume) and the 3-D map of regional wall functions (*e.g.* wall contractility and wall thickness). Moreover, the three-dimensional display of quantitative results such as percent shortening and percent wall thickening makes it possible to recognize the location and spread of wall motion abnormality. The figure shows the color encoded functional displays of wall thickness at the end-diastolic (ED) and end-systolic (ES) phases (upper two), percent thickening (lower left), and percent shortening (lower right).

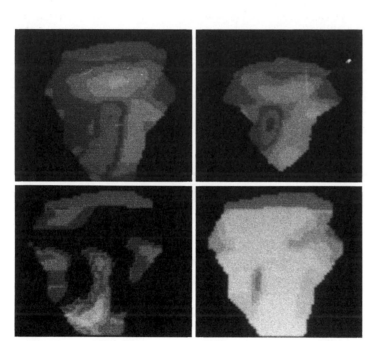

Functional 3-D images of the left ventricle: wall thickness at ED (upper left), at ES (upper right), percent thickening and percent shortening (below).

4.4   **Three-Dimensional Echocardiography**
4.4.5   **Sources of Error**

Before closing this section, it is necessary to address an important issue, namely sources of error in 3-D echocardiography. Errors in quantitative analysis arise mainly from spatial registration and boundary detection. The accuracy of spatial information recorded at image acquisition could be improved by developing a better transducer holding arm that can precisely locate the position and orientation of the cross sectional plane. Because of the ambiguity of boundary location in echocardiograms, the problem of boundary detection remains rather complex and will require further investigation before a definitive solution can be found.

1. Adam D, Harenveni O, Sidenan S. Semiautomated border tracking of cine echocardiographic ventricular images. IEEE Transactions on Medical Imaging 1987; 6: 266-271.

2. Chu CH, Delp EJ, Buda AJ. Detecting left ventricular endocardial and epicardial boundaries by digital two-dimensional echocardiography. IEEE Transactions on Medical Imaging 1988; 7: 81-90.

3. Eiho S, Kuwahara M, Asada N, Sasayana S, Takahasi M, Kawai C. Reconstruction of 3-D-images of pulsating left ventricle from two-dimensional sector scan echocardiograms of apical long axis views. Computers in Cardiology 1982: 19-24.

4. Eiho S, Kuwahara M, Asada N, Yamashita E. A microcomputerized image processor for 2-D-echocardiography and 3-D reconstruction of left ventricle. Computers in Cardiology (1985) 1986: 269-272.

5. Feng J, Lin FC, Chen CT. Automatic left ventricular boundary detection in digital two-dimensional echocardiography using fuzzy reasoning techniques. SPIE Biomedical Image Processing 1990; 1245: 192-205.

6. Geiser EA, Lupkiewicz SM, Christie LG, Ariet M, Conetta DA, Conti CR. A framework for three-dimensional time-varying reconstruction of the human left ventricle: sources of error and estimation of their magnitude. Computers in Biomedical Research 1980; 13: 225-241.

7. Han CY, Lin KN, Wee WG, Mintz RM, Porembka DT. Knowledge-based image analysis for automated boundary extraction of transesophageal echocardiographic left ventricular images. IEEE Transactions on Medical Imaging 1991; 10: 602-610.

8. Jensch P, Susanto H, Schneider W, Ameling W, Besen RV, Lambertz H, Grenner B, Effert S. Reconstruction of 3-D-images and selected cross sections of the heart. Computers in Cardiology (1983) 1984: 483-486.

9. Kuwahara M, Eiho S, Asada N, Osakada G, Kawai C. 3-D-images of left ventricular myocardium reconstructed from 2-D echocardiograms. Computers in Cardiology (1984) 1985: 505-508.

10. Moritz WE, Pearlman AS, McCabe DH, Medesa DK, Ainsworth ME, Boles MS. An ultrasonic technique for imaging the ventricle in three dimensions and calculating its volume. IEEE Transactions on Biomedical Engineering 1983; 30: 482-491.

11. Pini R, Costi M, Mensah GA, Masotti L, Novins KL, Greenberg PD, Greppi B, Cerotolini M, Devereox RB. Computed tomography of the heart by ultrasound. Computers in Cardiology (1991) 1992: 17-20.

12. Taxt T, Lundervold A, Angelsen B. Noise reduction and segmentation in time-varying ultrasound images. Proceedings 10th ICPR 1990: 591-596.

4.5	**Ultrasonic Tissue Characterization and Acoustic Microscopy**
4.5.1	**Ultrasonic Tissue Characterization**
	(Kurt J.G. Schmailzl)

Differentiating between healthy and abnormal cardiac tissue by analyzing the acoustic properties of the myocardium requires a completely different approach than that of clinical ultrasonic morphometry and wall motion analysis. Ultrasonic tissue characterization is based on some known and some assumed acoustic properties of biological material,

---

Biological determinants of myocardial acoustic properties

▸ Geometry and architecture of scatterers (fiber orientation)
▸ Scatter variations due to cardiac cycle and function
▸ Collagen content
▸ Water content and hematocrit

---

as well as on the physical properties and characteristic changes of ultrasound as it travels through or is reflected by different tissue volumes.

Physical parameters that change due to the interaction of ultrasound with body tissue

- Propagation velocity c
- Wavelength λ
  (Penetration, attenuation, reflection, scattering, absorption)

Techniques of ultrasonic tissue characterization are based on these interactions:

Techniques of ultrasonic tissue characterization

- Image data analysis
  - Gray-level statistics
  - Textural analysis
- Radiofrequency (RF) signal analysis (raw data analysis)

4.5.1   **Ultrasonic Tissue Characterization**
4.5.1.1   **Image Data Analysis**

The scatter properties of an object, attenuation processes that occur during ultrasound propagation, and variations in instrument settings give rise to differences in echo amplitude. In ultrasonic tissue characterization, the observer is usually interested in the visual differences observable on the display, which he or she would describe as differences in echogenicity. The best known example of this is the brilliant white color which, in clinical practice, is known as a "calcium-dense echo".

Qualitative visual descriptions such as echo-dense, echolucent, echo-free, and fine, coarse, homogeneous and inhomogeneous echo pattern, etc. are commonly used in clinical ultrasound. Although some diseases of the heart as well as of other organs can be described in this manner, such findings are unspecific. Although Doppler color flow mapping enables the observer to better distinguish gray level and textural differences with the naked eye, such diagnoses are based on inductive reasoning (*e.g.* white = calcium). Therefore, the method of qualitative visual assessment is open to criticism.

As an alternative to conventional qualitative visual assessment techniques, statistical techniques have been developed to quantify the differences between spatially localized regions, *e.g.*, differences between regions of infarcted and normal myocardium. The most commonly used statistical techniques are the amplitude histogram and differential gray-level distribution [1].

Generally, any data set can be analyzed with respect to certain individual characteristics of reflected ultrasound or their regional distribution pattern. In the former case, the most frequently occurring gray level value can be related directly to a specific tissue characteristic. In the second case, the spatial distribution of minimal gray level contrast differences are related to a particular tissue characteristic (textural analysis). Thus, not only the differences in total intensity (gray level) of an echo picture element (pixel), but also differences in the spatial distribution (texture) of the gray levels can be described.

Commonly used of gray levels parameters

▸ Gray-level histogram statistics
    Histogram limit values (minimal, maximal, most frequent gray-level value,
    variance, skewness, kurtosis) [12]

▸ Gray-level difference distribution
    Contrast
    Energy

▸ Gray-level run length statistics   Data measures

The gray-level difference distribution describes differences in pixels separated on the image by a constant distance. Gray-level run length statistics describes the frequency of occurrence at which two different gray levels that are separated by a specified distance on the image occur. Using gray-level histogram statistics, gray-level difference distributions, and the gray-level run length statistics, various characteristics of gray-level size, spatial and temporal distribution, etc. can be derived. For example, the minimum, maximum, and most frequent gray-level value can be derived from the gray-level histogram, and can be related to contraction-related changes in gray-level values [4].

Thus, it is possible to statistically analyze various parameters of texture and to compare the *spatial pattern of occurrence* of these texture parameters with those of a "healthy" reference frame. Alternatively, the data can be used do create a "mask frame", which can be subtracted from other frames. The temporal pattern of occurrence of one or more parameters can also be analyzed, *i.e.*, by observing diastolic to systolic variation during the cardiac cycle.

Textural Analysis
▸ Spatial pattern of occurrence ▸ Temporal pattern of occurrence

Many studies analyze individual parameters and/or the spatial and/or temporal relationships between two or more parameters. However, it is also possible to describe reflected signals using a variety of parameters and then study the set as a whole, using such statistical methods as discriminance analysis, factor analysis, and canonic analysis to determine which subset most selectively characterizes known or assumed tissue differences [5]. Image frames derived from A-mode spectra and their transformations, from which a set of parameters to describe individual wave forms can be established, are well suited for this purpose.

As long as ultrasonic tissue characterization is performed on the basis of image data instead of radiofrequency signal data, the results can only be viewed as a means of operationalizing a primarily qualitative assessment method. Standard echocardiographic image data is highly dependent on the instrument and instrument settings, and on the skill and experience of the operator. In raw data analysis, on the other hand, radio frequency signals are extracted before they are routed to the image processing circuits. At that stage, very little compression or distortion of the signal has occurred. Therefore, analysis of those signals is a more sensitive method for detecting changes in backscattered signal amplitude [10].

Ultrasound and tissue-related acoustic parameters

▸ Propagation velocity c
▸ Wavelength λ, nominal frequency f
(Penetration depth, attenuation, reflection, scatter, absorption)
▸ Acoustic impedance Z
▸ Backscatter η

The velocity at which a longitudinal wave travels through solid material is dependent on the density and compressibility of the material.

$$c = \sqrt{E/\rho} \; (p, T = \text{const.});$$
$$[c] = \text{m/s}$$

p	Pressure
T	Temperature
c	Velocity of ultrasound propagation
E	Elasticity module
ρ	Tissue density

In fat, water, and muscle, the propagation velocity of ultrasound is approximately 1540 m/s. For simplification, the algorithms implemented in commercial medical ultrasound machines assume a uniform propagation velocity of 1540 m/s, regardless of which type of soft tissue is being interrogated. There still is no analytical concept that accounts for tissue-specific differences in the propagation velocity or that would be of use for the purpose of tissue characterization.

Wavelength is defined as a product of the propagation velocity and the period length, or as the quotient of the propagation velocity and frequency.

$$\lambda = c \, T = c/f;$$
$$[\lambda] = \text{m}$$

λ	Wavelength
c	Propagation velocity
T	Period
f	Frequency

Thus, in 2.5, 30 and 400 MHz transducers, the backscatter of wavelength λ will equal 600 µm, 50 µm, and 4 µm, respectively. Sarcomeres are around 2 µm in size, myofibrils are around 0.5 to 1.0 µm thick, collagen fibrils are around 1 to 10 µm in size, and the diametric length of collagen fibrils is 0.2 to 0.4 µm.

Each transducer has a specific frequency bandwidth. For simplification, frequency is given as the nominal frequency f (center frequency) of the bandwidth.

As the frequency increases, resolution also increases. The amplitude of echoes from deeper structures is normally lower than that of echoes from structures closer to the transducer, because attenuation A increases as the path length s of ultrasound becomes longer.

Attenuation is a result of reflection, scatter, and absorption on the path from the transducer and back. The magnitude of attenuation can be determined *in vitro* by comparing the reduction in total ultrasound energy after interrogating a tissue sample with the reduction in ultrasound measured after interrogating a corresponding volume of saline solution.

Angle-dependence of the reflected signal is a problematic factor. The amplitude and amplitude transformations are reduced due to changes in the transducer position and to contraction and respiration-related changes in the position of the heart in the chest cavity. Angle deviations of around 6° reduce the amplitude and the corresponding amplitude transformations by one-tenth. This can be falsely interpreted as attenuation effects.

Acoustic impedance Z, which is the product of propagation velocity and tissue density, is modulated by statistical and dynamic physiological and pathological factors.

Z	=	$\rho\,c$;
$[Z]$	=	$kg\,/\,(m^2\,s)$

Z	Acoustic impedance
ρ	Tissue density
c	Propagation velocity

When interfaces are larger than the wavelength of ultrasound, the ultrasound wave is reflected by the interfaces between structures of different acoustic impedances, *i.e.*, between tissues of different densities and/or with different propagation velocities of sound. When the interfaces are smaller than the wavelength, a multidimensional overlapping pattern of scattered echoes occurs. Scattered echoes that return to the transducer are defined as backscatter η. The extent of backscatter and attenuation can be quantitated and used for purposes of tissue characterization. However, both exhibit a nonlinear relationship to the related frequency. When the Rayleigh condition is satisfied, the relationship between scatter and frequency is determined by the size of the scatterer. The smaller the scatterer as compared to the wavelength of ultrasound, the higher the intensity of backscatter. In scatters that are much larger than the wavelength, the intensity of backscatter is approximately equal to the transmission frequency.

$\eta \approx f^4$	(scatterer << wavelength) *Rayleigh scatter*
$\eta \approx f^3$	*backscatter*; e.g. normal myocardium
$\eta \approx f^0$	(scatterer >> wavelength) *specular scatter;*
	e.g. endocardium-blood interface

Therefore, backscatter is usually expressed as a function of transducer frequency. Phase cancellation effects can be minimized by averaging (integrating) backscatter across the total frequency bandwidth *(integrated backscatter)*.

The returning, frequency-dependent ultrasound energy or *power spectrum* $|E(f)|^2$ can be studied in various tissue samples, using a glass or steel plate as the reference reflector. The power spectrum of the plate (reference reflector) is determined at various transmission frequencies (*e.g.* 2.0 to 7.5 MHz).

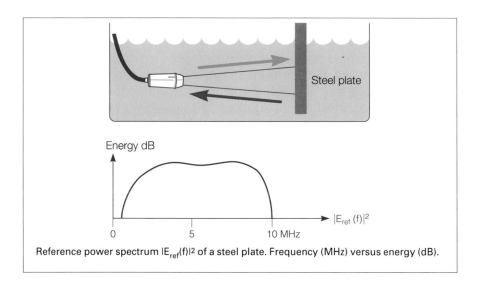

Reference power spectrum $|E_{ref}(f)|^2$ of a steel plate. Frequency (MHz) versus energy (dB).

Then, the power spectrum of a myocardial frame is related to the reference power spectrum of the perfect reflector.

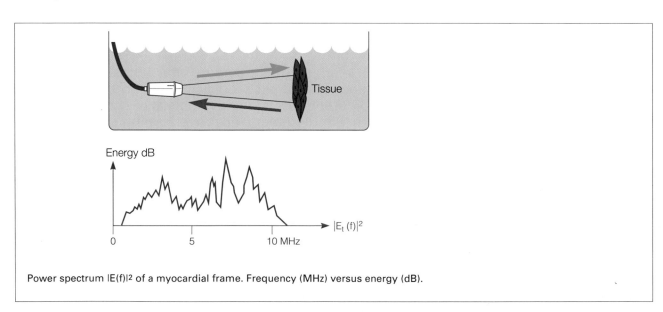

Power spectrum $|E(f)|^2$ of a myocardial frame. Frequency (MHz) versus energy (dB).

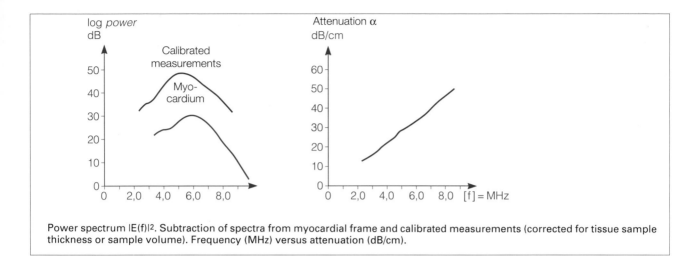

Power spectrum IE(f)I². Subtraction of spectra from myocardial frame and calibrated measurements (corrected for tissue sample thickness or sample volume). Frequency (MHz) versus attenuation (dB/cm).

The *backscatter transfer function* IB(f)I² describes the relationship between frequencies and energies and can be expressed in terms of energy (decibels) below the backscatter obtained from a perfect reflector (reference spectrum) [15].

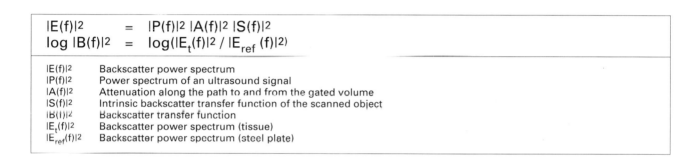

$$IE(f)I^2 = IP(f)I^2 \, IA(f)I^2 \, IS(f)I^2$$
$$\log IB(f)I^2 = \log(IE_t(f)I^2 / IE_{ref}(f)I^2)$$

IE(f)I²	Backscatter power spectrum
IP(f)I²	Power spectrum of an ultrasound signal
IA(f)I²	Attenuation along the path to and from the gated volume
IS(f)I²	Intrinsic backscatter transfer function of the scanned object
IB(f)I²	Backscatter transfer function
IE_t(f)I²	Backscatter power spectrum (tissue)
IE_ref(f)I²	Backscatter power spectrum (steel plate)

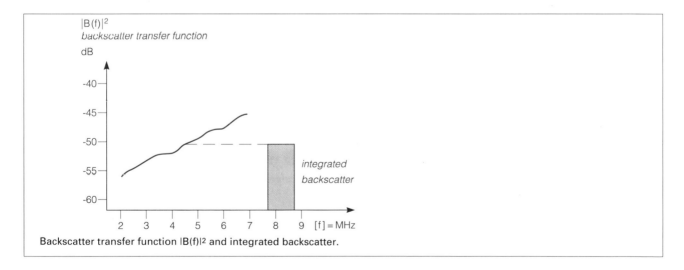

Backscatter transfer function IB(f)I² and integrated backscatter.

Integrated backscatter is the frequency-averaged backscatter over the total frequency band-width of the transducer [7]. Like the backscatter transfer function, integrated backscatter is dependent of the attenuation of ultrasound by tissue and on the aperture and focus of the transducer. The *backscatter transfer coefficient,* on the other hand, is an absolute measure of the scatter properties of tissue. It is derived by multiplying the backscatter transfer function by the appropriate correction factors.

Deriving the total energy of backscatter from data which were obtained from integrated backscatter data and the backscatter coefficient has certain advantages. For example, instrument setting dependence and phase cancellation effects are reduced, and follow-up and comparison studies can be performed based on the data.

New approaches can be achieved by using radio frequency data in instruments already designed for textural analysis. For example, cyclic variation in gray-level values, which is already used for textural analysis, can be reformulated with respect to the logarithmic relationship of diastolic to systolic backscatter. The attenuation of ultrasound in the interrogated tissue is contraction-dependent [2]. Therefore, the cyclic variation in backscatter can be interpreted as an individual expression of muscle function.

In order to pictorially display the derived measurement and calculation data, they could be reformatted into images by converting the integrated backscatter data as the basis for each sector scan line. The pixels in these images represent the local integrated backscatter.

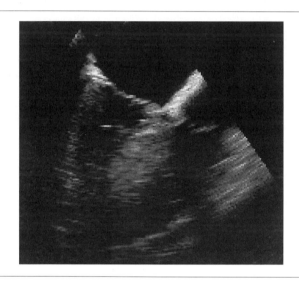

Hypertrophic obstructed cardiomyopathy (transesophageal short-axis 2-D echocardiogram). Image reconstructed from raw data.

Scatter occurs when ultrasound interacts with interfaces of structures of different acoustic impedances that are smaller than the wavelength of the ultrasound wave. Such structures are mycocytes (length 50 to 100 µm, diameter 10 to 20 µm) and collagen fibrils (transverse striation at a distance of 70µm, diameter 15 to 200µm). Scatter is dependent on the size, shape, density, and spatial orientation of scatterers, and is also dependent on the difference between the acoustic impedance of the scatters and their immediate surroundings.

The acoustic impedance, attenuation and scattering of ultrasound are affected by myocardial collagen, muscle tissue, and water content; furthermore, scattering is also dependent on the structural integrity of collagen fibrils and the tertiary structure of the tissue unit [9, 11].

Presently, the best studied biological determinants of the acoustic properties of tissue are collagen content, water content, and cardiac muscle fiber orientation. The focus of connective tissue content analysis is, primarily, to characterize scar tissue and heart diseases associated with hypertrophic changes. The focus of water content and hematocrit analyses is to characterize inflammatory heart diseases and cardiac diseases associated with edema formation.

Post-infarction scarring leads to variation in the frequency-dependent parameters of scatter and attenuation. When applying this for analysis of ischemic myocardium, it is assumed that the acoustic reflectance of infarcted myocardium is lower than that of healthy myocardium.

This has been demonstrated in several transmission experiments.

For example, if one compares the attenuation of ultrasound in normal and infarcted myocardium by placing a perfect reflector behind the respective tissue sample, the observed a scar tissue-related increase in attenuation [6]. This is even more marked in higher frequency ranges. A correlation can also be observed between the extent of necrosis and attenuation (-increase in attenuation) [8].

Reflection experiments have shown that an increase in backscattered energy occurs in the postinfarction phase (ca. four weeks after acute infarction). "Since scattering is one of the causes of attenuation, the increase in backscattered energy in chronic infarction is consistent with the increased attenuation noted in transmission studies" [3].

However, in the immediate postischemic phase (≤ two hours after acute ischemia), there is a decrease in attenuation, while backscatter increases.

A possible explanation is that the ischemia-induced edema reduces the magnitude of attenuation by dilution of protein constituents, but leaves the tissue ultrastructure, and hence scattering, intact [3]. A similar increase in backscatter occurs in acute transplant rejection and associated edema formation.

As an alternative to studies on the correlation between acoustic impedance, attenuation, and scatter of ultrasound and biological determinants of myocardial acoustic properties, the backscatter properties of characteristic organizational patterns of normal and pathological tissue can be studied at the microscopic level [3]. The idea behind this approach is that acoustically different targets within the tissue exhibit a characteristic and relatively consistent spatial orientation. Also, when they are struck by an ultrasound wave, they behave as a series of diffuse scatterers, which leads to selective reinforcement or cancellation of certain frequencies. These scatterers are small and regularly spaced. They produce interference patterns, which cause wavelengths within the frequency spectrum which are similar to the underlying organizational pattern.

Bragg scattering condition [adapted from 3]
$n \lambda \quad = 2 \, d \sin \theta$
λ Ultrasonic wavelength   n   Number of wavelengths   d   Distance between scatterers θ Angle from the horizontal to the scattered signal

When the Bragg scattering condition for the maxima of the amplitude quadrant is satisfied, tissue can be characterized by either finding the known wavelength (λ) and then by varying the angle or by using a constant angle and by varying the wavelength. The sequence of the largest amplitudes is characteristic of the organizational pattern of the studied tissue at the microscopic level. [3]

Study of the complex intramural organization of the heart muscle fibers in different diseases is of great importance. The specific fiber alignment at different transmural levels can be studied by measuring the dependence of integrated backscatter on the angle of insonification (anisotropy). When the angle of insonification is perpendicular to the normal fiber orientation, the integrated backscatter is greater than in a parallel angle of insonification [16]. In initial experiments, the physiological changes in the epicardium and endocardium were described [13, 14]. The anisotropy concept was later used to describe ischemic myocardium, stunned myocardium, scarring, and cardiomyopathy. By adjusting the depth of the gated volume, muscle is interrogated at different depths. The power spectral density data for each gated segment is then measured and stored off-line. In order to properly describe the fiber alignment, it is necessary to systematically insonificate the samples in very small angle increments, by proceeding in a stepwise fashion until the entire circumference of the sample has been interrogated. At the same time, the transmural depth must be varied incrementally in steps of a few millimeters each, to encompass the epicardium and endocardium. By measuring the integrated backscatter for each individual energy spectrum, the transmural shift in the alignment of fibers from epicardium to endocardium can be observed.

Radio frequency signal analysis appears to hold the key to the detection of myocardial perfusion after intravenous administration of transpulmonary echo contrast agents [10]. Radio frequency data sequences are edited and processed to produce a frequency spectrum for each frame obtained from the myocardium and ventricle (before and after contrast administration). The mean integrated backscatter is calculated, and the mean ultrasound frequency is also measured in order to detect any shifts in the spectral curve attributable to resonance of the contrast microspheres. The mean integrated backscatter and the mean ultrasound frequency values for both the ventricle and the myocardium are plotted for every frame of acquired data. Transpulmonary contrast agents lead to a resonance-related decrease in the mean frequency and, thus, to an increase in total energy [10]. This technique may some day make it possible to perform intravenous organ perfusion studies at rest and at exercise using ultrasound imaging.

References

1. Ameling W. Digitale Bildverarbeitung und Echokardiographie: 3D-Rekonstruktion und Texturanalyse. In: Erbel W, Meyer J, Brennecke R (eds). Fortschritte der Echokardiographie. Springer, Berlin 1985: 10.
2. Barzilai B, Madaras EI, Sobel BE, Miller JG, Perez JE. Effects of myocardial contraction on ultrasonic backscatter before and after ischemia. Am J Physiol 1984; 247: H478-H483.
3. Franklin TD jr, Brink JA, Cuddeback JL, Sanghvi NT, Weyman AE. Tissue parameter characterization by ultrasound: state-of-the-art in cardiology. In: Hanrath P, Bleifeld W, Souquet J (eds). Cardiovascular diagnosis by ultrasound. Martinus Nijhoff Publishers, The Hague 1982: 159.
4. Haendchen RV, Ong K, Fishbein MC, Zwehl W, Meerbaum S, Corday E. Early differentiation of infarcted and noninfarcted reperfused myocardium in dogs by quantitative analysis of regional myocardial echo amplitude. Circ Res 1985; 57: 718-728.
5. Jensch P, Kubalski W, De Araujo A, Ameling W, Essen R, Lambertz H, Effert S. Pattern analysis approaches to ultrasound tissue characterization using an image sequence processing system. Proc IEEE Computers in Cardiology, Aachen: 483-486.
6. Lele PP, Mansfield AB, Murphy AI, Namery J, Senapati N. Tissue characterization by ultrasonic frequency-dependent attenuation and scattering. In: Linzer M (ed). Ultrasonic tissue characterization. NBS Spec. Publ. No. 435, U.S. Government Printing Office, Washington, D.C. 1976: 153.
7. Miller JG, Perez JE, Mottley JG et al. Myocardial tissue characterization: An approach based on quantitative backscatter and attenuation. Proc IEEE Ultrasonics Symp 1983; 83CH1947-1: 782.

8. Mimbs JW, Yuhas DE, Miller JG, Weiss AN, Sobel BE. Detection of myocardial infarction in vivo based on altered attenuation of ultrasound. Circ Res 1977; 41: 192.

9. Mimbs JW, O'Donnell M, Bauwens D, Miller JG, Sobel BE. The dependence of ultrasonic attenuation and backscatter on collagen content in dog and rabbit hearts. Circ Res 1980; 47: 49-58.

10. Monaghan MJ, Metcalfe JM, Odunlami S, Waaler A, Jewitt DE. Digital radiofrequency echocardiography in the detection of myocardial contrast following intravenous administration of Albunex. Eur Heart J 1993; 14: 1200-1209.

11. O'Donnell M, Mimbs JW, Miller JG. The relationship between collagen and ultrasonic backscatter in myocardial tissue. J Acoust Soc Am 1981; 69: 580-588.

12. Skorton DJ, Melton HE jr, Pandian NG et al.Detection of acute myocardial infarction in closed-chest dogs by analysis of regional two-dimensional echocardiographic gray-level distributions. Circ Res 1983; 52: 36.

13. Streeter DDJ, Hanna WT. Engineering mechanics for successive states in canine left ventricular myocardium: II.Fiber angle and sarcomere length. Circ Res 1973; 33: 656-664.

14. Verdonk ED, Wickline SA, Miller JG. Quantification of the anisotropy of ultrasonic quasilongitudinal velocity in normal human and canine myocardium with comparison to anisotropy of integrated backscatter. IEEE Ultrason Sym 1990; 90CH2938-9: 1349-1352.

15. Wear KA, Milunski MR, Wickline SA, Perez JE, Sobel BE, Miller JG. Differentiation between acutely ischemic myocardium and zones of completed infarction in dogs on the basis of frequency-dependent backscatter. J Acoust Soc Am 1989; 85: 2634-2641.

16. Wickline SA, Verdonk ED, Miller JG. Quantification of the transmural shift of myofiber orientation in normal human heart with ultrasonic integrated backscatter. J Clin Invest 1991; 88: 438-446.

17. Wong AK, Verdonk ED, Hoffmeister BK, Miller JG, Wickline SA. Detection of unique transmural architecture of human idiopathic cardiomyopathy by ultrasound tissue characterization. Circulation 1992; 86: 1108-1115.

4.5	**Ultrasound Tissue Characterization and Acoustic Microscopy**
4.5.2	**Acoustic Microscopy**
	(P. Anthony N. Chandraratna)

Transducers used for conventional transthoracic echocardiography operate at 2 to 3.5 MHz. Higher frequency transducers employed in pediatric echocardiography and transesophageal echocardiography provide better resolution. A 20 or 30 MHz transducer mounted at the tip of a cardiac catheter enables visualization, in excellent detail, of the intima, media and adventitia of coronary arteries and peripheral vessels. Thus, a progressive increase in transducer frequency provides improved axial and lateral resolution. Transducer resolution is determined by the wavelength of ultrasound, which is a function of the transducer frequency, focal length and transducer diameter, as expressed by the equation:

$$\text{Resolution} = \text{wavelength} \times (\text{focal length} \div \text{diameter})$$

Thus, resolution can be improved by increasing transducer frequency,

$$\text{wavelength} = \text{velocity of sound} \div \text{frequency}$$

by shortening the focal length, or by increasing the diameter of the transducer. Acoustic microscopy employs very high frequency ultrasound transducers which permit visualization of cellular detail (ultrastructure).

Sokolov first proposed the use of very high frequency ultrasound for a system of microscopy in 1936 [13]. Lemons and Quate developed the scanning acoustic microscope and described some biomedical applications [10, 11].

They examined a variety of specimens and described the acoustic microscopic appearance of red blood cells, human lung tissue, human breast tissue, and malignant tumor of the human breast. Hildebrand et al. [9] performed acoustic microscopy on living chicken heart fibroblasts in tissue culture and noted that the cells exhibited normal motility patterns. Neild et al. [12] used a 600 MHz scanning acoustic microscope to image arterioles in connective tissue from the submucosa of the guinea pig small intestine. More recently, the acoustic microscopic appearance of neoplastic and inflammatory cutaneous tissue specimens was described by Barr et al. [1]. They were able to make a specific diagnosis in most neoplasms. In the inflammatory disorders, a specific diagnosis was possible in all but bullous pemphigoid and *lichen planus*.

The use of acoustic microscopy to detect myocardial pathology was first described by our group [3-6]. The wavelength of ultrasound at a frequency of 1000 MHz is approximately 1.5 µm and the resolution of the system approaches 1 µm, enabling the visualization of cardiac myocytes, cell membranes and myofibrils. Although light microscopy provides invaluable information about tissue pathology, this technique requires staining of specimens for visualization of abnormalities, and the method is not suitable for *in vivo* imaging. Apart from our preliminary reports, there have been no systematic studies of the myocardium using acoustic microscopy. We therefore conducted a series of experiments to assess the feasibility of *in vivo* acoustic microscopy. These studies will be summarized in the following.

A schematic of the acoustic microscope is shown in the following figure. An electromagnetic radio-frequency signal stimulates a piezoelectric crystal which emits ultrasound waves that are focused by a sapphire crystal. The ultrasound wave traverses the myocardial tissue specimen on the slide and is then reflected from the slide. On returning to the piezoelectric crystal, a radio-frequency (RF) signal is emitted and collected by a receiver. The acoustic signal intensity is converted to brightness for display as a point of light on a cathode ray tube. The specimen is scanned in the horizontal plane in a raster fashion, thus allowing point-by-point analysis of the elastic properties of a cross section of tissue. A 600 or a 1000 MHz transducer is used for this study. The acoustic image is displayed on a screen.

Ultrasound image contrast is produced by differing attenuation between various components of myocardial tissue [2]. Structures with the greatest attenuation appear black, while tissue components with the least attenuation appear white. When a section contains significant amounts of structural protein, particularly collagen, both attenuation and impedance play a role in the generation of the image [2]. The described system is also sensitive to changes in viscosity. Furthermore, no staining is required to generate the images.

The myocardium consists of myocytic cells, nonmyocytic cells, and interstitial tissue. Cardiac myocytes, which are the largest of these cells, occupy 75% of myocardial structural space, although they constitute only one-third of the total cell population. Other cell types found in the myocardial interstitium include:

1. endothelial cells, which line the coronary arteries and the endocardium;
2. vascular smooth muscle cells, which are found in the coronary arteries and arterioles;
3. fibroblasts, which produce and degrade collagen and elastin in the interstitium; and
4. macrophages.

Fibroblasts contain messenger RNA for type I and type III collagen, which are the major collagens that constitute the structural protein network of the heart. The studies performed by us were designed to assess the ability of acoustic microscopy to image normal and abnormal cardiac myocytes, interstitial inflammatory cell infiltration, and changes in the myocardial interstitium.

A comparison of myocardial pathology assessed by acoustic microscopy and light microscopy was performed. The observer interpreting the acoustic microscopic images was blinded to the results of light microscopy. Unstained, deparaffinized 5 μm sections of myocardial biopsy specimens from 10 patients were placed on a slide and imaged using an Olympus UH3 scanning acoustic microscope. For subsequent light microscopy, the section used for acoustic microscopy was stained with hematoxylin and eosin (H & E), and a serial section from the paraffin block was stained with phosphotungstic acid hematoxylin (PTAH), which specifically stains myofibrils. Myocytes, myofibrils and interstitial tissue were accurately imaged.

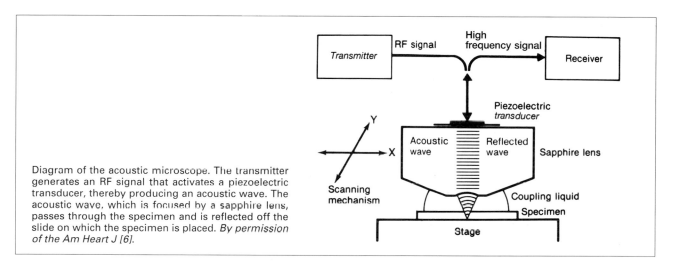

Diagram of the acoustic microscope. The transmitter generates an RF signal that activates a piezoelectric transducer, thereby producing an acoustic wave. The acoustic wave, which is focused by a sapphire lens, passes through the specimen and is reflected off the slide on which the specimen is placed. *By permission of the Am Heart J [6].*

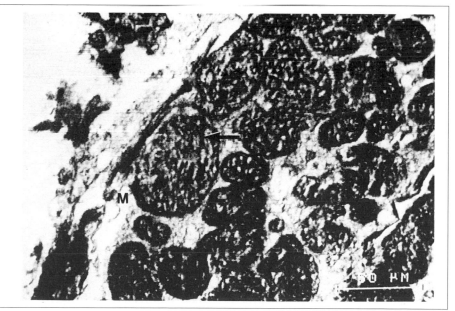

Acoustic microscopic picture of the myocardium illustrating cells of various sizes. The cell membrane (M) and myofibrils (horizontal arrow) can be seen. *By permission of the Am Heart J [6].*

Pathological phenomena such as cell fallout, interstitial fibrosis and lymphocytic infiltration were identified by acoustic microscopy. Intramural vessels, nuclei of endothelial cells and the media were clearly identified by this technique.

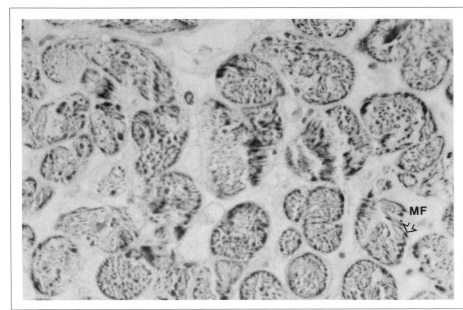

Light microscopic picture of the myocardium stained with PTAH to illustrate myofibrils (MF). *By permission of the Am Heart J [6].*

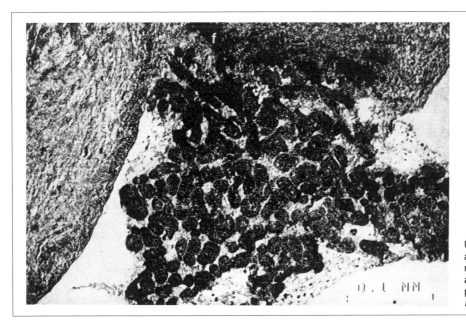

Ultrasound picture of the myocardium depicting an area with normal cells (lower right quadrant), an acellular area (left), and a dark zone probably representing fibrosis (f). *By permission of the Am Heart J [6].*

There was a close correlation between the findings of acoustic microscopy and light microscopy. In 9 out of 10 patients, normal and abnormal histological features (*i.e.*, cell dropout, fibrosis and lymphocytic infiltration) assessed by acoustic microscopy and light microscopy were identical. In one patient, acoustic microscopy failed to identify a focus of lymphocytic infiltration (seen on light microscopy), because the area of interest was not imaged [3].

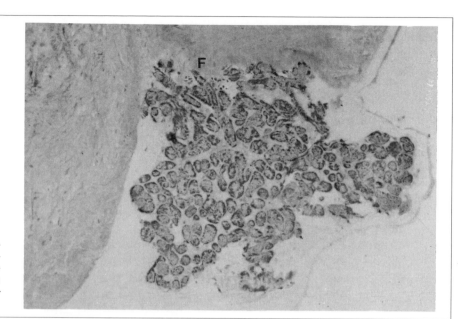

Light microscopic picture of specimen shown above. An area containing normal cells (lower right quadrant), an acellular area (left), and an area of fibrosis (F) are seen. *By permission of the Am Heart J [6].*

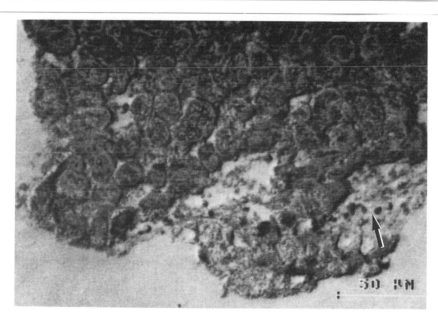

Ultrasound picture of the myocardium showing an area of normal cells (top half), a zone of cell fallout (bottom right), and discrete round echoes representing lymphocytes (arrowhead); confirmed by light microscopy. *By permission of the Am Heart J [6].*

4.5.2   **Acoustic Microscopy**

4.5.2.2 **Acoustic Microscopic Diagnosis of Homograft Rejection**

Acute transplant rejection is a serious complication associated with cardiac transplantation. Although the introduction of cyclosporine has reduced the incidence of this ominous complication, acute rejection still is the major cause of death in the early phase after cardiac transplantation. Serial myocardial biopsies are therefore performed after heart transplantation in an effort to detect rejection in its early stages.

One of the disadvantages of endomyocardial biopsy is the problem of sampling error. Both the cardiologist and the pathologist assume that samples obtained at biopsy are representative of the pathological process affecting the entire myocardium. The problem of sampling error also affects the diagnosis of acute myocarditis, a condition that may often be focal.

We believe that the development of *in vivo* acoustic microscopy will circumvent the problem of sampling error associated with endomyocardial biopsy. If it is possible to mount a very high frequency transducer at the top of a cardiac catheter and to perform *in vivo* imaging, multiple sites in both ventricles and atria could be sampled, thus minimizing sampling error.

We evaluated the role of acoustic microscopy in detecting homograft rejection [4]. In five patients, myocardial biopsy specimens were obtained at the time of acute rejection diagnosed by light microscopy and following recovery from rejection. All patients had moderate rejection as defined by lymphocytic infiltration and focal myocytolysis. The specimens were sectioned at 5 μm. Unstained, deparaffinized sections were used for acoustic microscopy. The acoustic microscopic images of all patients showed cell necrosis, cell fallout, and lymphocytic infiltration during the acute stage of rejection. However, in some patients, while one specimen showed severe myocytolysis, another specimen obtained from a different area on the same day showed normal myocytes. This clearly illustrates the problem of sampling error in myocardial biopsy specimens.

After recovery from rejection, the acoustic microscopic images showed cell fallout and areas of fibrosis.

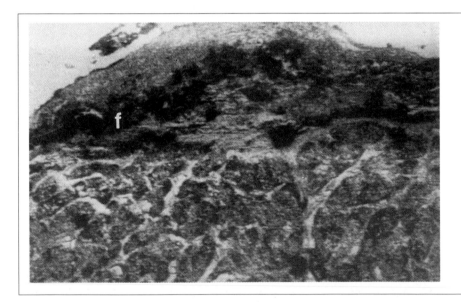

Ultrasound picture showing expansion of the subendocardial region with dense echoes representing fibrosis (f). *By permission of the Am Heart J [6].*

Two types of fibrous tissue were noted in the acoustic microscopic images. The first demonstrated a relatively hypoechoic fibrillar pattern, and the second was characterized by hyperechoic amorphous tissue. The acoustic microscopic findings both during acute rejection and with resolved rejection correspond closely with light microscopic findings.

Atherosclerosis produces characteristic changes in the coronary arteries. We studied the role of acoustic microscopy in imaging normal and atherosclerotic arteries. Fifteen blood vessels (12 coronary artery and 3 abdominal aorta specimens) obtained at the time of autopsy were sectioned at 5 μm. Unstained, deparaffinized sections were used for acoustic microscopy. Six vessels were normal and the rest contained atherosclerotic plaque. After acoustic microscopy was performed, the sections were stained with hematoxylin and eosin, and light microscopy was done.

Acoustic microscopy of normal coronary arteries revealed a thin intima, an echogenic internal elastic lamina, media, adventitia, and perivascular adipocytes. Expansion of the space between the internal elastic lamina and endothelium was identified in atherosclerotic vessels. Fatty plaque produced hypoechoic zones interspersed with collagen fibers (fibrous component). Large numbers of cholesterol crystals were seen in some fatty plaques. Fibrous plaques consisted mainly of collagen fibers. Calcific plaques were very echogenic. The acoustic microscopic findings were confirmed by light microscopy.

Intraluminal thrombus could be clearly differentiated from fatty plaque, a distinction that cannot be easily made by other forms of ultrasound imaging, including intravascular ultrasound. The thrombus consisted of clumps of dark, discrete echoes, which probably represented red blood cells and/or clumps of platelets. Vascular spaces and hemorrhage into the wall of the artery could be identified by acoustic microscopy.

4.5.2   **Acoustic Microscopy**
4.5.2.4   **Evaluation of Myocardial Microvasculature by High-Frequency Ultrasound**

Changes in myocardial microvasculature have been described in a variety of diseases such as diabetes mellitus and hypertension. These changes may account for abnormal coronary flow reserve, which occurs in these disease states. We therefore explored the role of high-frequency ultrasound in detecting abnormalities of the myocardial microvasculature. Twenty specimens of myocardium obtained by myocardial biopsy or at autopsy were sectioned 5 μm thick. The unstained sections were imaged with a 600 MHz transducer and an Olympus UH3 acoustic microscope [7]. The specimens were then stained with H & E and examined by light microscopy. Ultrasound images of 10 specimens had normal intramyocardial arterioles that were characterized by endothelial cells with elongated nuclei, an internal elastic lamina, and a thin media and adventitia. The diameter of normal arterioles was 93 μm ± 29; the vessel wall thickness was 12 ± 2 μm. Ten specimens showed abnormal intramyocardial arterioles. Marked thickening of the intima was seen in six patients. The diameter of these vessels was 93 ± 57 μm, and the vessel wall thickness was 52 ± 18 μm. In four patients with acute homograft rejection, thickening of the vessel was associated with intimal cellular infiltration.

4.5.2   **Acoustic Microscopy**
4.5.2.4   **Evaluation of Myocardial Microvasculature by**
          High-Frequency Ultrasound

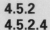

170

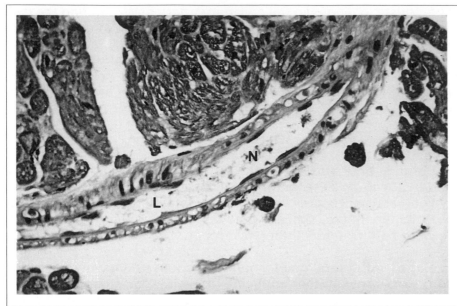

Light microscopic imaging showing an intramural vessel (arteriole) cut in its long axis. A clear lumen (L), endothelial cell nuclei (N), and media are seen. *By permission of the Am Heart J [6].*

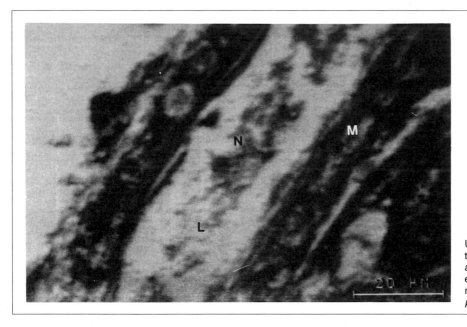

Ultrasound image corresponding to the light microscopic image above. Intramural vessel lumen (L), endothelial cell nuclei (N), and media (M) are clearly identified. *By permission of the Am Heart J [6].*

Focal intimal thickening was noted in one patient. Multiple intra-arteriolar thrombi were seen in four patients with myocardial infarction. Marked perivascular fibrosis was observed in three patients. These changes were confirmed by light microscopy. These preliminary data indicate that high-frequency ultrasound is capable of detecting histopathological changes in the myocardial microvascular.

We have demonstrated that the ultrastructure of myocardial cells can be exquisitely imaged with a 1000 MHz transducer. The cell membrane, myofibrils and interstitial tissue can be clearly identified. Pathological phenomena such as cell necrosis, fibrosis and lymphocytic infiltration can be detected with an accuracy comparable to that of light microscopy. Although the resolution of a 1000 MHz transducer is excellent, tissue penetration of ultrasound at this frequency is poor. Furthermore, significant technical difficulties have to be circumvented in order to build an ultrasound system for *in vivo* applications using a 1000 MHZ transducer. Thus, lower frequency transducers will provide better tissue penetration.

We have performed preliminary studies to determine the lowest frequency required to image cellular detail. To ascertain the lowest frequency at which adequate cellular detail can be obtained, we performed ultrasound imaging of 5 µm sections of five samples of myocardium and two coronary arteries. Each specimen was examined serially with a 600 MHz, 400 MHz, 200 MHz and 100 MHz transducer [2]. Normal cellular detail, including cardiac myocytes, interstitial tissue, vascular endothelium, internal elastic lamina, media, adventitia, and pathological phenomena such as interstitial fibrosis, cell necrosis, cell fallout, and expansion of the intima with hypoechoic zones suggestive of fatty plaque were clearly seen with a 600 MHz transducer. These findings were confirmed by light microscopy. Although there was a slight decrease in resolution, normal and pathological phenomena were also identified with a 400 and 200 MHz transducer.

However, cellular detail could not be adequately identified with a 100 MHz transducer. From these preliminary studies, we concluded that transducer frequencies of 600 to 200 MHz enable visualization of cell detail in the myocardium and coronary artery. A transducer frequency of at least 200 MHz is probably required for *in vivo* application of this technique.

4.5.2   Acoustic Microscopy
4.5.2.6   Imaging Subsurface Cellular Detail in Thick Myocardial Specimens

Preliminary work done by our group has demonstrated the feasibility of imaging cellular architecture in thick myocardial sections [8].

In a series of experiments, we imaged full thickness specimens of normal myocardium with a 600, 400, 200 and 100 MHz transducer. Only the 200 MHz transducer produced a satisfactory image.

The acoustic lens was positioned above the endocardial surface of the myocardial specimen with a drop of deionized water coupling the lens to the surface of the sample. The acoustical pulse was focused within the tissue.

Once the tissue sample was acoustically imaged, it was embedded in paraffin and sectioned 5 µm thick in a plane parallel to the scanning plane, which was in fact parallel to the endocardium. The sections were stained with H & E and examined by light microscopy. By making serial fine adjustments of the focal plane, it was possible to image cardiac myocytes with reasonable clarity. The cardiac myocytes in ultrasound images of thick sections were mostly arranged longitudinally, and their appearance was similar to that obtained by light microscopy.

In summary, we were able to demonstrate that normal cardiac myocytes, the interstitium and a variety of pathological abnormalities can be imaged in exquisite detail using high-frequency ultrasound. Preliminary data generated in our laboratory suggest that in vivo imaging of cellular detail is probably feasible. Further development of this technique for *in vivo* use appears warranted.

References

1. Barr RJ, White GM, Jones JP, Shaw LB, Ross PA. Scanning acoustic microscopy of neoplastic and inflammatory cutaneous tissue specimens. J Invest Dermatol 1991; 96: 38-41.

2. Chandraratna PAN, Awaad MI, Khan M, Choudhary S, Jones JP, Gallet J. Myocardial imaging with high frequency ultrasound: observations on the minimum frequency required for imaging cellular detail. Circulation 1992; 86: 1-189.

3. Chandraratna PAN, Choudhary S, Jones J, Chandrasoma P, Rahimtoola SH, Gallet J: Imaging of normal and atherosclerotic coronary arteries by acoustic microscopy. Circulation 1991; 84: 11-371.

4. Chandraratna PAN, Choudhary S, Jones J, Kapoor A, Gallet J, Rahimtoola SH. Role of acoustic microscopy in detecting cardiac homograft rejection. Circulation 1991; 84: 11-373.

5. Chandraratna PAN, Choudhary S, Jones J. Visualization of isolated myocardial cells by acoustic microscopy. Circulation 1990; 82: 111-169.

6. Chandraratna PAN, Choudhary S, Jones JP, Chandrasoma P, Kapoor A, Gallet J. Acoustic microscopy of the myocardium. *Mit freundlicher Druckgenehmigung:* Am Heart J 1992; 124: 1358-1364.

7. Chandraratna PAN, Khan M, Chandrasoma P, Jones JP, Gallet J. Evaluation of myocardial microvasculature by high frequency ultrasound. Circulation 1992; 86: 1-575.

8. Chandraratna PAN, Mushtaq K, Awaad MI, Jones JP, Gallet J. Comparison of backscatter images of myocardial cells generated by high frequency ultrasound with light microscopic findings. Circulation 1992; 86: 1-575.

9. Hildebrand JA, Rugar D, Johnston RN, Quate Cl. Acoustic microscopy of living cells. Proc Natl Acad Sci U.S.A. 1981; 78: 1656-1660.

10. Johnston RN, Atalar, A, Heiserman J, Jipson V, Quate Cl. Acoustic microscopy: resolution of subcellular detail. Proc Natl Acad Sci U.S.A. 1979; 76: 3325-3329.

11. Lemons RA, Quate CF. Acoustic microscope - scanning version. Appl Phys Letter 1974; 24: 163-165.

12. Neild TO, Attal J, Saurel JM. Images of aterioles in unfixed tissue obtained by acoustic microscopy. J Micros 1985; 139: 19-25.

13. Sokolov. USSR patent no. 49 (August 31, 1936), British patent no. 477 139, 1937, und US patent no. 21 64, 125: 1939.

In cardiac ultrasound different image textures result from different acoustic properties of the examined structures. Theoretically, any substance with variable echogeneity can be used as an echo contrast agent.

For clinical use, the echo contrast agent must meet the following requirements:

1. Must be well tolerated
2. Must form stable solutions and have uniform particle size.
3. Must provide uniform opacification
4. Must be reproducible
5. Must be suitable for intravascular administration
   (intravenous, intra-arterial, intraaortic, intracoronary)

Contrast echocardiography is used to detect and assess the following diseases and to achieve the following clinical goals:

Indications for Contrast Echocardiography

Applicable Echocardiographic Techniques

▸ *2-D and M-mode echocardiography*
▸ Transthoracic and transesophageal echocardiography
▸ In combination with conventional (CW/PW) Doppler
▸ In combination with Doppler color flow imaging

Diseases and Clinical Goals

▸ Tricuspid insufficiency, pulmonary insufficiency
▸ Atrial septal defect
▸ Ventricular septal defect, ventricular septal rupture
▸ Patent foramen ovale

▸ Complex congenital heart diseases
▸ Suspected cardiac origin in cerebral embolism
▸ Patent ductus arteriosus
▸ Pulmonary valvular disease
▸ Persistent left upper vena cava

▸ Identification and topographic localization of questionable structures

▸ Improved detection of left and right ventricular endocardial contours

▸ Myocardial perfusion

The materials required for contrast echocardiography are listed in the table below.

Materials for Contrast Echocardiography

▸ Echo contrast agent
▸ Cannula suitable for peripheral venous access (*e.g.* Abboth®, Braunüle®, Butterfly®), or other access (*e.g.* intravenous, intra-arterial, intra-aortic, or intracoronary)
▸ Materials for fixation of cannula
▸ 50 to 100 ml of 0.9% NaCl as flush solution
▸ 10 or 20 ml syringes
▸ Three-way cock to connect syringes to the cannula

The examination procedure can be summarized as follows:

Examination Procedure
1. History, particularly any history of allergies (previous allergic reaction to echo contrast agents, radiographic contrast agents, albumin, saccharides, or infusions?).
2. Children: Written parental consent must be obtained beforehand.
3. A rapid injection of ca. 5 to 10 ml of contrast agent is injected (peripheral venous injection) is immediately followed by an injection of 5 to 10 ml of 0.9% NaCl flush solution. The procedure is repeated approx. 4 to 5 times from different imaging views, depending on the diagnostic questions to be clarified.
The entire examination sequence is recorded on video tape.

5.1   Contrast Echocardiography
5.1.1   Physical Characteristics of Echo Contrast Agents

Spontaneous contrast effects are often observed in the left atrium and left ventricle of patients with mitral valve defects or prosthetic mitral valves and in patients with poor left ventricular function. Similar to the „sludge" phenomena observed in gallbladder sonography, *echocardiographic „smoke"* may extend through the left atrium or ventricle, even through no contrast agent has been injected. This is thought to occur primarily due to the interaction of erythrocytes and plasma proteins during low flow states and in dead water zones, and in conjunction with low kinematic viscosity, *i.e.*, low shear forces [21]. Spontaneous contrast effects are thought to be an indicator of patients at risk for clot formation and other thrombo-embolic conditions. Anticoagulatory treatment must therefore be taken into consideration when this observation is made.

Echo contrast effects were more or less accidentally discovered by Gramiak, Shah, and Kramer, who observed these effects while rinsing an inserted cardiac catheter with saline solu-tion with the echocardiograph in operation [12, 13]. Many experimental trials with various echo contrast agents were to follow [17, 22].

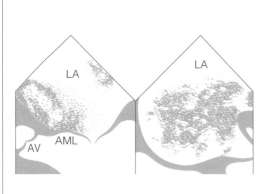

Spontaneous contrast effects in the left atrium.

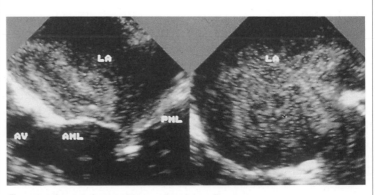

Transesophageal short and long-axis echocardiograms.

Echo contrast agents can be roughly grouped as follows:
1. Aqueous solutions
2. Emulsions
3. Colloid suspensions
4. Free gas bubbles (usually microbubbles)
5. Encapsulated gas bubbles (usually microbubbles)

The echogeneic properties of echo contrast agents are due to the inclusion of air micro-bubbles in a more or less stable carrier substance. Microbubbles in the solution are created by means of *sonication, i.e.* by application of high-frequency ultrasound, or by manually shaking and agitating the solution with or without the help of syringes.

Experimental studies have shown that the reflection of ultrasound from air bubbles plays a minor role in producing the desired contrast effects, as compared with the summation of scatter on the surface of the microbubbles due to acoustically effective inhomogeneities in the substance. The sudden change in impedance at the gas-liquid interface is extreme. The particle size and the transmitter frequency to be used are determined by the degree of im-pedance difference. When, for example, the impedance difference is only slight, larger par-ticles and a higher transmitter frequency must be used [11].

Various physical factors such as gas pressure, temperature, and viscosity affect the density, size, and distribution of the microbubbles in a given carrier substance.

A multitude of substances have been tested for right and left-heart contrast effects. They include microfoam from agitated or sonicated solutions, gas-filled hollow microspheres from pretreated human serum albumin, and microbubble-containing suspensions produced with α-D(+)-galactose microparticles.

Echo contrast agents

- 0.9% NaCl, with and without CO_2
- Agitated 0.9% NaCl solution
- 5-10% glucose
- Fat emulsions
- Agitated gelatine solutions (such as oxypolygelatines, Gelifundol®)
- H_2O_2
- Patient's own blood mixed with saline solution
- Radiographic contrast agents (such as meglumine diatrizoate® and Renografin®)
- Dyes (such as *indocyanine green*)
- Perfluorocytylbromide
- Pretreated human serum albumin, 5% (such as Albunex®)
- α-D(+)-galactose microparticles (such as Echovist®, or Laevovist® – galenically modified for lung passage)

The best documented and commercially most readily available echo contrast agents are the one containing air-filled human serum albumin microspheres and saccharide microparticles with entrapped microbubbles in an aqueous solution. In around two-thirds of all cases, Albu-nex® leads to complete or partial opacification of the left heart cavities. Echovist® provides isolated right-heart opacification, and Laevovist® provides sequential right and left-heart o-pacification. None of the lung-specific echo contrast agents provide reproducible opacifica-tion of the myocardium when administered via peripheral venous injection. Therefore, a cen-tral injection site or another method of signal analysis must be used is those cases.

Most of the currently available echo contrast agents opacify only the right heart. This is because they do not traverse the pulmonary capillary bed, but dissolve within a few seconds due to the drop in concentration that occurs when they are diluted in plasma [4]. A substance capable of isolated opacification of the left-heart cavities would be desirable.

Tricuspid Insufficiency

Tricuspid insufficiency can be diagnosed by either Doppler or contrast echocardiographic studies. With contrast echocardiography, the diagnosis is made using two-dimensional or M-mode echocardiograms obtained from multiple views. Microbubbles that circulate between the right atrium and ventricle, or the cloud of contrast medium below the tricuspid valve closed in systole can be observed on these echocardiograms. In severe tricuspid insufficiency, retrograde flow extends as far as the inferior vena cava and/or the hepatic veins. In these cases, echo contrast effects can also be observed in these veins in echocardiograms obtained from the subcostal route.

The specificity and sensitivity of contrast echocardiography for diagnosis of tricuspid insufficiency shows a wide range of variation [3, 20, 25]. Furthermore, the introduction of Doppler ultrasound has made it possible to obtain direct proof of tricuspid insufficiency [6]. Therefore, contrast echocardiography is now almost exclusively reserved for special diagnostic problems, to enhance the Doppler signal, or in hospitals without Doppler systems.

Atrial Septal Defects

Atrial septal defects are classified according to their location:
• Ostium primum defects (ASD-I), located near the atrioventricular canal
• Ostium secundum defects (ASD-II), located in the mid to upper atrial septum
• Sinus venosus defects, located high in the atrium septum
• Patent foramen ovale.

Sinus venosus defects cannot be visualized from a transthoracic access. Atrial septal defects of the ostium primum and secundum type (ASD-I and II) are also difficult to detect 1) because they are very small, and 2) because it is difficult to distinguish between true defects and dropout in images of the interarterial septum obtained from tangential apical projections. Contrast echocardiography therefore plays an important role in the diagnosis of these defects. Method-related problems make color Doppler echocardiography very unreliable for this task.

In patients without concomitant Eisenmenger's syndrome, the majority of shunts flow from left to right. The defects can then be identified as a zone of *negative contrast effect* or „washout". The left-to-right shunt causes washout of contrast medium in a part of the right atrium adjacent to the interatrial septum. This area of washout, or negative contrast effect, corresponds to the site of the atrial septal defect. However, since a small right-to-left shunt usually coexists, the contrast agent „leaks" into the other cavity. This leakage is intensified by early diastolic suction phenomena. Therefore, the atrial septal defect can be detected, even in the absence of a negative contrast effect. A temporary increase in right ventricular pressure can be provoked by having the patient cough, or by performing Valsalva's maneuver. This enhances contrast agent leakage effects.

However, depending on the site of the defect, it sometimes is impossible to identify the location of the defect, even with the help of contrast echocardiography [2, 10].

Contrast transesophageal echocardiography (contrast TEE) is the most precise method for obtaining morphological proof of an atrial septal defect. Contrast TEE usually permits direct visualization and assessment of the defect [14]. The diagnostic results can be optimized by combining contrast TEE with Doppler color flow imaging.

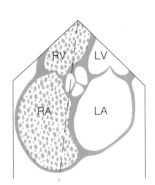

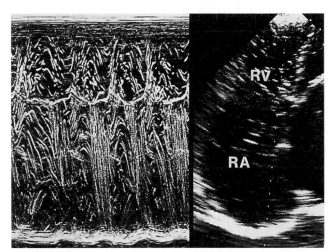

Tricuspid insufficiency. Opacification of the right ventricle (RV) and right atrium (RA) (right panel). Systolic contrast effects below the tricuspid valve (left panel).

M-mode (left) and 2-D echocardiograms (right); apical four-chamber view.

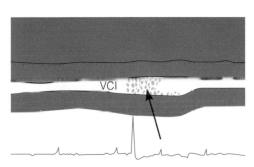

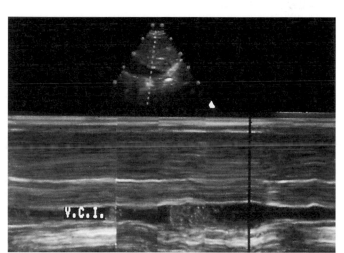

Opacification of the inferior vena cava (VCI) and a hepatic vein demonstrating severe tricuspid insufficiency.

Subcostal 2-D echocardiogram through the inferior vena cava (V.C.I.) and a hepatic vein.

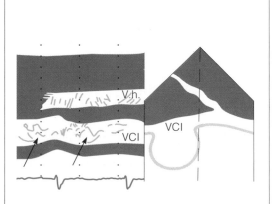

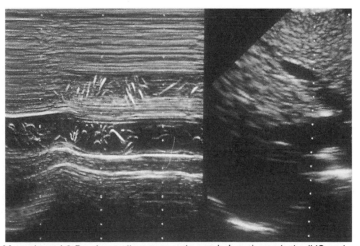

Tricuspid insufficiency. Systolic contrast effects are seen as fine white lines in venous vessels.

M-mode and 2-D echocardiograms; subcostal view through the IVC and a hepatic vein (HV).

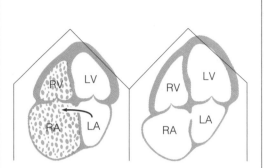

Negative contrast effect in ostium primum defect (ASD-I). The interatrial septum is hardly recognizable. Homogeneous opacification of dilated right heart cavities. The small zone of negative contrast effect above the atrioventricular valve plane corresponds to the location of the ASD-I.

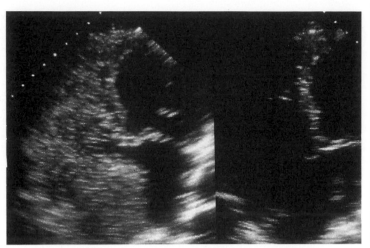

Apical four-chamber views. Before and after contrast injection.

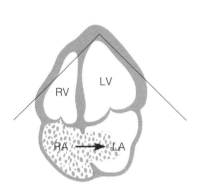

Ostium secundum defect (ASD-II) with right-to-left shunt (positive contrast effect). Isolated microbubbles also detected in left ventricle.

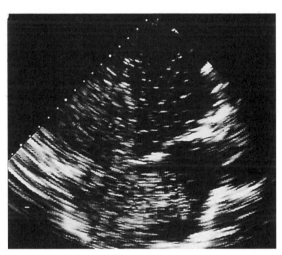

Apical four-chamber view. Injection of contrast agent (oxypolygelatine).

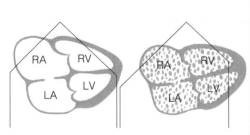

ASD-II with crossed shunt. Left panel: Suspicion of atrial septal defect. Right atrium dilated. Right panel: Uniform opacification of all four heart cavities.

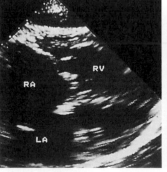 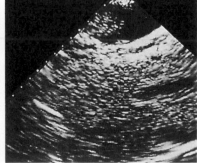

Subcostal four-chamber 2-D echocardiograms before and after injection of contrast agent (oxypolygelatine).

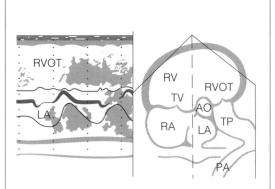

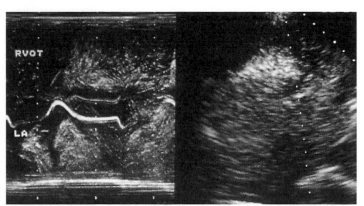

ASD-II. Left: Intense opacification of right ventricular outflow tract and left atrium; contrast agent also passes through the mitral valve. Right: Opacification of all four heart cavities.

Contrast M-mode and 2-D echocardiograms, parasternal short axis view, with M-mode cursor placed in the right ventricular outflow tract and left atrium.

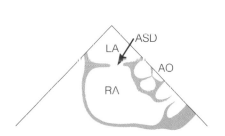

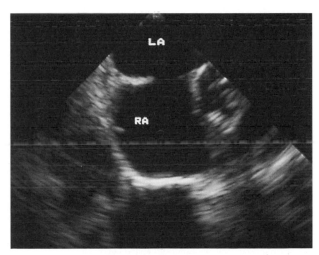

ASD-II. Defect in the medial part of the interarterial septum.

Transesophageal short-axis (transverse) view through both atria.

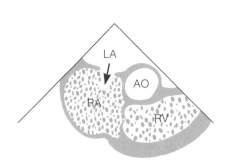

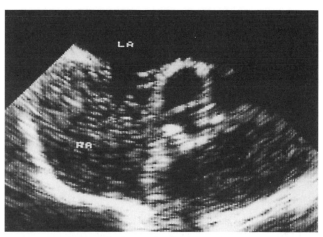

ASD-II. Opacification of the right atrium with negative contrast effect proximal to the septum.

Contrast transesophageal short-axis (transverse) scan through both atria.

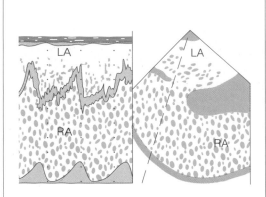

ASD-II. Left panel: Interatrial septum appears as a bold echo line dividing the uniformly opacified right and left atria. Isolated microbubbles detected in the left atrium. Right panel: Uniform opacification of the right cardiac cavities; contrast agent also detected in the left atrium.

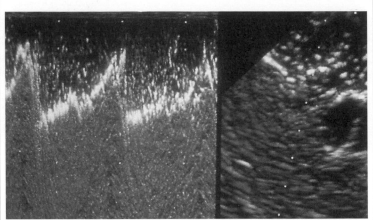

Contrast transesophageal short-axis M-mode and 2-D echocardiograms.

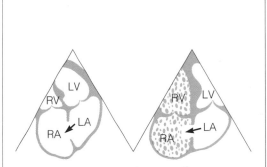

Aneurysm of the interatrial septum. Left panel: Marked discontinuity of the interatrial septum and dilated atria. After the injection of contrast agent, right-sided aneurysmal dilation of the interatrial septum is observed, but no contrast agent leakage. Atrial septal defect can therefore be excluded.

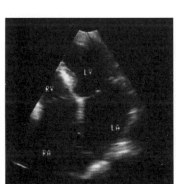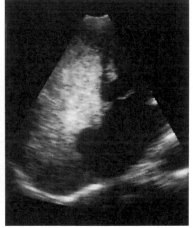

Apical four-chamber echocardiograms before and after contrast injection.

Ventricular Septal Defects

Contrast echocardiography can also be used to detect a shunt at the level of the ventricle [8]. However, it is often very difficult to identify negative contrast effects in this case. Furthermore, right-to-left shunts usually occur only in very large shunts.

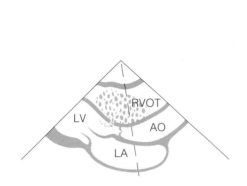

Ventricular septal defect (VSD). Opacification of the right ventricle. No contrast agent leakage.

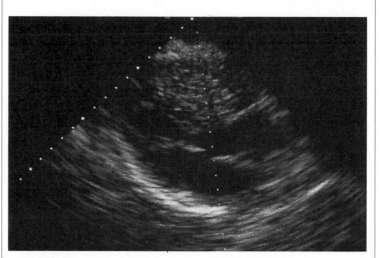

Contrast echocardiography with parasternal long-axis 2-D echocardiogram.

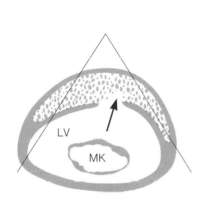

VSD. Opacification of the right ventricle. In the presence of a left-to-right shunt, a negative contrast effect occurs at the junction of the anterior wall and the lateral wall proximal to the septum.

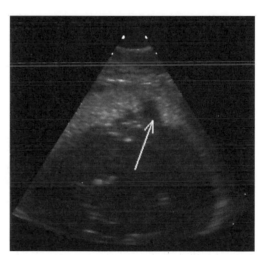

Contrast echocardiography with parasternal short-axis 2-D echocardiogram.

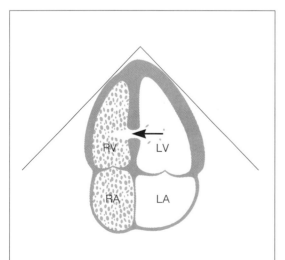

Negative contrast effect: „washout" phenomenon characteristic of VSD.

When Valsalva's maneuver is performed, contrast agent leakage should occur immediately after the contrast injection, because subsequent slight opacification of the left atrium almost always occurs due to the physiological intrapulmonary shunt. Since the significance of the finding of patent foramen ovale is still being debated, larger scale studies must be performed to clarify this issue [7, 15, 17, 26].

Patent Foramen Ovale

A patent foramen ovale is found at autopsy in 25% of all cases. The incidence of patent foramen ovale is significantly higher in patients with cerebral ischemia. An unexplained cerebral embolism always raises the question of a crossed embolism through a patent foramen ovale. One can attempt to make the diagnosis of patent foramen ovale from the transesophageal route. However, it frequently is not possible to determine whether the foramen ovale is patent, not even with the help of Doppler color flow imaging.

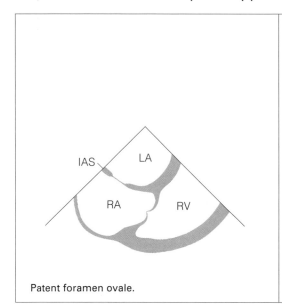

Patent foramen ovale.

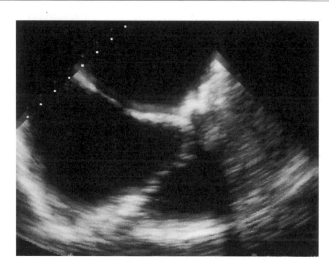

Transesophageal short-axis (transverse) echocardiogram.

Contrast transesophageal echocardiography (contrast TEE) can provide an unequivocal diagnosis: After performing an obligatory Valsalva's maneuver, the contrast agent immediately leaks from the fossa ovalis into the left atrium.

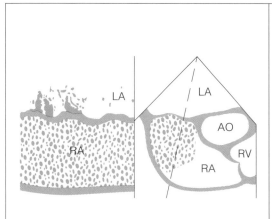

Patent foramen ovale. Right panel: Slice through the interatrial septum in the region of the fossa ovalis. Left panel: Intense opacification of the right atrium and immediate but slight leakage of contrast agent into the left atrium.

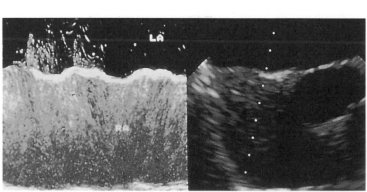

Transesophageal short-axis M-mode and 2-D echocardiograms.

In order for an echo contrast agent to be capable of crossing the pulmonary vascular bed, its microbubbles must be much more stable that those suitable for right-heart opacification. Transpulmonary contrast agents such as Levovist® provide opacification of both right and left heart cavities and, when administered in low doses, only increase the Doppler signal intensity.

| 5.1 | Contrast Echocardiography |
| 5.1.4 | Myocardial Contrast Echocardiography |

Contrast enhancement of the myocardium can be achieved by injecting a contrast agent into the pulmonary capillary bed or into the aortic root. However, none of the myocardial contrast agents on the market to date have been approved for routine use in humans [5, 18, 23]. Impressive defects in myocardial perfusion could be demonstrated in animal experiments. Further experiments must be performed in order to determine whether peripheral venous injections of transpulmonary echo contrast agents will be able to provide sufficiently uniform enhancement of the myocardium [9].

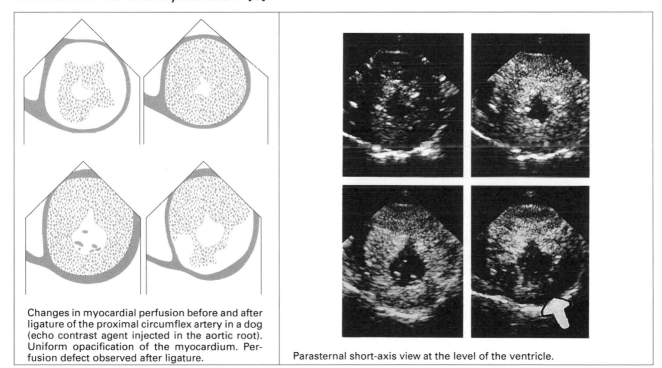

Changes in myocardial perfusion before and after ligature of the proximal circumflex artery in a dog (echo contrast agent injected in the aortic root). Uniform opacification of the myocardium. Perfusion defect observed after ligature.

Parasternal short-axis view at the level of the ventricle.

5.1	Contrast Echocardiography
5.1.5	Future Perspectives of Contrast Echocardiography
	(Kurt J.G. Schmailzl)

Contrast echocardiography primarily expands the means of diagnosing right-heart defects and complex congenital heart diseases that otherwise must be diagnosed indirectly using conventional M-mode and two-dimensional echocardiographic techniques. An extremely low rate of severe side effects has been reported [1].

Although introduction of Doppler echocardiography has reduced the range of indications for contrast echocardiography, it is still a powerful tool for diagnosing shunts and complex congenital heart defects. Contrast echocardiography is even more effective when combined with transesophageal echocardiography and color Doppler techniques.

The future perspectives for contrast echocardiography include evaluation of myocardial perfusion and calculation of blood flow [16]. The quantitation of tissue perfusion according to the principles of contrast agent dilution methodologies assume the observed tissue passage time is constant as long as the volume of injectate and flow remain unchanged. This has led to some unsolved method-related problems. With currently available ultrasound technologies, instrument settings and output must be varied according to the individual acoustic conditions in order to obtain optimal images. The result of this, however, is that low contrast agent concentrations may be overlooked and that this will have an effect on the observed tissue passage time. An unsolved question is how to most reliably perform contrast echocardiographic quantitation of relative flow - by contrast agent dilution curve analysis, videodensitometry, radiofrequency signal analysis, or Doppler audio signal analysis? The degree of mixation of blood and echo contrast agent and, thus, the flooded cross-sectional area may have significant effects which are more favorable in the case of smaller vessels such as the coronary arteries, and less favorable in larger vessels such as the aorta.

Further potentials lie in the combination of echo contrast agents with direct intraluminal injections. The lumen or the cavity then becomes highly echo-dense, and measurements of vessel and cavity diameters could be improved by the better visualization conditions.

References

1. Bommer WJ, Shah PM, Allen H, Meltzer R, Kisslo J. The safety of contrast echocardiography. J Am Coll Cardiol 1984; 3: 6-13.
2. Bourdillon PDV, Foale RA, Rickards AF. Identification of atrial septal defects by cross-sectional contrast echocardiography. Br Heart J 1980; 44: 401-405.
3. Brown AK, Anderson V. The value of contrast cross-sectional echocardiography in the diagnosis of tricuspid regurgitation. Eur Heart J 1984; 5: 62-66.
4. Butler BD, Hills BA. The lung as a filter for microbubbles. J Appl Physiol 1979; 47: 537-543.
5. Corday E, Shah PM, Meerbaum S. Seminar on contrast two-dimensional echocardiography: application and new developments. Part I. J Am Coll Cardiol 1984; 3: 1-5.
6. Curtius JM, Thyssen M, Breuer HM, Loogen F. Doppler versus contrast echocardiography for diagnosis of tricuspid regurgitation. Am J Cardiol 1985; 56: 333-336.
7. Decodt P, Kacenelenbogen R, Heuse D. Detection of patent foramen ovale in stroke by transoesophageal contrast echocardiography. Circulation 1989; 80: II-339.
8. Detrano R, Salcedo EE, Yiannikas J, Moodie DS. Contrast two-dimensional echocardiography in the diagnosis of adult congenital heart disease. Cleve Clin 1985; 52: 229-238.
9. Feinstein SB, Cheirif J, Ten Cate FJ, Sivermann PR, Heidenreich PA, Dick C, Desir RM, Armstrong WF, Quinones MA, Shah PM. Safety and efficacy of a new transpulmonary ultrasound contrast agent: initial multicenter clinical result. J Am Coll Cardiol 1990; 16: 316-324.
10. Fraker TD, Harris PJ, Behar VS, Kisslo JA. Detection and exclusion of interatrial shunts by two-dimensional echocardiography and peripheral venous injection. Circulation 1979; 59: 379-384.
11. Fritsch T, Schartl M, Siegert J. Kontrast-Echokardiografie des rechten und linken Herzens nach intravenöser Injektion standardisierter Mikrobläschen. In: Grube E (ed). Farbdoppler und Kontrast-Echo- kardiografie 1988; 354-367.
12. Gramiak R, Shah PM. Echocardiography of the aortic root. Invest Radiol 1968; 3: 356-366.
13. Gramiak R, Shah PM, Kramer DH. Ultrasond cardiography. Contrast studies in anatomy and function. Radiology; 92: 939-948.
14. Hanrath P, Schlüter M, Langenstein BA. Detection of ostium secundum atrial septum defects by transoesophageal cross-sectional echocardiography. Br Heart J 1983; 49: 350-358.
15. Hausmann D, Muegge A, Becht I, Daniel WG. Patent foramen ovale diagnosed by echocardiography: high prevalence in young adults with stroke or peripheral embolism. Am J Cardiol 1991; 17: 143A.

16. Heidenreich PA, Wieneck JG, Zaroff JG, Aronson S, Segil LJ, Harper PV, Feinstein SB. In vitro calculation of flow by use of contrast ultrasonography. J Am Soc Echo 1993; 6: 51-61.
17. Lechat PH, Mas JL, Lascout G. Prevalence of patent foramen ovale in patients with stroke. N Engl J Med 1988; 318: 1148-1152.
18. Lim YJ, Nanto S, Masuyama T, Kodama K, Ikeda T, Kitabatake A, Kamada T. Visualization of subendocardial myocardial ischemia with myocardial contrast echocardiography in humans. Circulation 1989; 79: 223-244.
19. Meltzer RS, Tickner EG, Sahines TP, Popp RL. Source of ultrasond contrast effect. J Clin Ultrasound 1980; 8: 121-127.
20. Meltzer RS, van Hoogehuyze D, Serruys PW, Haalebos MMP, Hugenholz PG, Roelandt J. Diagnosis of tricuspid regurgitation by contrast echocardiography. Circulation 1981; 63: 1093-1099.
21. Merino A, Hauptmann P, Badimon L, Badimon JJ, Cohen M, Fuster V, Goldman M. Echocardiographic 'smoke' is produced by an interaction of erythrocytes and plasma proteins modulated by shear forces. J Am Coll Cardiol 1992; 20: 1661-1668.
22. Ophir J, Parker KJ. Contrast agents in diagnostic ultrasound. Ultrasound Med Biol 1989; 15: 319-333.
23. Shapiro JR, Reisner SA, Amico AF, Kelly FP, Meltzer RS. Reproducibility of quantitative myocardial contrast echocardiography. J Am Coll Cardiol 1990; 15: 602-609.
24. Willard GW. Ultrasonically induced cavitation in water. J Acoust Soc Am 1953; 25: 669-686.
25. Wise NK, Myers S, Fraker TD, Stewart JA, Kisslo JA. Contrast m-mode ultrasonography of the inferior vena cava. Circulation 1981; 63: 1100-1103.
26. Zhu W, Khandheria BK, Click RL. Patent foramen ovale detected by contrast transoesophageal echo; a lack of association with systemic events. Circulation 1989; 84: II-694.

5.	**Interventional Echocardiography**
5.2	**Stress Echocardiography**
	(Ursula Wilkenshoff)

Stress echocardiography is a relatively new method for detection and assessment of coronary artery disease [65]. *Exercise electrocardiography* frequently cannot be performed in patients with vascular, neurologic, and orthopedic diseases, and unsatisfactory results are obtained in patients with such primary ECG limitations as pre-excitation syndrome, mitral valve prolapse, left bundle-branch block, left heart hypertrophy, and digitalis-related repolarization disturbances. In these cases, stress echocardiography often provides a very helpful supplementary technique [12, 70].

5.2	**Stress Echocardiography**
5.2.1	**Pathophysiology of Ischemia**

Myocardial ischemia leads to dysfunction in the undersupplied region. Contractile dysfunction arises as a result of the reduced systolic wall thickness. Since echocardiography makes it possible to visualize and evaluate regional wall motion, ischemia can be detected as a wall motion disturbance [6].

The temporal sequence of myocardial ischemia has been described as a hierarchically ordered cascade of various markers of ischemia [28, 43]. According to this model, heterogeneity of subendocardial and subepicardial perfusion occurs, followed by metabolic changes and diastolic dysfunction. As the muscle becomes increasingly ischemic, systolic dysfunction with regional contractile dysfunction occurs, followed by typical ECG changes, global left ventricular dysfunction, and angina pectoris symptoms.

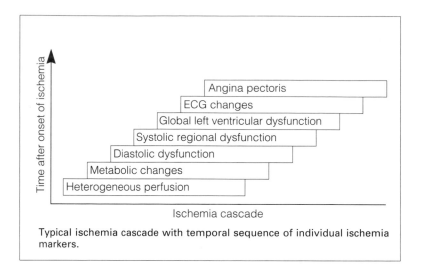

Typical ischemia cascade with temporal sequence of individual ischemia markers.

In experimental ischemia, a close correlation between the extent of transmural blood flow and myocardial wall thickening was found [31, 60]. It was shown that wall motion abnormalities can be detected by echocardiography when the blood flow in more than 5% of the myocardial mass is reduced by 50% [6].

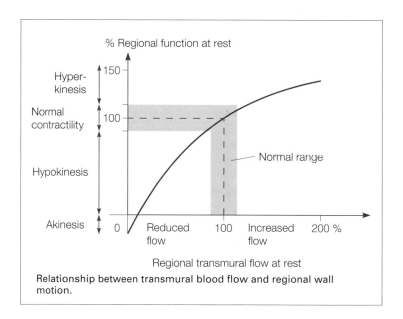

Relationship between transmural blood flow and regional wall motion.

Post-ischemic recovery is dependent on the duration of ischemia and the degree of reperfusion. When transient ischemia is caused by severe coronary stenosis, underperfusion and myocardial dysfunction may persist even after ischemia has disappeared. In some cases, contractile dysfunction may persist for hours, days, or even weeks after perfusion has been restored. The reperfused but still dysfunctional postischemic myocardium is referred to as the *stunned myocardium* [13]. In contrast, in the *hibernating myocardium* myocardial perfusion is chronically reduced but still able to maintain myocardial viability and reduced but sufficient myocardial function. In both stunned and hibernating myocardium, positively inotropic substances have been shown to improve reduced myocardial function [14]. However, in myocardial infarction with subsequent tissue necrosis, neither positively inotropic substances, nor a blood flow increase, nor a blood flow decrease had a direct effect on myocardial function.

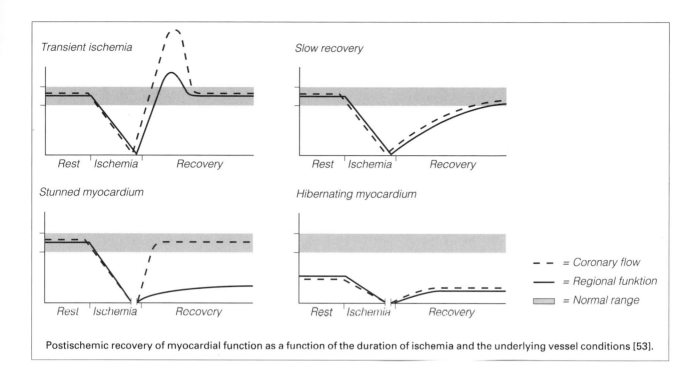

Postischemic recovery of myocardial function as a function of the duration of ischemia and the underlying vessel conditions [53].

5.2 Stress Echocardiography
5.2.2 Echocardiographic Detection of Ischemic Response

According to Picano [53], an ischemic response in the left ventricle can be detected by echocardiography as follows:

- Systolic dysfunction expressed as wall motion abnormality on 2-D echocardiograms.
- Systolic dysfunction expressed as reduced aortic flow velocity on CW Doppler recordings.
- Diastolic dysfunction expressed as a change in the mitral inflow profile (E/A ratio) in PW Doppler recordings.
- Global left ventricular dysfunction expressed as a new mitral regurgitant jet in Doppler color flow images.

Normal myocardial contractions are characterized by systolic thickening and endocardial inwards motion towards the center of the ventricle. Ischemic myocardial muscle is characterized by the following wall motion abnormalities at rest and during exercise :

- Hypokinesis
- Akinesis
- Dyskinesis

Wall thickening and inward motion of the endocardium are significantly decreased in hypokinesis, and completely fail to occur in akinesis. Dyskinesis is marked by systolic outward motion of the endocardium. In hyperkinesis, on the other hand, both systolic wall thickening and inward motion of the endocardium are more pronounced.

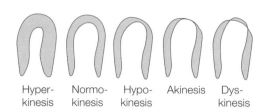

Hyper-kinesis   Normo-kinesis   Hypo-kinesis   Akinesis   Dys-kinesis

Myocardial contractility: *normokinesis* = normal inward motion and thickening of the myocardium; *hyperkinesis* = increased inward motion and thickening; *hypokinesis, akinesis, dyskinesis* = regional wall motion abnormality with regionally reduced, absent, or reversed wall motion).

Wall motion abnormalities that are present even in a resting state (*e.g.* nonuniform or abnormal septal motion after surgery or in patients with left bundle-branch block) may limit the use of inward motion of the endocardium as a criterion for ischemic muscle. However, this usually does not limit the use of wall thickening [73]. Furthermore, a hypokinetic wall segment may remain undetected when influenced by the movement of normally contracting adjacent segments.

Left ventricular size is another criterion for ischemic muscle. Pronounced ventricular dilation occurs in severe ischemia with global left ventricular dysfunction. However, left ventricular dysfunction occurs relatively late in the ischemia cascade, and is preceded by regional localized wall disturbances. Left ventricular size is therefore a less specific marker.

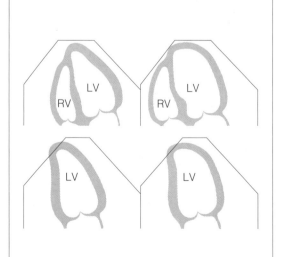

Postischemic dilation of the left ventricle in dipyridamole echocardiograms.

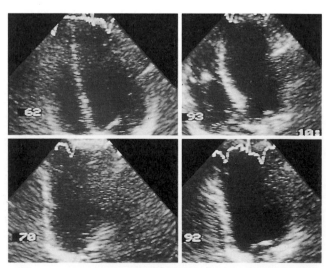

Apical four-chamber (upper panels) and two-chamber echocardiograms (lower panels) before (left) and after (right) dipyridamole injection.

During ischemia the peak aortic flow velocity and the velocity integral are reduced as an expression of systolic left ventricular function [45]. The change in heart rate also affects the aortic flow velocity.

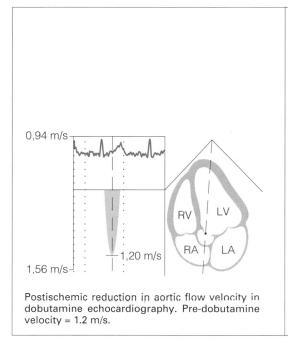

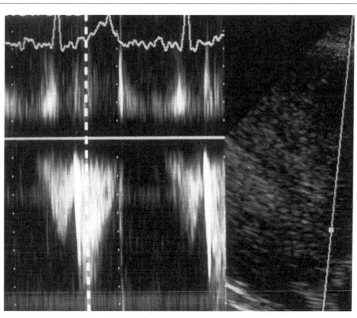

Postischemic reduction in aortic flow velocity in dobutamine echocardiography. Pre-dobutamine velocity = 1.2 m/s.

CW Doppler recording and apical four-chamber 2-D echocardiogram.

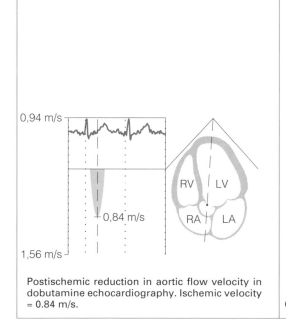

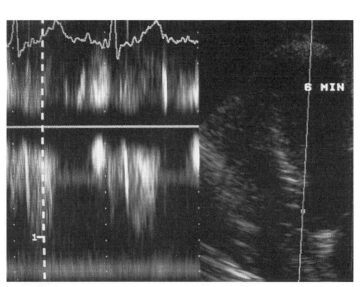

Postischemic reduction in aortic flow velocity in dobutamine echocardiography. Ischemic velocity = 0.84 m/s.

CW Doppler recording and apical four-chamber 2-D echocardiogram.

The mitral inflow profile may also be affected by an ischemic response: the E wave then decreases as the A wave increases, thereby reducing the E/A ratio [45, 55, 72]. Although diastolic dysfunction and an altered E/A ratio occur relatively early (see ischemia cascade), this marker is influenced by a number of factors and is, thus, limited in predictive value. First, the E to A wave velocity varies when the position of the sample volume changes. Second, an increase in heart rate unites both waves, and hemodynamic changes (compliance vs. relaxation disturbances) also affect the E/A ratio even in absence of ischemia.

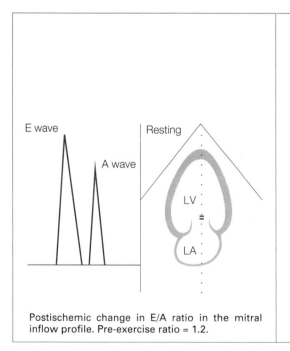

Postischemic change in E/A ratio in the mitral inflow profile. Pre-exercise ratio = 1.2.

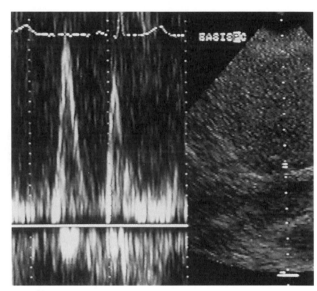

PW Doppler recording.

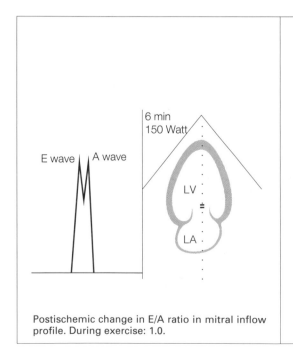

Postischemic change in E/A ratio in mitral inflow profile. During exercise: 1.0.

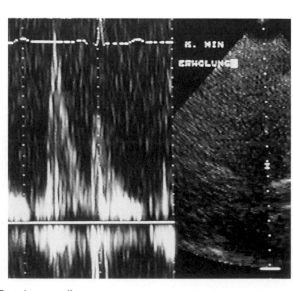

PW Doppler recording.

E wave

A wave

6 min recovery

LV

LA

Postischemic change in E/A ratio in mitral inflow profile. Postischemic value > 1.0.

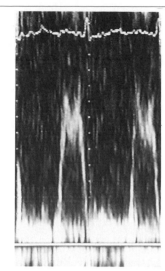

PW Doppler recording.

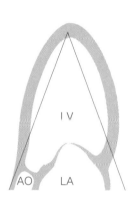

New region of ischemic mitral regurgitation after exercise-induced global systolic dysfunction of the left ventricle: resting state.

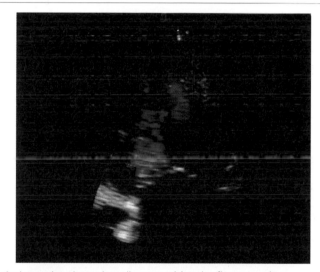

Apical two-chamber echoardiogram with color flow mapping.

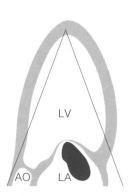

New region of ischemic mitral regurgitation after exercise-induced global systolic dysfunction of the left ventricle: mitral insufficiency.

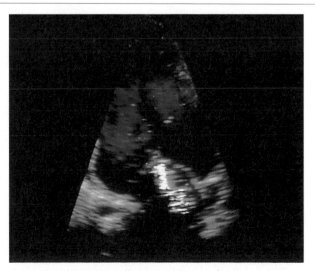

Apical two-chamber echoardiogram with color flow mapping.

Relative mitral insufficiency, which can be detected using CW Doppler and color Doppler techniques, may also occur when global systolic dysfunction occurs in severely ischemic muscle. Several studies have shown that Doppler examinations do not improve the effectiveness of stress echocardiography in diagnosing ischemia [8, 71].

However, Doppler measurements do provide additional diagnostic information. Only two-dimensional echocardiography, which provides visualization of ischemia-related wall motion abnormalities, is capable of identifying ischemia *per se.*

| 5.2 | Stress Echocardiography |
| 5.2.3 | Left Ventricular Wall Motion Analysis |

The advantage of two-dimensional echocardiography is that the left ventricle can be visualized from multiple views, anatomic levels, and angles. Parasternal long and short axis views and two and four-chamber views have proven to be the best scanning planes for stress echocardiography. The short axis should be scanned at the level of the papillary muscles. The *American Society of Echocardiography* recommends a 16 segment model for assessment of the left ventricle [22].

As is shown in the figure below, the anterior, lateral and inferior walls of the left ventricle are divided into apical, medial (distal), and basal segments. From the ventricular long axis, the posterior and anteroseptal walls are divided into basal and medial segments only.

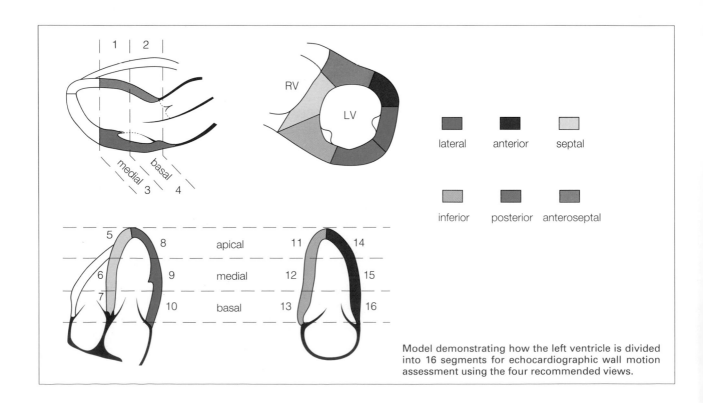

Model demonstrating how the left ventricle is divided into 16 segments for echocardiographic wall motion assessment using the four recommended views.

In cases where the posterior wall cannot be adequately assessed from the parasternal long-axis view, we recommend imaging the posterior wall from the apical long-axis view.

The *American Society of Echocardiography* makes the following recommendations for 2-D echocardiographic quantitation of left ventricular wall motion at rest and during exercise [64].

1 = Normokinesis
2 = Hypokinesis
3 = Akinesis
4 = Dyskinesis

The *wall motion index* is calculated by summing the scores determined for all the individual wall segments and dividing this figure by the number of segments studied. For example: in normal left ventricular contractility, the total motion score (16) is divided by the sum of evaluated segments (n=16) to yield an index score of 1. A wall motion index score greater than 1 is an indicator of abnormal left ventricular contractility.

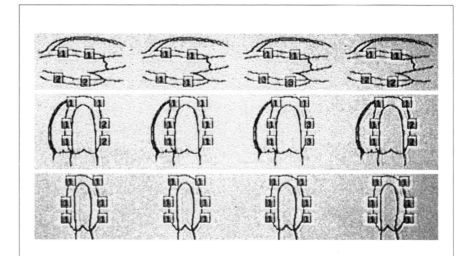

Echocardiographic calculation of the wall motion index at various stages of stress.

Stage 1: At rest, there is reduced LV contractility with hypokinesis (= 2) of the basal and posterolateral segments (index = (4 x 2 + 12 x 1)/16 = 1.25.
Stage 2: A low dose of dobutamine normalizes contractility (index = 1.0).
Stage 3: The maximum dose of dobutamine provokes akinesis in the posterolateral segment (index = 1.5).
Stage 4: In the recovery phase the baseline contractility is reached with hypokinesis of the posterolateral wall (index = 1.25).

The wall motion indices for pre-stress (resting), peak stress, and other stages of stress can be compared. The extent and severity of ischemia can be assessed by comparing resting and stress indices. Step-by-step documentation of the development of ischemia can be obtained by making multiple determinations of the wall motion index during stress conditions. The resting wall motion index provides information as to global LV function. It is also a suitable parameter for following left ventricular dysfunction before and after interventional revascularization and particularly when conservative treatment of acute myocardial infarction is preferred. In order to properly assess the results of stress echocardiography, the physician must understand the distribution of coronary arteries supplying each segment of the left ventricle.

The following figure demonstrates the 16 left ventricular wall segments and their corresponding supply vessels [20]. There is some overlap, which must be considered when making assessments.

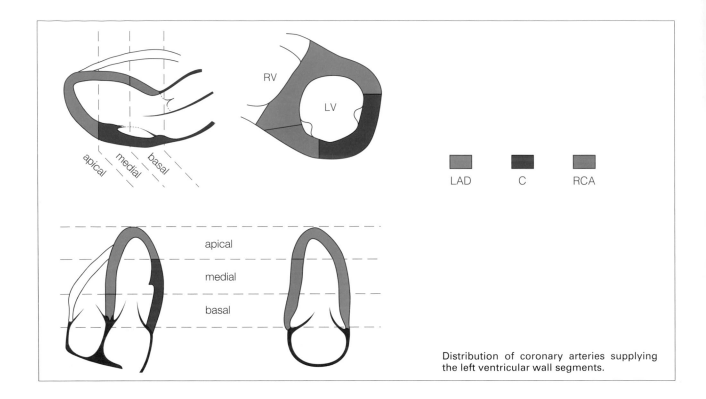

Distribution of coronary arteries supplying the left ventricular wall segments.

5.2 Stress Echocardiography
5.2.4 Interpretation of Stress Echocardiograms

In a resting normal left ventricle, the dobutamine test is negative when hypercontractility is provoked under stress, and is positive when the contractility of a given wall segment remains normal under stress, *i.e.,* when there is not a sufficient increase in contractility. In the dipyridamole test, the contractility is not expected to increase. The dipyridamole test is negative when contractility under stress remains normal in patients with normal contractility before stress. In both tests, the occurrence of hypokinesis, akinesis, or dyskinesis under stress means that the test is positive. When pre-stress hypokinesis is observed in a given segment, and akinesis or dyskinesis occurs under stress, the test is positive only if new areas of akinesis or dyskinesis remote from the previous zone are found. The test is negative if only the original pre-stress hypokinetic zone becomes akinetic under stress. The test is also negative when originally akinetic or dyskinetic segments remain so under stress.

| **Transthoracic and Transesophageal Accesses** |
| Active Stress |
| ▸ Exercise echocardiography
(Bicycle exercise, supine or upright; treadmill exercise) |
| Passive Stress |
| ▸ Pharmacologic agents
(adenosine, dipyridamole, dobutamine) |
| ▸ Pacing
(transesophageal/venous atrial/ventricular stimulation) |

The above modalities can be implemented in transthoracic echocardiography as well as in transesophageal echocardiography [1, 26, 76].

Bicycle and Treadmill Echocardiography

Dynamic physical exercise is the most physiological form of stress testing. Exercise electrocardiograms are routinely performed for assessment of myocardial ischemia [2]. Exercise testing can also be used for echocardiographic detection of wall motion abnormalities characteristic of ischemia [5, 38]. The exercise-related increase in heart rate produces ischemia primarily by means of increasing the myocardial oxygen demand. The increase in atrial blood pressure and the degree of inotropism plays a lesser role [61]

Adenosine and Dipyridamole

The administration of adenosine and dipyridamole induces vasodilation in normal subjects with nonsclerotic arteries, in the coronary arteries. Adenosine has a direct vasodilatory effect on the vessel wall, whereas dipyridamole acts indirectly by blockage of the cellular uptake of adenosine [7]. In the presence of coronary artery disease, both adenosine and dipyridamole lead to redistribution of blood flow and dilation of healthy vessels, to the disadvantage of poststenotic vessel segments. This vasodilator-induced „coronary steal" is the method by which these pharmacologic agents provoke ischemia [47, 50]. The heart rate and the degree of inotropism are only slightly increased, and arterial blood pressure is decreased.

Dobutamine

By means of α and β-adrenoreceptor stimulation, dobutamine causes positively chronotropic and positively inotropic effects, which are accompanied by an increase in heart rate, arterial blood pressure, and inotropism. Ischemia results from the inability of coronary perfusion to properly compensate for the higher myocardial oxygen demand.

Considering its positively inotropic effects, the normal reaction to dobutamine would be an increase in left ventricular contractility. The absence of such a reaction is interpreted an indication of ischemia.

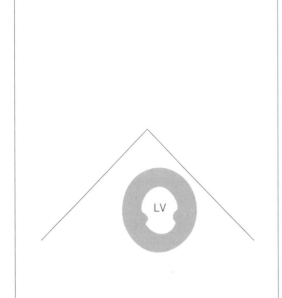

Dobutamine echocardiography: resting frame.

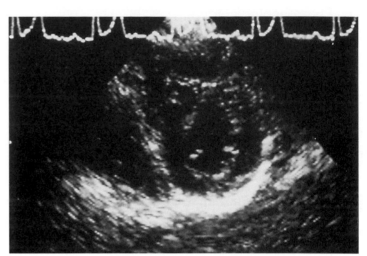

Parasternal short-axis 2-D echocardiogram.

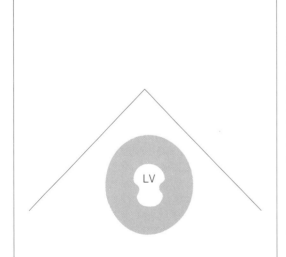

Dobutamine echocardiography: Increase in contractility during dobutamine stimulation, *i.e.*, the normal reaction.

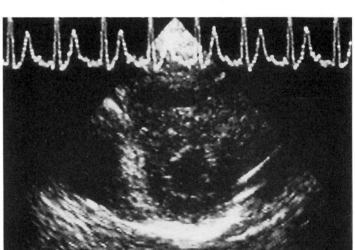

Parasternal long-axis 2-D echocardiogram.

Pacing (Atrial and Ventricular Stimulation)

Pacing is performed by means of an atrial or ventricular electrode. The resulting increase in heart rate correspondingly raises the cardiac oxygen demand. Inotropism also increases in the presence of a slight drop in blood pressure.

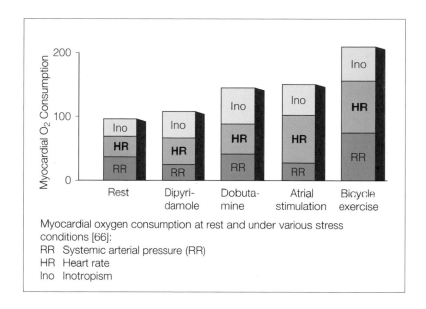

Myocardial oxygen consumption at rest and under various stress conditions [66]:
RR   Systemic arterial pressure (RR)
HR   Heart rate
Ino Inotropism

Clinical Applications

The safety requirements for stress echocardiography are the same as those for exercise electrocardiography. Emergency resuscitation personnel and equipment, including a defibrillator, must be on hand. The physician performing the examination must be trained in emergency medicine. The patient must be monitored by continuous ECG. A 12-lead ECG should be performed at rest and once per minute during stress testing. As in exercise electrocardiography, blood pressure should also be measured each minute. We also recommend having an assistant write the test protocol and make notes of ECG and pressure measurements, angina pectoris symptoms, side effects, etc.

Stress echocardiography is usually performed with the patient in the left lateral decubitus position with the upper body slightly raised. The left ventricle should be interrogated from the parasternal long and short-axis views and from apical two and four-chamber views. Images are documented at various times, depending on the stress protocol.

The images are recorded on videotape, and the ECG-triggered, synchronized frames are simultaneously digitized and stored in the computer. One complete cardiac cycle is recorded from each of the four recommended views. Eight single frames are stored and are later reviewed off-line as a cine-loop on a quad screen (split into four sections). The quad-screen display of these ECG-triggered frames makes it possible to directly compare resting and stress frames before and after peak stress.

In order to precisely reproduce the transducer position at different times during the examination, a mark should be made on the patient's chest to indicate the transducer position.

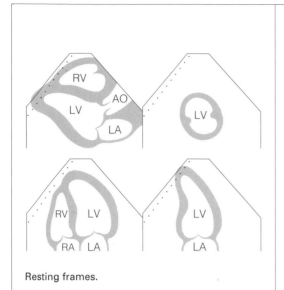

Resting frames.

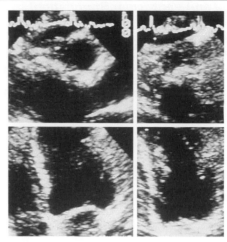

Quad-screen display. Synchronized, simultaneous frames obtained from the four standard views (parasternal long and short-axis views, apical two and four-chamber views).

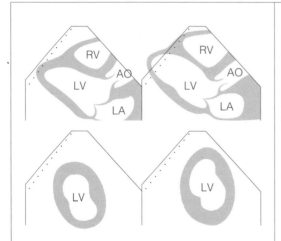

Exercise testing: Resting frames (left) and directly after exercise (right). The heart rate is given in the lower left corner of each frame.

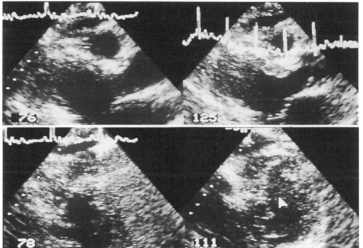

Quad-screen display: Synchronized, simultaneous frames from obtained from two standard views (parasternal long and short-axis views).

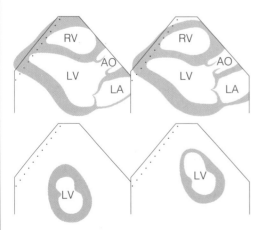

Dipyridamole echocardiograms before (left) and after (right) administration of dipyridamole. anteroseptal ischemia in the supply region of the LAD artery.

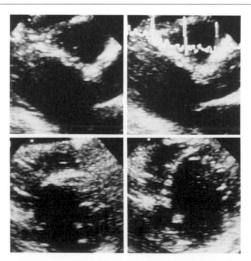

Quad-screen display: Synchronized, simultaneous frames from obtained from two standard views (parasternal long and short-axis views).

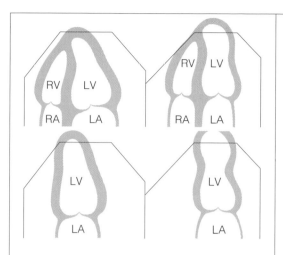

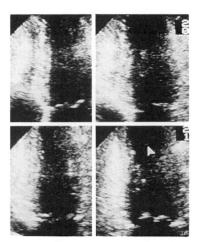

Dobutamine echocardiograms before (left) and after (right) administration of dobutamine. Apical akinesis to dyskinesis after 2 min of stress.

Quad-screen display: Synchronized, simultaneous frames obtained from apical four-chamber (top) and two-chamber (bottom) view.

A peripheral venous access is needed when performing pharmacologic stress echocardiography. The end point of any stress echocardiographic examination is achieved when significant wall motion abnormalities, severe angina pectoris, significant ECG changes, complex arrhythmias, or severe side effects occur.

Specialized computer software for pharmacologic stress echocardiography makes it possible to simultaneously display frames at rest, with high and low doses of the pharmacologic agent, and after recovery. The frames can then be compared at a glance. Quad-screen displays are especially helpful in identifying viable myocardial tissue after acute myocardial infarction. As would be expected, the viable myocardium shows improved contractility after administration of low doses of dobutamine, whereas the contractility of the jeopardized myocardium decreases, even with the maximum dose.

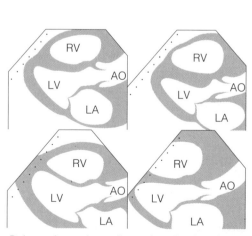

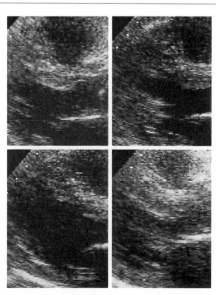

Dobutamine echocardiography: Resting frame with septal hypokinesis; reduced contractility 6 min after dobutamine injection (low dose); septal akinesis after maximum stimulation (high dose); return to initial condition in recovery phase. Viable but jeopardized myocardium.

Quad-screen display: Synchronized frames (parasternal long-axis 2-D echocardiograms).

Examination Protocol

In addition to physical exercise, stress echocardiography is also performed using such pharmacologic agents as dipyridamole and dobutamine as well as atrial stimulation. Stress echocardiography is usually performed from the transthoracic route. When conditions are poor for transthoracic echocardiography, the transesophageal route can be used instead. In that case, pharmacologic stress echocardiography or atrial pacing must then be performed. It is not feasible to perform transesophageal stress echocardiography in patients who are performing physical exercise.

Exercise Echocardiography

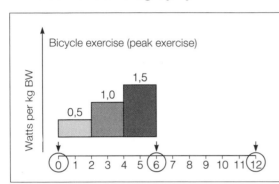

Exercised echocardiography with a peak exercise protocol. Exercise level is increased incrementally from 0.5 to 1.5 W per kg body weight or is sustained until the target level for the patient's age group has been achieved. The circles indicate the times at which echocardiographic images were obtained: 0 = at rest; 6 = directly after termination of exercise; 12 = after 6 min of recovery. The submaximum stress protocol that is used in patients after acute myocardial infarction is similarly performed with 0.33, 0.66, and 0.99 W/kg BW.

The criteria for performing bicycle exercise echocardiography are the same as those for exercise ECG. All echocardiographic images are recorded with the patient in the left lateral decubitus position. After initial resting images have been obtained, the patient gets into position and performs exercise, then reassumes the left lateral decubitus position in order for the peak exercise recording to be made. A third recording is made after the patient has rested for 6 min.

Controversy exists over the optimum timing of the peak exercise recording. The method described above seems to be the most practical. However, one study has shown that a loss of information occurs from the time of peak exercise until postexercise imaging [19].

Dobutamine Echocardiography

On the day of the examination the patient should abstain from nitrates and beta blockers. My own personal experience has shown beta blockers prevent the desired increase in heart rate, even with supplementary doses of atropine. However, other authors have reported that neither the continued use of beta blockers nor anti-ischemic medications has an influence on the results of dobutamine echocardiography [21, 35].

A perfusor is used to ensure continuous intravenous infusion of dobutamine, starting at a dose of 10 µg/kg BW/min. The dose is increased by 10 µg/kg BW/min every three minutes to obtain doses of 20, 30, and a maximum of 40 µg/kg BW/min.

If this does not achieve the desired heart rate (220 - age x 0.85), a supplementary fractionated dose of atropine is given (1 mg maximum) while still infusing 40 µg/kg BW/min until the maximum recommended infusion time of 20 minutes. Adding atropine increases the heart rate, and is reported to increase the sensitivity of dobutamine echocardiography for detecting coronary disease [24].

Images are obtained before starting the infusion (resting), before each incremental increase, at the end of the infusion, and after 2 and 6 min of recovery (postinfusion).

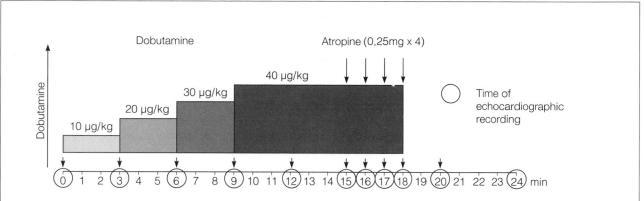

Protocol for dobutamine echocardiography: Incremental increase in infusion rate (10 to 40 µg/kg BW/min). Images are recorded: at rest; every 3 min from beginning to end of infusion; immediately following cessation of infusion; 2 and 6 min after cessation of infusion. Four 0.25 mg doses of atropine can also be administered as needed to achieve the desired heart rate.

Dipyridamole Echocardiography

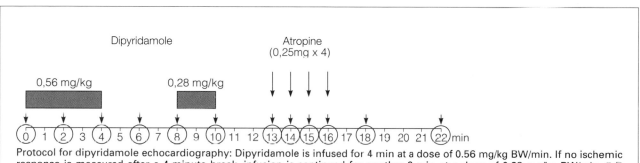

Protocol for dipyridamole echocardiography: Dipyridamole is infused for 4 min at a dose of 0.56 mg/kg BW/min. If no ischemic response is measured after a 4-minute break, infusion is continued for another 2 min at a dose of 0.28 mg/kg BW/min. 2-D images are recorded: at rest, every 2 min from the beginning to the end of infusion, immediately after cessation of infusion, and 2 and 6 min after cessation of infusion. Four 0.25 mg doses of atropine can also be administered as needed to achieve the desired heart rate.

On the day of the examination, the patient should abstain from coffee, tea, chocolate, and medicines containing xanthines (*e.g.* theophylline), which all reduce the effects of dipyridamole [52].

A perfusor is used to infuse dipyridamole in two phases. First, it is infused for 4 min at a rate of 0.56 mg/kg BW/min. If no ischemic reaction has been noted after a 4-min break, a second infusion of 0.28 mg/kg BW/min is given for 2 min. This yields a maximum dipyridamole dose of 0.84 mg/kg body weight. A fractional dose of up to 1 mg adenosine (4 x 0.25 mg) can also be administered as needed, 3 min after termination of the dipyridamole infusion, in order to achieve the desired heart rate.

Echocardiographic images are recorded at the beginning of infusion, every two minutes during infusion, immediately post-infusion, and 2 and 6 min post-infusion.

Because the effects of dipyridamole begin after a slight latency period, it is a good idea to give the patient a fractional dose. On the other hand, the post-infusion phase is just as important for detecting the ischemic reaction as the actual infusion phase. In view of dipyridamole's protracted effects, the peripheral access should be maintained for ca. 15 min after the end of infusion, during which time the patient is kept under medical supervision.

Atrial Pacing Echocardiography

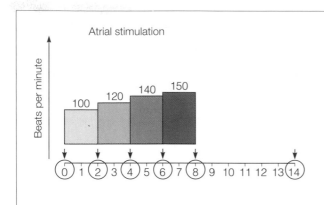

Protocol for atrial pacing echocardiography: Electrical stimulation is performed to achieve a heart rate of 100 beats/min, which is incrementally increased every 2 min until maximum heart rate of 150 beats/min is achieved. Echocardiographic images are recorded after every incremental increase in heart rate and 6 min after cessation of pacing.

In transesophageal atrial pacing, the probe is introduced transnasally or transorally. Pacing should start at a heart rate of 100 beats/min, which should be increased in increments of 20 beats/min every 2 min until a maximum heart rate of 150 beats/min is achieved. The optimum result is to achieve a rate of 150 beats/min within 5 minutes. However, heart blocks often make it impossible to achieve this heart rate. Echocardiographic images are recorded before initiation of pacing, before and after each increase in heart rate, after cessation of pacing, and 6 min after cessation of pacing.

Feasibility and Tolerance of the Stress Echocardiographic Protocols

Exercise Echocardiography

The requirements of exercise echocardiography are the same as for exercise ECG. The limited ability to perform physical exercise due to vascular, orthopedic, or muscular diseases can limit use of this method. Increased and deepened respiration under exercise can also make it more difficult to obtain suitable echocardiographic images.

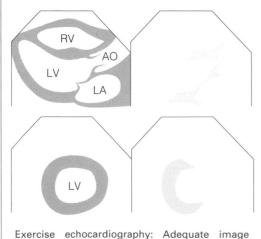

Exercise echocardiography: Adequate image quality in resting image (left). Immediately after starting exercise (right), image quality degrades, and wall contours become hardly recognizable.

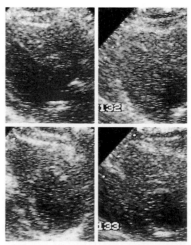

Quad-screen display: Synchronized simultaneous display of two standard views (parasternal long (top) and short-axis (bottom) views).

Dobutamine and Dipyridamole

The requirements and restrictions of dobutamine and dipyridamole echocardiography are also similar to those of exercise echocardiography. The examination is prematurely terminated if significant wall motion abnormality, angina pectoris, complex arrhythmias, and other nontolerable side effects occur. The side effects usually cease when the examination is terminated. Sublingual glycerol trinitrate can be administered if angina pectoris persists.

Although both of these pharmacologic agents are well tolerated, some side effects still may occur. Listed in order of frequency, they are:

Potential Side Effects	
Dobutamine	**Dipyridamole**
Arrhythmias	Hypotension
Headache	Bradycardia
Tremor	Headache
Hypertension/Hypotension	Dizziness/Stupor
Dizziness/Stupor	Abdominal pain
Restlessness	Arrhythmias

The most serious side effects, particularly with dobutamine, are supraventricular and ventricular arrhythmias. AV heart block has also been reported. Clinically significant arrhythmias (atrial fibrillation, persistent bigeminy, volleys, and ventricular tachycardia) occur infrequently. In our comparison study of 144 dobutamine and dipyridamole examinations, the incidence of such sides effects under dobutamine was 5%; no significant side effects occurred with dipyridamole [74]. All arrhythmias occurring with dobutamine were kept under control. Intravenous administration of beta blockers is recommended for treatment of dobutamine-induced tachycardia or hypertension. Occasionally a significant drop in blood pressure occurs with dobutamine. However, in contrast with the occurrence of hypotension during exercise echocardiography, this has no diagnostic or prognostic relevance [36, 59]. Such side effects as palpitations, headache, and tremor were observed in around 25 to 30 % of all patients, probably due to the physiological effects of dobutamine. In the published literature, dobutamine echocardiography is generally determined to be safe [36, 62, 74].

Whereas only a few arrhythmias are to be expected with dipyridamole, bradycardia and hypotension are more frequent side effects. However, they can usually be controlled well by interrupting the examination and by intravenous theophylline [53]. When theophylline is given as an antidote to dipyridamole, its effects can be observed after 1 to 2 min, and it immediately terminates the ischemic response. Other side effects such as headache, stupor, and dizziness can also be easily reversed. Some authors recommend administering theophylline at the end of every dipyridamole test, regardless of the severity of the ischemic response [62]. However, a differential approach to theophylline administration is probably safer. Glycerol trinitrate can be used to treat persistent wall motion abnormality or angina pectoris. An Italian study group has documented the safety of dipyridamole echocardiography in almost 20,000 cases [48].

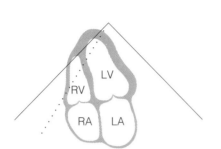

Dipyridamole echocardiography: resting frame.

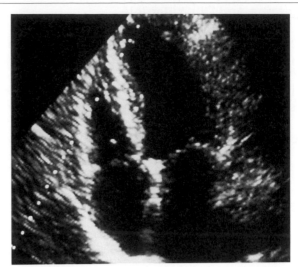

Apical four-chamber 2-D echocardiogram.

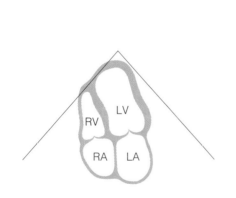

Dipyridamole echocardiography: apical akinesis 10 min after infusion.

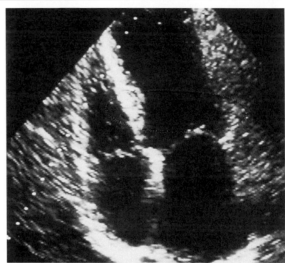

Apical four-chamber 2-D echocardiogram.

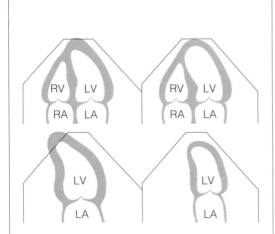

Apicoseptal and apical akinesis (different depth in lower right frame).

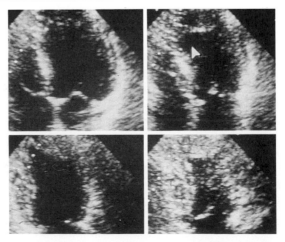

Quad-screen display: Synchronized simultaneous display of two standard projections. Apical four (top) and two-chamber echocardiograms (bottom), before (left) and after (right) dipyridamole infusion.

Atrial Pacing Echocardiography

Transesophageal pacing cannot be performed in 15 to 20% of all cases, primarily due to technical limitations or because the test is not tolerated by the patient. Other reasons include impaired impulse conduction and AV heart block [16, 30]. A major drawback is that this technique is semi-invasive. In other words, the test can only be performed in patients who cannot perform physical exercise, or when theophylline treatment cannot be interrupted (in patients with obstructive respiratory tract diseases), or in patients with a history of complex arrhythmias.

Validity of Each of the Stress Echocardiographic Protocols

Echocardiographic stress testing was originally performed using exercise echocardiography. This test, like dobutamine and dipyridamole echocardiography, now plays an important role in is highly valued, because it not only provides information as to the coronary status, but also makes it possible to simultaneously test the patient's general cardiopulmonary exercise tolerance.

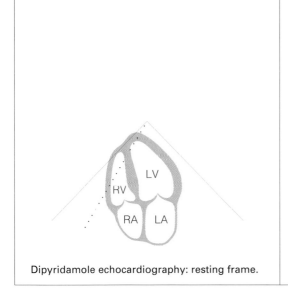

Dipyridamole echocardiography: resting frame.

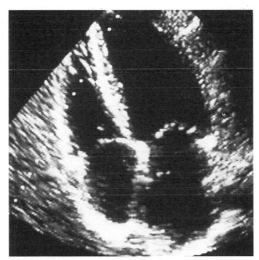

Apical four-chamber 2-D echocardiogram.

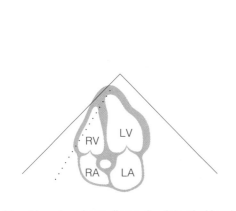

Dipyridamole echocardiography: lateral akinesis in the circumflex artery supply region.

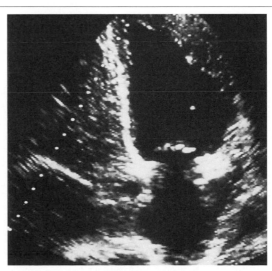

Apical four-chamber 2-D echocardiogram.

According to various authors, the sensitivity of exercise echocardiography (EE) ranges from 80 to 90 % [3, 4, 18, 23, 25, 38, 56]. EE reportedly has a sensitivity over 90% for detecting multivessel disease, which is therefore higher than the ca. 80% sensitivity reported for single vessel disease. The specificity of EE, which was reported to be 85%, is comparably high. Several studies demonstrated the significant superiority of EE over exercise ECG, which is reported to have a sensitivity of only around 65%. A study comparing the effectiveness of EE and 201-TI single-proton emission computed tomography (201-TI SPECT) in the evaluation of coronary artery disease reported good results for both methods, which were improved by combined use of the two methods [57]. A study comparing pharmacologic stress echocardiography with EE reported similar sensitivities and specificities [17, 32].

An important factor when performing exercise echocardiography is the timing of echocardiographic image recording. A comparison of peak exercise versus immediate postexercise images demonstrated the higher sensitivity of peak exercise images [27, 30]. However, it is often difficult to obtain images at that time. A compromise can be made by obtaining the stress images with the patient in a semirecumbent position. After the cessation of exercise, he simply rolls over to more quickly reassume the left lateral decubitus position for postexercise recording.

As in exercise ECG, exercise echocardiography also is greatly limited by the patient's physical exercise tolerance. The higher the patient's exercise tolerance, the greater the sensitivity of the EE [30]. Studies performed at our hospital have shown that the sensitivity of EE at submaximum exercise levels (78%) is significantly lower than EE at peak exercise levels [65]. As a rule, one should generally strive to fully exercise the patient to obtain the necessary 85% of the age-appropriate heart rate. This, however, is not possible in some cases (*e.g.* shortly after myocardial infarction), and the text must be performed at submaximum, ergo less effective, exercise levels [65].

A further drawback in exercise echocardiography is the difficulty in properly documenting the left ventricle at peak levels of exercise. However, the previously mentioned computer software mitigates this problem somewhat, in that it is able to take four consecutive frames from the same transducer position and view and select the qualitatively superior image for storage in memory.

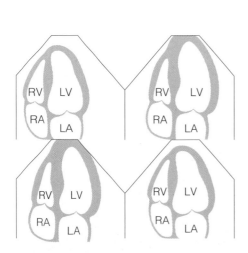

Dipyridamole echocardiography: Resting (upper left); after 5 min at low-dose level (upper right); after 10 min at high-dose level (lower left); after recovery (lower right). The reaction of the left ventricular wall segments is adequate.

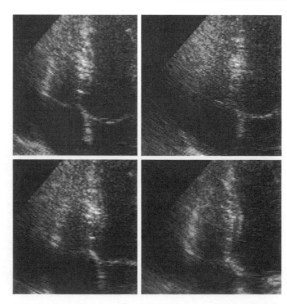

Quad-screen display: Synchronized simultaneous display of 2-D images obtained from the apical four-chamber view.

A number of studies have documented the diagnostic utility of dipyridamole and dobutamine echocardiography for detection of significant coronary stenosis (> 50%). The reported sensitivity of dobutamine echocardiography ranged from 60 to 80 %, and the specificity ranged from 80 to 90 % [34, 40, 41, 68]. In patients with multivessel disease the sensitivity increases to over 90% [63]. Similar figures were reported for the sensitivity and specificity of dipyridamole echocardiography [10, 11, 15, 39, 50, 51].

Comparison studies of dobutamine versus dipyridamole echocardiography have shown that the sensitivity of dobutamine and dipyridamole ranges from 60 to 80 %, and that specificity ranges from 80 to 90 % [9, 62]. These figures correlate well with our own data [74].

Several study groups have reported that dipyridamole and dobutamine echocardiography is well tolerated [48].

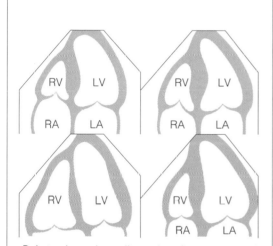

Dobutamine echocardiography after anteroseptal infarction: Resting with septal hypokinesis; contractility improves under low-dose dobutamine; septal akinesis occurs under high-dose dobutamine. Diagnosis: viable but jeopardized myocardium.

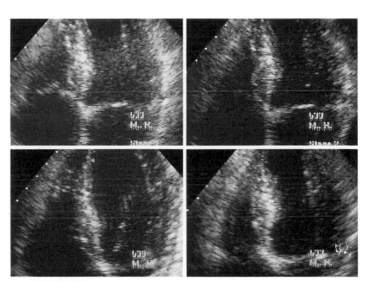

Quad-screen display: Synchronized display of apical four-chamber 2-D echocardiograms.

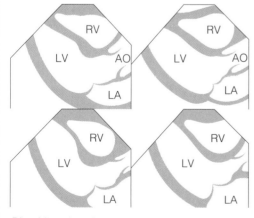

Dipyridamole echocardiography: normal at rest; onset of wall motion abnormalities (WMA) with low-dose dipyridamole; WMA increase as dole level increases; WMA improve after cessation of infusion and recovery.

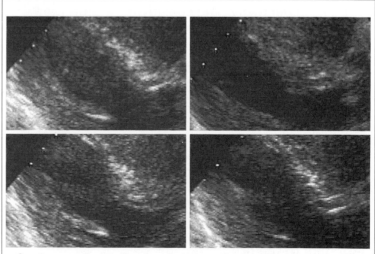

Quad-screen display: Synchronized display of parasternal long-axis 2-D echocardiograms.

Individual studies have shown that dipyridamole echocardiography can safely be performed as soon as some days after acute myocardial infarction, in order to plan the further course of treatment [70]. It is safe to perform low-dose dobutamine echocardiography for identification of viable myocardium as early as three days after acute myocardial infarction [42]. Most centers do not usually perform high-dose dobutamine echocardiography until one to two weeks after acute myocardial infarction [34, 54]. According to the most recent reports, dipyridamole echocardiography is also helpful in identification of viable myocardium [49, 75]. Besides in the detection and assessment of coronary artery disease, both of the pharmacologic stress protocols and exercise echocardiography have proven their value in risk stratification [67] and prognostic assessment [46, 70].

In all previous studies, the diagnostic value of adenosine echocardiography has been shown to be similar to that of dobutamine and dipyridamole echocardiography. The sensitivity and specificity of adenosine echo are 85% and 92%, respectively [77].

Transesophageal atrial pacing echocardiography also has a high sensitivity and specificity, namely 91% and 88%, resp. [30]. This semi-invasive method is not tolerated well in all patients, as experience in our hospital has shown [66].

Transesophageal atrial pacing also makes it possible to perform exercise echocardiography in patients who cannot be imaged echocardiograpically from the transthoracic route. The technique is reported to be well tolerated and safe. Preliminary results have also shown that this is a very safe technique for detecting myocardial ischemia [29, 33]. The advantage of using a biplane or multiplane probe instead of a single plane probe is improved visualization and assessment of apical and basal segments of the left ventricle. A disadvantage is the semi-invasive nature of the technique.

5.2   Stress Echocardiography
5.2.6   Comparison of Stress Echocardiography with Other Diagnostic Techniques

In three studies, stress echocardiography was compared with such established nuclear cardiologic imaging methods as 201-Tl myocardial scintigraphy, technetium MIBI SPECT, and 201-Tl SPECT, respectively. The sensitivity of both methods for detecting ischemic reactions was high [37, 54, 57]. The sensitivity of scintigraphy and SPECT appears to be lower, but their specificity is higher. The overall advantage of stress echocardiography is that these techniques are radiation-free, they save time and money, and can be performed by the cardiologist.

A number of studies have documented the diagnostic superiority of various stress echocardiographic techniques over exercise electrocardiography [10, 58, 69].

Although coronary angiography provides information on morphological changes in the coronary arteries, only a functional test can provide information on the functional effects of coronary stenosis. Studies performed before and after PTCA and CABG were able to document the value of stress echocardiography in this application [41, 50, 54, 74]. Stress echocardiographic techniques provide answers to important questions concerning coronary artery disease. Stress echocardiographic methods are very valuable not only in the diagnosis of coronary artery disease, but also in risk stratification after acute myocardial infarction and in assessment of the prognosis.

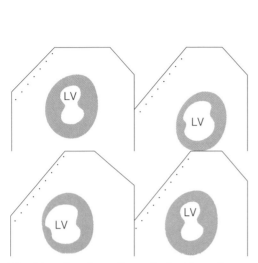

Dipyridamole echocardiography is able to detect anteroseptal akinesis that remained undiagnosed by exercise ECG.

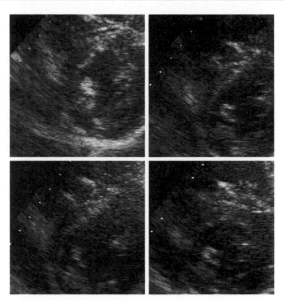

Quad-screen display: Synchronized simultaneous display of parasternal short-axis 2-D echocardiograms.

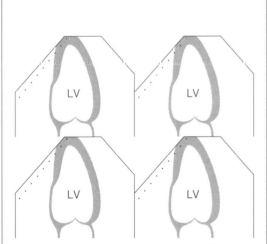

Dobutamine echocardiography: detection of inferior akinesis. Contractility in the infarcted area increases under dobutamine administration, and wall motion disturbances do not spread to infarcted zones. The test is negative: scar tissue, completed infarction. The RCA is angiographically occluded.

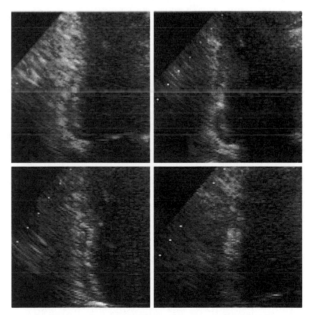

Quad-screen display of synchronized 2-D images obtained from the apical two-chamber view.

A decisive factor for successful performance of stress echocardiography is the experience of the echocardiographer. In order to master the technique, the physician must independently perform and interpret around 80 to 100 examinations, the results of which are checked by an invasive examination. This training period must be completed to ensure the high validity of stress echocardiographic diagnosis. In clinical practice, the following diagnostic schema is recommended for patients with suspected coronary artery disease.

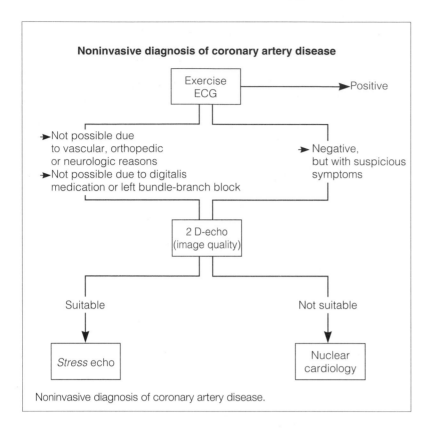

Noninvasive diagnosis of coronary artery disease

Noninvasive diagnosis of coronary artery disease.

References

1. Agati L, Renzi M, Sciomer S, Vizza DC, Voci P, Penco M, Fedele F, Dagianti A. Transesophageal dipyridamole echocardiography for diagnosis of coronary artery disease. J Am Coll Cardiol 1992; 19: 765-770.
2. American College of Cardiology/American Heart Accociation Task Force on Assessment of Cardiovascular Procedures. Guidelines for exercise testing. J Am Coll Cardiol 1986; 8: 725-738.
3. Armstrong FW. Clinical validation and application of exercise echocardiography. Learning center, Highlights 1988; 4: 1-5.
4. Armstrong WF, O'Donnell M, Dillon JC, McHenry PL, Morris SN, Feigenbaum H. Complementary value of two-dimensional exercise echocardiography to routine treadmill exercise testing. Ann Int Med 1986; 105: 829-835.
5. Armstrong WF. Exercise echocardiography: Phase II, convincing the sceptics. J Am Coll Cardiol 1992; 19: 82-83.
6. Armstrong WF. Stress echocardiography for the detection of coronary artery disease. Circulation 1991; 84 (suppl I): 43-49.
7. Becker LC. Conditions for vasodilatator-induced coronary steal in experimental myocardial ischemia. Circulation 1978; 57: 1103-1110.
8. Blasini R, Theisen T, Töpfer M, Lutilsky L, Blömer H. Streßechokardiographie: Stellenwert zusätzlicher Doppler-echokardiographischer Messungen. Z Kardiol 1992; 81 (suppl I): 187.
9. Boccanelli A, Pontillo D, Greco C, Zanchi E, Carboni GP, Cecchetti C, Risa AL. Comparison of exercise stress test, dipyridamole and dobutamine stress echocardiography for the detection of multivessel disease after myocardial infarction. J Am Coll Cardiol 1992; 19 (suppl A): 359A.
10. Bolognese L, Sarasso G, Aralda D, Bongo AS, Rossi L, Rossi P. High dose dipyridamole echocardiography early after uncomplicated acute myocardial infarction: correlation with exercise testing and coronary angiography. J Am Coll Cardiol 1989; 14: 357-363.
11. Bolognese L, Sarasso G, Bongo AS, Rossi L, Aralda D, Piccinino C, Rossi P. Dipyridamole echocardiography test. Circulation 1991; 84: 1100-1106.
12. Borer JS, Brensike JF, Redwood DR. Limitations of the electrocardiographic response to exercise in predicting coronary artery disease. New Engl J Med 1975; 293: 367-371.

13. Braunwald E, Kloner RA. The stunned myocardium: prolonged, postischemic ventricular dysfunction. Circulation 1982; 66: 1146-1151.
14. Braunwald E, Rutherford JD. Reversible ischemic left ventricular dysfunction: evidence for the hibernating myocardium. Am J Cardiol 1986; 8: 1467-1470.
15. Casanova R, Parrocini A, Guidalotti PL, Capacci PF, Jacopi F, Fabbri M, Maresta A. Dose and test for dipyridamole infusion and cardiac imaging early after uncomplicated acute myocardial infarction. Am J Cardiol 1992; 70: 1402-1406.
16. Chapman PD, Doyle TP, Troup PJ, Gross CM, Wann LS. Stress echocardiography with transesophageal atrial pacing: preliminary report of a new method for detection of ischemic wall motion abnormalities. Circulation 1984; 70: 445-455.
17. Cohen JL, Duvvuri S, George A, Ottenweller J, Wilchfort SD, Binenbaum SZ, Kim CS. Dobutamine versus exercise digital echocardiography for detecting coronary artery disease. J Am Coll Cardiol 1992; 19 (suppl A): 39A.
18. Crouse LJ, Harbrecht JJ, Vacek JL, Rosamond TL, Kramer PH. Exercise echocardiography as a screening test for coronary artery disease and correlation with coronary arteriography. Am J Cardiol 1991; 67: 1231-1218.
19. Deutsch HJ, Curtius JM, Klaer R, Schenkel C. Streflechokardiographie: Ein Vergleich von Peak- versus Post-Exercise-Auswertung. Z Kardiol 1992; 81 (suppl I): 188.
20. Edwards WD, Tajik AJ, Seward JB. Standardized nomenclature and anatomic basis for regional tomographic analysis of the heart. Mayo Clin Proc 1981; 56: 479-497.
21. Epstein M, Gin K, Sterns L, Pollick C. Dobutamine stress echocardiography: Diagnosis of CAD with continuation of anti-anginal medication. Circulation 1991; 84 (suppl): II704.
22. Feigenbaum H. Coronary artery disease. In: Feigenbaum H (ed). Echocardiography, 4th ed. Lea and Febiger, Philadelphia, 462-513.
23. Feigenbaum H. Exercise echocardiography. In: Visser C, Kan G, Meltzer R (eds). Echocardiography in coronary artery disease. Kluver, Bosten 1988; 1-64.
24. Fioretti PM, McNeill AJ, El-Said ESM, Salustri A, Brace MJ, Roelandt JR TC. Adding Atropine to dobutamine Echocardiography increases sensitivity for detecting coronary disease. Circulation 1991; 84 (suppl): II704.
25. Fshman EZ, Ben-Ari E, Pines A, Drory Y, Motro M, Kellermann JJ. Usefulness of heavy isometric exercise echocardiography for assessing left ventricular wall motion pattern late (> 6 month) after acute myocardial infarction. Am J Cardiol 1992; 70: 1123-1128.
26. Geiser EA. Transesophageal echocardiographic stress testing: feasible, but place and accuracy still in question. J Am Coll Cardiol 1992; 15: 771-772.
27. Hecht HA, DeBord L, Shaw RE, Ryan C, Chin H. Supine bicycle stress echocardiography: evaluation of coronary disease and comparison with post exercise imaging. Echocardiography; in press.
28. Heyndrick CR, Baic H, Nelkins P, Leusen K, Fishbein MC, Vatner SF. Depression of regional blood flow and wall thickening after brief coronary occlusion. Am J Physiol 1978; 234: H653-H660.
29. Hoffmann R, Lambertz H, K‰smacher H, Liebich I, Flachskampf FA, Plum M, Hanrath P. Transesophageal stress echocardiography for pre-operative detection of patients at risk of intra-operative myocardial ischemia. Eur Heart J 1992; 13: 1482-1488.
30. Iliceto S, Sorino M, D'Ambrosio G, Papa A, Favale S, Biasco G, Rizzon P. Detection of coronary artery disease by two-dimensional echocardiography and transesophageal atrial pacing. J Am Coll Cardiol 1985; 5 (5): 1188-1197.
31. Kaul S. Echocardiography in coronary artery disease. Curr Probl Cardiol 1990; 15: 235-287.
32. Klaer R, Curtius JM, Deutsch HJ, Schenkel C. Vergleich der Wertigkeit der Dipyridamol-Echokardiographie und der Ergometer-Echokardiographie bei koronarer Herzerkrankung. Z Kardiol 1992; 81 (suppl I): 188.
33. Lambertz H, Kreis A, Tr.mper H, Hanrath P. Simultaneous transesophageal atrial pacing and transesophageal two-dimensional echocardiography: a new method of stress echocardiography. J Am Coll Cardiol 1990; 16: 1143-1153.
34. Mrcovitz PA, Armstrong WF. Dobutamine stress echocardiography: diagnostic utility. Herz 1991; 16: 372-378.
35. Marcovitz PA, Bach DS, Markarian M, Armstrong WF. Beta blockade blunts heart rate and blood pressure response but not contractility augmentation during incremental dobutamine infusion. J Am Coll Cardiol 1992; 19 (suppl A): 278A.
36. Marcovitz PA, Bach DS, Markarian M, Mathias WS, Armstrong WF. Implications of a hypotensive response during dobutamine stress echocardiography. J Am Coll Cardiol 1992; 19 (suppl A): 360A.
37. Marwick TH, D'Hondt AM, Melin J, Willemart B, DeKock M, Wyns W, Detry JM. Detection of myocardial ischemia by dobutamine stress with echocardiography and TcMIBI SPECT: comparison of accuracy and defect size. J Am Coll Cardiol 1992; 19 (suppl A): 40A.
38. Marwick TH, Nemec JJ, Pashkow FJ, Stewart WJ, Salcedo EE. Accuracy and limitations of exercise echocardiography in a routine clinical setting. J Am Coll Cardiol 1992; 19: 74-81.
39. Mazeika PK, Nihoyannopoulos P, Joshi J, Oakley CM. Uses and limitations of high dose dipyridamole stress echocardiography for evaluation of coronary artery disease. Br Heart J 1992; 67: 144-149.
40. Mazeika PK, Nadazdin A, Oakley CM. Dobutamine stress echocardiography for detection and assessment of coronary artery disease. J Am Coll Cardiol 1992; 19: 1203-1211.

41. McNeill AJ, Fioretti PM, El-Said EM, Salustri A, de Feyter PJ, Roeland JR. Dobutamine stress echocardiography before and after coronary angioplasty. Am J Cardiol 1992; 69: 740-745.
42. Mertes, H Sawada SG, Segar DS, Feigenbaum H, Bates JR, Ryan T. Dobutamine vs. bicycle stress echocardiography in the assessment of patients following acute myocardial infarction: A prospective study. Circulation 1993, 88 (suppl): I-121.
43. Nesto RW, Kowalchuk GJ. The ischemic cascade: Temporal sequence of hemodynamic, electrocardiographic and symptomatic expressions of ischemia. Am J Cardiol 1987; 57: 23C-30C.
44. Nishimura RA, Abel MD, Hatle LK, Tajik AJ. Assessment of diastolic function of the heart: background and current application of Doppler echocardiography: II. Clinical studies. Mayo Clin Proc 1989; 64: 181-204.
45. Pandian NG, Wang SS, Thanikachalam S. Role of Doppler echocardiography in ischemic heart disease. In: Kerber RE (ed). Echocardiography in coronary artery disease. Futura, Mount Kisco 1988; 259-277.
46. Pellikka PA, Oh JK, Bailey KR, Nichols BA, Rooke TW, Tajik AJ. Prognostic role of Dobutamine stress echocardiography before noncardiac surgery. J Am Coll Cardiol 1992; 19 (suppl A): 100A.
47. Picano E, Lattanzi F, Masini M, Distantd A, L'Abbate A. High dose dipyridamole echocardiography test in effort angina pectoris. J Am Coll Cardiol 1986; 8: 848-854.
48. Picano E, Marini C, Pirelli S, Maffei S, Bolognese L, Chiriatti G, Chiarella F, Orlandini A, Seveso G, Colosso MQ et al (EPIC study group). Safety of intravenous high-dose dipyridamole echocardiography. Am J Cardiol 1992; 70 (2): 252-258.
49. Picano E, Marzullo P, Gigli G, Reisenhofer B, Parodi O, Distante A, L'Abbate A. Identification of viable myocardium by dipyridamole-induced improvement in regional left ventricular function assessed by echocardiography in myocardial infarction and comparison with thallium scintigraphy at rest. Am J Cardiol 1992; 70: 703-710.
50. Picano E, Pirelli S, Marzilli M, Faletra F, Lattanzi F, Campoplo L, Massa D, Alberti A, Gara E, Distante A, L'Abbate A. Usefulness of high-dose dipyridamole echocardiography test in coronary angioplasty. Circulation 1989; 80: 807-815.
51. Picano E, Severi S, Michelassi C, Lattanzi F, Masini M, Orsini E, Distante A, L'Abbate A. Prognostic importance of dipyridamole-echocardiography test in coronary artery disease. Circulation 1989; 80: 450-457.
52. Picano E. Dipyridamole-echocardiography test. In: Visser C, Kan G, Meltzer R (eds). Echocardiography in coronary artery disease Kluver, Bosten 1988; 65-75.
53. Picano E. Stress Echocardiography, Springer, Berlin/Heidelberg/New York 1992.
54. Pierard LA, de Landsheere C, Berthe C, Rigo P, Kulbertus HE. Identification of viable myocardium by echocardiography during dobutamine infusion in patients with myocardial infarction after thrombolytic therapy: comparison with positron emission tomography. J Am Coll Cardiol 1990; 15: 1021-1031.
55. Plotnick GD. Changes in diastolic function - difficult to measure, harder to interpret. Am Heart J 1989; 118: 637-641.
56. Previtali M, Lanzarini L, Ferrario M, Tortorici M, Mussini A, Montemartini C. Dobutamine versus dipyridamole echocardiography in coronary artery disease. Circulation 1990; 83 (suppl III): 27-31.
57. Quinones MA, Verani MS, Haichin RM, Mahmarian JJ, Suarez J, Zoghbi WA. Exercise echocardiography versus 201 Tl single-photon emission computed tomography in evaluation of coronary artery disease. Circulation 1992; 85: 1026-1031.
58. Reisenhofer B, Moscarelli E, Zanchi M, Picano E, Distante A. Dobutamine echocardiography in coronary artery disease: comparison with coronary angiography and exercise electrocardiography. J Am Coll Cardiol 1992; 19 (suppl A): 359A.
59. Rosamund TL, Vacek JK, Hurwitz A, Rowland AJ, Beauchamp GD, Crouse LJ. Hypotension during dobutamine stress echocardiography: initial description and clinical relevance. Am Heart J 1992; 123: 403-407.
60. Ross J jr, Gallagher KP, Matzusaki M, Lee JD, Guth B, Goldfarb R. Regional myocardial blood flow and function in experimental myocardial ischemia. Can J Cardiol 1986; 1 (suppl A): 9A-18A.
61. Ross J jr. Factors regulating the oxygen consumption of the heart. In: Russek HI, Zoham BL (eds). Changing concepts in cardiovascular disease. Williams and Wilkins, Baltimore, 20-31.
62. Salustri A, Fioretti PM, McNeill AJ, Pozzoli MMA, Roeland JR. Pharmacological stress echocardiography in the diagnosis of coronary artery disease and myocardial ischemia: a comparison between dobutamine and dipyridamol. Eur Heart J 1992; 13: 1356-1362.
63. Sawada SG, Segar DS, Ryan T, Brown SE, Dohan AM, Williams R, Fineberg NS, Armstrong WF, Feigenbaum H. Echocardiographic detection of coronary artery disease during dobutamine infusion. Circulation 1991; 83: 1605-1614.
64. Schiller NB, Shah PM, Crawford M, DeMaria A, Devereux R, Feigenbaum H, Gutgesell H, Reichek N, Sahn D, Silverman AH, Tajik AJ. Recommandations for quantification of the left ventricle by two-dimensional echocardiography. J Am Soc Echocardiography 1989; 2: 358-367.

65. Schröder K, Völer H, Hansen B, Levensen B, Wilkenshoff U, Schr^der R. Strefl-Echokardiographie als Routine-Untersuchung bei koronarer Herzkrankheit. Dtsch Med Wschr 1992; 117: 1583-1588.
66. Schröder K, Völler H, Hansen B, Linderer T, Spielberg C, Münzberg H, Schr^der R. Which stress-echocardiographic test is best suitable to identify jeopardized myocardium shortly after myocardial infarction? Circulation 1991; 84 (suppl II): II208.
67. Schröder K, Völler H, Hansen B, Schröder R. Can stress induced changes in the wall motion score indicate the necessity for an intervention in patients with coronary artery disease? A stress echocardiographic study. J Am Coll Cardiol 1992; 19 (suppl A): 101A.
68. Segar DS, Brown SE, Sawada SG, Ryan T, Feigenbaum H. Dobutamine stress echocardiography: correlation with coronary lesion as determined by quantitative angiography. J Am Coll Cardiol 1992; 19: 1197-1202.
69. Severi S, Michelassi C, Picano E, Lattanzi F, Landi P, L'Abbate A. The prognostic value of dipyridamole-echocardiography exercise stress, electrocardiography and coronary angiography test in previous myocardial infarction. J Am Coll Cardiol 1992; 19 (suppl A): 100A.
70. Seveso G, Chiarella F, Previtali M, Bolognese L et al, on behalf of the EPIC study group. The prognostic value of dipyridamole-echocardiography early after uncomplicated acute myocardial infarction: Updated results of the EPIC study. J Am Coll Cardiol 1992; 19: 100A.
71. Völler H, Schröder K, Köhler T, Spielberg C, Linderer T, Schröder R. Dipyridamol-Strefl-Echokardiographie: Kein diagnostischer Gewinn durch gepulste Doppler-Echokardiographie. Z Kardiol 1992; 81 (suppl I): 187.
72. Völler H, Spielberg C, Schröder K, Wilkenshoff U, Schröder R. Exercise Doppler Echocardiography: Do diastolic flow patterns identify patients with myocardial ischemia? Eur Heart J 1990; 11 (suppl): 73.
73. Wann DL, Glllam LD, Weyman AE. Cross-sectional echocardiographic assessment of regional left ventricular performance and myocardial perfusion. Prog Cardiovasc 1986; 29: 1-52.
74. Wilkenshoff U, Schröder K, Völler H, Dissmann R, Linderer T, Schröder R. Validity and tolerance of dobutamine and dipyridamole stress echocardiography before and after PTCA. Am Soc Echocardiography 1993; 6 (abstract issue): S38.
75. Wilkenshoff U, Schröder K, Völler H, Münzberg H, Dissmann R, Spielberg C, Linderer T, Schröder R. Detection of jeopardized myocardium after acute myocardial infarction with dipyridamole stress echocardiography test. Europ Heart J 1993; 14 (suppl): 281.
76. Zabalgoitia M, Gandhi DK, Mansour P, Rosenblum J. Transesophageal stress echocardiography: a new method for detection of coronary artery disease. Circulation 1991; 84 (suppl): II705.
77. Zoghbi WA, Cheirif J, Kleiman NS, Verani MS, Trakhtenbroit A. Diagnosis of ischemic heart disease with adenosine echocardiography. J Am Coll Cardiol 1991; 18: 1271-1279.

5.3 Transluminal Cardiac Ultrasound Diagnosis
5.3.1 Transesophageal Echocardiography
(Kurt J.G. Schmailzl)

The transesophageal approach has several advantages. It provides better imaging quality, there is no interference from the chest wall and, because of the shorter distance to the target object, higher frequency transducers can be used for increased resolution.

In transthoracic echocardiography, some target structures cannot be visualized at all (*e.g.* atrial appendage), or only with great difficulty (*e.g.* small vegetations. Transesophageal echocardiography is now routinely used for diagnosis and assessment of such cases and in other typical situations (*e.g.* paraprosthetic leaks and aortic dissection).

In these cases, transesophageal echocardiography (TEE) is used to confirm the presence or absence of the suspected vegetation, leak, dissection, etc. in order to obtain the information necessary for treatment planning. For example, when the source of cardiac embolism is determined by TEE, anticoagulant or surgical treatment must be initiated. When vegetations are found in a patient with clinical symptoms of active endocarditis, a 4-6 week-long antibiotic treatment regime must be started. If TEE demonstrates the presence of a paraprosthetic leak, reoperation must be considered; proof of type A aortic dissection indicates a critical need for surgery.

Indications for transesophageal echocardiography

▸ Inadequate transthoracic image quality

▸ Intensive care or emergency medicine

▸ Intraoperative and perioperative monitoring

▸ Congenital heart disease

▸ Native valve disease and prosthetic valve dysfunction

▸ Determination of the source of embolism

▸ Intra- and extracardiac masses

▸ Aortic disease

5.3.1   **Transesophageal Echocardiography**
5.3.1.1   **Technique and Practice of TEE**

The technique and practice of TEE encompasses details such as the proper instrumentation, personnel, patient preparation, knowledge of premedication considerations, insertion of the echoscope, its operation, the examination procedure, and post-examination patient observation.

Equipment required by echocardiography laboratory in order to perform transesophageal echocardiography

▸ Oral suction apparatus
▸ ECG monitoring equipment
▸ Pulsed oximeter
▸ Automatic interval blood pressure measurement
▸ Peripheral venous access with three-way cock
▸ Several 10 ml syringes
▸ 0.9% NaCl
▸ Echo contrast agent
▸ Resuscitation personnel and equipment

This list was made while keeping in mind that, although complications seldom occur during endoscopic examinations, TEE is usually performed in the echocardiography laboratory, not in the endoscopy suite itself. Those who have frequently had to examine unstable patients will appreciate these requirements better than those who have never been confronted with such complications.

The cardiologist-echocardiographer will need a trained assistant to observe and sedate the patient, to operate the oral suction apparatus, and to execute other duties that may arise, such as administration of echo contrast agent and attending to complications. At our laboratory, we have not found it helpful to let a second assistant adjust the controls of the echocardiograph.

As in any operation with a statistically relevant risk factor, TEE may not be performed before receiving the informed consent of the patient. In our experience, TEE can usually be performed without sedatives or short-term hypnotics. In contrast with gastroscopy or bronchoscopy, TEE is a relatively „blind" procedure. In other words, the physician is unable to see obstructions, etc. while inserting the echoscope. Topical anesthesia of the oropharynx is often recommended to facilitate insertion (*e.g.* lidocaine spray or gargle, lidocaine gel to lubricate the echoscope). Lidocaine is applied a few puffs etc. at a time until sufficient effects are observed, *i.e.* until pressure on the back of the tongue does not evoke gagging. Although this provides adequate anesthetization, the drawback is that swallowing is impaired, and the patient cannot follow swallowing commands as well. Aside from local anesthetics, intravenous sedation, and short-term hypnotics, it is even more important to psychologically prepare the patient to ensure his or her cooperation in the performance of the procedure. If sedatives or short-term hypnotics must be used, the physician should select one whose effects can be controlled well. The effects should be short-term, and the appropriate antidote should be on hand. The sedatives most commonly used in TEE are midazolam, propofol, fentanyl, and diazepam. However, one should be aware that a substantial part of the risk associated with the procedure is due to the effects of these substances.

In addition to sedatives, parasympatholytic substances can also be used to reduce salivary secretions and undesired vagus reflexes. The physician should be assured of the absence of contra-indications such as glaucoma, myasthenia syndrome, and enlargement of the prostate. Either the substance cannot be used in these patients, or the patient must receive the appropriate antagonist after completion of TEE.

In most cases, special endocarditis prophylaxis is considered unnecessary. Since no biopsy samples are removed during TEE, bacteremia can occur only if the oropharynx mucosa is traumatized due to overly forceful insertion and advancement of the echoscope. The best endocarditis prophylaxis, then, is gentle guidance of the echoscope. Opinions vary whether this will suffice in high-risk patients.

During insertion of the echoscope, the patient should lie in a left lateral position with the neck slightly flexed. The tip of the echoscope is advanced through the mouth guard and across the dorsum of the tongue. Some operators insert their index finger over the middle of the patient's tongue to help guide the echoscope. However, this may evoke gagging if the patient has not received adequate local anesthesia. Some resistance may be encountered when the echoscope reaches the cricopharyngeus muscle. This resistance can be overcome by having the patient swallow, which relaxes the muscle and makes it possible to advance the tip of the echoscope further distal. When the index finger is withdrawn, the mouth guard then rests in its final position, and the echoscope can be advanced into the fundus of the stomach or to the mid-esophageal region. During the entire insertion procedure, one should avoid using excessive force or pressure in order to prevent injury to the delicate mucous membranes or the piriform sinuses. Between the inferior constrictor muscle of the pharynx and the esophagus is a weak muscular triangle through which the upper esophageal diverticulum may herniate. The operator should always advance the echoscope into the esophagus with caution. Any resistance encountered while blindly inserting the echoscope may lead to perforation of the diverticulum. As in bronchoscopy, a lateral contrast chest x-ray of the esophagus should be displayed within view during the TEE examination.

When the echoscope rests in the primary position, the video recorder is activated and the entire examination is taped. It does not matter whether the examination is started with the echoscope in the fundus of the stomach or in the mid-esophagus. When starting from the esophagus, one should consider that insertion of the echoscope in the lower esophageal sphincter may cause the patient some discomfort. Therefore, this step should be reserved for the end of the examination in unanesthetized patients. In patients under general anesthesia, the TEE examination is usually started with the probe in the stomach.

Many operators use an external tape recorder to tape their remarks during the examination. The total examination time should not exceed 10 to 15 minutes. This should be adequate time for a thorough and complete examination if the operator proceeds systematically.

Systematic examination procedure

1. Transgastric short and long-axis views of the left ventricle
   35 to 40 cm from the incisors, with anteflection of the echoscope tip
   ▸ Short-axis view at papillary muscle and mitral valve levels
   ▸ Long-axis views: transgastric 2-chamber and long-axis views

2. Mid-esophageal short and long-axis views
   30 cm from the incisors, with retroflection if necessary
   ▸ Short-axis views: four and five-chamber views
   ▸ Long-axis views: two-chamber view, and view through left atrial appendage

3. Basal short and long-axis views
   25 to 30 cm from the incisors (landmarks: aorta, left atrium), with increasing cranialization of the echoscope tip or slight withdrawal
   ▸ Short-axis views:
     – Aortic valve, atria with interatrial septum, right ventricle and RVOT,
     – Proximal ascending aorta, proximal coronary arteries, right atrial appendage, superior vena cava, left atrium, proximal inferior pulmonary veins, superior vena cava
     – Proximal ascending aorta, superior vena cava, left atrium, left atrial appendage; and proximal superior pulmonary veins, left atrial appendage, and pulmonary valve
     – Proximal ascending aorta, superior vena cava, pulmonary trunk, and proximal pulmonary arteries, left atrium, and left superior pulmonary vein
   ▸ Long-axis views:
     – LV inflow tract and left superior pulmonary vein
     – RVOT and pulmonary trunk
     – Proximal ascending aorta
     – Superior vena cava and atrial septum
     – Right superior pulmonary vein
     – LVOT
     – Aortic valve

4. Aortic short and long-axis views
     – From the midthoracic region (25 to 30 cm), with counter-clockwise rotation
     – Through the descending aorta and aortic arch, with supra-aortic branches

---

At the end of the examination, the patient should be observed for 15 to 60 min, depending on whether and which sedatives were used and on the patient's clinical condition.

Since the successful preliminary trials with transesophageal M-mode and 2-D echocardiography in the mid-seventies [4, 8, 10, 11], and most of all since the introduction of phased array transducer systems in the late seventies [9, 13, 25, 36, 27], transesophageal echocardiography (TEE) has won secure standing in clinical cardiac diagnosis. TEE has become an invaluable tool for demonstration of vegetations on native and prosthetic cardiac valves [3, 7], for assessment of the morphological features of the cardiac valves and the intra-atrial septum in patients with embolism, for assessment of prosthetic valve function, for detecting thrombi in the right atrium, right ventricle, and especially in the (right) pulmonary artery after pulmonary artery embolization, and, more recently, in the diagnosis of aortic dissection [5, 18, 19]. Moreover, transesophageal echocardiography is a useful diagnostic tool in all patients in whom transthoracic diagnosis is not possible - be it due to obesity, pulmonary emphysema, or in ventilated intensive care patients [6].

In the early eighties, many echocardiographers realized that since conventional single-array transesophageal endoscopes allowed imaging only in the horizontal (transverse) plane, their diagnostic usefulness was limited. Although the work groups around Hanrath and Souquet described trials using miniaturized phased array systems and parallel experiences with biplane TEE in the early eighties [9, 29], the first usable biplane transesophageal probes were not available until the late eighties [14, 15, 21, 22, 23, 24]. The first multiplane probes were developed in the early nineties; they have again broadened the scope of diagnostic possibilities with TEE.

In transesophageal two-dimensional echocardiography, scan planes are defined according to their anatomic orientation with respect to the heart [3, 28].

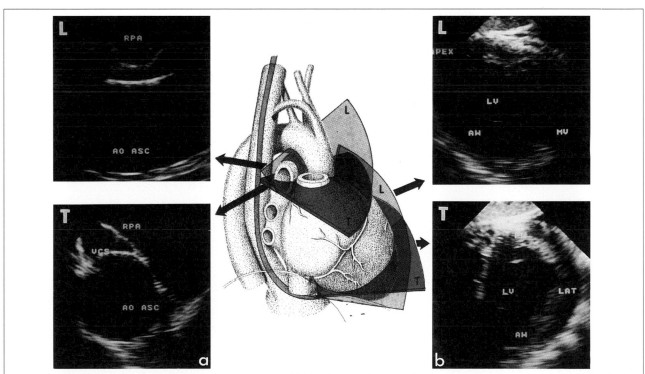

a. Ascending aorta (AO ASC) and right pulmonary artery (RPA). **b.** Long and short-axis views through the left ventricle (LV), mitral valve (MV), anterior (AW), lateral wall (LAT), superior vena cava (VCS). L = longitudinal, T = transverse plane.

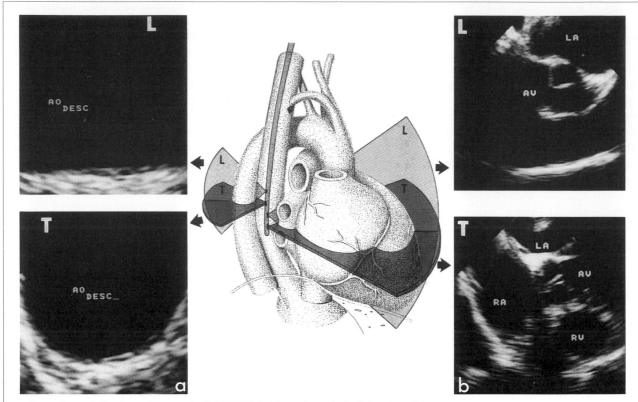

a. Plane through the descending aorta (AO DESC). **b.** Plane through the left atrium (LA), aortic valve (AV), right atrium (RA), right ventricle (RV). In the long-axis view, the pulmonary trunk is below the aortic valve.

First, the transducer is positioned in the fundus of the stomach to obtain the transgastric-transhepatic view of the heart, and transgastric short-axis scans are uniformly obtained. The operator then switches to the longitudinal array or, when using a biplane probe, the transducer is rotated into the longitudinal plane, and transgastric long-axis scans are obtained.

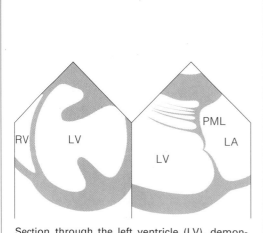

Section through the left ventricle (LV), demonstrating posterior (HW), anterior (VW), and lateral (LAT) walls, interventricular septum (IVS), and papillary muscles (PAP MUSC).

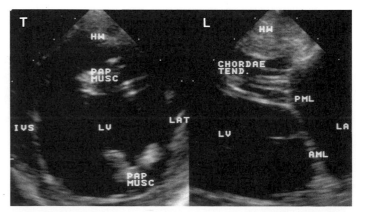

Transesophageal transverse (left) and longitudinal (right) echocardiograms.

The operator should ensure that the imaged structure is centered exactly on the middle axis of the display screen. The papillary muscles and the mitral valve apparatus can be assessed from the longitudinal plane. By rotating the tip of the echoscope clockwise, transgastric short and long-axis views of the right ventricle can be obtained. Unfortunately, due to the anatomic orientation of the heart and the stomach, the transgastric long-axis view of the ventricle is somewhat off-center. The operator can attempt correct the off-axis position by angulating the probe. However, this usually results in a loss of contact between the gastric wall and the echoscope and, thus, insufficient image quality. By retracting the transducer into the esophagus and by rotating the it along the conventional transverse axis, the four-chamber view of the heart can be obtained. When positioned properly, the left atrium should be directly in front of the transducer. These scans image the atrioventricular valves, the intra-atrial septum, the interventricular septum, and the lateral walls of the ventricle. From the longitudinal axis, the mitral valve and the left atrial appendage can be assessed in addition to the left heart cavities.

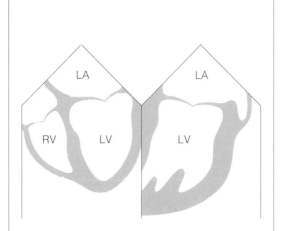

Four and two-chamber views. Left (LA) and right (RA) atria, left (LV) and right (RV) ventricles, tricuspid valve (TK), interventricular septum (IVS), anterior (AMS) and posterior (PMS) mitral leaflets, left atrial appendage (LHO).

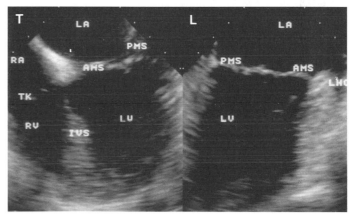

Transesophageal 2-D transverse (left) and longitudinal (right) echocardiograms.

The mitral valve can be scanned in its entirety by incrementally rotating the transducer 180° along its axis. This permits better color flow mapping of both normal [30] and pathological flow. Furthermore, the risk of overestimating regurgitations can be minimized [2].

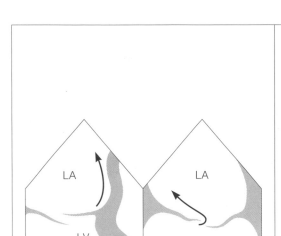

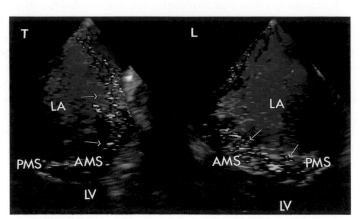

Mitral regurgitation (arrow). Jet can be recognized more easily in the long-axis view.

Transesophageal 2-D transverse (left) and longitudinal (right) echocardiograms with color flow mapping.

As in transthoracic echocardiography, TEE can also demonstrate the left ventricular walls in their entirety.

The long-axis view of the interatrial septum is obtained by rotating the transducer clockwise. The septum secundum is then clearly visible above the fossa ovalis.

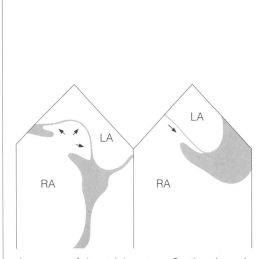

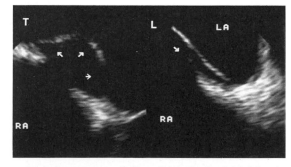

Aneurysm of the atrial septum. Section through the atrial septum demonstrating septum secundum (arrow).

Transesophageal transverse (left) and longitudinal (right) echocardiograms.

Atrial septal defects are easily detected from this view [16]. The tricuspid valve, the right ventricular in- and outflow tracts, the normally very fragile pulmonary valve, and the pulmonary trunk are demonstrated below the atrial septum.

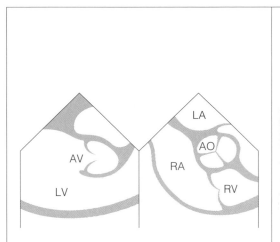
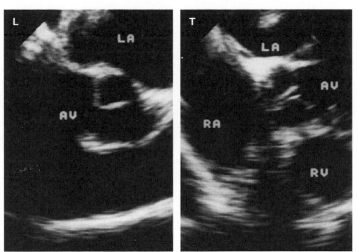

Plane through the left atrium (LA), aortic valve (AV), right atrium (RA), right ventricle (RV). In the long-axis view, the pulmonary trunk is located underneath the aortic valve.

Transesophageal longitudinal and transverse echocardiograms.

By rotating the transducer further clockwise, the view of the right atrium with the junctions of the superior and inferior vena cavae is obtained.

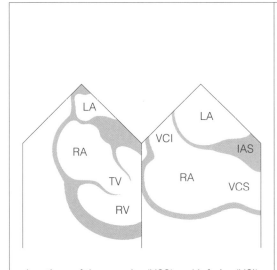
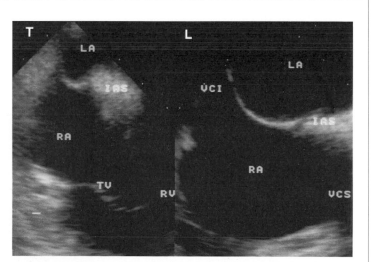

Junctions of the superior (VCS) and inferior (VCI) vena cavae in the right atrium (RA).

Transesophageal transverse (left) and longitudinal (right) echocardiograms.

Starting from the four-chamber short-axis position, the probe can be angulated to obtain the five-chamber view for visualization of the left ventricular outflow tract and the aortic valve. By rotating the multiplane transducer ca. 70 to 90°, it is possible to transsect the aortic valve for morphological assessment and planimetry [12].

5.3.1   **Transesophageal Echocardiography**
5.3.1.2 **Transesophageal and Transgastric Single and Multiplane Imaging**

222

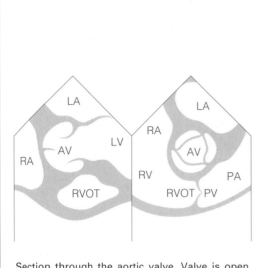

Section through the aortic valve. Valve is open during systole.

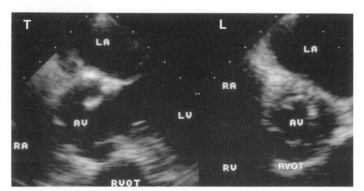

Transesophageal transverse (left) and longitudinal (right) echocardiograms.

The left atrial appendage can be visualized by slightly retracting the transducer a bit further into the esophagus [1]. The inflow of the left pulmonary veins into the left atrium can be seen more dorsally.

Next, the ascending aorta and the right pulmonary artery are visualized by again slightly retracting the transducer [31]. The first 10 cm of the ascending aorta can be assessed in cross section by rotating the transducer 90° around its axis.

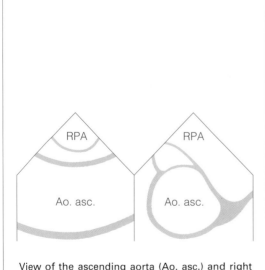

View of the ascending aorta (Ao. asc.) and right pulmonary artery (RPA).

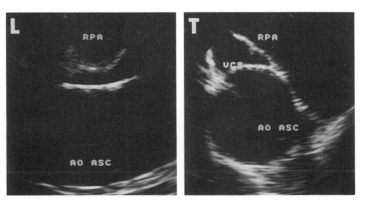

Transesophageal longitudinal and transverse echocardiograms.

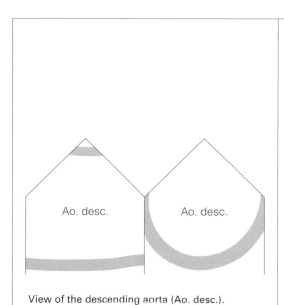

View of the descending aorta (Ao. desc.).

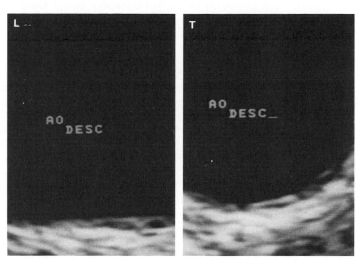

Transesophageal longitudinal and transverse echocardiograms.

The descending aorta is routinely scanned at the end of the examination.
The long-axis view of the descending aorta can be obtained from the longitudinal plane. By incrementally retracting the echoscope, the descending aorta can be viewed in its entirety. Long and short-axis views of the aortic arch can also be obtained from the longitudinal plane [18, 19].

References

1. Aschenberg W, Schlüter M, Kremer P, Schröder E, Siglow V, Bleifeld W. Transesophageal two-dimensional echocardiography for the detection of left atrial appendage thrombus. Am Coll Cardiol 1986; 7: 163-166.
2. Bolger AF, Eigler NL, Maurer G. Quantifying valvular regurgitation, limitations and inherent assumptions of Doppler techniques. Circulation 1988; 78: 1316-1318.
3. Daniel WG, Schröder E, Mügge A, Lichtlen PR. Transesophageal echocardiography in infective endocarditis. Am J Cardiac Imaging 1988; 2: 78-85.
4. DiMagno E, Regan PT, Wilson DA, Buxton JL, Hattery RR, Suarez JR, Green PS. Ultrasonic endoscope. Lancet, March 22, 1980.
5. Erbel R, Daniel WG, Visser C, Engberding R, Roeland J, Rennollet H, European Cooperative Study Group for Echocardiography. Echocardiography in diagnosis of aortic dissection. Lancet, March 1989; 4: 457-461.
6. Erbel R, Mohr-Kahaly S, Wittlich N, Drexler M, Henrichs KJ, Darius H, Meyer J. Indikation zur transösophagealen Echokardiographie. Ultraschall Klin Prax 1989; 4: 60-75.
7. Erbel R, Rohmann S, Drexler M, Mohr-Kahaly S, Gerharz CD, Iversen S, Oelert H, Meyer J. Improved diagnostic value of echocardiography in patients with infective endocarditis by transesophageal approach. A prospective study. Eur Heart J 1988; 9: 43-53.
8. Frazin L, Talano JV, Stephanides L, Loeb HS, Kopel L, Gunnar RM. Esophageal echocardiography. Circulation 1976; 54.
9. Hanrath P, Schlüter M, Langenstein BA, Polster J, Engel S. Transesophageal horizontal and sagittal imaging of the heart with a phased array system, initial clinical results. In: Hanrath P, Bleifeld W. Cardiovascular diagnosis by ultrasound. The Hague: Nijhoff, 1982.
10. Hanrath P, Schlüter M, Langenstein BA, Polster J, Engel S, Kremer P, Krebber HJ. Detection of ostium secundum atrial septal defects by transesophageal cross-sectional echocardiography. Br Heart J 1983; 49: 350-358.

11. Hisanaga K, Hisanaga A, Hibi N, Nishimura K, Kambe T. High speed rotating scanner for transeso-phageal cross-sectional echocardiography. Am J Cardiol 1980; 46: 837-842.

12. Hofmann T, Kasper W, Meinertz T, Spillner G, Schlosser V, Just HJ. Determination of aortic valve orifice area in aortic valve stenosis by two-dimensional transesophageal echocardiography. Am J Cardiol 1987; 59: 330-335.

13. Lancée CT, De Jong N, Gussenhoven WJ, Taams M, Bom N, Brommersma P, Roelandt JRTC. Techno-logical Developments of transesophageal echocardiography in a historical perspective. In: Erbel R, Khanderia K (eds). Transesophageal echocardiography. Berlin, Heidelberg: Springer, 1989

14. Leischik R, Curtius JM, Deutsch HJ, Arnold G, Sander C, de Vivie R, Hilger HH. Vorteile der biplanen transösophagealen Echokardiographie. Z Kadiol 1990; 79: 850-857.

15. Makowski T, Erbel R, Nixdorff U, Zotz R, Meyer J. Diagnostic value of biplane transesophageal color Doppler echocardiography. Eur Heart J 1990; 11 (suppl): 111.

16. Makowski T, Erbel R, Zotz R, Wittlich N, Nixdorff U, Meyer J. Diagnostische Wertigkeit biplaner trans-ösophagealer Echokardiographie bei Krankheiten des Vorhofseptums. Z Kardiol 1991; 80 (suppl I): 130.

17. Matsamura M, Kyo S, Shah PM, Adachi H, Yokote J, Omoto R. A new look at mitral valve pathology with biplane color Doppler transesophageal probe. J Am Soc Echo 1989; 2: 215.

18. Mohr-Kahaly S, Erbel R, Renollet H, Wittlich N, Drexler M, Oelert H, Meyer J. Ambulatory follow-up of aortic dissection by transesophageal two-dimensional and color-coded Doppler echocardiography. Circulation 1989; 80: 24-33.

19. Mohr-Kahaly S, Erbel R, Steller D, Börner N, Drexler M, Meyer J. Aortic dissection detected by transeso-phageal echocardiography. Int J Cardiac Imag 1987; 2: 31-35.

20. Mügge A, Daniel WG, Klöpper J, Lichtlen PR. Visualization of patent foramen ovale by transesophageal color-coded Doppler echocardiography. Am J Cardiol 1988; 62: 837-838.

21. Omoto R, Kyo S, Matsumura M, Shah PM, Adachi H, Matsunaka T, Miura K. Bi-plane color transeso-phageal Doppler echocardiography (color TEE): Its advantages and limitations. Int J Cardiac Imag 1989; 4: 57-58.

22. Omoto R, Kyo S, Matsumura M, Shah PM, Adachi H, Matsunaka T. Biplane color Doppler transeso-phageal echocardiography: Its impact on cardiovascular surgery and further technological progress in the probe, a matrix phased-array biplane probe. Echocardiography 1989; 6: 423-430.

23. Omoto R, Kyo S, Matsumura M, Shah PM, Maruyama M, Adachi H, Yokote Y. New on line real-time bi-plane transesophageal imaging technique. Circulation 1989; 80 (suppl II): 475.

24. Omoto R, Kyo S, Matsumura M, Shah PM, Adachi H, Matsunaka T, Tachikawa K. Recent technological progress in transesophageal color Doppler flow imaging with special reference to newly developped biplane and padiatric probes. In: Erbel R, Khandheria K (eds). Transesophageal echocardiography. Berlin, Heidelberg: Springer, 1989.

25. Schlüter M, Langenstein BA, Polster J, Kremer P, Souquet J, Engel S, Hanrath P. Transesophageal cross-sectional echocardiography with a phrased array transducer system. Technique and initial clinical results. Br Heart J 1982; 48: 67-72.

26. Schlüter M, Langenstein BA, Hanrath P, Kremer P, Bleifeld W. Transösophageale Doppler-Echokardi-ographie. Erste klinische Ergebnisse. Z Kardiol 1981; 70: 797-802.

27. Schlüter M, Thier W, Hinrichs A, Kremer P, Siglow V, Hanrath P. Klinischer Einsatz der transösopha-gealen Echokardiographie. Dtsch med Wschr 1984; 109: 722-727.

28. Seward JB, Khanderia BK, Edwards WD, Oh JK, Freeman WK, Tajik AJ. Biplanar transesophageal echo-cardiography. Atomic correlations, image orientation and clinical applications. Mayo Clin Proc 1990; 65: 1193-1213.

29. Souquet J. Phased array transducer technology for transesophageal imaging of the heart: Current status and future aspects. In: Hanrath P, Bleifeld W. Cadiovascular diagnosis by ultrasound. Nijhoff, The Hague: Nijhoff,1982.

30. Wittlich N, Siemens J. Transesophageal Color-Doppler flow mapping in normal subjects. Circulation 1988; 78 (suppl II): 297.

31. Wittlich N, Erbel R, Eichler A, Jakob H, Iversen S, Oelert H, Meyer J. Detection of pulmonary artery thrombi by transesophageal echocardiography in patients with pulmonary embolism. J Am Soc Echo 1990; 3: 225.

As in transthoracic echocardiography, oblique imaging planes are the most common source of error in transesophageal echocardiography. This affects volumetry of the cardiac cavities and wall motion analyses. Furthermore, the ideal transducer-to-mucous-membrane-contact does not always exist due to the topography of the heart and its cavities. Image dropout can occur when an attempt is made to better visualize certain segments of the heart by angulating the tip of the echoscope, because of loss of contact between the echoscope and the mucous membrane.

Misinterpretation of natural structures or of artifactual images can lead to false-positive findings of intracardiac masses. Oblique views of the cardiac valves can lead to false-positive findings of thickening or vegetations.

Trivial (normal) regurgitation, which is usually found in all four cardiac valves directly before or after valve closure, should not be mistakenly diagnosed as pathological regurgitation.

Limitations that apply for (semi-) quantitation of regurgitations using color jet assessments in transthoracic echocardiography also apply in monoplane transesophageal echocardiography. Although multiplane echoscopes create a good spatial impression of the geometric extent of a regurgitant jet, the method still has not been validated using 3-D reconstructions from well-defined sectional planes.

When diagnosing aortic dissection, false-positive findings can have catastrophic consequences. Atheromatous deposits on the aortic wall, and thickening and calcification that result in surface irregularities can be misinterpreted as a thrombotic dissection. In contrast with chronic thrombosis, only freshly thrombosed false lumina indicate an urgent need for surgery in connection with acute aortic dissection. Freshly thrombosed false lumina do not exhibit calcific echoes, but have uniform echo density. Atherosclerotic lesions, as compared with acute dissections, never demonstrate either torn intimal flaps nor flow signals in color flow imaging.

The major advantage of multiplane transesophageal echocardiography is its ability to provide continuous interrogation of suspicious structures from multiple angles.

An immediate practical goal for research and development teams is the development of continuous transducer-to-mucous-membrane-contact systems. This would finally make it possible to avoid image dropout, even in extreme transducer angulation. It would also ensure the reproducibility of oblique imaging planes and of volumetric calculations of the cardiac cavities.

More fundamental limitations of current transesophageal echocardiography technology are
1. the need for further miniaturization to open potentials for perspective transvascular access,
2. the lack of a wide range of interventional possibilities as compared with bronchoscopy and gastrointestinal endoscopy, and
3. the not yet fully developed potentials for 3-D reconstruction from different sectional planes that prevents perspectively complete imaging of the mediastinum, as is possible in established radiological techniques such as computed tomography and magnetic resonance imaging.

The past five years have witnessed remarkable developments in visualizing human arteries from within, thus bringing the „Fantastic Voyage"[1] of science fiction a step closer to our daily life [39]. Although angioscopy provides a colorful picture of the book cover, intravascular ultrasound allows us to read inside the book. It allows the examination of features within the vessel wall of living humans never before possible except in a microscopic specimen. New developments like three-dimensional (3-D) reconstruction promise to enhance the images by offering projections of the vessel that can be rotated or sliced in any plane we choose. Intravascular ultrasound imaging is already providing important information for planning and monitoring endovascular interventions. This chapter reviews the historical development and design features of the various ultrasound catheters, describes the appearance of normal and abnormal vessels and discusses the applications of this new technology.

5.3.2 Intravascular Ultrasound
5.3.2.1 Rationale for Development

The limitations of angiography in the diagnosis of coronary disease are well known. Angiography underestimates the severity and extent of atherosclerosis as compared to pathological examination or to epicardial ultrasound performed at the time of surgery [19]. Since intravascular ultrasound can usually define the internal elastic membrane, a definition of stenosis similar to the histologic one is used, *i.e.*, the percent of area bounded by the internal elastic membrane that is occupied by atheroma. Angiography, on the other hand, compares the lumen to an adjacent, apparently normal area. If that area is not normal, as is often the case, the severity of stenosis is underestimated. Furthermore, intra- and interobserver variability in interpreting the angiogram is high, and the correlation with physiological measures of severity (flow reserve) is suboptimal. In the context of vascular interventions, the „luminogram" provided by angiography at the site of intervention does not reveal fine details that are necessary to optimize the results. Residual atherosclerotic plaque cannot be directly visualized and therefore cannot be targeted by ablation or atherectomy techniques. The extent and depth of dissection and the presence of clot often cannot be determined with accuracy.

Several alternative means of imaging have been tried to overcome these limitations. It was well known that high-frequency ultrasound has the ability to produce high-resolution images through tissue planes, but the capacity to miniaturize a transducer and successfully image from within an artery was a difficult engineering feat. Although the first real-time intravascular ultrasound catheter (for intracardiac imaging) was described twenty years ago, the major advances in miniaturization occurred only over the past five years.

Three major factors helped to make this possible: First, the widespread use of balloon angioplasty and the advances in guide wire technology made the idea of the introduction of ultrasound catheters into the coronary arteries on a routine basis conceivable and safe. Second, the limitations of angiography in guiding, monitoring and understanding the effects of the various endovascular interventions created a need for the kind of information that intravascular ultrasound can provide. third, significant advances in technology allowed the miniaturization, increased flexibility and improved image quality of the catheters.

---

[1] Title of a 1966 science Fiction movie where the actors are miniaturized and taken through an adventure inside the heart and circulation.

Early Development

Early attempts at intracardiac imaging date back to the early 1950's [1]. Progress was slow until 1988 when several groups described their initial experiences with a variety of ultrasound catheters. Catheter design and image quality have undergone striking improvements. Like other ultrasonic transducers, two basic designs are available: mechanical and electronic array. The term „electronic array" is adopted in this chapter to indicate electronic control of the number, sequence and timing of activation of the transducer elements. This definition encompasses the phased array and the so-called „synthetic aperture array" transducers, as described later.

The Mechanical Catheter

Several groups have developed catheters that contain a single transducer element at the tip. Three basic configurations exist. In the first, the transducer is mechanically rotated to sweep the ultrasonic beam 360°. In the second configuration, the transducer is stationary and the beam is reflected by an acoustic reflector which is mechanically rotated. This again results in a beam that rotates 360°, thereby producing an image perpendicular to the catheter. In the third configuration, the relationship of the transducer and reflector remains constant as the whole catheter rotates along its axis. The purpose of the reflecting mirror is to permit imaging right up to the surface of the catheter without creating any dead space.

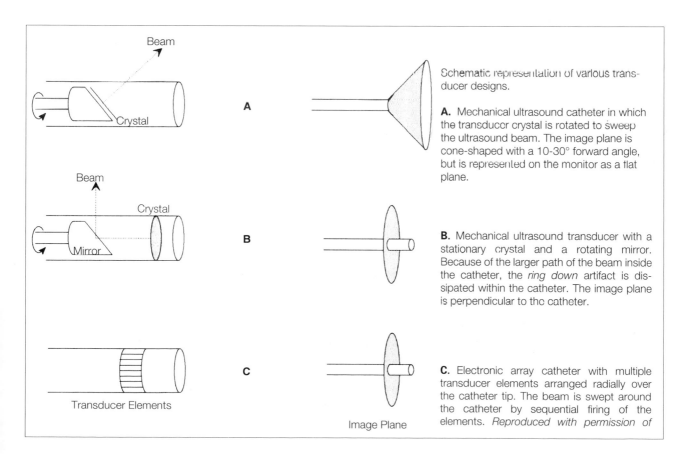

Schematic representation of various transducer designs.

A. Mechanical ultrasound catheter in which the transducer crystal is rotated to sweep the ultrasound beam. The image plane is cone-shaped with a 10-30° forward angle, but is represented on the monitor as a flat plane.

B. Mechanical ultrasound transducer with a stationary crystal and a rotating mirror. Because of the larger path of the beam inside the catheter, the *ring down* artifact is dissipated within the catheter. The image plane is perpendicular to the catheter.

C. Electronic array catheter with multiple transducer elements arranged radially over the catheter tip. The beam is swept around the catheter by sequential firing of the elements. *Reproduced with permission of*

Certain designs employ a thin plastic sheath in which the catheter is inserted. The sheath is introduced into the coronary artery over a guide wire and remains there during the procedure. It allows the catheter to rotate freely and also permits the catheter to be passed repeatedly inside the sheath for repeated imaging without risking increased injury to the artery. The various catheters are rotated at speeds of up to 1,800 RPM by a small, hand-held external motor to produce cross-sectional images at 30 frames per second in real-time.

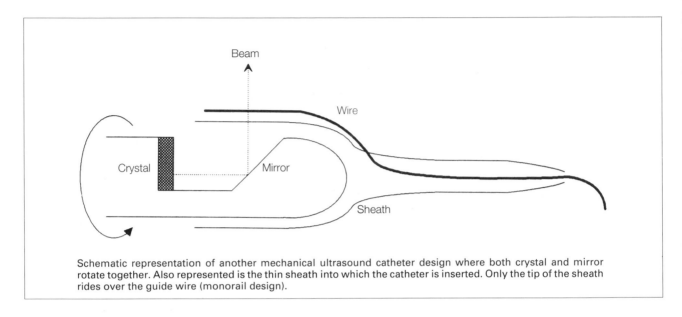

Schematic representation of another mechanical ultrasound catheter design where both crystal and mirror rotate together. Also represented is the thin sheath into which the catheter is inserted. Only the tip of the sheath rides over the guide wire (monorail design).

The Electronic Array Catheter

The catheter introduced in 1972 for cardiac imaging consisted of 32 elements arranged circumferentially near to the tip of the catheter [1]. The *phased array* technique (sequential firing of groups of elements) was used to sweep the ultrasonic beam 360° in a plane perpendicular to the catheter. The catheter was relatively large (3.2 mm) and the image quality was suboptimal. The only electronic array catheter currently available uses a polymeric 64-element transducer [10]. Four integrated circuits incorporated at the tip serve to digitize, amplify and multiplex the signal for transmission to an external computer. This reduces the number of wires running through the catheter and enhances its flexibility. A complex algorithm termed „*synthetic aperture array*" is used for image reconstruction. Ultrasound signals are transmitted from single (or multiple elements, and the reflected signals are received by all available elements. Multiple elements are available for reception of points far from the catheter (wide aperture), whereas only one or two elements may be available for near points (narrow aperture). Thus, theoretically, the beam remains focused for all points. The image is updated at 10 frames per second, which is slower than the *phased array* and mechanical catheters.

The Ultrasound Transducer

Current transducers (both single and multi-element) range in size from 1 to 1.4 mm for coronary applications to up to 2.7 mm for peripheral vascular applications. Most transducers operate at a center frequency of 20 to 25 MHz, and some are set at 30 or 40 MHz. These high frequencies, compared to 2.5 to 3.5 MHz for transthoracic echocardiography, result in very high resolution images but unfortunately have a small depth of field. Axial resolution (parallel to the ultrasonic beam) is about 0.1 mm. Lateral resolution (perpendicular to the beam) varies with the distance from the catheter but averages 0.2 to 0.5 mm.

The penetration of the ultrasound beam at these high frequencies is about 1 cm, which is adequate since the width of the arteries is comparable to the ultrasound penetration. The higher frequency transducers (30 to 40 MHz) offer better resolution at the cost of less penetration and backscatter from flowing blood particles. Transducers of 5 to 12 MHz may be more suitable for intracardiac imaging.

A Comparison of Mechanical and Electronic Array Catheters

Although each catheter system has its advantages and disadvantages, we believe that the image quality of the mechanical catheters is superior to that achieved with the electronic array devices. miniaturization of the ultrasonic transducer to below 1 mm is an important technical goal for all the systems. In the electronic array catheter, which uses multiple elements, this is more complicated and may require new transducer materials which could be costly. The electronics involved are also quite complex. The incorporation of integrated circuits at the tip of these catheters avoids the earlier problem of having multiple wires running the length of the catheter. Since there is no need for a rotating cable, the electronic array catheter is more flexible and easier to manipulate in tortuous arteries. It is also possible to incorporate a movable 0.014 inch angioplasty guide wire in a central lumen, which facilitates tracking in tortuous segments. Instead of a central guide wire, the newer mechanical catheters have utilized monorail designs where the catheter or its sheath rides over the wire for only a short distance (1 to 3 cm) at its tip.

This has greatly improved their ease of use and flexibility. The major technical challenges with the mechanical systems are the miniaturization of the moving parts and the maintenance of smooth rotation in tortuous segments.

A physical property of ultrasonic transducers is that the area immediately adjacent to the transducer cannot be imaged. This results from *amplifier saturation* at the time of pulse transmission. Once this dissipates, signal reception can take place. This amplifier saturation produces a very bright signal at the transducer interface, the so-called „*ring down artifact*". This is a problem with side viewing catheters, since they may lie immediately adjacent to the structure to be imaged. In mechanical catheters that employ an acoustic reflector, the initial path of the beam occurs within the catheter. Therefore, the imaging window starts at the surface of the catheter and there is no *ring down artifact*. This is a major advantage when imaging small arteries. In the electronic catheter, this artifact is electronically subtracted to improve the image, however, it is not clear that the subtraction algorithm is adequate.

In summary, each catheter design has advantages and limitations. Furthermore, technology is evolving at a rapid pace. The various designs will find specific applications for which they are best suited.

| 5.3.2 | Intravascular Ultrasound |
| 5.3.2.3 | Imaging of Systemic Arteries |

Vessel Dimensions

Intra- and Inter-observer Variabilities

Measurements performed on intravascular ultrasound images have shown excellent reproducibility. *In vitro* measurements of luminal cross-sectional area showed a good correlation coefficient of 0.99 for the same observer and 0.98 between two observers [20]. Another group of investigators found and intra and inter-observer variability of 0.5 ± 5% and 2.8 ± 7%, respectively [30].

Reliability of Quantitative Measurements

For phantoms of known dimensions, the luminal area measured by intravascular ultrasound is practically identical to the known area of the phantom [9, 22]. In a study of phantoms with irregular (tear-shaped) narrowing, the mean cross-sectional area at the stenosis was 6.6 ± 2.4 mm^2 by direct measurement, 7.2 ± 2.6 mm^2 by intravascular ultrasound, and 10.9 ± 3.9 mm^2 by radiography [20]. Therefore, when the image quality is adequate, the available catheters yield very accurate measurements.

Numerous studies have correlated measurements made by intravascular ultrasound to histological measurements. For luminal area and atherosclerotic plaque thickness, the correlation coefficients are generally above 0.9 [6, 18, 22, 38]. In some studies, the ultrasound measurements were higher than the histologic ones by a small and predictable magnitude [27]. This may be due to shrinkage of the pathological specimens during formalin fixation [6, 38]. When the luminal areas are compared to anatomic photographs obtained at the same time (arteries previously formalin fixed), the correlation is very high (r = 0.98) with minimal overestimation by intravascular ultrasound [27].

Luminal areas (cross-sectional) measured by intravascular ultrasound and by quantitative angiography in vivo have shown excellent correlation when the lumen is circular (r = 0.92) [24]. However, in the presence of eccentric plaque and following angioplasty when the lumen is irregular, the correlations are lower (r = 0.77 and 0.86, resp.) [23, 24]. A recent study of patients with saphenous vein graft stenoses showed a high correlation (r = 0.96) between the minimal luminal dimensions measured by intravascular ultrasound and by angiography both before and after angioplasty [22].

Arterial Wall Morphology

One of the most exciting features of intravascular ultrasound is its ability to visualize the vessel wall and characterize its structure and dimensions. Numerous studies have directly compared the ultrasonic appearance of the walls of various vessels to their corresponding histologic sections.

Layers of the Arterial Wall

The ultrasonic appearance of systemic arterial wall arteries varies with the composition of their layers. Even within the broad histological classification into elastic, transitional and muscular arteries, enough variation exists to produce different ultrasonic patterns in arteries of the same class [22].

Two basic patterns are seen with intravascular ultrasound [6, 18]. First, a characteristic three layer appearance where the innermost and the outermost layers are highly echo reflective (white) and are separated by an echolucent (black) layer. Second, some arteries demonstrate a single echo reflective (white) ring. Some authors [22] describe a variation of the above patterns where the two echo reflective layers can be distinguished by different echo densities, but are not separated by an echolucent layer and their interface is not distinct.

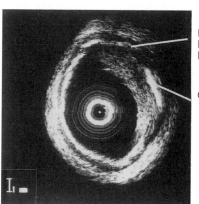
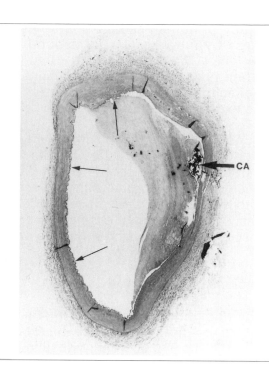

Ultrasound image and the corresponding histologic section of a human carotid artery demonstrating an eccentric atheromatous plaque with calcification at its base. The calcium causes dropout of the image behind it. The echolucent media is seen circumferentially. The internal elastic membrane (thin arrows) is highly echo reflective and its thickness is overestimated by ultrasound.

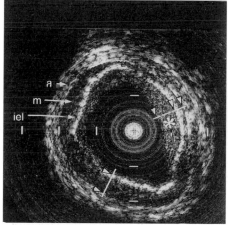
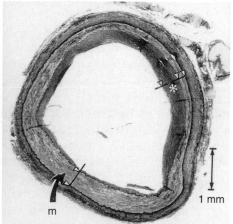

Ultrasound image and histologic sections of a renal artery. Bright echoes of the internal elastic lumina (iel) and adventitia (a) circumscribe the echolucent media. At 7 o'clock the intima and media appear normal. Intimal thickening at 2 o'clock is associated with medial thinning. [6].

Controversy exists in the literature regarding what each of the three characteristic layers (-especially the middle one) represents [6, 10]. Contributing to the disagreement are several factors including the experimental design, type of vessel and the varying capabilities of the catheters used. We will present the interpretation which is now shared by most researchers [6,7, 30, 37].

When imaging muscular arteries (*e.g.* coronary or femoral arteries) the three layer pattern is most evident. In a normal artery, the inner echo reflective layer results from the highly echo reflective internal elastic membrane separating intima and media. The thickness of this innermost layer often exceeds that of the intima due to blooming or broadening or a „trailing edge" effect caused by the highly reflective elastin fibers of the internal elastic membrane [7, 37].

In a study of human cadaveric arteries (coronary, carotid and femoral) the average intimal thickness by intravascular ultrasound overestimated the histological measurement by 0.3 mm or 33% (1.2 ± 0.8 versus 0.9 ± 0.8) [18]. Similar numbers were reported in another study [6]. When fibrous atheroma is present, the thickened plaque corresponds to the innermost band of echo reflectance and the internal elastic membrane can be demonstrated behind the plaque exactly corresponding to the position on histology [37].

Surrounding the first echo reflective layer is an echolucent layer of about 0.5 ± 0.2 mm in cadaveric arteries (0.4 ± 0.2 by histology [18]. This layer represents the media which in muscular arteries lacks concentric elastin fibers and is therefore hypoechoic [6]. Surrounding the echolucent layer is another echo reflective layer representing the external elastic membrane and adventitia. This three layer appearance is present in muscular and in some elastic arteries. As the content of elastic fibers in the media increases (as in elastic arteries) the entire wall becomes equally echo reflective and is represented by a single ring [6].

Dimensions of Vessel Wall Layers

A study of eight presumably normal adults (studied for atypical chest pain) and 43 patients with coronary disease was recently reported [24]. In the normal subjects, the innermost layer measured 0.18 ± 0.06 mm with a maximal thickness of 0.3 mm. The echolucent layer measured 0.11 ± 0.04 mm. the thickness of the outermost layer usually cannot be measured *in vivo* because its outer border is not distinct from the surrounding tissues. In patients with coronary disease, the innermost layer was thickened (> 0.3 mm) in 31% of angiographically normal sites.

Visualization of Atherosclerotic Plaque

The characteristic three layer appearance is a very valuable feature because it allows definition of the intimal thickness between the echolucent media and the lumen. Therefore, intravascular ultrasound can identify the location, extent and eccentricity of the atheromatous plaque and permits quantitative measurement of its thickness or volume. Visualization of the hypoechoic media (which delineates the intima) is possible in 75% of segments [24]. At the time of this study, this could be improved by catheter manipulation, by using the moving video image rather than a still frame, and by extrapolation from adjacent segments. The media underlying atherosclerotic plaques is usually thinned and sometimes absent. This has also been documented by intravascular ultrasound in pathological specimens and in living humans [6]. Even when the media cannot be visualized (*e.g.* in elastic arteries or because the media is absent), the presence and location of atheroma can often be deduced from the reduction in size and the eccentricity of the normally circular lumen.

Ultrasound Characterization of Components of Atherosclerotic Plaque

1. *Calcification:* Intravascular ultrasound is much more sensitive than fluoroscopy for the presence of calcium, a common component of plaque [37]. Calcification is usually patchy and occurs in the deeper layers of the intima. However, it can occur superficially or be very extensive.

   The presence of calcium results in shadowing or dropout of the image behind it and, when extensive, can make measurements or further interpretation of the image difficult or impossible. Even in these cases, however, the lumen can still be defined and measured. Defining the location and extent of calcification may prove very helpful for selecting patients for various catheter interventions. For example, laser and directional atherectomies are less effective if the fibrous cap is calcified [43].

2. *Atheroma:* Early atheroma is identified as a thickened intima of medium echodensity [37]. A fibrous cap with a brighter echodensity may be seen overlying a fibromuscular plaque of medium density [6]. Dense fibrous tissue can have an echo brightness approaching that of calcified tissue. The latter is determined by the presence of shadowing. Lipid deposits within the plaque appear as hypoechoic (black) holes surrounded on all sides by more echo-dense plaque [6, 30]. As the diseased intima thickens, it may encroach upon or totally replace the echolucent media [7]. In a prospective, double-blind *in vitro* study [30], 96% of areas of fibrous plaque were correctly identified. Of the lipid plaques, 78% were correctly identified and 22% were misinterpreted as areas of dropout. All calcific areas were correctly identified. The overall accuracy was 95%.

3. *Thrombus:* Thrombus has a medium echodensity close to that of fibromuscular plaque, but characteristically has a speckled appearance. Small or layered thrombus may be impossible to differentiate from plaque. The thrombus is easier to recognize when it is large, globular, pedunculate and/or mobile. This may explain the differences in the reported sensitivities of intravascular ultrasound to identify thrombus *in vitro* from 92% [40] to 57% [34].

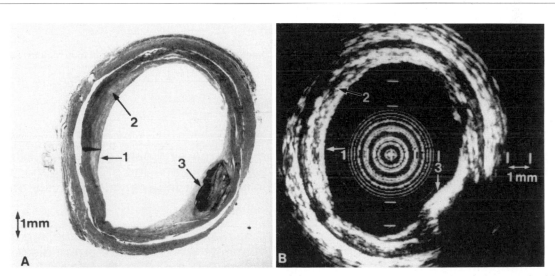

Histologic and echographic sections from an iliac artery. Bright echoes (arrow 1) correspond to dense organized fibrous cap; calcified base. Calcium causes shadowing of image. Hypoechoic zones correspond to lipid deposits. Very bright echoes causing a shadowing effect behind them correspond to the calcific plaque on the histologic section [6].

Tissue Characterization

Analysis of the reflected ultrasound signals can provide information beyond that available on the visual image of the artery. This information can enhance our ability to characterize the components of the vessel wall [20]. Because of the proximity of the transducer to the tissues and the high frequencies utilized, intravascular ultrasound is well suited for this purpose. However, much experiment work still needs to be done before this becomes clinically useful.

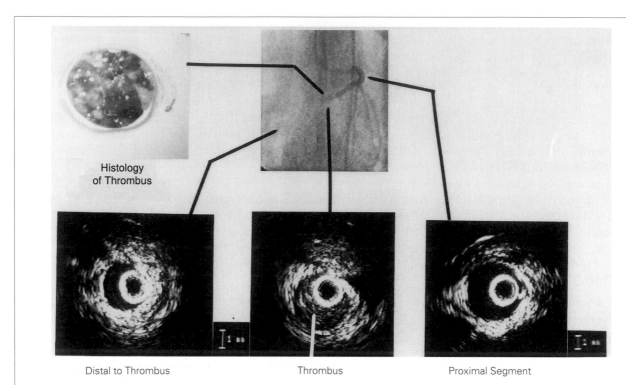

| Distal to Thrombus | Thrombus | Proximal Segment |

Experimentally induced thrombus in porcine coronary artery. Differentiation from fibromuscular plaque may be quite difficult [20].

Arterial Wall Compliance

Accurate and continuous measurement of the luminal area by means of intravascular ultrasound requires a determination of global arterial wall compliance and of intracoronary pressure [16]. The local *compliance* of one sector of the circumference can alternatively be calculated.

Even without measuring the pressure, changes in the diameter between systole and diastole can be measured. In a study of 8 normals and 18 patients with coronary artery disease [23], the mean change in the lumen between systole and diastole was 23 ± 6% in healthy subjects and 8 ± 3.4% in patients at angiographically normal sites. The variation between segments along the circumference of the vessels was significantly higher in the patients.

Coronary Blood Flow

Intravascular Doppler permits measurement of blood flow velocity and relative changes in flow.

The addition of cross-sectional area measurements using an imaging ultrasound catheter allows measurement of volumetric (absolute) coronary flow. The recent availability of miniaturized 0.036 cm (0.014 inch) Doppler wires [35] allows the introduction of the imaging catheter over the Doppler wire to obtain simultaneous measurements of flow velocity and cross-sectional area. This makes it possible to measure changes in volumetric blood flow occurring in response to pharmacologic intervention [35].

Imaging During and After Endovascular Intervention

Angiography provides a „roadmap" of the intervention site and is very useful in guiding the placement of intervention catheters. It has, however, several shortcomings in its ability to detect and differentiate dissection and thrombus, to define a successful result, and to predict or help us advance our knowledge of re-stenosis. Angiography is suboptimal in guiding plaque-directed interventions such as directional atherectomy and laser. Intravascular ultrasound has potential benefits in all of these areas.

Balloon Angioplasty

The effects of balloon angioplasty have been investigated by intravascular ultrasound. The atherosclerotic plaque is often torn at its thinnest region or at its junction with a normal segment [38]. The outer layers of the artery are stretched, resulting in separation of the torn ends of the plaque. A dissection plane is frequently seen separating the diseased intima from the internal elastic membrane, thereby creating an intimal flap that may protrude into the lumen. In experimental *in vitro* and in vivo studies [28, 38], the sensitivity of intravascular ultrasound in detecting tears and flaps ranged from 83% to 100%. In one *in vitro* study, it detected 81% of such disruptions compared to 73% by angiography [34]. After *successful* human coronary angioplasty, the mean residual atheroma occupied 63% of the available lumen (within the boundaries of the media) [37]. Due to the complicated post-angioplastic anatomy, the measurements of the luminal cross-sectional area measured from orthogonal angiograms correlated poorly with the intravascular ultrasound images [37].

The data from 66 coronary lesions imaged immediately after balloon angioplasty have resulted in a morphological classification of the effects of balloon dilatation as they are viewed by intravascular ultrasound [11]. In Type A, there is partial tear in the plaque which does not extend to the media. Type B is characterized by a tear that extends to the media and usually occurs at the thinnest region in eccentric plaque. Although the torn ends of the plaque may be separated, there is no extension of the tear behind the plaque to form a dissection plane. The presence of such a dissection plane at an arc of up to 180° around the circumference characterizes Type C dissection. In Type D, there is no apparent tear in the plaque, but there is a dissection between the atheroma and the media extends around most of the circumference. The plaque wavers with the blood flow, but remains attached to the media proximal and distal to the dissection and is distinguished from an arterial flap. Finally, in Type E, balloon dilatation results in stretching of the artery without tear or dissection. Two subtypes are recognized.

In the first, E1, there is a concentric thick plaque which stretches but does not crack.

These plaques frequently contain less calcium than plaques that fracture. In the second type, E2, there is very eccentric plaque, and dilatation results in stretching of the normal vessel wall opposite the plaque.

Twenty out of the original 100 patients had clinical ischemia and showed re-stenosis by angiography. The luminal area and atheroma area following the initial angioplasty did not predict re-stenosis. However, 50% of the patients with an E1 morphology developed re-stenosis, compared to an average of only 12% of the patients with other morphological types [11]. We believe this classification system may provide a method of differentiating the mechanical effects of balloon dilation which, in turn, will have prognostic significance for the long-term result of the intervention. In addition, this system may prove useful as a means to identify which interventional device would be the most appropriate for a given plaque architecture.

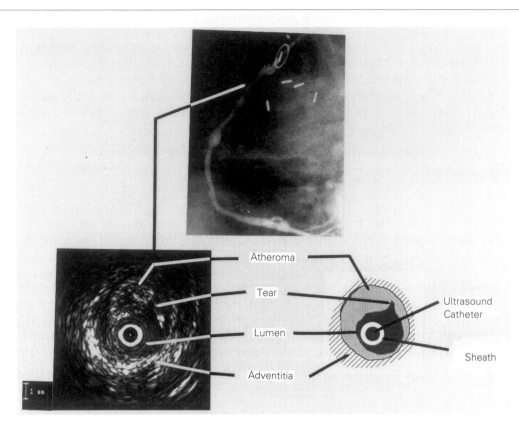

Type A morphology. Ultrasound image following balloon angioplasty (lower left) and schematic presentation (lower left). The area in the coronary artery where the image was obtained is indicated on the angiogram. A linear partial tear of the atheroma that does not extend into the media (Type A) is shown. *Reproduced with permission of the American Heart Association.*

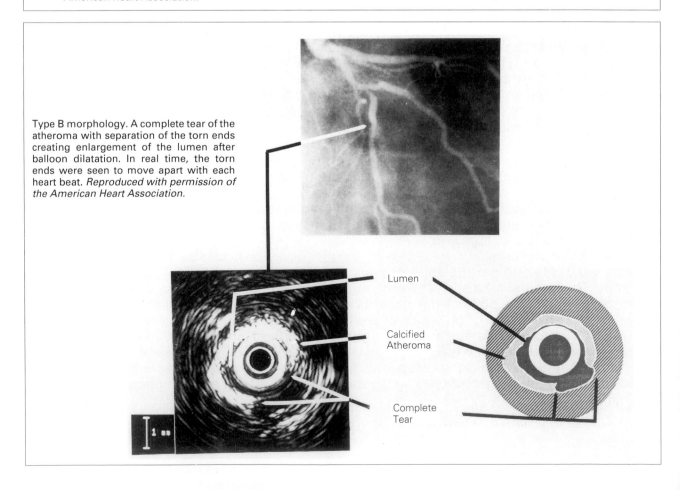

Type B morphology. A complete tear of the atheroma with separation of the torn ends creating enlargement of the lumen after balloon dilatation. In real time, the torn ends were seen to move apart with each heart beat. *Reproduced with permission of the American Heart Association.*

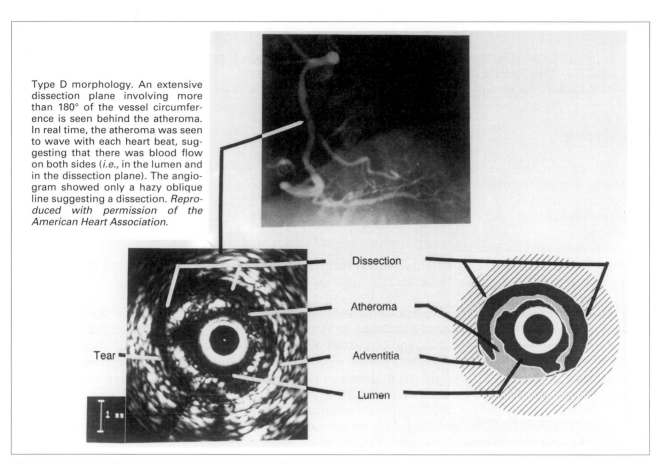

Type D morphology. An extensive dissection plane involving more than 180° of the vessel circumference is seen behind the atheroma. In real time, the atheroma was seen to wave with each heart beat, suggesting that there was blood flow on both sides (*i.e.*, in the lumen and in the dissection plane). The angiogram showed only a hazy oblique line suggesting a dissection. *Reproduced with permission of the American Heart Association.*

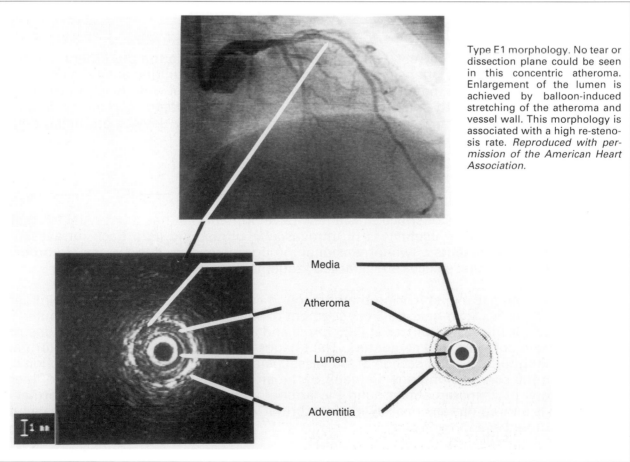

Type F1 morphology. No tear or dissection plane could be seen in this concentric atheroma. Enlargement of the lumen is achieved by balloon-induced stretching of the atheroma and vessel wall. This morphology is associated with a high re-stenosis rate. *Reproduced with permission of the American Heart Association.*

Incorporating an ultrasound imaging transducer inside the balloon of an angioplasty catheter allows imaging in real time before, during and after balloon inflation [13]. The catheter was used in peripheral arteries to document the onset of plaque fracture and the immediate partial recoil of the artery after balloon deflation. A coronary balloon/ultrasound imaging catheter has also been developed.

Atherectomy

Although angiography provides a very useful „roadmap" for the placement of intravascular catheters, it does not provide optimum guidance for interventions that must be directed to the sector containing the plaque such as during atherectomy. An ultrasound transducer that has been integrated into the Simpson atherectomy catheter appears to be helpful in guiding the procedure.

This makes it possible to achieve maximum removal of atheroma while avoiding the removal of subintimal tissue and vessel perforation [5, 43].

For coaxial (non-directional) atherectomy catheters such as the Rotablator® or the TEC® devices, intravascular ultrasound can help select the optimum catheter size. Furthermore, since some atherectomy catheters can cut calcified plaque while others cannot, intravascular ultrasound can help select which atherectomy device should be used [43]. In a clinical series, intravascular ultrasound detected small areas of calcification in 82% of the arteries at the site of angioplasty, whereas fluoroscopy detected by ultrasound only 8% [36]. Although calcification usually occurs at the base of the atheroma, it occasionally occurs in the fibrous cap. The location of calcification as defined by intravascular ultrasounds impacts the various atherectomy devices differently.

Other Interventional Devices

Intravascular ultrasound is currently being investigated as an aid to the placement of intravascular stents and seems to offer substantial benefits [15]. It has a unique ability to document the degree of expansion of the stent and its contact with the vessel wall. Also, protrusion of tissue and intimal regrowth can be seen. Several „hybrid" catheters combining imaging ultrasound with laser, *spark erosion* or various other atherectomy devices are being developed [2].

3-D Reconstruction

Three-dimensional (3-D) reconstruction is a new development that has a potential to significantly enhance the clinical usefulness of intravascular ultrasound [32]. Each intravascular ultrasound image represents a two-dimensional tomographic slice of the vessel. In order to produce a 3-D image, these slices are „stacked" together using computer software.

The slices are obtained by advancing the ultrasound catheter into the vessel, then imaging during a timed pullback. To image a 5 cm segment of vessel takes less than four minutes for the automated (or manual) pullback at 0.25 mm/s and another 15 to 90 s for 3-D reconstruction with current software and computers. The images are presented in three basic formats. The first is a longitudinal hemi-section of the vessel. The plane of this longitudinal section can be chosen on the screen along any diameter of the artery. This offers visualization of longitudinal sections in 2° increments around the arterial circumference. The second format of presentation is a three-dimensional, cylindrical format where the artery is projected as a tube that can be rotated around any axis.

Rather than examine the tube from the outside, one can also bisect it and look at the endoluminal surface. The third format permits subtracting the wall of the artery and projecting a „cast" of the lumen as a solid tube. Three-dimensional reconstruction has recently been applied to images obtained by a prototype foward-looking ultrasound catheter [21]. Instead of examining many individual longitudinal vessel sectors, these are reconstructed in a 3-D image. Preliminary data showed a good correlation of these 3-D forward images with histology [21].

Available software allows great flexibility in image manipulation. For example, any target structure or layer can selectively displayed in its entirety and its volume determined. *In vivo* human studies indicate that the longitudinal section format facilitates analysis of dissections and the bisected cylindrical format facilitates analysis of endovascular stents [32]. One problem, however, is that the current systems for 3-D reconstruction assume a straight path of the catheter and thus erroneously project the artery as a straight structure. Some loss of resolution also occurs. Corrections for these problems are currently being developed.

| 5.3.2 | Intravascular Ultrasound |
| 5.3.2.4 | Imaging of Veins and Vein Grafts |

Veins are normally seen as a homogeneous, echo-dense ring. *In vitro* intravascular ultrasound images clearly demonstrate the abnormal thickening of the walls of excised vein grafts. A good correlation with histology is reported in distinguishing between normal intima, intimal hyperplasia, venous wall fibrosis and atheromatous plaque [41]. In a recent study of patients with saphenous vein transplants imaged before and after angioplasty, intravascular ultrasound was more sensitive than angiography in detecting calcification and intimal dissection [14].

| 5.3.2 | Intravascular Ultrasound |
| 5.3.2.5 | Imaging of the Heart and Great Vessels |

Background

Although ultrasound was first conceived as a method of intracardiac imaging, this application has lagged behind other intravascular applications. The current expansion of catheter-based interventions for the treatment of various congenital and acquired cardiac diseases is the major impetus for the resurgence of active research in this area. The scope of applications, however, extends into improving our diagnostic abilities in a variety of disorders.

Potential Applications

Many potential applications in the area of catheter-based interventions exist [17, 26].

During balloon valvuloplasties, intravascular ultrasound can be used in guiding the transseptal catheterization, defining the valvular morphology and suitability of the valve for the intervention, selecting the balloon size, and assessing the result and complications. During closure of intracardiac defects, defining the size and shape of the defects and therefore the appropriate size of the occluder may prove very helpful. Moreover, proper placement can be confirmed. Continuous imaging, *e.g.* from a right atrial position, may be useful in monitoring ventricular function and to discover complications like hemopericardium during the intervention. In coarctation of the aorta, intravascular ultrasound can be helpful in sizing the balloon and assessing the results and complications (dissection).

Where the placement of intravascular stents is required, *e.g.* after dilation of peripheral pulmonary artery stenosis, intravascular ultrasound permits confirmation of the placement and expansion of the stent.

In the area of diagnosis, several potential applications exist, especially when transthoracic and transesophageal imaging is suboptimal or not feasible. It is possible to define valvular anomalies, aortic dissections, intracardiac defects, tumors and clots [26]. Imaging vascular grafts and shunts may help detect malfunction. Intravascular ultrasound may also prove useful in investigating pulmonary hypertension and its etiology, *e.g.*, chronic thrombo-embolism [31].

Catheter and Transducer Designs

The catheters used for investigation have ranged from transesophageal probes (5 MHz) inserted into the right atrium (in animals) to small intravascular ultrasound catheters (20 MHz) designed for intracoronary use. Catheters designed specifically for intracardiac imaging are currently being developed. Optimum transducer frequency will depend on the patient's size and the type of application, but 5 to 20 MHz appears to provide sufficient depth of field in adults at the best possible resolution. Incorporating Doppler capabilities into the catheters and incorporating ultrasound transducers into various interventional catheters are expected future developments.

Imaging of the Aorta

The aorta can easily be visualized throughout its entire length by retrograde introduction of a catheter from a femoral artery. Normally, one, two or three layers may be visualized in the aortic wall [26].

In the atherosclerotic aorta, calcification may range from a few patches to extensive circumferential calcification. Fibrotic, echo-dense plaques and fatty, less dense plaques as well as ectasia, thrombi and dissections may also be seen [26]. Recently case reports have described the detection of aortic dissection (both spontaneous [25] and following angioplasty for coarctation [8]) by intravascular ultrasound.

Imaging of the Aortic Valve

Since the pathological substrate of the stenotic aortic valve (congenital bicuspid vs. degenerative tricuspid) can influence the success and the complications of balloon valvuloplasty, the ability of intravascular ultrasound to distinguish between the two types was recently investigated [12].

In 15 post mortem examinations and in 7 patients whose valves were later available for pathological investigation, intravascular ultrasound accurately classified all the valves into bicuspid or tricuspid. This distinction is often difficult or impossible by transthoracic echocardiography or contrast aortography. For these examinations, the intravascular ultrasound catheter was introduced through a sheath which was placed retrograde into the left ventricle. By placing the transducer midway across the valve. Also, the presence of median raphe calcification and the mobility of each of the leaflets can be determined.

Imaging the Left and Right Sides of the Heart

The various catheters can be introduced retrograde from the femoral artery and positioned at various planes from just above the aortic valve to the left ventricular apex. Views analogous to various short-axis views, the two and four-chamber views plus a number of other different views can thereby be obtained [26]. Catheters shaped specifically for certain applications and those steerable by a variety of mechanisms allow more control of the imaging plane. Miniaturization of transesophageal echocardiography probes with their Doppler and steering capabilities is also being pursued. Introducing the catheters through the femoral or jugular vein permits imaging of the vena cava, the right atrium and ventricle, the tricuspid valve and the pericardial cavity. In addition, a lower frequency catheter (5-10 MHz) positioned in the right atrium or ventricle can visualize the left atrium and ventricle as well as the aortic and mitral valves.

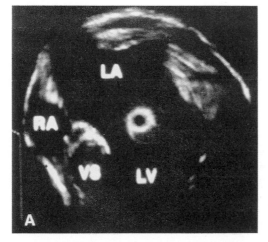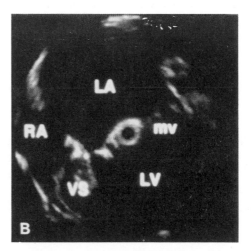

Intracardiac ultrasound image from the left ventricular cavity of a dog obtained with a 12.5 MHz transducer. The right atrium (RA), left atrium (LA), left ventricle (LV), mitral valve (mv) and ventricular septum (VS) are seen. **A**. Diastolic frame. **B**. Systole frame showing the mitral valve closed [26].

Imaging of the Pulmonary Arteries

From the right ventricle, the catheter may then be directed to the right ventricular outflow tract and pulmonary artery. A balloon-tipped catheter has recently been described which potentially could be used at the bedside without fluoroscopy [33]. Imaging of the pulmonary artery and its branches has been performed in healthy probands [29] and in patients with chronic thrombo-embolic disease [31]. Evaluation of wall thickness can be difficult in normals, but is facilitated in the presence of thickening due to organized thrombi. Intravascular ultrasound correctly identified 10 out of 11 segments with thrombi as well as 9 normal segments (all confirmed at the time of surgery) [31].

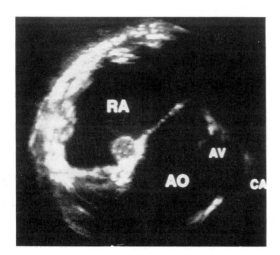

Intracardiac ultrasound image obtained with a 12.5 MHz catheter. The catheter is positioned in the right atrium (RA) of a dog. Aortic valve (AV), aortic root (AO), coronary ostium (CA) [26].

5.3.2   **Intravascular Ultrasound**
5.3.2.6 **Limitations of Intravascular Ultrasound**

Like any diagnostic techniques, intravascular ultrasound also has its specific limitations. The inability to image the area immediately adjacent to the catheter due to the *ring down artifact* is still a limitation with the electronic array catheters. The inability to image behind calcified areas *(drop out)* sometimes limits measurements of plaque thickness, although the lumen can still be measured. Also, *drop out* of the image can be misinterpreted as a „lipid pool". Blooming of the echoes from the internal elastic membrane leads to overestimation of its thickness, but the magnitude of this is small and its effect on relevant measurements is negligible.

In the coronaries, many severe narrowing cannot be imaged prior to intervention because their diameter is smaller than that of the catheter. Also, because of the size of current catheters, there is a possibility of distending the narrowed segment (Dotter effect) and thus underestimating its severity.

Inserting the catheter through a severe coronary stenosis may reduce blood flow and cause ischemia. It may also lead to partial collapse of the distal artery, resulting in underestimation of its diameter. A special problem that occurs after angioplasty is that the catheter or its sheath may cause „stenting" of an intimal flap resulting in underestimation of damage to the lumen. Further miniaturization and development of forward-looking intravascular ultrasound catheters may help solve this problem. A prototype forward-looking catheter was recently described [4]. This catheter images a longitudinal sector of the vessel and provides accurate images up to 14 mm in front of the catheter tip.

An eccentric position of the catheter may result in deterioration of the image of the arterial wall furthest away from the catheter. An off-axis (non-coaxial) position produces an oblique cross section of the artery with a larger lumen and is recognized by its elliptical shape. These problems with positioning can often be corrected by catheter and guide wire manipulation. Sometimes an ultrashort „weblike" lesion occurs in the coronaries and may difficult or impossible to visualize with angiography.Although we have found intravascular ultrasound to be helpful in such circumstances, it is possible to overlooked these lesions by rapid movement of the catheter [3]. The recently introduced automated timed pullback of the catheters may prevent this.

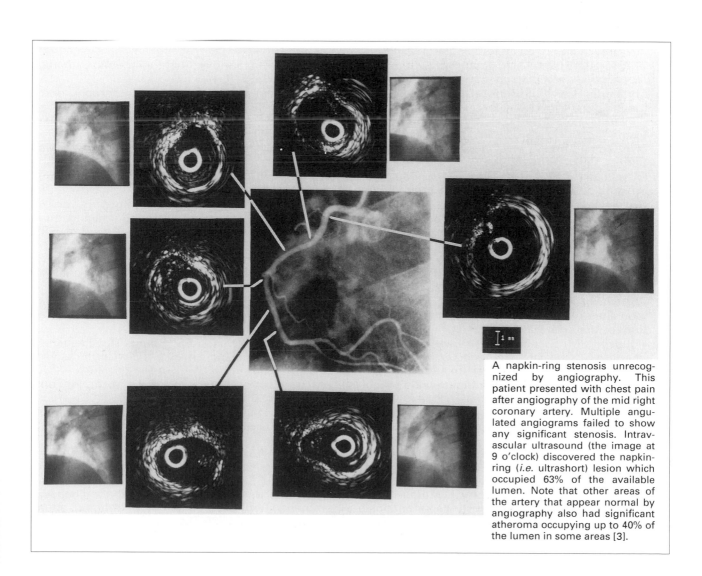

A napkin-ring stenosis unrecognized by angiography. This patient presented with chest pain after angiography of the mid right coronary artery. Multiple angulated angiograms failed to show any significant stenosis. Intravascular ultrasound (the image at 9 o'clock) discovered the napkin-ring (*i.e.* ultrashort) lesion which occupied 63% of the available lumen. Note that other areas of the artery that appear normal by angiography also had significant atheroma occupying up to 40% of the lumen in some areas [3].

Intravascular ultrasound represents an important new imaging modality which provides unique diagnostic information. We believe it will replace angiography as the „golden standard" for quantification of the severity and extent of atherosclerosis. Its main clinical application is likely to be as an aid to endovascular interventions as well as improving the diagnostic capability of standard angiography.

The contribution of intravascular ultrasound may, however, go beyond being an adjunct to the mechanical aspects of cardiovascular medicine. Its major important contribution may be in improving our understanding of the pathogenesis and pathophysiology of atherosclerosis and in monitoring the effects that diet and drug interventions on this disease process.

Judging from the remarkable advances in the hardware and image processing that occurred with transthoracic echocardiography, it stands to reason that intravascular ultrasound, which is still in its infancy, will undoubtedly go through and equally remarkable journey.

References

1. Bom N, ten Hoff H, Lancee CT, Gussenhoven WJ, Bosch JG. Early and recent intraluminal ultrasound devices. Int J Cardiac Imaging 1989; 4: 79-88.
2. Crowley RJ, Hamm MA, Joshi SH, Lennox CD, Roberts GT. Ultrasound guided therapeutic catheters: recent developments and clinical results. Int J Cardiac Imaging 1991; 6: 145-156.
3. Ehrlich S, Honye J, Mahon D, Bernstein R, Tobis JM. Unrecognized stenosis by angiography documented by intravascular ultrasound imaging. *Reproduced with permission of:* Catheterization and Cardiovascular Diag 1991; 23: 198-201.
4. Evans JL, Ng KH, Vonesh MJ, Kramer BL, Mills TA, Kane BJ, Aldrich WN, Jang YT, Yock PG, et al. Arterial imaging utilizing a new forward viewing intravascular ultrasound catheter: initial studies. J Am Coll Cardiol 1992; 19: 140A.
5. Fitzgerald PJ, Sudhir K, Gupta M, Honda G, Belef WM, Yock PG. Combined atherectomy/ultrasound imaging device reduces subintimal tissue injury. J Am Coll Cardiol 1992; 19: 223A.
6. Gussenhoven EJ, Essed CE, Lancee CT, Mastik F, Frietman P, van Egmond FC, Reiber J, Bosch H, van Urk H, Roelandt J, et al. Arterial wall characteristics determined by intravascular ultrasound imaging: an in vitro study. *Reproduced with permission of the American Heart Association in:* J Am Coll Cardiol 1989; 14: 947-952.
7. Gussenhoven EJ, Frietman PA, The SH, van Suylen RJ, van Egmond FC, Lancee CT, van Urk H, Roelandt JR, Stijnen T, Bom N. Assessment of medial thinning in atherosclerosis by intravascular ultrasound. Am J Cardiol 1991; 68: 1625-1632.
8. Harrison JK, Sheikh KH, Davidson CJ, Kisslo KB, Leithe ME, Himmelstein SI, Kanter RJ, Bashore TM. Balloon angioplasty of coarctation of the aorta evaluated with intravascular ultrasound imaging. J Am Coll Cardiol 1990; 15: 906-909.
9. Hodgson JM, Graham SP, Savakus AD, Dame SG, Stephens DN, Dhillon PS, Brands D, Sheehan H, Eberle MJ. Clinical percutaneous imaging of coronary anatomy using an over-the-wire ultrasound catheter system. Int J Cardiac Imaging 1989; 4: 187-193.
10. Hodgson JMcB. Coronary imaging and angioplasty with an electronic array catheter system. In: Tobis JM, Yock PG, eds. Intravascular Ultrasound Imaging. Edinburgh: Churchill Livingston, 1992: 161-170.
11. Honye J, Mahon DJ, Jain A, White CJ, Ramee SR, Wallis JB, Alzarka A, Tobis JM. Morphological effects of coronary balloon angioplasty in vivo assessed by intravascular ultrasound imaging. Circulation 1992; 85: 1012-1025.
12. Isner JM, Losordo DW, Rosenfield K, Ramaswamy K, Kelly S, Pastore JO, Kosowsky BD. Catheter-based intravascular ultrasound discriminates bicuspid from tricuspid valves in adults with calcific aortic stenosis. J Am Coll Cardiol 1990; 15: 1310-1317.
13. Isner JM, Rosenfield K, Losordo DW, Rose L, Langevin RE, Razvi S, Kosowsky BD. Combination balloon-ultrasound imaging catheter for percutaneous transluminal angioplasty - Validation of imaging, analysis of recoil, and identification of plaque fracture. Circulation 1991; 84: 739-754.
14. Jain SP, Roubin GS, Nanda NC, Dean LS, Agrawal SK, Pinheiro L. Intravascular ultrasound imaging of saphenous vein graft stenosis. Am J Cardiol 1992; 69: 133-136.

15. Keren G, Bartorelli AL, Bonner RF, Douek PC, Leon MB. Intravascular ultrasound examination of coronary stents. In: Tobis JM, Yock PG, eds. Intravascular Ultrasound Imaging. Edinburgh: Churchill Livingston, 1992: 219-230.

16. Linker DT, Yock PG. Tissue characterization in intra-arterial ultrasound: potential methods and clinical implications. In: Tobis JM, Yock PG, eds. Intravascular Ultrasound Imaging. Edinburgh: Churchill Livingston, 1992: 85-92.

17. Ludomirsky A, Ricou F, Weintraub RG, Sahn DJ. Applications of intravascular scanning in congenital heart disease. In Tobis JM, Yock PG, eds. Intravascular Ultrasound Imaging. Edinburgh: Churchill Livingston, 1992: 247-253.

18. Mallery JA, Tobis JM, Griffith J, Gessert J, McRae M, Moussabeck O, Bessen M, Moriuchi M, Henry WL. Assessment of normal and atherosclerotic arterial wall thickness with an intravascular ultrasound imaging catheter. Am Heart J 1990; 119: 1392-1400.

19. McPherson DD, Hiratzka LF, Lamberth WC, Brandt B, Hunt M, Kieso RA, Marcus ML, Kerber RE. Delineation of the extent of coronary atherosclerosis by high-frequency epicardial echocardiography. N Engl J Med 1987; 316: 304-309.

20. Moriuchi M, Gordon I, Honye J, Yen R, Tobis JM. Validation of intravascular ultrasound images. In: Tobis JM, Yock PG, eds. Intravascular Ultrasound Imaging. *Reproduced with permission of:* Edinburgh: Churchill Livingston, 1992: 57-70.

21. Ng KH, Evans JL, Vonesh MJ, Meyers SN, Mills TA, Kane BJ, Aldrich WN, Jang YT, Yock PG, et al. Three-dimensional reconstruction and display of forward viewing intravascular ultrasound data. J Am Coll Cardiol 1992; 19: 383A.

22. Nishimura RA, Edwards WD, Warnes CA, Reeder GS, Holmes DR Jr, Tajik AJ, Yock PG. Intravascular ultrasound imaging: in vitro validation and pathologic correlation. J Am Coll Cardiol 1990; 16: 145-154.

23. Nissen SE, Grines CL, Gurley JC, Sublett K, Haynie D, Diaz C, Booth DC, DeMaria AN. Application of a new phased-array ultrasound imaging catheter in the assessment of vascular dimensions. In vivo comparison to cineangiography. Circulation 1990; 81: 660-666.

24. Nissen SE, Gurley JC, Grines CL, Booth DC, McClure R, Berk M, Fischer C, DeMaria AN. Intravascular ultrasound assessment of lumen size and wall morphology in normal subjects and patients with coronary artery disease. Circulation 1991; 84: 1087-1099.

25. Pande A, Meier B, Fleisch M, Kammerlander R, Simonet F, Lerch R. Intravascular ultrasound for diagnosis of aortic dissection. Am J Cardiol 1991; 67: 662-664.

26. Pandian NG, Hsu TL, Schwartz SL, Weintraub AR. Intracardiac ultrasound imaging: rationale, current developments, and future directions. In Tobis JM, Yock PG, eds. Intravascular Ultrasound Imaging. *Reproduced with permission of:* Edinburgh: Churchill Livingston, 1992: 231-246.

27. Pandian NG, Kreis A, Brockway B, Isner JM, Salem D, Sacharoff A, Boleza E, Caro R. Ultrasound angioscopy: feasibility and potential. Echocardiography 1989; 6: 1-7.

28. Pandian NG, Kreis A, Brockway B, Sacharoff A, Caro R. Intravascular high frequency two-dimensional ultrasound detection of arterial dissection and intimal flaps. Am J Cardiol 1990; 65: 1278-1280.

29. Pandian NG, Weintraub A, Kreis A, Schwartz SL, Konstam MA, Salem DN. Intracardiac, intravascular, two-dimensional, high-frequency ultrasound imaging of pulmonary artery and its branches in humans and animals. Circulation 1990; 81: 2007-2012.

30. Potkin BN, Bartorelli AL, Gessert JM, Neville RF, Almagor Y, Roberts WC, Leon MB. Coronary artery imaging with intravascular high-frequency ultrasound. Circulation 1990; 81: 1575-1585.

31. Ricou F, Nicod PH, Moser KM, Peterson KL. Catheter-based intravascular ultrasound imaging of chronic thromboembolic pulmonary disease. Am J Cardiol 1991; 67: 749-752.

32. Rosenfield K, Losordo DW, Ramaswamy K, Pastore JO, Langevin RE, Razvi S, Kosowsky BD, Isner JM. Three-dimensional reconstruction of human coronary and peripheral arteries from images recorded during two-dimensional intravascular ultrasound examination. Circulation 1991; 84: 1938-1956.

33. Schwartz S, Pandian N, Katz S, Humar R, Crowley R, Aronovitz M, Hsu TL. Flow-directed, balloon-floatation intravascular ultrasound catheter for percutaneous pulmonary artery imaging and intracardiac echocardiography. J Am Coll Cardiol 1991; 17: 216A.

34. Siegel RJ, Ariani M, Fishbein MC, Chae JS, Park JC, Maurer G, Forrester JS. Histopathologic validation of angioscopy and intravascular ultrasound. Circulation 1991; 84: 109-117.

35. Sudhir K, MacGregor JS, Barbant S, Foster E, Fitzgerald PJ, Chatterjee K, Yock PG. Simultaneous intravascular two-dimensional and Doppler ultrasound: a new technique for in vivo assessment of coronary flow and vascular dynamics. J Am Coll Cardiol 1992; 19: 140A.

36. Tobis JM, Mahon DJ, Moriuchi M, Honye J, McRae M. Intravascular ultrasound imaging following balloon angioplasty. Int J Cardiac Imaging 1991; 6: 191-205.

37. Tobis JM, Mallery J, Mahon D, Lehmann K, Zalesky P, Griffith J, Gessert J, Moriuchi M, McRae M, Dwyer ML, et al. Intravascular ultrasound imaging of human coronary arteries in vivo. Analysis of tissue characterizations with comparison to in vitro histological specimens. *Reproduced with permission of the American Heart Association in:* Circulation 1991; 83: 913-926.

38. Tobis JM, Mallery JA, Gessert J, Griffith J, Mahon D, Bessen M, Moriuchi M, McLeay L, McRae M, Henry WL. Intravascular ultrasound cross-sectional arterial imaging before and after balloon angioplasty in vitro. Circulation 1989; 80: 873-882.

39. Tobis JM. Intravascular ultrasound: a fantastic voyage. Circulation 1991; 84: 2190-2192.
40. Weintraub A, Schwartz S, Pandian N. How reliable are intravascular ultrasound and fiberoptic angioscopy in the assessment of the presence and duration of intraarterial thrombosis in atheromatous vessels with complex plaques? J Am Coll Cardiol 1990; 15: 17A.
41. Willard JE, Netto D, Demian SE, Haagen DR, Brickner ME, Eichhorn EJ, Grayburn PA. Intravascular ultrasound imaging of saphenous vein grafts in vitro: comparison with histologic and quantitative angiographic findings. J Am Coll Cardiol 1992; 19: 759-764.
42. Yock PG, Linker DT, Angelsen BA. Two dimensional intravascular ultrasound: Technical development and initial clinical experience. *Reproduced with permission of:* J Am Soc Echo 1989; 2: 296-304.
43. Yock PG, Fitzgerald PJ, Sudhir K, Ports TA. Intravascular ultrasound guidance during atherectomy. In: Tobis JM, Yock PG, eds. Intravascular Ultrasound Imaging. Edinburgh: Churchill Livingston, 1992: 149-159.

5.3	**Transluminal Cardiac Ultrasound Diagnosis**
5.3.3	**Coronary Doppler Catheters**
	(Robert F. Wilson)

Since the recognition of coronary artery lesions as the cause of angina pectoris and acute myocardial infarction, concepts of ischemic heart disease have been shaped by the methods available to assess the coronary circulation. The demystification of coronary artery disease together with the ready availability of coronary arteriography focused attention on the anatomy of the epicardial conduit arteries while often excluding considerations of hemodynamics and flow regulation by the remainder of the downstream circulation. Recent advances, however, have made clear that arteriographic anatomy (particularly visually assessed anatomy) can be a misleading indicator of coronary arteries to appropriately conduct blood flow to the myocardium (coronary flow reserve) [41]. Consequently, ultrasound transducer-tipped „Doppler" catheters have been developed to directly assess the blood flow in coronary arteries. Application of this method has brought about a new understanding of the coronary circulation in humans.

| 5.3.3 | **Coronary Doppler Catheters** |
| 5.3.3.1 | **Measurement of Coronary Blood Flow** |

Several methods of measuring coronary blood flow in humans have been developed previously. Some can be used only during surgery (*e.g.* electromagnetic flow meters) and thus are of limited utility for clinicians and researchers [40, 41]. While various other methods can be used in the catheterization laboratory, they cannot provide exact measurement of regional blood flow (*e.g.* coronary sinus thermodilution method). They are therefore unable to relate abnormalities in perfusion to a specific artery or perfusion field [23, 40, 46].

Doppler ultrasound transducers were developed previously to measure blood flow velocity in individual arteries of animals or in humans undergoing open heart surgery. Doppler technology is advantageous for use in the catheterization laboratory, because instantaneous, on-line blood flow velocity can be obtained and the method lends itself to miniaturization. Consequently, we and others developed coronary Doppler catheters and wires to measure blood flow in individual arteries at the time of cardiac catheterization [2, 7, 8, 15, 36, 43].

Two types of coronary Doppler catheter designs have been developed for use in humans - those with an end-mounted transducer and others with a transducer mounted into the catheter's side wall. All use pulsed Doppler methodology and have a single piezoelectric crystal to send and receive the ultrasound signal. A catheter with a crystal mounted on the catheter tip was used first by Benchimol et al. [2]. Later, the catheter design was modified by Hartley and Cole and again by Sibley et al. [7, 36]. In its presently available form, a circular 20 MHz piezoelectric crystal is mounted on the tip of a 1 mm diameter Rentrop reperfusion catheter [36].

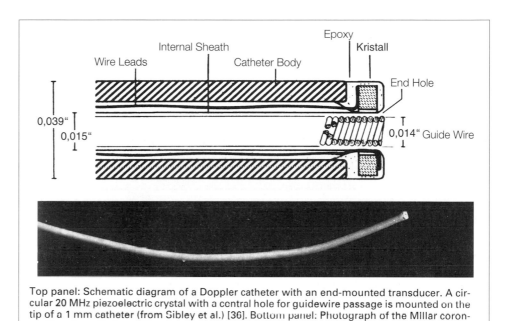

Top panel: Schematic diagram of a Doppler catheter with an end-mounted transducer. A circular 20 MHz piezoelectric crystal with a central hole for guidewire passage is mounted on the tip of a 1 mm catheter (from Sibley et al.) [36]. Bottom panel: Photograph of the Millar coronary Doppler catheter with end-mounted transducer.

The crystal has a hole in the center to allow for passage of an angioplasty guidewire. The catheter transducer system is passed into the coronary artery through a standard angioplasty guide catheter with the use of an angioplasty guidewire that is ≥ 0.36 mm (0.014") in diameter.

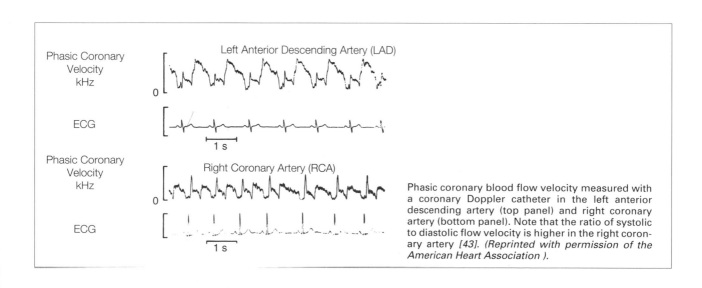

Phasic coronary blood flow velocity measured with a coronary Doppler catheter in the left anterior descending artery (top panel) and right coronary artery (bottom panel). Note that the ratio of systolic to diastolic flow velocity is higher in the right coronary artery [43]. (Reprinted with permission of the American Heart Association).

To measure blood flow, the crystal is connected to a 20 MHZ pulsed Doppler meter with an adjustable range gate. The catheter is positioned in the artery to obtain an acceptable signal of phasic coronary flow velocity, which is usually characterized by predominantly diastolic flow, brief zero flow or flow reversal in early systole, and a mean velocity of at least 1 kHz shift. The range gate is adjusted to the maximum returned frequency shift (*e.g.* near center-line velocity).

We developed another type of Doppler catheter by mounting a piezoelectric crystal into the side of a 1 mm coronary catheter [43].

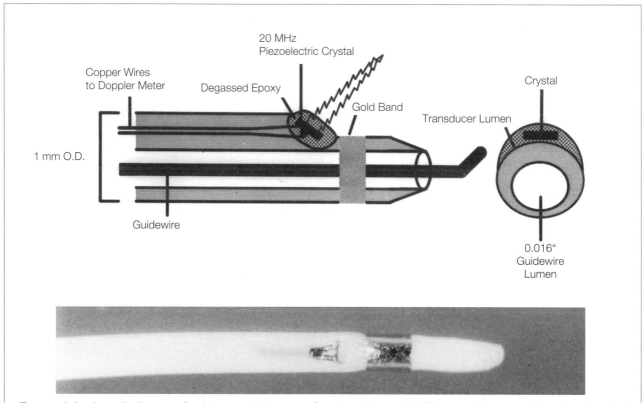

Top panel: A schematic diagram of a side-mounted coronary Doppler catheter. A 20 MHz crystal is mounted into the side of a 1 mm two-lumen catheter. The lower lumen is reserved for a steerable angioplasty guidewire. Bottom panel: Close-up view of the tip of a NuMed side-mounted crystal Doppler catheter.

Using this catheter, the ultrasound field cuts across the stream of blood flow, intersecting the center line. The size of the sample volume in side-mounted catheter systems is relative to the arterial area. In validation studies, the catheter was placed into the coronary arteries of calves (50-70 kg), and the range gate was adjusted to the maximum returned frequency shift. Coronary blood flow varied over a wide range (0.1 to 5.7 times resting blood flow).

Measurement of the change in blood flow velocity assessed using the catheter correlated closely with simultaneous measurements of blood flow velocity obtained with an epicardial Doppler probe and with timed-volume collections of coronary sinus blood flow [43]. In additional studies, we demonstrated that the 1 mm catheter did not reduce maximal coronary hyperemia when placed in a major coronary artery (*e.g.* > 2.0 mm diameter). However, catheters with an outer diameter of ≥ 1.4 mm slightly reduced maximal hyperemia in some animals, suggesting that flow measurement catheters should not exceed 1.0 to 1.3 mm in diameter.

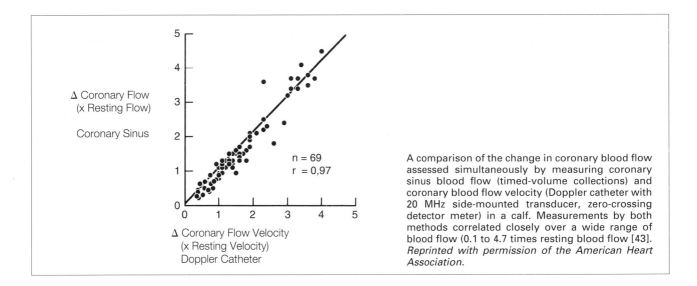

Δ Coronary Flow
(x Resting Flow)

Coronary Sinus

n = 69
r = 0,97

Δ Coronary Flow Velocity
(x Resting Velocity)
Doppler Catheter

A comparison of the change in coronary blood flow assessed simultaneously by measuring coronary sinus blood flow (timed-volume collections) and coronary blood flow velocity (Doppler catheter with 20 MHz side-mounted transducer, zero-crossing detector meter) in a calf. Measurements by both methods correlated closely over a wide range of blood flow (0.1 to 4.7 times resting blood flow [43]. *Reprinted with permission of the American Heart Association.*

More recently, two new devices have been developed. Doucette et al. developed a small guidewire (0.46 mm diameter) with a 12 MHz piezoelectric transducer at the tip of the wire [8]. The advantage of the wire transducer is that it can be advanced through standard diagnostic angiography catheters into small coronary arteries without the wire itself causing flow obstruction. Additionally, the wire can be passed through angioplasty catheters and used to monitor coronary blood flow during angioplastic procedures. Validation studies in animals demonstrated that *average peak velocity* assessed using the wire correlated closely with changes in coronary blood flow over a wide range of flows [8].

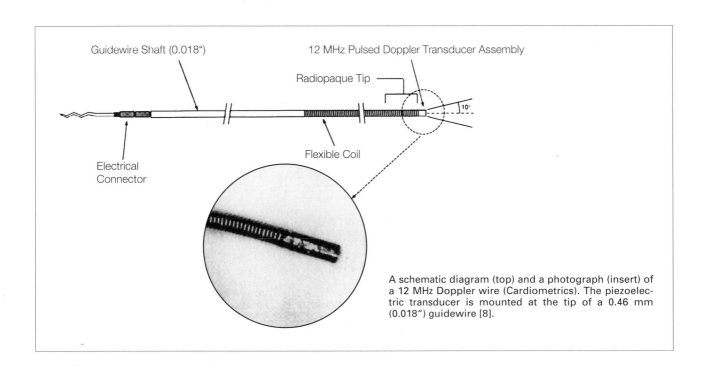

Guidewire Shaft (0.018")

12 MHz Pulsed Doppler Transducer Assembly

Radiopaque Tip

10°

Electrical
Connector

Flexible Coil

A schematic diagram (top) and a photograph (insert) of a 12 MHz Doppler wire (Cardiometrics). The piezoelectric transducer is mounted at the tip of a 0.46 mm (0.018") guidewire [8].

In contrast to the Doppler wire, Kern et al. [15] recently developed an angiographic Doppler catheter by placing a 20 MHz piezoelectric crystal at the tip of a standard Judkins-type coronary catheter. The advantage of this catheter design is that the blood flow velocity in the left main left coronary artery can be monitored without the need for intracoronary cannulation. When subselective Doppler blood flow velocity measurements are not needed, this catheter could simplify the procedure and reduce both cost and risk.

| 5.3.3 | **Coronary Doppler Catheters** |
| 5.3.3.2 | **Signal Analysis** |

Several factors that affect the accuracy of Doppler catheter measurement of flow velocity must be taken into consideration. The most important is the method of signal analysis. Two broad methods of signal analysis are the zero crossing detector method and the more complicated fast Fourier transform series method (FFT). The first pulsed Doppler meters were developed by Franklin and Peronneau in the 1960's and utilized a zero crossing method of detection to measure the mean frequency shift of the returned signal [9, 30]. These inexpensive meters detect the direction and frequency at which the returned signal is shifted from the carrier signal (*i.e.* the rate at which the returned signal crosses „zero velocity"). However, the reflected signal contains a broad spectrum of returned frequencies that represent, in part, the different flow velocities that exist within a blood vessel lumen.

More recently, faster electronic analysis has permitted the real-time measurement of the spectral nature of the returned signal using FFT ($\geq$ 100 spectra/s).

The method of signal analysis can be important. Johnson et al. proved that catheters with an end-mounted transducer require FFT signal analysis for accurate measurement of changes in blood flow velocity [14]. When returned signals from end-mounted transducers were analyzed using a zero crossing method, changes in *mean* flow velocity (*i.e.* kHz shift) from the Doppler meter consistently underestimated the true change in flow in an *in vitro* tube system. In *in vivo* studies, the changes in frequency shift detected by the zero crossing method consistently underestimated changes in coronary blood flow by 20 to 30% [36]. However, changes in the *average peak velocity* assessed from FFT analysis of the spectral signal correlated closely with true changes in blood flow. *Hence, when end-mounted transducer are used, FFT signal analysis is important.*

Side-mounted transducers appear to accurately measure changes in blood flow when either zero crossing detectors or FFT analysis is utilized. One reason for the difference between end and side-mounted transducers may be that the signal from the side-mounted transducer slices across the flow profiles of the arterial stream, while the ultrasound field of the end-mounted transducer encompasses more of the flow stream along the vessel wall. Although the returned signal from the end-mounted transducer may contain elements of the center line velocity, reflections from the center of the vessel might account for a smaller fraction of the total spectrum of returned signal. If this is true, the mean peak velocity (assessed by FFT) might be more representative of mean flow velocity within the artery. For side-mounted transducers, the ultrasound field usually encompasses the center line, which may obviate the need for spectral analysis and signal selection.

A second important factor in signal analysis is impedance matching between the catheter and the Doppler meter. This can be difficult because all transducer and connector wires have slightly different impedances. Presently, connecting cables containing a single toroid are utilized to isolate the Doppler meter from the individual catheter and to increase the ultrasound power from the crystal transducer. This empirical method usually improves the signal-to-noise ratio, but does not offer optimal impedance matching. One system (FloWire®, Cardiometrics) provides more accurate impedance matching adjusted to each Doppler wire and optimizes the acoustic power output. In general, if the measured frequency shift from a coronary artery is less than 1 kHz, one should consider the signal unreliable (possibly due to poor impedance matching) and use another cable or catheter.

The accuracy of the Doppler signal in reflecting blood flow velocity in the artery can be affected by several technical factors. The position of the catheter within the artery is the most important. If a large portion of the ultrasound field is directed against the vessel wall, none of the reflected signal will originate from the vessel center line. Typically, the returned signal frequency shift is low and the audio output has been described as a „wall glop" sound. The Doppler wire can be rotated into the velocity stream, but the small catheters are difficult to rotate and they must usually be moved to a different portion of the vessel to obtain an adequate signal.

A second important caveat is that the relationship of the frequency shift is proportional to the cosine of the angle of the transducer relative to blood flow, which is expressed in the Doppler equation itself. In most cases, the true angle between the transducer and flow velocity is not known accurately. This is of lesser importance for end-mounted transducers, because the cosine changes little when the angle is approximately 90°. However, even when using end-mounted transducers, inhomogeneities in the ultrasound field may occur. As a result, transducers may not sample the vessel center line in all axial positions. Rotation of the catheter may cause a marked change in the returned frequency shift. *Hence, it is presently not possible to derive the absolute coronary blood flow velocity in humans from currently available catheters* [32].

A third factor is that Doppler devices measure changes in blood flow velocity, but not changes in flow. Changes in the diameter of the artery at the site of the transducer will alter the relationship between velocity and flow. Consequently, if changes in blood flow are to be assessed using a Doppler device, the artery must be maximally dilated (*e.g.* with nitroglycerin) or the vessel caliber must be measured during each velocity measurement (*e.g.* using quantitative angiography or intravascular sonography).

Blood flow to the myocardium is usually regulated by the microcirculation (*i.e.* vessels < 400 µm in diameter). The tone of the resistance vessels is closely linked to the metabolic needs of the surrounding tissue and to the blood pressure in the epicardial coronary artery.

As the blood pressure changes, the microcirculation autoregulates its resistance to compensate and maintain blood flow at levels appropriate for tissue needs. Under normal circumstances, complete dilation of the microcirculation can reduce coronary resistance to less than one-fourth of the resting resistance.

It is important to emphasize that the large arteries that can be seen on the arteriogram are conduit vessels that provide little resistance to the blood flow, even during maximal coronary hyperemia [6, 21]. However, once stenosis has developed in the epicardial arteries, the resistance of the large vessels becomes important. To compensate for the drop in blood pressure across the epicardial lesion, the microcirculation dilates and maintains resting blood flow. However, once the stenosis has induced microvascular dilation, the inability of the microcirculation to dilate further (*e.g.* in reaction to increased oxygen demand or changes in perfusion pressure) can lead to stress-induced ischemia.

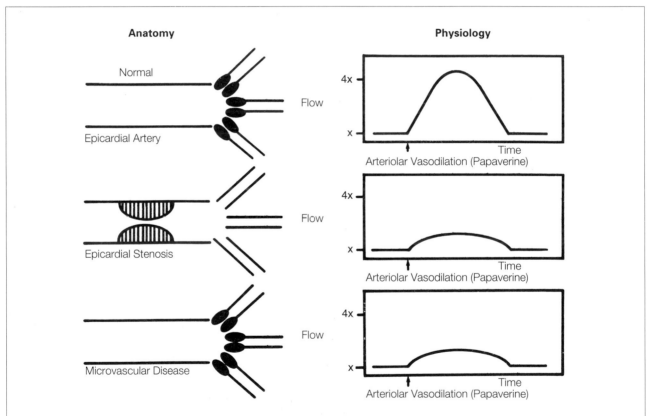

A schematic of coronary anatomy (left panel) and coronary flow reserve (right panel) in patients with normal coronary arteries (top), an epicardial stenosis (middle panel), and microvascular obstruction (bottom panel). In normal arteries resting microvascular tone is relaxed with exercise or vasodilating drugs, resulting in a large increase in blood flow. Arteries with an epicardial stenosis compensate with microvascular dilation; a further microvascular dilation is limited. Vasodilating stimuli are ineffective in patients with microvascular disease.

The function of the microcirculatory resistance vessels can be impaired by a number of diseases. These include arterial hypertension, hypertrophy, collagen vascular diseases (systemic lupus erythematosis, scleroderma), and ischemic injury [3, 4, 16, 29].

Many other etiologies probably exist, but have not yet been described. When microcirculatory impairment coexists with epicardial stenotic lesions, the effects can be additive. Epicardial stenoses that might cause only minimal impairment in hyperemic blood flow (through compensation by the microcirculation) might lead to significant symptoms.

Since factors that accelerate atherosclerosis (*e.g.* hypertension) may also cause microcirculatory injury, many patients with ischemic heart disease have impairment of both large conduit arteries and the microcirculation. *One should remember that Doppler derived measurements of blood flow velocity reflect the resistance of the entire coronary bed, not just the portion imaged by the angiogram.*

5.3.3   Coronary Doppler Catheters
5.3.3.5   Measurement of Coronary Reserve

Coronary flow reserve is a measurement of maximal coronary conductance (or its inverse minimal vascular resistance). It can be defined in absolute terms (maximal blood flow/gram myocardium) or in relative terms (ratio of peak blood flow to resting blood flow). Doppler catheters can be used only to measure relative coronary flow reserve because absolute coronary blood flow and myocardial mass perfused by the artery under study cannot be determined presently.

Coronary Vasodilators

Measurement of coronary flow reserve with a Doppler catheter requires the use of a maximal coronary vasodilator. Three agents are available for use in humans: papaverine, adenosine, and dipyridamole. Each produces maximal coronary dilation independent of endothelial function. The kinetics and side effects, however, are different.

Papaverine causes maximal coronary dilation, but only when given by the intracoronary route [49]. When administered in a maximally dilating dose of 12 mg in the left coronary (8 mg in the right coronary), blood flow velocity increases 4.8 ± 1.0 (mean $\pm$ SD, range 3.5 to 8.2 peak/resting velocity at sinus heart rate 74 ± 3 beats/min). The duration of hyperemia is fairly brief (111 ± 17 s). The main drawback of papaverine is that it lengthens the QT interval on the ECG and can cause *Torsade de Pointes* in about 1 to 2 % of patients [50].

Adenosine causes maximal coronary hyperemia in 90% of patients, has a very brief duration of action and minimal side effects [51]. When given by the intracoronary route, ≥ 16 µg boluses in the left coronary cause hyperemia that is intense (4.6 ± 0.7, peak/resting ratio at heart rate of 76 ± 3 beats/min, mean $\pm$ SD) but brief (37 ± 7 s). Continuous infusions of (80 µg/min in the left coronary cause sustained regional hyperemia. Intracoronary administration usually causes no significant changes in heart rate or blood pressure, although brief heart block is infrequently seen in patients with predisposing factors (*e.g.* concomitant use of drugs that depress sinoatrial or atrioventricular node function) or when large doses are given (> 24 µg/min). Intravenous infusions of 140 µg/kg/min cause maximal coronary hyperemia in 84% of patients.

Systemic administration causes a moderate increase in heart rate ($+24 \pm 14$ beats/min) and a slight drop in blood pressure (-6 ± 7 mmHg). Patients often have a feeling of flushing and chest discomfort, but the effects of the drug dissipate within 145 ± 67 seconds of stopping the infusion.

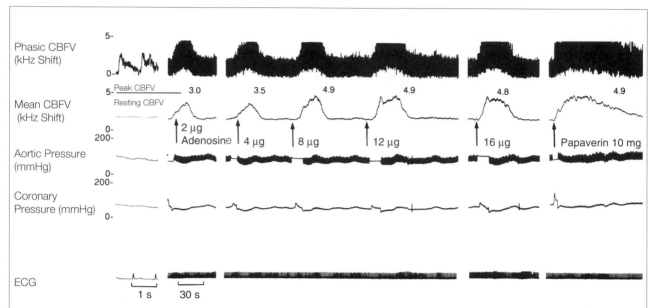

The effect of adenosine and papaverine on coronary blood flow velocity (CBFV) measured in the left anterior descending coronary of a patient with normal coronary arteries [51]. The two top panels show phasic and mean flow velocity. The middle panels show aortic and mean intracoronary blood pressure. The bottom panels show the heart rate and electrocardiogram. Progressively larger doses of adenosine cause a stepwise increase in CBFV, peaking at 4.8 peak/resting velocity. Maximal coronary hyperemia after adenosine was similar to that caused by papaverine. *Reprinted with permission of the American Heart Association.*

Dipyridamole, an agent that indirectly increases the adenosine concentration in tissue, has also been used for measurement of coronary flow reserve [33, 43]. Intravenous doses (≥ 0.56 mg/kg) of dipyridamole cause maximal hyperemia in about 90% of patients. However, it has a long duration of action (> 30 min), which makes it impractical for measuring coronary flow reserve in the catheterization laboratory.

Effects of Systemic Hemodynamics

The coronary flow reserve is affected by systemic hemodynamics [24, 39]. Heart rate and ventricular preload increase the resting blood flow velocity, but do not significantly change the hyperemic peak flow velocity. As a result, the coronary flow reserve decreases as these two parameters increase.

Arterial blood pressure increases both the resting flow velocity (through increased metabolic demand) and the hyperemic peak flow velocity (through increased coronary perfusion pressure). When arterial pressure lies within the range of autoregulation, these effects are cancelled and coronary flow reserve measurements are not affected significantly.

To interpret coronary flow reserve measured as a ratio of peak-to-resting flow velocity, it is important that the resting flow velocity be standardized during measurement of coronary flow reserve. When possible, coronary flow reserve measurements should therefore be obtained using a standardized heart rate (*e.g.* 100 beats/min) at which laboratory normal values have been determined.

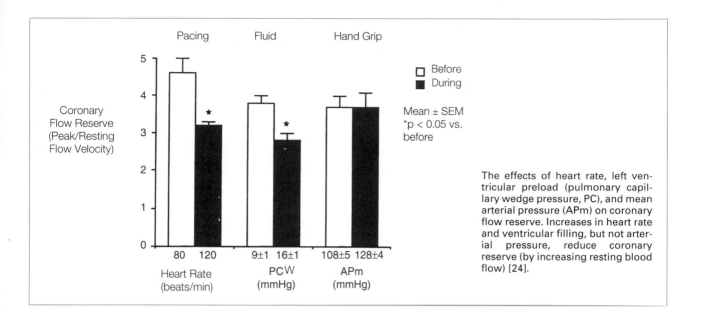

The effects of heart rate, left ventricular preload (pulmonary capillary wedge pressure, PC), and mean arterial pressure (APm) on coronary flow reserve. Increases in heart rate and ventricular filling, but not arterial pressure, reduce coronary reserve (by increasing resting blood flow) [24].

The preload should be taken into account when interpreting the measurements. When the heart rate is constant, repeat measurements of coronary reserve over time (mean interval 11±3 months) are remarkably reproducible (r=0.95, mean absolute difference = 0.3±0.1 peak/resting ratio).

Assessment of the Microcirculation

The most important clinical use of Doppler catheters today is the assessment of microcirculation in patients with angina pectoris, but no significant obstruction in the epicardial arteries visualized on the angiogram. Since blood flow is regulated by the microcirculation, a reduction in coronary flow reserve without larger vessel stenosis can be viewed as *a priori* evidence of microcirculatory disease.

Microcirculatory insufficiency in patients with angina pectoris symptoms and normal coronary arteries is not uncommon. In our laboratory, 34% of patient undergoing angiography for chest pain and who are found to have normal or minimally narrowed coronary arteries have reduced coronary reserve. Cannon et al. report microcirculatory disease in nearly 75% of patients with essentially normal coronary angiograms who were referred for evaluation of chest pain [5].

Recent studies have demonstrated that many patients with microcirculatory insufficiency and angina pectoris also have endothelial dysfunction [34, 37]. Acetylcholine or *substance P*, both of which normally elicit coronary dilation (through endothelial release of endothelial-dependent relaxing factor, EDRF), frequently cause subnormal microvascular dilation or constriction (acetylcholine) in patients with microvascular angina.

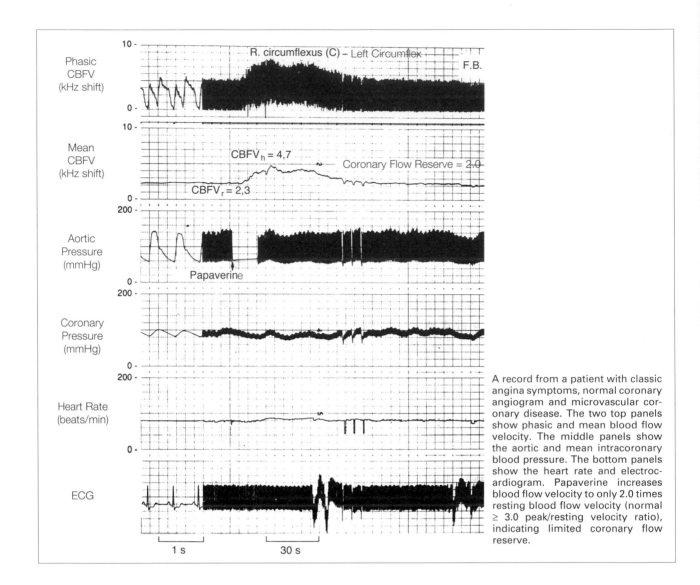

A record from a patient with classic angina symptoms, normal coronary angiogram and microvascular coronary disease. The two top panels show phasic and mean blood flow velocity. The middle panels show the aortic and mean intracoronary blood pressure. The bottom panels show the heart rate and electrocardiogram. Papaverine increases blood flow velocity to only 2.0 times resting blood flow velocity (normal $\geq$ 3.0 peak/resting velocity ratio), indicating limited coronary flow reserve.

Since coronary reserve measured with an endothelial-independent vasodilator such as adenosine tests only the maximal conduit capacity of the artery (*i.e.* the minimal fixed resistance), normal coronary reserve measurements do not necessarily exclude abnormal *function of* the microcirculation. As more is learned about the mechanisms of microcirculatory disease, it may become possible to test for *functional* abnormalities of coronary flow regulation (*e.g.* endothelial dependent agents and pacing) as well as by simply measuring coronary reserve.

Defining the Physiologic Significance of Coronary Arterial Stenosis

Another potential use of Doppler catheters is the assessment of the physiological significance of epicardial coronary lesions. Analysis of coronary angiograms using simple hydraulic formulae to predict the degree of flow impairment caused by a single lesion was shown in animal models, but their application in patients has been problematic. Although maximal coronary conductance in dogs with normal coronary arteries decreases when arterial stenosis exceeds 50% (75% cross-sectional area stenosis), similar studies in humans with extensive atherosclerosis showed a poor correlation between angiographically assessed luminal stenosis and maximal coronary conductance (as assessed by coronary flow reserve) [11, 41].

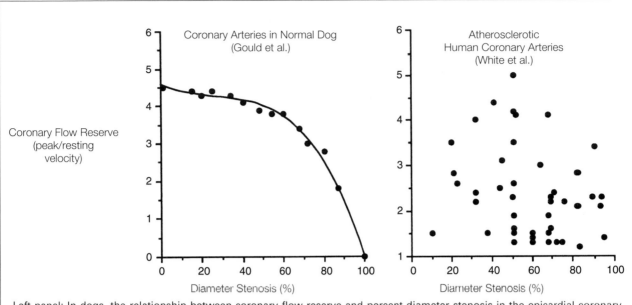

Left panel: In dogs, the relationship between coronary flow reserve and percent diameter stenosis in the epicardial coronary artery (redrawn from Gould et al. [11]). Right panel: In humans with atherosclerosis, the relationship between coronary flow reserve and percent diameter epicardial stenosis (redrawn from White et al. [14].

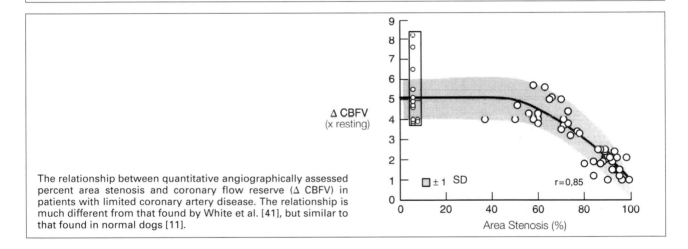

The relationship between quantitative angiographically assessed percent area stenosis and coronary flow reserve (Δ CBFV) in patients with limited coronary artery disease. The relationship is much different from that found by White et al. [41], but similar to that found in normal dogs [11].

The primary difference between studies in animals and those in humans is that humans have atherosclerosis, a disease that usually involves the entire coronary arterial tree with diffuse luminal narrowing in some areas and luminal dilation in others [10, 26]. Angiographic measurements of percent lumen stenosis compare the caliber of stenosis with the adjacent „normal" segment. In patients with atherosclerosis, however, the adjacent segment is not normal [22].

Percent luminal stenosis measurements thus compare one abnormal area to another. Hence, the more extensive the atherosclerosis, the less predictive angiographic measurements are of the physiological importance of individual lesions.

This concept is borne out by studies from our laboratory. In patients with one-vessel coronary artery disease, angiographic measurements of stenosis geometry correlated closely with coronary reserve [47, 54]. In patients undergoing coronary artery bypass surgery for widespread, multi-vessel coronary disease, angiographically defined lesion geometry no longer correlated with coronary reserve [41].

The relative inaccuracy of angiography in defining the functional significance of epicardial stenoses has led to the implementation of hemodynamic measurements. The Doppler catheter can be used to measure the significance of coronary lesions by two methods. Coronary flow reserve measurements can be helpful in determining whether a lesion is flow limiting, providing that the lesion is discrete, there is no branch point directly proximal to the lesion, and the patient has normal microcirculatory function.

The finding of normal coronary flow reserve despite what appears to be severe luminal stenosis has prognostic importance [18]. Of 26 patients in whom we deferred angioplasty because the lesion to be dilated did not cause hemodynamic obstruction (normal coronary flow reserve and/or translesional pressure gradient < 20 mmHg), 25 were asymptomatic or minimally symptomatic (Canadian Heart Association class 0 or 1) at follow-up 22 ± 11 months later. No patient suffered a myocardial infarction, and only one returned later for angioplasty. He was found to have a new severe lesion. The lesion previously found to be hemodynamically insignificant was unchanged.

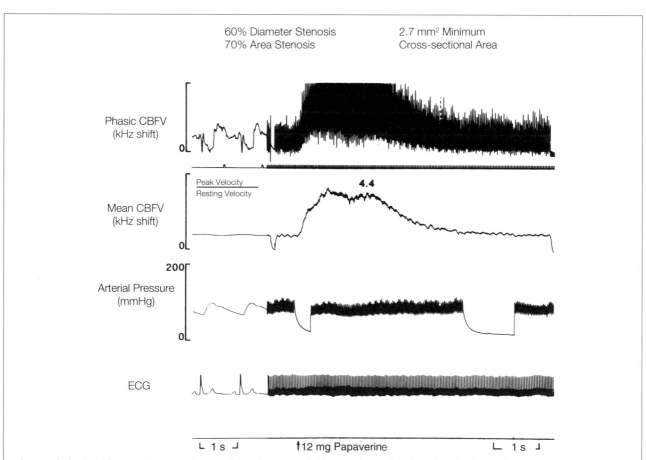

A record obtained from a 48-year-old man with a three-month history of exertional angina. Angiography demonstrated a stenosis in the left anterior descending artery causing 73% area stenosis. The top two panels show phasic and mean blood flow velocity. The bottom panels show aortic pressure and the electrocardiogram. Despite the angiographic severity of the lesion, papaverine caused coronary blood flow to increase 4.4-fold resting blood flow, indicating normal coronary flow reserve. At follow-up 4 years later, the patient was asymptomatic.

The primary problem in using coronary flow reserve measurements to define the physiological significance of individual lesions is the coexistence of microcirculatory anomalies. If coronary flow reserve is used to assess lesion significance, one should measure the coronary flow reserve in an adjacent, unobstructed artery and be certain that the vessel under study perfuses normally contracting myocardium (*i.e.* no evidence of focal microvascular disease). If the distal vascular system is not normal, lesion significance probably is better defined by a translesional pressure gradient. A mean translesional pressure gradient > 15 mmHg (using a 1.0 mm catheter) corresponds to a lesion that reduces coronary reserve in patients with normal microvascular function [42, 47].

A second method for assessing lesion significance was described by Johnson et al. and utilizes the continuity equation [41]. First, an end-mounted catheter is placed in a normal portion of the artery and the peak blood flow velocity is measured (using FFT signal analysis). A time velocity integral (TVI) for one cardiac cycle is then measured. The transducer is then advanced to a position immediately proximal to the lesion and aimed into the stenosis. Percent area stenosis is computed as follows:

$$A = (1 - TVI_{norm}/TVI_{sten}) \times 100$$

A	*Percent area stenosis*
TVI_{norm}	*time velocity integral in the normal segment*
TVI_{sten}	*time velocity integral in the stenosis*

Nakatani et al. recently validated this method in humans by demonstrating a close correlation between area stenosis defined by quantitative angiography and Doppler catheter derived assessment of luminal stenosis ($r=0.83$; area stenosis$_{Doppler}$ = 0.92 Area stenosis$_{angiography}$ - 0.45) [27].

The disadvantage of these methods is that, while they assess the flow impairment caused by the stenosis, none define the nature of the arterial lesion. Although other methods like intravascular ultrasound and coronary angioscopy may better define the presence of diffuse thickening (and calcification) of the arterial wall and intraluminal thrombus [38], they do no provide any direct physiological information relative to obstruction. Of significance is the fact that slight to moderate, diffuse narrowing, seen frequently after transplantations and in patients with generalized atherosclerosis, usually does not become impaired in maximal coronary hyperemia [19, 25, 31, 48].

Coronary Doppler Catheters in Coronary Interventions

Assessment of the residual lesion after coronary angioplasty has been difficult. Angiographic evaluation of the residual lesion is complicated by an inability to define precisely the vascular edges, dissection of the arterial wall with multiple flow channels, and intraluminal protrusions or filling defects [35].

Many investigators have attempted to utilize Doppler catheter derived pre- and post-interventional flow velocity measurements as a criterion for determining whether significant improvement has been achieved. In many patients with successful coronary dilation, coronary flow reserve normalizes immediately after the procedure [44, 53].

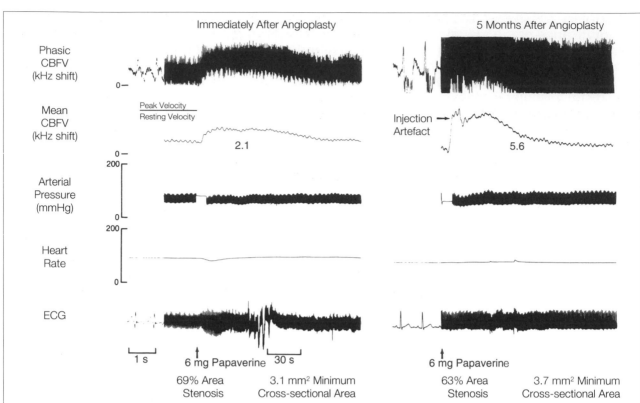

A record obtained immediately after (left) and five months after coronary angioplasty (right) [44]. The top two tracings show phasic and mean blood flow velocity. The middle tracings show the aortic and mean intracoronary blood pressure. The bottom tracings show the heart rate and electrocardiogram. Coronary flow reserve immediately after angioplasty remains depressed (2.1 times peak/resting blood flow velocity). Five months later, lesion geometry had not changed significantly, but coronary reserve had normalized (5.6 times peak/resting ratio).

Unfortunately, although the coronary flow reserve improves immediately after dilation in around 40% of all patients, it still remains low. Follow-up studies six months after angioplasty show that coronary flow reserve normalizes eventually [44]. Other studies in humans show transient defects in thallium scintigraphy soon after apparently uncomplicated dilation, and studies in animals show transient reductions in regional hyperemia in the dilated artery [1, 17, 20]. The mechanism of this temporary reduction in coronary flow reserve after angioplasty is not entirely certain, but it is probably related to transient dysfunction or micro-embolic obstruction of the microcirculation distal to the dilated lesion. In dogs, the platelet-released factors (especially serotonin and thromboxane A_2) released after angioplasty cause transient distal coronary constriction [17]. Receptor blockade or aspirin reduce angioplasty-induced microvascular constriction [1, 17]. From these studies and from the knowledge that many patients undergoing angioplasty have pre-existing microcirculatory impairment, it has become apparent that measurement of coronary flow reserve immediately after coronary dilation is a poor method of assessing the success of dilation.

Two other Doppler catheter methods might be useful in this regard. Assessment of the residual lesion using the continuity equation (see above) may provide a simple method of determining whether the lesion causes hemodynamic impairment. Before this method can be used clinically, however, validation will be required.

The second method uses the 0.46 mm (0.018") Doppler flow wire (Cardiometrics) that can be used during angioplasty for as a guidewire for balloon placement and as a continuous, on-line monitor of blood flow during the procedure.

In the presence of a severe coronary lesion, the blood pressure drops in the artery distal to stenosis. As a result, there is continuous blood flow through the stenosis and the ratio of systolic to diastolic blood flow increases. It has been suggested that monitoring the ratio of systolic to diastolic blood flow velocity ratio might also provide a way to determine when the significant obstruction in the epicardial vessel was removed. The normalization of the ratio would imply removal of low obstruction. In a preliminary study, the systolic-to-diastolic velocity ratio increased from 1.5±0.7 before angioplasty to 1.9±0.8 after dilation [28]. However, several other factors might also affect the systolic:diastolic ratio (*e.g.* hypertrophy, microcirculatory constriction or embolization). Additionally, the sensitivity of the systolic-to-diastolic ratio for assessing the severity of the residual lesion has not been adequately validated. Nonetheless, use of the wire in monitoring blood flow during angioplasty has promise.

One of the more exciting methods for assessing lesions after angioplasty is intravascular ultrasound. Recent studies demonstrate impressive imaging of the arterial wall of dilated lesions [12, 52]. The value of these imaging in determining when significant obstruction has been removed remains unclear. It is possible, however, that the morphological information obtained from imaging (presence of intramural calcium, balloon-induced fracture of the wall) may be very useful in determining the most appropriate method for angioplasty and when angioplasty is sufficiently successful to stop.

5.3.3   Coronary Doppler Catheters
5.3.3.7   Other Uses

Perhaps the most important uses of coronary Doppler catheters are in studies of coronary pathophysiology in humans. Because Doppler catheters provide beat-by-beat measurement of blood flow in individual coronary vessels, rapidly occurring changes in coronary hemodynamics can be studied „on-line".

The Doppler catheter has made possible studies of neural reflex control of the coronary circulation [45], assessment of coronary endothelial function, definition of the direct effects of the intra-aortic balloon pump on coronary blood flow [13], and investigation of the impact of a variety of disease states on the coronary circulation [25]. Further refinement of these devices should permit easier and more accurate methods for assessing the coronary circulation in humans.

References

1. Bates ER, McGillem MJ, Beals TF. Effect of angioplasty induced endothelial denudation compared with medial injury on coronary flow reserve. Circulation 1987; 76: 710-716.
2. Benchimol A, Stegall HF, Gartlan JL. New method to measure phasic coronary blood velocity in man. Am Heart J 1971; 81: 93-101.
3. Bolli R, Triana JF, Jeroudi MO. Prolonged impairment of coronary vasodilation after reversible ischemia: evidence for microvascular stunning. Circ Res 1990; 67: 332-343.
4. Brush JE, Cannon RO, Schenke WH, Bonow RO, Leon MB, Maron BJ, Epstein SE. Angina due to coronary microvascular disease in hypertensive patients without left ventricular hypertrophy. N Engl J Med 1988; 319: 1302-1307.

5. Cannon RO, Cattau EL, Yakshe PN, Maher K, Schenke WH, Benjamin SB, Epstein SE. Coronary flow reserve, esophageal motility, and chest pain in patients with angiographically normal coronary arteries. Am J Med 1990; 88: 217-222.

6. Chilian WM, Layne SM, Klausner EC, Eastham CL, Marcus ML. Redistribution of coronary microvascular resistance produced by dipyridamole. Am J Physiol 1989; 256: H383-H390.

7. Cole JS, Hartley CJ. The pulsed Doppler coronary artery catheter: preliminary report of a new technique for measuring rapid changes in coronary artery blood flow velocity in man. Circulation 1977; 56: 18-25.

8. Doucette JW, Corl D, Payne HM, Flynn AE, Goto M, Nassi M, Sejal J. Validation of a Doppler guide wire for intravascular measurement of coronary artery blood flow velocity. Circulation 1992; 85: 1899-1911.

9. Franklin DL, Schlegel W, Rushmer RF. Blood flow measured by Doppler frequency shift of backscattered ultrasound. Science 1961; 134: 564-655.

10. Glagov S, Weisenberg E, Zarins CK, Stankunavicius R, Kolettis GJ. Compensatory enlargement of human atherosclerotic coronary arteries. N Engl J Med 1987; 316: 1371-1375.

11. Gould KL, Lipscomb K, Hamilton GW. Physiologic basis for assessing critical coronary stenosis: instantaneous flow response and regional distribution during coronary hyperemia as measures of coronary flow reserve. Am J Cardiol 1974; 33: 87-94.

12. Hoyne J, Mahon DJ, Jain A, White CJ, Ramee SR, Wallis JB, Al-Zarka A, Tobis JM. Morphological effects of balloon angioplasty in vivo assessed by intravascular ultrasound imaging. Circulation 1992; 85: 1012-1025.

13. Ishihara M, Sato H, Tateishi H, Kawagoe T, Muraoka Y, Yoshimura M. Effects of intraaortic balloon pumping and coronary blood flow in acute myocardial infarction. J Am Coll Cardiol 1992; 19; 137A.

14. Johnson EL, Yock PG, Hargrave VK, Srebro JP, Manubens SM, Seitz W, Ports TA. Assessment of the severity of coronary stenoses using a Doppler catheter: validation of a method based on the continuity equation. Circulation 1989; 80: 625-635.

15. Kern MJ, Courtois M, Ludbrook P. A simplified method to measure coronary blood flow velocity in patients: validation and application of a Judkins-style Doppler-tipped angiographic catheter. Am Heart J 1990; 120: 1202-1212.

16. Klein LW, Agarwal JB, Schneider RM, Herman G, Weintraub WS, Helfant RH. Effects of previous myocardial infarction on measurements of reactive hyperemia and coronary vascular reserve. J Am Coll Cardiol 1986; 8: 357-363.

17. Laxson DD, Homans DC, Pavek T, Crampton M, Zhang XW. PTCA causes microvascular constriction. Circulation (in press).

18. Lesser JL, Wilson RF, White CW. Can a physiologic assessment of coronary stenoses of intermediate severity facilitate patient selection for coronary angioplasty? Coronary Artery Dis 1990; 1: 697-705.

19. Mallory JA, Tobis JM, Griffith J, Gessert J, McRae M, Moussabeck O, Bessen M, Moriuchi M, Henry WL. Assessment of normal and atherosclerotic arterial wall thickness using an intravascular ultrasound imaging catheter. Am Heart J 1990; 119: 1392-1400.

20. Manyari DE, Knudtson MR, Kloiber R, Roth D. Sequential thallium-201 myocardial perfusion studies after successful percutaneous transluminal coronary artery angioplasty: delayed resolution of exercise induced scintigraphic abnormalities. Circulation 1988; 77: 86-95.

21. Marcus ML, Chilian WM, Kanatsuka H, Dellsperger KC, Eastham CL, Lamping KG. Understanding the coronary circulation through studies at the microvascular level. Circulation 1990; 82: 1-7.

22. Marcus ML, Harrison DG, White CW, McPherson DD, Wilson RF, Kerber RE. Assessing the physiologic significance of coronary obstructions in patients: importance of diffuse undetected atherosclerosis. Prog Cardiovasc Dis 1988; 31: 39-56.

23. Marcus ML, Wilson RF, White CW. Methods of measuring coronary blood flow in humans: a critical review. Circulation 1987; 76: 245-257.

24. McGinn AL, White CW, Wilson RF. Interstudy variability in coronary flow reserve: the importance of heart rate, arterial pressure, and ventricular preload. Circulation 1990; 81: 1319-1330.

25. McGinn AL, Wilson RF, Olivari MT, Homans DC, White CW. Coronary vasodilator reserve after human orthotopic cardiac transplantation. Circulation 1988; 78: 1200-1209.

26. McPherson DD, Hiratzka LF, Lamberth WC, Brandt B, Hunt M, Kieso RA, Marcus ML, Kerber RE. Delineation of the extent of coronary atherosclerosis by high frequency epicardial echocardiography. N Engl J Med 1987; 316: 304-308.

27. Nakatani S, Yamagishi M, Tamai J, Takaki H, Haze K, Miyatake K. Quantitative assessment of coronary artery stenosis by intravascular Doppler catheter technique: application of the continuity equation. Circulation 1992; 85: 1786-1791.

28. Ofili EO, Kerm MJ, Segal J, St Vrain JA, Castello R, Labowitz AJ. Improvement of coronary flow dynamics after angioplasty: analysis by guidewire spectral Doppler. J Am Coll Cardiol 1992; 19: II-703.

29. Opherk D, Schwartz F, Mall G, Manthey J, Baller D, Kubler W. Coronary dilatory capacity in idiopathic dilated cardiomyopathy: analysis of 16 patients. Am J Cardiol 1983; 51: 1657-1662.

30. Peronneau PA, Leger F. Doppler ultrasonic pulsed blood flow meter. Proc 6th ICMBE 1969; 10-11.

31. Pinto FJ, St Goar FG, Chiang M, Popp RL, Valentine HA. Intracoronary ultrasound evaluation of intimal thickening in cardiac transplant recipients: correlation with clinical characteristics.

32. Qin JJ, Kuban BD, Freidman MH, Van Fossen DB. Accuracy of intravascular Doppler catheter system - assessment by an in-vitro coronary cast model. Circulation 1991; 84: II-722).

33. Rosen JD, Simonetti I, Marcus ML, Winneford MD. Coronary dilation with standard dose dipyridamole and dipyridamole combined with handgrip. Circulation 1989; 79: 566-572.

34. Ryan TJ, Treasure CB, Yeung AC, Klein JL, Selwyn AP, Ganz P. Impaired endothelium-dependent dilation of the coronary microvasculature in patients with atherosclerosis.

35. Serruys PW, Reiber HJC, Wijns W, Brand VDM, Kooijman CJ, tenKaten HJ, Hugenholtz PG. Assessment of percutaneous transluminal coronary angioplasty by quantitative coronary angiography: diameter versus densitometric area measurements. Am J Cardiol 1984; 54: 482-487.

36. Sibley DH, Millar HD, Hartley CJ, Whitlow PL. Subselective measurement of coronary blood flow velocity using a steerable Doppler catheter. J Am Coll Cardiol 1986; 8: 1332-1340.

37. Vrints CJM, Bult H, Hitter E, Herman AG, Snoeck J. Impaired endothelium-dependent cholinergic coronary vasodilation in patients with angina and normal coronary arteriograms. J Am Coll Cardiol 1992; 19: 21-31.

38. Waller BF, Pinkerton CA, Slack JD. Intravascular ultrasound: a histological study of vessels during life - the new 'gold standard' for vascular imaging. Circulation 1992; 85: 2305-2310.

39. Watson KR, Foley B, Chisholm RJ, Armstrong PW. The effect of physiologic variables on coronary flow reserve. J Am Coll Cardiol 1990; 17: II-64.

40. White CW, Wilson RF, Marcus ML. Measurement of coronary blood flow in humans. Prog Cardiovasc Dis 1988; 31: 79-94.

41. White CW, Wright CB, Doty D, Eastham C, Harrison DG, Marcus ML. Does visual interpretation of the coronary arteriogram predict the physiologic importance of a coronary stenosis? N Engl J Med 1984; 310: 819-823.

42. Wijns W, Serruys PW, Reiber JHC, Van Den Brand M, Simoons ML, Kooijman CJ, Balakumaran K, Hugenholtz PG. Quantitative angiography of the left anterior descending coronary artery: correlation with pressure gradients and results of exercise thallium scintigraphy. Circulation 1986; 73: 286-295.

43. Wilson RF, Laughlin DE, Ackell PH, Chilian WM, Holida MD, Hartley CJ, Armstrong ML, Marcus ML, White CW. Transluminal, subselective measurement of coronary artery blood flow velocity and vasodilator reserve in man. Circulation 1985; 72: 82-92.

44. Wilson RF, Marcus ML, Aylward PE, Talman CT, White CW. The effect of coronary angioplasty on coronary flow reserve. Circulation 1988; 77: 873-885.

45. Wilson RF, Marcus ML, Laughlin DE, White CW. The pulmonary inflation reflex: Its physiologic significance in man. Am J Physiol 1988; 255: H866-H871.

46. Wilson RF, Marcus ML, White CW. Coronary flow reserve after coronary bypass surgery or angioplasty. Prog Cardiovasc Dis 1988; 31: 95-114.

47. Wilson RF, Marcus ML, White CW. Prediction of the physiologic significance of coronary arterial lesions by quantitative lesion geometry in patients with limited coronary artery disease. Circulation 1987; 75: 723-732.

48. Wilson RF, White CW. Does coronary bypass surgery restore normal coronary flow reserve?: The effect of diffuse atherosclerosis and focal obstructive lesions. Circulation 1987; 76: 653-571.

49. Wilson RF, White CW. Intracoronary papaverine: an ideal vasodilator for studies of the coronary circulation. Circulation 1986; 73: 444-451.

50. Wilson RF, White CW. Serious ventricular dysrythmias after intracoronary papaverine. Am J Cardiol 1988; 62: 1301-1302.

51. Wilson RF, Wyche K, Christensen BV, Zimmer S, Laxson DD. The effects of adenosine on the human coronary circulation. Circulation 1990; 82: 1595-1606.

52. Yorck PG, Fitzgerald PJ, Sykes C, Rowe MH, Hinohara T, Robertson GC, Selmon MR, Simpson JB. Morphological features of successful coronary atherectomy determined by intravascular ultrasound imaging. Circulation 1990; 82: III-676.

53. Zijlistra J, Reiber JC, Julliere Y, Serruys PW. Normalization of coronary flow reserve by percutaneous transluminal coronary angioplasty. Am J Cardiol 1988; 61: 55-60.

54. Zijlstra F, van Ommeren J, Reiber JHC, Serruys PW. Does the quantitative assessment of coronary artery stenosis dimensions predict the physiologic significance of a coronary stenosis? Circulation 1987; 75: 1154-1161.

5.   **interventional Echocardiography**   **264**
5.4   **Principles of Intra- and Perioperative Echocardiography**
(Christian Detter, Bruno Reichart)

For many years, the use of echocardiography in cardiac surgery was limited to preoperative diagnosis and postoperative follow-up examinations. Only after the development of high-resolution transducers, two-dimensional echocardiography, and, in particular, Doppler echocardiography was it possible to make highly reliable echocardiographic assessments of the results of surgery in the immediate postoperative phase [39, 53]. The major limitation of transthoracic echocardiography (TTE) is the difficulty in obtaining good images when the patient has is a fresh thoracotomy scar and is ventilated artificially. Patient positioning, bandages, drainage tubes, and monitor cables are further limitation of transthoracic echocardiography.

The advent of transesophageal echocardiography (TEE) has provided new possibilities for intra- and postoperative echocardiographic evaluation of cardiac surgeries (for example, surgical management of aortic dissection) [11, 24, 25, 43]. Easy to use, sterile epicardial transducers has expanded the realm of intraoperative cardiac ultrasound diagnosis [63]. However, in contrast to intraoperative epicardial echocardiography, surgery must not be interrupted in order to perform intraoperative transesophageal echocardiography. TEE therefore permits continuous monitoring of surgery.

TEE also permits intraoperative assessment of the results of valve reconstruction surgery and assessment of prosthetic valve function subsequent to valve replacement. When combined with Doppler color flow imaging, the physician can intraoperatively detect, quantitate, and repair regurgitations and paravalvular leaks during a single session.

By intraoperatively monitoring left ventricular wall motion, ischemia can be detected after early occlusion of aortocoronary bypass. Moreover, the risk of imminent myocardial infarction can be reduced by early intervention.

The various applications of echocardiography in cardiac surgery will be detailed in the following.

5.4   **Principles of Intra- and Perioperative Echocardiography**
5.4.1   **Monitoring Ventricular Function**

In view of its noninvasive nature, peri- and intraoperative echocardiography is an ideal means of assessing left ventricular function. Echocardiography is quick and can be performed at any time with a minimum of effort. Unlike some other methods, it is also free of radiation effects and contrast agents.

In light of its excellent spatial and temporal resolution, one-dimensional (M-mode) echocardiography is still a highly valued technique for assessment of left ventricular function. M-mode echocardiography permits measurement of wall thicknesses, left ventricular end-diastolic and end-systolic diameters, and of left ventricular fractional shortening (LVFS). This is an important parameter for assessment of left ventricular contractility; a comparison of pre-, intra-, and postoperative measurements is of particular clinical interest. However, the value of LVFS is severely restricted under the following conditions.

1. Nonsynchronized contraction of the interventricular septum and LV anterior wall, which can occur in left bundle-branch block or paradoxical septal motion after cardiac surgery.
2. Segmental contraction abnormality due to coronary artery disease.

In contrast with M-mode echocardiography, 2-D (B-mode) echocardiography permits assessment of the entire left ventricle and a complete analysis of left ventricular wall motion.

Apical and transesophageal transducer positions are preferred for intra- and postoperative echocardiographic monitoring of ventricular function.

In transthoracic echocardiography (TTE), the standard scan planes for regional functional analysis of the left ventricle are the parasternal long and short-axis views at papillary muscle level and apical two and four-chamber views. The standard TEE plane is the long-axis views of the left ventricle. These views usually permit detection and assessment of asynchronous contractions, *e.g.* after myocardial infarction, or in myocardial ischemia due to inadequate bypass supply, or due to bypass occlusion [31, 55]. Contractile abnormalities of ischemic myocardial segments are described according to the *American Society of Echocardiography's* recommendations for segmental analysis.

Acute myocardial infarction produces contraction abnormalities that can be detected within minutes by echocardiography. Systolic wall thickness, the motion amplitude, and the excursion velocity are reduced. The affected region becomes either hypokinetic, akinetic, or dyskinetic in the absence of systolic wall thickening.

Reduced systolic wall thickening is the most important parameter in the functional assessment of ischemic myocardial segments. Since akinesis of a particular segment can be masked by normal contractile motion of adjacent segments, the results of wall motion analysis alone can be misleading.

If there is a possibility of acute bypass occlusion, coronary angiography should be performed and bypass revision surgery must be considered.

Echocardiography also permits early detection and differentiation of infarction-related complications such as ventricular aneurysm and ischemia-related papillary muscle dysfunction or rupture.

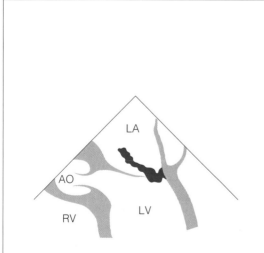

Ischemic mitral incompetence due to a post-infarction tear in the posteromedial papillary muscle.

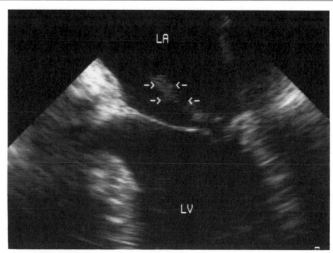

Transesophageal short-axis view of the left cardiac cavities demonstrating the mitral valve.

Echocardiography is also useful for excluding intracavitary thrombi or tumors as the source of embolism.

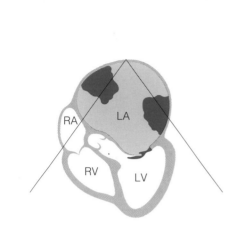

Dilated left atrium in mitral stenosis. Two large thrombi are located in the left atrium.

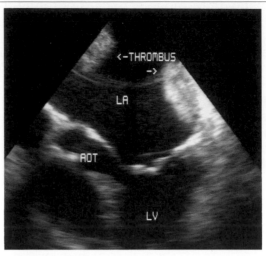

Transesophageal short-axis view of the left heart cavities and left ventricular outflow tract.

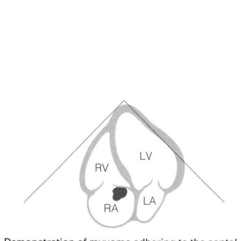

Demonstration of myxoma adhering to the septal tricuspid valve leaflet.

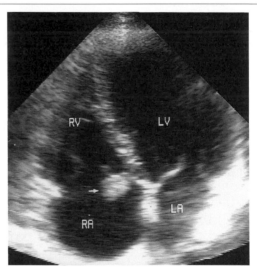

Two-dimensional apical four-chamber view.

Because it can be performed quickly even at the bedside of intensive care patients, echocardiography is very helpful in the differential diagnosis of low cardiac output syndrome. Low cardiac output syndrome is characterized by reduced cardiac output, which in turn causes a reduction in peripheral arterial pressure, an increase in central venous pressure, peripheral vasoconstriction, and reduced urine output. The consequence is insufficient organ blood supply with secondary organ dysfunction. Other possible causes include pericardial tamponade, severely impaired pump function due to perioperative myocardial infarction, incomplete myocardial revascularization, coronary embolism, and insufficient bypass blood flow. Noncorrected residual defects can be reliably excluded.

In addition to left ventricular fractional shortening, the cardiac output (heart rate times stroke volume) is another important parameter in intra- and postoperative monitoring of ventricular function. Cardiac output is of great diagnostic value in the assessment of critical circulatory conditions such as shock and sepsis. It is therefore an indispensable tool in perioperative monitoring of patients undergoing cardiac surgery.

Cardiac output is generally measured by indicator dilution methods, using dye or temperature as the indicator. In thermodilution techniques, cardiac output is determined by injecting cold saline solution into the right atrium, then measuring the rise in temperature in the pulmonary artery with the help of a special catheter (*e.g.* Swan-Ganz catheter) and a cardiac output computer.

When using the aortic flow curve for echocardiographic calculation of cardiac output, the diameter of the aorta is measured from the left parasternal position in order to determine the aortic valve area (AVA). Next, the peak velocity in the aortic annulus and the time-velocity integral (TVI) are determined using an apical pulsed Doppler scan. The cardiac output is then calculated by multiplying the time-velocity integral by the aortic valve area and the heart rate.

Various studies have shown a very good correlation between simultaneous determinations of cardiac output using invasive thermodilution methods versus noninvasive Doppler echocardiography [35, 62]. However, in difficult to manage cardiac surgery patients, cardiac output is determined by means of cardiac catheterization using a Swan-Ganz catheter. Catheterization also permits measurement of such diagnostically important parameters as systemic and pulmonary resistance.

5.4   **Principles of Intra- and Perioperative Echocardiography**
5.4.2   **Functional Assessment of Prosthetic Valves.**
               Intraoperative Transesophageal and Epicardial Echocardiographic Evaluation
               of the Results of Valve Reconstruction

All prosthetic cardiac valves are associated with valve-related or valve-induced complications. Hemorrhage is the primary complication in mechanical prostheses (tilting disk, bileaflet, caged ball, and caged disk prosthesis), which require continued anticoagulation treatment for the remainder of the patient's life. Thrombo-embolism and/or valvular dysfunction may also occur due to thrombogeneity of the prosthetic valve.

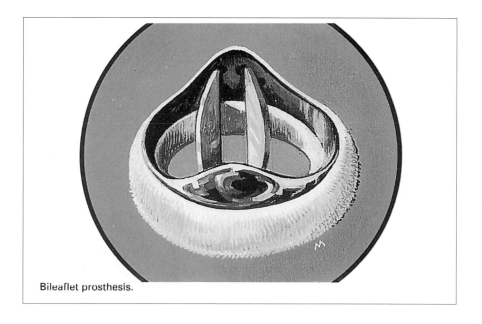

Bileaflet prosthesis.

5.4   **Principles of Intra- and Perioperative Echocardiography**
     268

5.4.2   **Functional Assessment of Prosthetic Valves.**
          Intraoperative Transesophageal and Epicardial Echocardiographic
          Evaluation of the Results of Valve Reconstruction

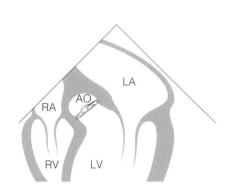

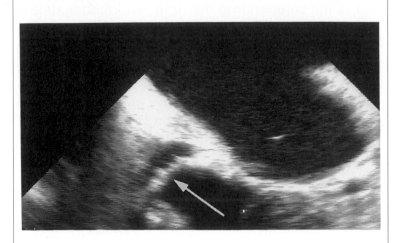

Sorin bileaflet aortic valve prosthesis. Prosthetic valve incompetence occurred in the immediate postoperative phase. Only one leaflet moves, the other remains stuck in the open position. Diastolic frame.

2-D transesophageal short-axis view

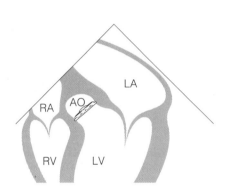

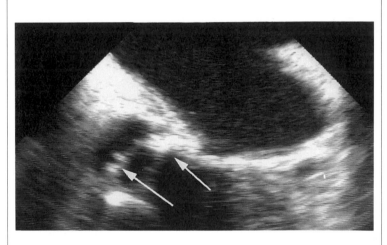

Sorin bileaflet aortic valve prosthesis. Prosthetic valve incompetence occurred in the immediate postoperative phase. Only one leaflet moves, the other remains stuck in the open position. Systolic frame.

2-D transesophageal short-axis

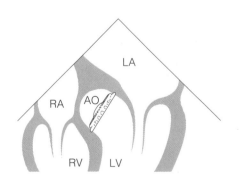

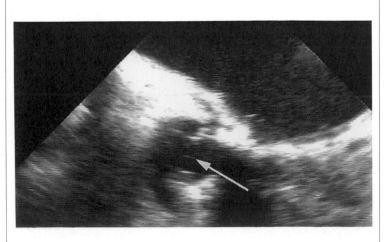

Sorin bileaflet aortic valve prosthesis. Prosthetic valve incompetence occurred in the immediate postoperative phase. After it is rotated slightly, the prosthesis opens and closes properly. Diastolic frame.

2-D transesophageal short-axis view.

5.4   **Principles of Intra- and Perioperative Echocardiography**   **269**
5.4.2   **Functional Assessment of Prosthetic Valves.**
             Intraoperative Transesophageal and Epicardial Echocardiographic
             Evaluation of the Results of Valve Reconstruction

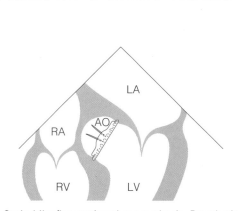

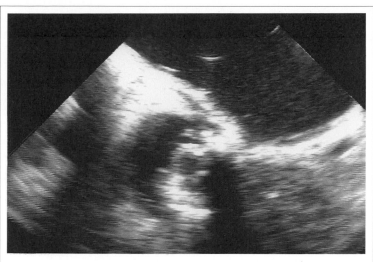

Sorin bileaflet aortic valve prosthesis. Prosthetic valve incompetence occurred in the immediate postoperative phase. Only one leaflet moves, the other remains stuck in the open position. After it is rotated slightly, the prosthesis opens and closes properly. Systolic frame.

2-D transesophageal short-axis view of the left atrium, aorta, and left ventricular outflow tract.

The major drawback of bioprosthetic valves (porcine valves, bovine pericardial valve) is their limited durability due to the occurrence of degenerative changes and calcification. This leads to increasingly restricted leaflet mobility which, in turn, leads to obstruction or tissue defects, and tearing or perforation of the leaflets. The durability of bioprosthetic valve is reported to range between 7 and 15 years. The homograft is an alternative that is gaining increasing influence today (see below).

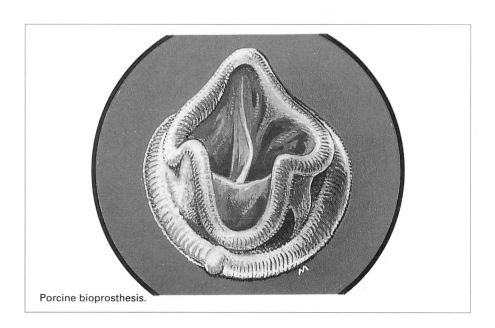

Porcine bioprosthesis.

Although bioprosthetic and mechanical cardiac valves are being continuously improved, they still are inferior to the endogenous native valve. Corrective surgery to preserve the native valve is most commonly performed in atrioventricular valves, and less commonly in the aorta, with the exception of commissurotomies performed in congenital stenosis.

5.4	Principles of Intra- and Perioperative Echocardiography	270
5.4.2	Functional Assessment of Prosthetic Valves.	
	Intraoperative Transesophageal and Epicardial Echocardiographic	
	Evaluation of the Results of Valve Reconstruction	

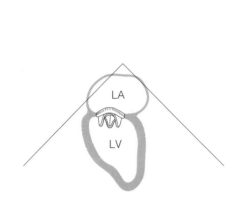

Carpentier-Edwards mitral valve bioprosthesis, demonstrating proper prosthetic valve function.

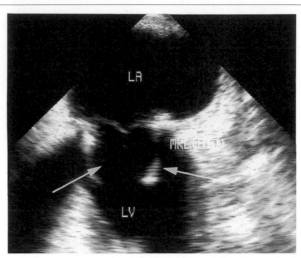

2-D transesophageal long-axis scan through the left atrium, mitral valve, and left ventricle.

Due to its anatomic relationships, the valvular apparatus, especially that of the mitral valve, is particularly suitable for reconstructive surgery.

In our experience, valvular reconstruction can be performed in up to 90% of all children with congenital mitral incompetence, and in up to 50% of all adults with acquired mitral incompetence. In mitral incompetence secondary to degenerative disease, reconstruction can be performed in 95% of all cases. In stenotic but noncalcified mitral valves, reconstruction can be performed in 90% of all cases with good long-term results.

Heavy calcium deposits and severe leaflet thickening that impairs leaflet function are contraindications for reconstruction of stenotic or regurgitant valves. In either case, valvular replacement would be the better choice.

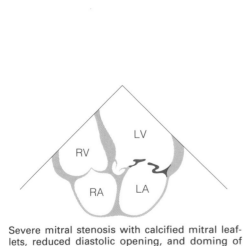

Severe mitral stenosis with calcified mitral leaflets, reduced diastolic opening, and doming of the valve.

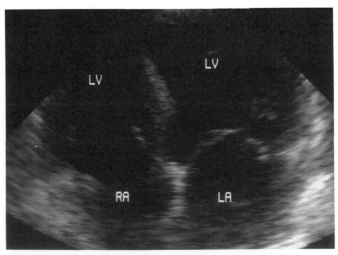

Two-dimensional apical four-chamber view.

5.4   **Principles of Intra- and Perioperative Echocardiography**   271
5.4.2   **Functional Assessment of Prosthetic Valves.**
Intraoperative Transesophageal and Epicardial Echocardiographic
Evaluation of the Results of Valve Reconstruction

In numerous works, such investigators as Carpentier, Duran, Lessana and Kreuzer and their respective co-workers were able to demonstrate good long-term results after mitral valve reconstruction [6, 7, 8, 17, 44, 46]. The major advantages of valvular reconstruction versus valvular replacement are its low rate of operative mortality and thrombo-embolism and better long-term survival [12, 57]. Another advantage is that, when there is no atrial fibrillation, anticoagulation is not required. Preservation of the mitral valve apparatus also has a beneficial effect on left ventricular geometry and function. One study [44] that evaluated mitral valves reconstructed using the „first-pass technique" versus prosthetic mitral valves demonstrated that, due to their central diastolic inflow, the reconstructed valves achieved physiological, functional flow patterns that hardly differed from the left ventricular flow patterns in normal subjects. Therefore, it is not surprising that an increasing number of valve-preserving reconstructive surgeries are being performed today.

The final decision to perform either valvular reconstruction or replacement is basically determined by pathophysiological changes in the valvular apparatus, which is a functional unit consisting of six anatomical elements: the left atrium, valvular annulus, both valve leaflets, the chordae tendineae, the papillary muscles, and the left ventricular wall. Each of these components should be assessed individually with respect to its respective function or dysfunction, and the underlying lesion causing the dysfunction.

Using this functional approach, Carpentier [7] classifies pure mitral incompetence into three types according to various characteristics of leaflet motion. Type I incompetence is characterized by normal leaflet motion; the cause of dysfunction may be annular dilatation, calcification, or leaflet tearing or shrinkage. Type II incompetence is characterized by increased leaflet motion and prolapse, i.e., one or both free edges of the leaflet override the plane of the orifice, thereby extending into the left atrium during systole. The underlying lesions associated with type II incompetence are chordal rupture or elongation and papillary muscle rupture or elongation.

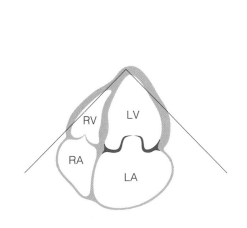

Severe mitral incompetence with prolapse of both mitral leaflets and annular dilatation.

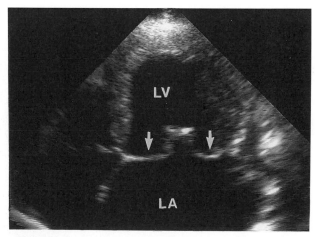

Two-dimensional apical four-chamber view.

5.4   **Principles of Intra- and Perioperative Echocardiography**   272
5.4.2   **Functional Assessment of Prosthetic Valves.**
            Intraoperative Transesophageal and Epicardial Echocardiographic
            Evaluation of the Results of Valve Reconstruction

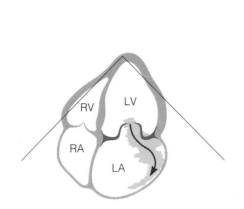

Severe mitral incompetence with prolapse of both mitral leaflets and annular dilatation.

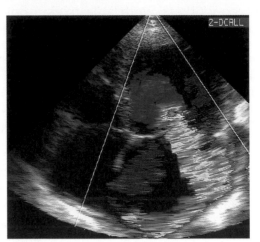

Apical four-chamber view with color flow mapping.

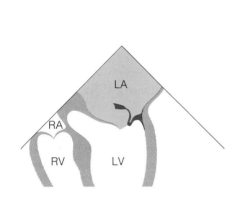

Severe mitral incompetence with prolapse of the posterior mitral leaflet.

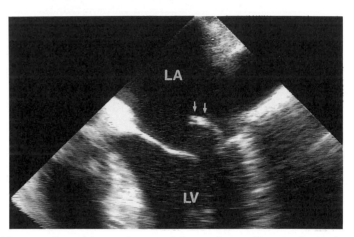

Transesophageal long-axis scan of the cardiac cavities at mitral valve level.

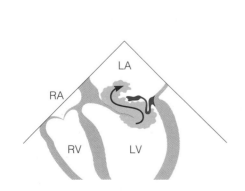

Severe mitral incompetence with prolapse of the posterior mitral leaflet.

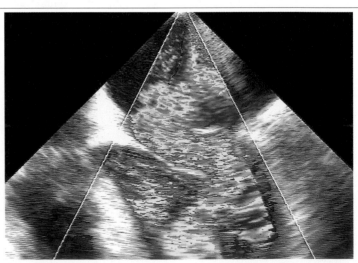

Color flow map of the transesophageal long-axis scan of the left heart cavities at mitral valve level.

5.4 **Principles of Intra- and Perioperative Echocardiography** **273**
5.4.2 **Functional Assessment of Prosthetic Valves.**
Intraoperative Transesophageal and Epicardial Echocardiographic
Evaluation of the Results of Valve Reconstruction

Type III mitral incompetence is characterized by restricted leaflet motion. The underlying lesions affects either the leaflet (leaflet thickening, commissural fusion) or the subvalvular apparatus (chordal thickening or fusion).

Prolapse of the anterior leaflet is sometimes associated with restricted function of the posterior leaflet; this is classified as *mixed type* incompetence.

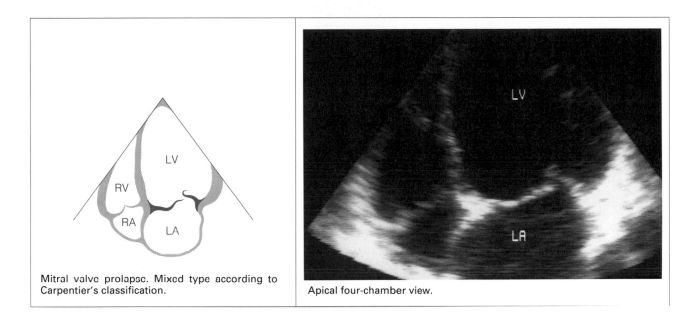

Mitral valve prolapse. Mixed type according to Carpentier's classification.

Apical four-chamber view.

When using this functional approach to assessment, one evaluates only the motion of the leaflets (normal, prolapsed, or restricted). This tricuspid valve is similarly evaluated in order to make the decision of whether to perform valvular reconstruction or replacement.

In mitral stenosis, valvular dysfunction is caused by restricted motion of the valvular or subvalvular apparatus.

Echocardiography is a virtually ideal method for preoperative assessment and description of pathomorphological changes.

For cardiac surgeons, it is a very useful tool for planning surgery. The standard projections for echocardiographically describing valvular morphology are the left parasternal and apical transducer positions. Transesophageal echocardiography (TEE) is indicated when transthoracic studies are insufficient and when special clinical questions must be addressed. Because of the proximity of the esophagus to the mitral valve apparatus, TEE is especially effective in visualizing valvular morphology.

A good understanding of the physiopathological changes in the valve and a standardized surgical procedure are two decisive factors in the functional success of valvular reconstruction. An experienced heart surgeon can perform valve reconstruction in about the same time as valve replacement. Different reconstructive procedures are used to correct different pathoanatomical changes in the valve. For instance, chordal elongation is corrected by means of Carpentier's shortening plastic repair; mural leaflet prolapse is repaired by extensive rectangular resection of the prolapsed portion; and chordal rupture of the aortic leaflet is repaired by partial resection [7]. The final step in valve reconstruction surgery is usually prosthetic ring annuloplasty (*e.g.* using Carpentier's ring). This is necessary to remodel and stabilize the dilated mitral valve annulus.

5.4   **Principles of Intra- and Perioperative Echocardiography**   274
5.4.2   **Functional Assessment of Prosthetic Valves.**
          Intraoperative Transesophageal and Epicardial Echocardiographic
          Evaluation of the Results of Valve Reconstruction

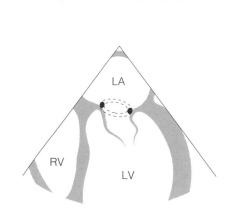

Intraoperative transesophageal scan demonstrating the results of mitral valve reconstruction with additional prosthetic ring annuloplasty.

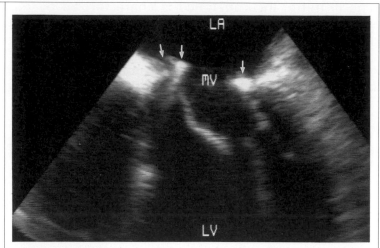

Transesophageal long-axis view of the cardiac cavities at mitral valve level.

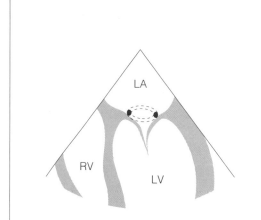

Intraoperative transesophageal scan demonstrating the results of mitral valve reconstruction with additional prosthetic ring annuloplasty. No signs of residual regurgitation.

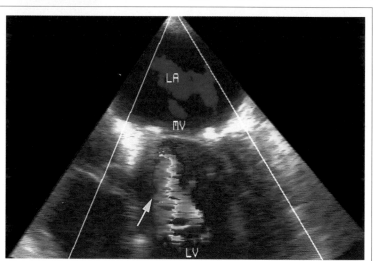

Transesophageal long-axis view of the cardiac cavities at mitral valve level with color flow mapping.

After completing the final steps of valvular reconstruction, the results are checked intraoperatively by means of transesophageal Doppler echocardiography. In addition to providing morphological data, transesophageal Doppler is also able to semiquantitate residual regurgitation. The position of the leaflet as well as its ability to close should also be assessed. The repair is judged satisfactory when both free edges of the leaflet form a horizontal contact line, and when no residual regurgitation can be detected. When the images are recorded on videotape, they can be used as baseline images for comparison with long-term follow-up images.

If the repair has been judged unsatisfactory, the heart surgeon must decide whether to perform valvular replacement or repeat reconstruction at that time. In modern medicine this approach is justifiable, because improved myocardial protection and systemic hypothermia give the surgeon enough time for a second attempt. In most cases, cardiopulmonary bypass time is no longer a limiting factor. This is another reason why intraoperative transesophageal or epicardial monitoring should become standard procedure for evaluating the results of valvular reconstruction surgeries: it could save the patient from having to undergo a second operation.

Homograft valve replacement, *i.e.* the implantation of autologous cardiac valves, has gained increasing interest and significance in the past decade. As early as 1962, two independent researchers, Ross and Barrat-Boyes, performed the first homograft transplantations in London and New Zealand, respectively. In contrast with autologous bioprostheses, homografts are not fixed in glutaraldehyde, but are stored at 4°C in culture medium immediately after collection.

This ensures the preservation of intact and vital cell and tissue structures. This will hopefully retard the degeneration of homografts in order to provide better long-term clinical results. Clinical echocardiographic studies have shown another important advantage of homograft valves, namely their good hemodynamic properties [37].

At our hospital most homograft material is sterilely removed from the explanted hearts of transplant recipients or from donor hearts not used for transplantation. The excised valve is placed in our valve bank for long-term storage at -196°C. Another source of homograft valve material is autopsy material obtained from the pathology or autopsy department. This material must be removed within 24 hours post mortem, and must be sterilized for 3 days in an antibiotic solution.

Besides providing the preoperative diagnosis, echocardiography can also be used to determine the valve diameter and, thus, the required homograft size. This is a necessary step in surgical planning, because a suitable homograft must be ordered in advance from the valve bank at the surgeon's own or another hospital.

From the left parasternal long-axis view, we measure aortic valve diameter at the narrowest site in the aortic annulus, from the inner boundary of the anterior aortic root to the leading edge of the posterior aortic root (leading edge methodology). However, this may be problematic when the aortic valve is heavily calcified. Our experience has shown that valve measurements using leading edge methodology are accurate to within ±0.5 mm, as compared with intraoperative measurements.

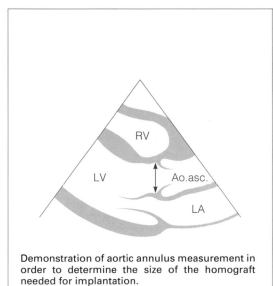

Demonstration of aortic annulus measurement in order to determine the size of the homograft needed for implantation.

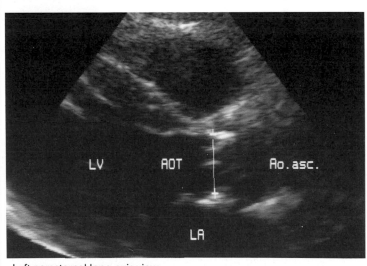

Left parasternal long-axis view.

During the echocardiographic examination, the presence of extensive transmural annular calcification, a contra-indication for homograft implantation, should be excluded. Coronary anomalies can also make it difficult to impossible to implant a homograft.

Homograft implantation is a very difficult procedure. Therefore, the risk of intraoperative valvular insufficiency due to homograft distortion is higher than in prosthetic ring annuloplasties.

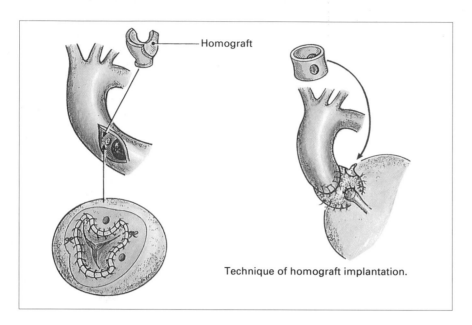

Technique of homograft implantation.

To improve this risk, we systematically perform intraoperative transesophageal echocardiography at our hospital. This permits immediate identification and correction of valvular incompetence during the actual operation.

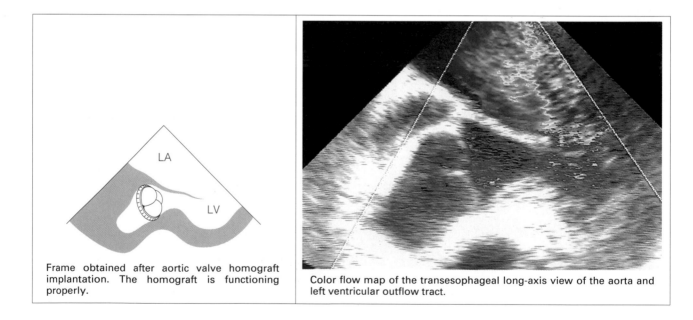

Frame obtained after aortic valve homograft implantation. The homograft is functioning properly.

Color flow map of the transesophageal long-axis view of the aorta and left ventricular outflow tract.

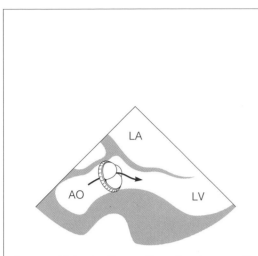

Frame obtained after aortic valve homograft implantation. There is a slight amount of prosthetic valve regurgitation.

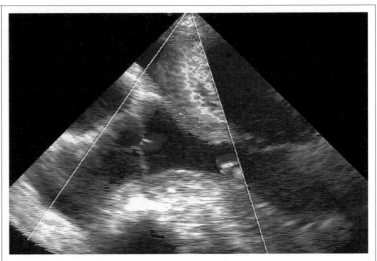

Color flow map of the transesophageal long-axis view of the aorta and left ventricular outflow tract.

The aortic valve can be visualized especially well using the new biplane and multiplane TEE transducers. The proximity of the transducer to the imaged structures provides higher resolution of valve morphology. This permits precise assessment of leaflet thickness and valve opening and closure motion.

5.4   **Principles of Intra- and Perioperative Echocardiography**
5.4.4   **Aortic Valve Replacement in Active Endocarditis**

Infective endocarditis, with an overall mortality rate of 20 to 30 %, still is a serious complication. After a temporary decline, the frequency of infective endocarditis has risen within the past few years, due mainly to the longer life expectancy, the wider use of invasive diagnostic and therapeutic methods, and drug use [32].

When a tentative diagnosis of infective endocarditis is made on the basis of clinical symptoms, the diagnosis must be confirmed by repeated blood cultures. Then, a specific antibiotic regimen must be begun immediately.

If complications occur despite treatment, valve replacement is indicated [33].

Surgical intervention is necessary, because progressive myocardial insufficiency can occur as a result of valvular insufficiency or obstruction. The removal of foci such as abscesses and infected tissue and the prevention of embolism are mandatory measures, particularly in annular abscess formation.

The extent of the valvular defect is a decisive factor in deciding whether surgery is indicated and in planning the timing of surgery. Echocardiography is very helpful in this regard. Echocardiography can diagnose such morphological changes as valve destruction, and can detect vegetations as small as 2-3 mm in size, which are echocardiographically visualized as irregularly delimited, moving and sometimes floating echo-dense structures. Doppler echocardiography furthermore provides visualization and semiquantitation of the endocarditic regurgitations.

5.4   **Principles of Intra- and Perioperative Echocardiography**
5.4.4   **Aortic Valve Replacement in Active Endocarditis**

278

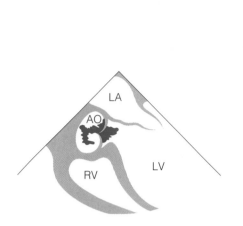

Extensive endocarditic vegetation on the destroyed aortic valve.

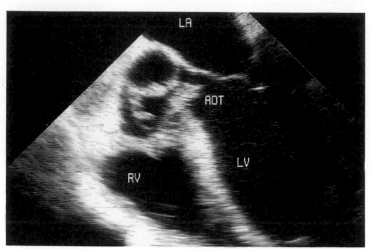

Transesophageal long-axis scan of the left atrium, the aorta, and the ventricle.

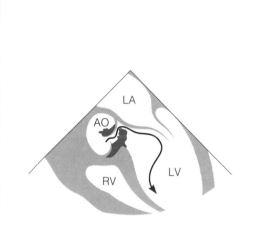

Severe aortic regurgitation.

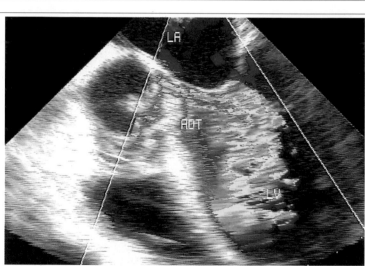

Color flow map of the transesophageal long-axis scan of the left atrium, the aorta, and the ventricle.

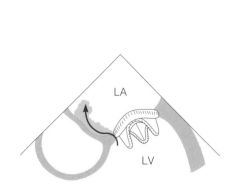

Mitral prosthetic valve endocarditis, with para-valvular leak.

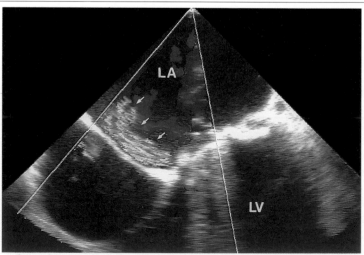

Color flow map of the transesophageal long-axis scan of the heart cavities at mitral valve level.

Large vegetations, particularly those located on the aortic valve, are associated with a high risk of embolism. These vegetations are therefore an absolute indication for prosthetic valve replacement.

Abscess formations and mycotic aneurysms, which usually remain relatively uninfluenced by antibiotic or antimycotic treatment, also require immediate surgical treatment.

Prosthetic valve endocarditis with prosthetic valve dysfunction is also an indication for immediate valve replacement.

The prosthesis should preferably be composed of biological tissue, which has a lower reinfection rate than nonbiological tissue. Homograft valve replacement is the ideal choice in patients with infective endocarditis. One advantage of homografts is their flexibility. The homograft can be custom cut, and can be used to cover ring abscesses. Cryopreserved valves made of vital valvular tissue are significantly more durable and resistant to reinfection, especially when they have been impregnated with antibiotics [23, 68].

5.4   **Principles of Intra- and Perioperative Echocardiography**
5.4.5   **Surgical Management of Aortic Dissection**

Aortic dissection or dissecting aneurysm of the aorta is characterized by longitudinal splitting of the aortic wall, which produces a tear in the intima and establishes communication with the lumen. In nondissecting aneurysms, on the other hand, only localized dilation of the aorta occurs.

Aortic dissections are most commonly described using the DeBakey classification scheme (types I, II, II), or the simpler Stanford classification scheme (types A and B) [13, 15]. The DeBakey scheme classifies aortic dissections according to the location of the primary tear and the longitudinal extent of the dissection. The Stanford scheme entails classification solely according to the extent of the double aortic lumen.

Classification of Aortic Dissection		
DeBakey		Stanford
Type I	The dissection arises in the ascending aorta and extends distally through the aortic arch as far as the ascending aorta.	Type A
Type II	The dissection arises in the ascending aorta and remains limited to the ascending aorta.	Type A
Type III	The dissection arises distal to the origin of the left subclavian artery, and remains limited to the descending aorta.	Type B

An aortic dissection is classified according to onset as acute (less than two weeks) or chronic (longer than two weeks). Since the mortality rate for untreated acute aortic dissection is 50% within the first 48 hours, a quick diagnosis and immediate surgery are decisive factors in the prognosis [16].

The two recommended methods for surgical management of dissecting aneurysm of the ascending aorta with clinically significant aortic regurgitation are the techniques of Wheat and Bentall, respectively.

Using *Wheat's technique* [66], the aneurysm is resected immediately above aortic valve level, leaving two tongue-shaped aortic wall segments containing the coronary ostia. The ascending aorta is replaced using a vascular graft, and an aortic valve prosthesis is sutured in separately. Coronary anastomosis is not necessary.

Bentall's technique [3], on the other hand, is a method for complete replacement of the ascending aorta (including the coronary ostia) in cases of aneurysm of the ascending aorta with aortic valve ectasia. The ring of a Starr valve is sutured to an aortic prosthesis (conduit), and the prostheses are inserted *en bloc*. The ostia of the coronary arteries are then anastomosed to the side of the aortic prosthesis.

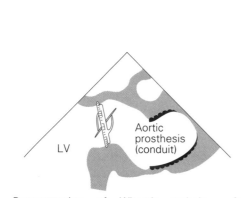

Demonstration of Wheat's technique for resection of ascending aortic aneurysm and implantation of an vessel prosthesis and a valve bioprosthesis. Arrows identify the leading edges of the vessel prosthesis.

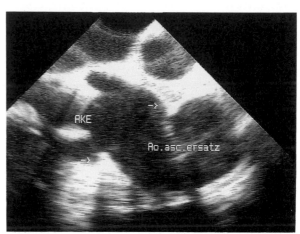

Transesophageal echocardiogram from the sagittal plane of the ascending aorta (biplane technique).

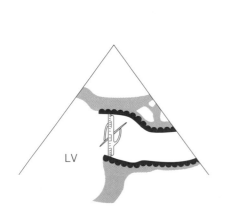

Demonstration of Bentall's technique for resection of ascending aortic aneurysm, implantation of an aortic prosthesis (conduit), and anastomosis of coronary ostia to the prosthesis.

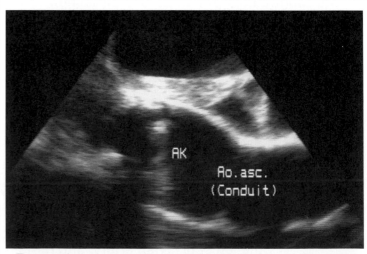

Transesophageal echocardiogram from the sagittal plane of the ascending aorta (biplane technique).

Particularly in acute dissection, aortic valve replacement frequently is not necessary, *i.e.*, reconstruction suffices. In this case, the affected segment of the aorta is excised and is replaced by a vessel prosthesis.

All the above techniques must be performed using an extracorporal circulation system under artificially induced cardioplegia. If the aortic arch must also be replaced, the patient's circulation must be briefly interrupted under conditions of deep hypothermia (15-19°C). The patient's head is additionally embedded in ice packs in order to prevent hypoxic brain damage.

In addition to such time-consuming and high-priced techniques as computed tomography (CT), magnetic resonance imaging (MRI), venous digital subtraction angiography, and conventional angiography, echocardiography has increasingly been utilized for diagnosis of diseases of the thoracic aorta.

In light of the rapid advances in imaging technology, it is important to determine which of these methods has the highest diagnostic value, while being the least time-consuming and least stressful to the patient. In our experience, and according to studies performed by other authors, combined transthoracic and transesophageal echocardiography has been shown to be highly sensitive and specific for aortic dissection as compared with computer tomography and angiography [20].

Value of various techniques for diagnosis of aortic dissection

Method	Sensi- tivity	Site of tear	Extent	Aortic valve	Coronary arteries	Availa- bility
Echo	95%	++	+++	+++	+	+++
Angio	95%	++	+++	+++	+++	++
CT	90%	++	+++	-	+	++
MRI	90%	++	++	-	-	+

-	diagnosis not possible	++	sufficient diagnostic value
+	slight diagnostic value	+++	high diagnostic value

Last but not least, the course of disease and the patient' hemodynamic situation also play a major role in the selection of the diagnostic technique. The more critical the situation, the more important it is for the technique to be quickly and readily available.

Such diagnostic techniques as CT and MRI can be used to assess chronic and questionable dissections.

With MRI it is possible to demonstrate the plane of dissection as well as the origin of dissection with more than 90% reliability [61]. However, MRI cannot be used in patients with a pacemaker or assisted ventilation.

CT also does not achieve the same diagnostic reliability as echocardiography and angiography. Involvement of aortic branches in not always reliably detected. In this case, and in every elderly patient, cardiac catheterization should be performed at the end of the CT examination in order to exclude coronary artery disease [29].

A quick and reliable diagnosis is imperative in acute aortic dissection. In this case, echocardiography is the method of choice, because it can be utilized in acute emergency situations, in hemodynamically unstable patients, and even at the patient's bedside. In artificially ventilated patients who cannot undergo comprehensive diagnostic studies, cardiac ultrasound diagnosis can be performed relatively quickly at the bedside. Moreover, echocardiography is capable of detecting concomitant aortic insufficiency. This is an important decision-making factor when considering aortic valve replacement in addition to replacement of the affected aortic segment.

Echocardiography permits assessment of the primary intimal tear and of the linear extent of the dissection [15]. Due to the intrapericardial position of the proximal ascending aorta, an acute rupture can lead to hemorrhage into the pericardium, which can lead to life-threatening symptoms of pericardial tamponade. This situation can also be diagnosed echocardiographically.

All four heart cavities, the proximal segment of the ascending aorta, the aortic arch, and the supra-aortic vessel origins can be visualized well in transthoracic scans. However, scans should be made from as many views as possible in order to avoid false-positive or false-negative diagnoses of aortic dissection [36, 60, 65], and in order to properly visualize the dissected membrane.

Due to the proximity of the esophagus to the aorta, and in patients with poor transthoracic window conditions, transesophageal echocardiography is the method of choice for assessing dissecting aneurysms of the aorta [5]. The dissected membrane can thereby be visualized throughout the entire ascending and descending aortic segments.

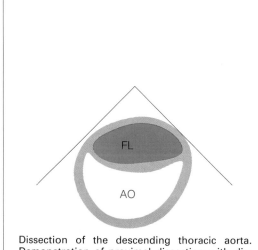

Dissection of the descending thoracic aorta. Demonstration of proximal dissection with dissected membrane.

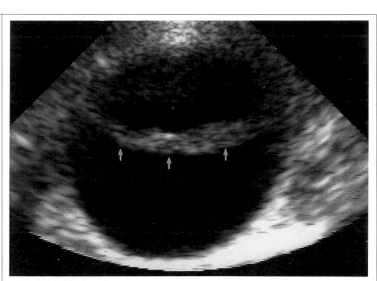

Transesophageal short-axis (transverse) view.

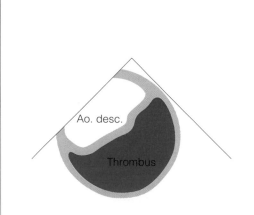

Dissection of the descending aorta. Demonstration of distal dissection above the diaphragm with thrombotic false lumen.

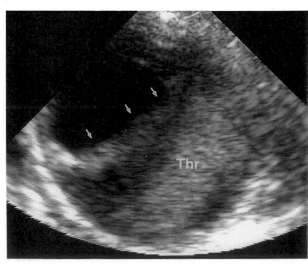

Transesophageal short-axis (transverse) view.

Particularly in the diagnosis of dissection of the descending aorta, transesophageal echocardiography is superior to its transthoracic counterpart [18]. The origins of the coronary arteries can also be visualized by transesophageal echocardiography.

For the heart surgeon, it is important to know whether the dissection involves the aortic arch. This information is important, not only for the DeBakey classification, but also for further clinical decision-making, since a primary intimal tear must be surgically excised. Due to the interposition of the trachea, the aortic arch cannot be completely visualized from the esophagus. Therefore, suprasternal views have proven to be the most effective in this case.

In order to adequately assess the anatomy of the entire aorta, combined transthoracic and transesophageal echocardiographic studies should always be performed [5, 18, 19, 48, 49]. Aneurysms and dissections in the entire aortic arch can then be visualized.

The following images demonstrate an old dissection at the aortic arch to descending aorta junction.

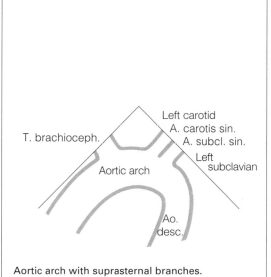

Aortic arch with suprasternal branches.

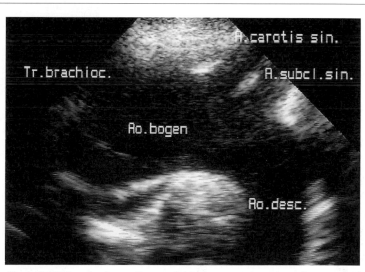

Two-dimensional echocardiogram from the suprasternal notch.

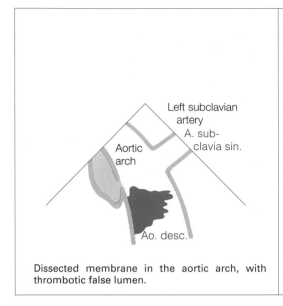

Dissected membrane in the aortic arch, with thrombotic false lumen.

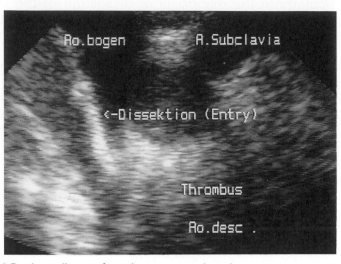

2-D echocardiogram from the suprasternal notch.

Biplane TEE transducers provide visualization of a sagittal plane in addition to the transverse plane. This permits assessment of nearly the entire ascending aorta, including the aortic valve.

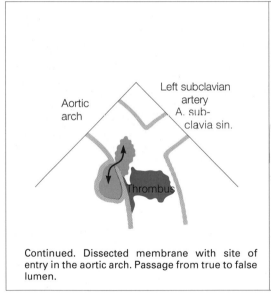

Continued. Dissected membrane with site of entry in the aortic arch. Passage from true to false lumen.

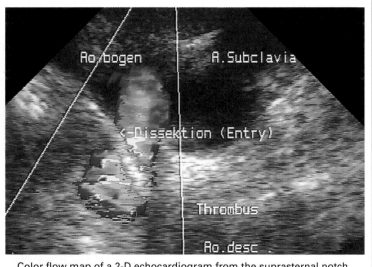

Color flow map of a 2-D echocardiogram from the suprasternal notch.

Doppler color flow imaging makes it possible to differentiate between the true lumen and the false lumen, and facilitates localization of the site of entry of the dissection [48]. Color Doppler is also helpful in detecting associated aortic insufficiency. Differentiation between true and false lumina is made on the basis of color differences on the color flow map and proof of systolic dilation of the true lumen.

Systolic or pendular flow in the region of the intimal tear indicates the location of the dissection site.

Thrombus in the false lumen is visualized as a weak echo-producing structure. Spontaneous echo contrast in a nonthrombotic lumen are attributable to „sludge" caused by reduced blood flow.

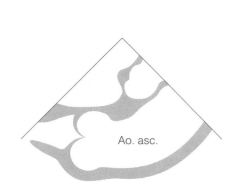

Ascending aorta, aortic valve, and sinuses of Valsalva. Valve closed in diastole.

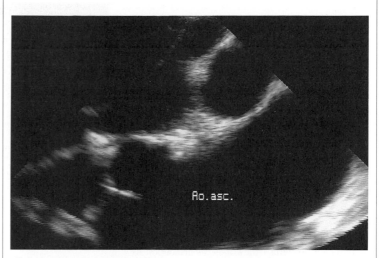

Transesophageal echocardiogram from the sagittal plane.

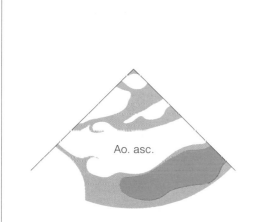

Tear immediately distal to the valve, and dissected membrane.

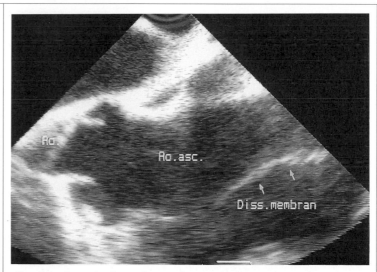

Transesophageal echocardiogram from the sagittal plane.

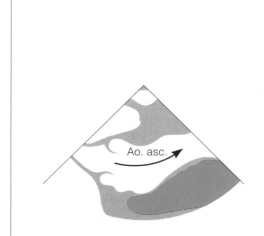

Identification of true lumen.

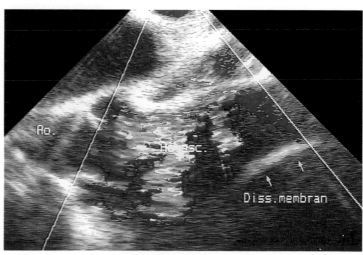

Color flow map from the sagittal plane.

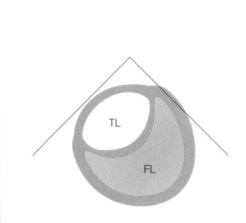

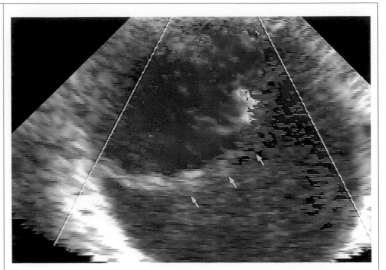

Identification of the true lumen in dissection of the descending aorta.

Transesophageal transverse scan (biplane technique). Color coded.

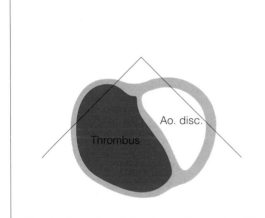

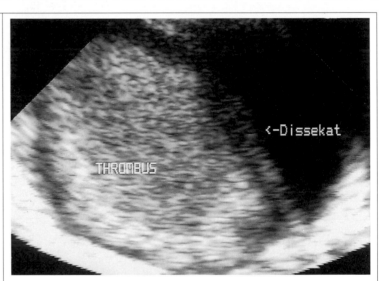

Chronic dissection of the descending aorta with thrombus in the false lumen.

Transesophageal short-axis view.

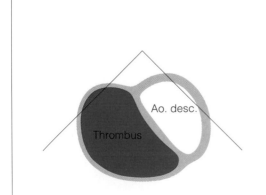

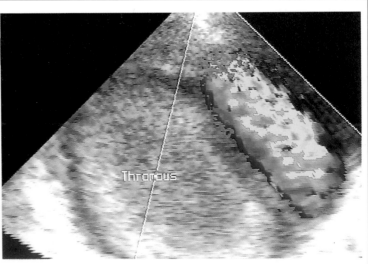

Continued. Corresponding scan with color flow mapping.

Color flow map of the transesophageal short-axis (transverse) scan.

Transesophageal and epicardial echocardiography are important methods for intraoperative evaluation of repair of aortic dissection [45].

Both methods can accurately detect residual aortic dissection and permit immediate evaluation of repair before closing the chest. As compared with epicardial echocardiography, an additional advantage of TEE is that it does not require interruption and delay of surgery.

In most acute type I and type III dissections, a new dissection or new aneurysm with imminent risk of perforation can develop distal to the segment that has been surgically resected. These patients must therefore be followed at semi-annual intervals. Because of their quick, readily available, and noninvasive nature, combined TTE and TEE studies can also be performed. The proximity of the transducer to the aorta makes it possible to clearly visualize details such as the entry or re-entry point of dissection.

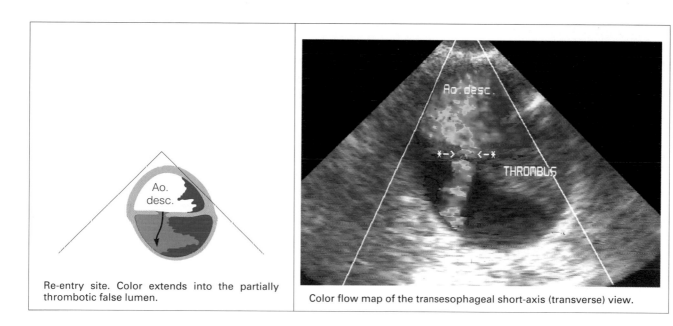

Re-entry site. Color extends into the partially thrombotic false lumen.

Color flow map of the transesophageal short-axis (transverse) view.

Other diagnostic techniques (*e.g.* digital subtraction angiography or CT) are indicated only when extrapericardial aortic rupture or acute obstruction of the vital, larger branches of the aorta (*e.g.* carotid artery, celiac trunk, superior mesenteric artery) are suspected.

Reoperation is indicated when the aortic diameter increases to at least 6 cm with clinically significant symptoms (*e.g.* chest or abdominal pain).

Due to the scarcity of donor hearts, around 20% of all candidates for cardiac transplantation die before a suitable donor heart can be procured. Hospital regulations sometimes make it impossible to assign highest priority to high-risk candidates with severe cardiac decompensation. Circulatory support with univentricular and biventricular assist devices or total artificial hearts has been proven effective in such patients who would otherwise die while waiting for a donor heart [21, 47, 50, 56]. In addition to providing bridging to transplantation, these devices can also be used in patients with postoperative low-output syndrome and cardiogenic shock of other origin that does not respond to therapy. Their use is also indicated in patients with acute myocardial infarction or acute myocarditis who continue to deteriorate, despite maximum pharmacologic therapy.

Transesophageal echocardiography is particularly suited for assessing left and right ventricular function when monitoring patients with mechanical ventricular assist devices and artificial hearts. Transesophageal Echocardiography is useful in:
- selecting the proper circulatory support system. The decision of whether to use a uni- or biventricular assist device is based on whether the patient has left, right, or global cardiac decompensation.
- treatment assessment and optimization of pump function.
- monitoring ventricular function after removing the ventricular assist device. For wall motion analysis, to determine which time to disconnect the device, determination of left ventricular end-diastolic and end-systolic diameters and fractional shortening as an expression of heart muscle recovery.

At the Cardiosurgery Department of the University of Munich Hospital, we have used the Novacor® system for bridging to transplantation since February 1992. The Novacor system supports the pump function of the left ventricle in patients with terminal circulatory failure. The system consists of an electromagnetically driven pump that is transplanted in the left upper abdominal wall. It is connected to a portable, extracorporal control unit by means of a subcutaneous tunnel-like connection cable. The inflow tract to the pump is anastomosed to the apex of the left ventricle, and the outflow tract is anastomosed to the ascending aorta (end-to-side).

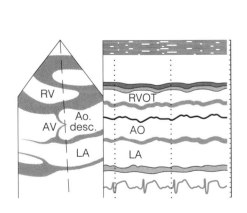

Novacor® left ventricular assess system. The aortic valve remains permanently closed.

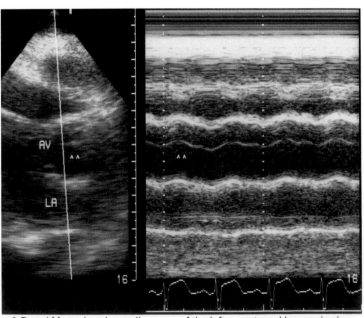

2-D and M-mode echocardiograms of the left parasternal long-axis view.

5.4   **Prinziples of Intra- and Perioperative Echocardiography**
5.4.6   **Transesophageal Echocardiography Assessment of Ventricular Assist Device and Artificial Heart Function**

289

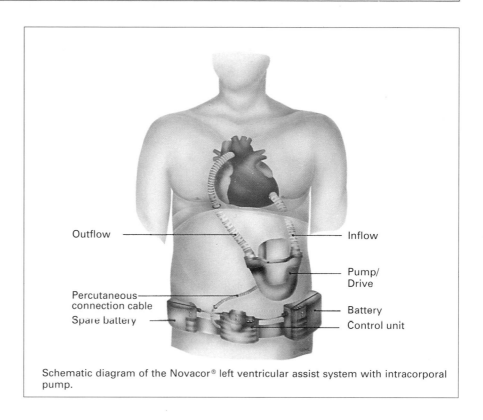

Outflow

Inflow

Pump/ Drive

Percutaneous connection cable

Battery

Spare battery

Control unit

Schematic diagram of the Novacor® left ventricular assist system with intracorporal pump.

This makes it possible to bypass the left ventricle, while reducing left ventricular pressure. The native aortic valve remains permanently closed.

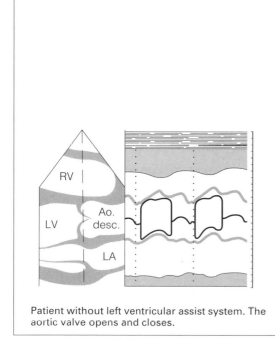

RV

LV

Ao. desc.

LA

Patient without left ventricular assist system. The aortic valve opens and closes.

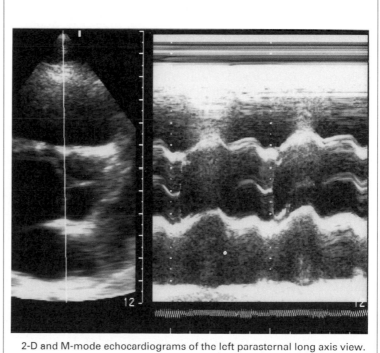

2-D and M-mode echocardiograms of the left parasternal long axis view.

A study at our hospital demonstrated that the Novacor® system also significantly improves right ventricular function by reducing the afterload [64]. Echocardiography is helpful in the assessment of ventricular function and ventricular filling conditions. Pericardial effusion must be excluded when pump function is reduced. The Novacor system produces demonstrable heart muscle recovery. After overall cardiac compensation has been restored, the assist device can be removed and the patient can be placed back on the transplantation list.

References

1. Angermann CE, Spes C, Hart RJ, Kemkes BM, Gokel M, Theisen K. Echokardiografische Diagnose akuter Abstoflungsreaktionen bei herztransplantierten Patienten unter Cyclosporintherapie. Z Kardiol 1989; 78: 243-252.
2. Barnard CN. The operation. A human cardiac transplantation: An interim report of the successful operation performed at the Groote Schuur Hospital, Cape Town. South African Med J 1967; 41: 1271-1274.
3. Bentall H, de Bono A. A technique for complete replacement of the ascending aorta. Thorax 1968; 23 (4): 338-339.
4. Billingham ME, Cary NR, Hammond ME, Kemnitz J, Marboe C, McCallister HA, Snovar DC, Winters GL, Zerbe A. A working formulation for the standardization of nomenclature in the diagnosis of heart and lung rejection: Heart Rejection Study Group. The International Society for Heart Transplantation. J Heart Transplant 1990; 9 (6): 587-593.
5. Börner N, Erbel R, Braun B, Henkel B, Meyer J, Rumpelt J. Diagnosis of aortic dissection by transesophageal echocardiography. Am J Cardiol 1984; 54: 1157-1158.
6. Carpentier A, Chauvaud S, Fabiani JN, Deloche A, Relland J, Lessana A, D'Allaines C, Blondeau P, Piwnica A, Dubost C. Reconstructive surgery of mitral valve incompetence - ten-year appraisal. J Thorac Cardiovasc Surg 1980; 79 (3): 338-348.
7. Carpentier A. Cardiac valve surgery - the „French correction". J Thorac Cardiovasc Surg 1983; 86 (3): 323-337.
8. Carpentier A. Mitral valve reconstructive surgery. In: Operative Surgery. Butterworth, London 1977.
9. Caves PK, Stinson EB, Billingham ME, Shumway NE. Serial transvenous biopsy of the transplanted human heart - improved management of the acute rejection episodes. Lancet 1974; 1 (862): 821-826.
10. Caves PK, Stinson EB, Billingham ME, Rider AK, Shumway NE. Diagnosis of human cardiac allograft rejection by serial cardiac biopsy. J Thorac Cardiovasc Surg 1973; 66: 461-466.
11. Clements FM, de Bruijn NP. Perioperative Evaluation of Regional Wall Motion by Transesophageal Two-Dimensional Echocardiography. Anaesth Analg 1987; 66: 249-261.
12. Cosgrove DH. Current Heart Valve Prostheses. In: Crawford FA (ed). Current Heart Valve Diseases. Henley & Belfus, Philadelphia 1987.
13. Dailey PD, Trueblood HW, Stinson EN, Eurtglin TF, Shumway NE. Management of acute aortic dissections. Ann Thorac Surg 1970; 10: 237-241.
14. Dawkins KD, Jamieson SW, Oldershaw PJ et al. Changes in diastolic function as a noninvasive marker of cardiac allograft rejection. Heart Transplant 1984; 3: 286-294.
15. DeBakey ME, Henley WS, Cooley DA, Morris GC, Crawford S, Beall AC. Surgical management of dissecting aneurysms of the aorta. J Thorac Cardiovasc Surg 1965; 49: 130-149.
16. Doroghazi RM, Slater EE. Aortic dissection. McGraw-Hill, New York 1983.
17. Duran CG, Ubago JL. Clinical and hemodynamic performance of a totally flexible prosthetic ring for atrioventricular valve reconstruction. Ann Thorac Surg 1976; 22 (5): 458-463.
18. Engberding R, Bender F, Grofle-Heitmeyer W, Most E, M.ller US, Bramann HU, Schneider S. Identification of dissection and aneurysms of the descending thoracic aorta by conventional and transesophageal two dimensional echocardiography. Am J Cardiol 1987; 59 (1): 717-719.
19. Engberding R, Bender F, Grofle-Heitmeyer W, M.ller US, Schneider D. Diagnose thorakaler Aortenaneurysmen durch kombinierte transthorakale und trans^sophageale 2-D-Echokardiografie. Z Kardiol 1986; 75: 225-230.
20. Erbel R, Mohr-Kahaly S, Brunier J, Rennollet H, Wittlich N, Drexler N, Iversen S, Oelert H, Thelen M, Meyer J. Value of trans-thoracic and transesophageal echocardiography in the preoperative dianosis of aortic dissection. Thorac Cardiovasc Surg 1987; 35: 69-70.
21. Farrar DJ, Hill JD, Gray LA, Pennington DG, McBride LR, Pierce WS, Pae WE, Glenville B, Ross D, Galbraith TA, Zumbro GL. Heterotopic prosthetic ventricles as a bridge to cardiac transplantation. A multi-center study in 29 patients. Ne Engl J Med 1988; 318: 333-340.

22. Furniss SS, Murray A, Hunter S, Dougenis V, McGregor CGA. Value of Echocardiographic Determination of Isovolumic Relaxation Time in the Detection of Heart Transplant Rejection J Heart Lung Transplant 1991; 10: 557-561e.

23. Glazier JJ, Verwilghen J, Donaldson RM, Ross DN. Treatment of Complicated Prosthetic Aortic Valve Endocarditis with Annular Abscess Formation by Homograft Aortic Root Replacement. J Am Coll Cardiol 1991; 17: 1177-1182.

24. Goldman ME, Guarino T, Mindich BP. Localization of Aortic Dissection Intimal Flap by Intraoperative Two-Dimensional Echocardiography. J Am Coll Cardiol 1985; 6: 1155-1159.

25. Goldman ME, Mindich BP. Intraoperative Two-Dimensional Echocardiography: New Application of an Old Technique. J Am Coll Cardiol 1986; 7: 374-382.

26. Haberl R, Weber M, Reichenspurner H, Kemkes BM, Osterholzer G, Anthuber M, Steinbeck G. Frequency analysis of the surface electrocardiogram for recognition of acute rejection after orthotopic cardiac transplantation in man. Circulation 1987; 76: 101-108.

27. Hammer C, Reichenspurner H, Ertel W, Lersch C, Plahl M, Prendel W, Reichart B, ‹berfuhr P, Welz A, Kemkes BM, Reble B, Funccius W, Gokel M. Cytological and immunological monitoring of cyclosporin - treated human heart recipients. J Heart Transplant 1984; 3: 228-231.

28. Haverich A, Scott WC, Dawkins KD, Billingham ME, Jamieson SW. Asymmetric pattern of rejection following orthotopic cardiac transplantation in primates. J Heart Transplant 1984; 3: 280-285.

29. Herter M, Harder TH, Leipner N, Krahe TH, Orellano L. Computertomografie und Angiografie bei der Aortendissektion. Fortschr Rˆntgenstr 1987; 147: 124-131.

30. Hetzer R, Warnecke H, Sch‚ler S, S‚thoff U, Borst HG. Heart transplantation - a two year experience. Z Kardiol 1985; 74 (6): 51-58.

31. Horowitz RS, Morganroth J, Parrotto C, Chen CC, Soffer J, Pauletto FJ. Immediate diagnosis of acute myocardial infarction by two-dimensional echocardiography. Circulation 1982; 65 (2): 323-329.

32. Horstkotte D, Bircks W, Loogen F. Infective endocarditis of native and prosthetic valves - the case for prompt surgical intervention? A retrospective analysis of factors affecting survival. Z Kardiol 1986; 75 (suppl II): 168-182.

33. Horstkotte D, Kˆrfer R, Loogen F, Rosin H, Bircks W. Prosthetic valve endocarditis: clinical findings and management. Europ Heart J 1984; 5 (suppl C): 117-122.

34. Hunt SA. Complications of heart transplantation: J Heart Transplant 1983; 3: 70-74.

35. Huntsman LL, Stewart DK, Barnes SR, Franklin SB, Colocousis JS, Hessel EA. Noninvasive Doppler determination of cardiac output in man clinical validation. Circulation 1983; 67 (3): 593-602.

36. Iliceto S, Antonelli G, Biasco G, Rizzon P. Two-dimensional echocardiographic evaluation of aneurysms of the descending thoracic aorta. Circulation 1982; 66: 1045-1049.

37. Jaffe WM, Coverdale HA, Roche AHG, Whitlock RML, Neutze JM, Barratt-Boyes BG. Rest and exercise hemodynamics of 20 to 23 mm allograft, Medtronic Intact (porcine), and St. Jude Medical valves in the aortic position. J Thorc Cardiovasc Surg 1990; 100: 167-174.

38. Jamieson SW, Oyer PE, Reitz BA, Baumgartner WA, Bieber CP, Stinson EB, Shumway NE. Cardiac transplatation at Stanford. Heart Transpl 1981; 1: 86.

39. Kavey REW, Krongrad E, Gersony WM. Perioperative echocardiographic evaluation of cardiovascular function: Assessment of changing hemodynamic state. Circulation 1980; 62: 773-782.

40. Kaye MP, Kriett JM. Heart Registry Report 1991. 11th Annual Meeting of the International Society for Heart Transplantation. Paris, April 7-9, 1991.

41. Kaye MP. The Registry of the International Society for Heart and Lung Transplantation: Tenth Official Report - 1993. Meeting of the International Society for Heart and Lung Transplantation, Boca Raton, USA, March 31 - April 3, 1993.

42. Kemkes BM, Reichenspurner H, Osterholzer G, Erdmann E, Lersch C, Schad N, Gokel JM, Klinner W. Herztransplantation. Internist 1986; 27: 322-330.

43. Konstadt SN, Thys D, Mindich BP, Kaplan JA, Goldman ME. Validation of Quantitative Intraoperative Transesophageal Echocardiography. Anesthesiology 1986; 65: 418-421.

44. Kreuzer E, Schad N, Peters D, Reichart B. Plastic and reconstructive surgery on the mitral-valve-long-term - follow-up with the 1st-pass-technique. Herz Kreislauf 1984; 16: 461-469.

45. Kyo S, Takamoto S, Adachi H, Matsumura M, Kimura S, Yokote Y, Omoto R. Intraoperative evaluation of repair of aortic dissection: surgical decision making. Int J Card Imaging 1989; 4: 49-50.

46. Lessana A, Tran Viet T, Ades F, Kara SM, Ameur A, Ruffenach A, Guerin F, Herreman F, Degeorges M. Mitral reconstructive operations. A series of 130 consecutive cases. J Thorac Cardiovasc Surg 1983; 86 (4): 553-561.

47. Miller CA, Pae WE, Pierce WS. Combined registry for the clinical use of mechanical ventricular assist pumps and the total artificial heart in conjunction with heart transplantation: Fourth official report 1989. J Heart Transplant 1990; 9: 453-458.

48. Mohr-Kahaly S, Erbel R, Bˆrner N, Drexler M, Wittlich N, Iversen S, Oelert H, Meyer J. Kombination von Farb-Doppler- und transˆsophagealer Echokardiografie in der Notfalldiagnostik bei Aortendissektionen vom Typ I. Z Kardiol 1986; 75: 616-620.

49. Mohr-Kahaly S, Erbel R, Steller D, Bˆrner N, Drexler M, Meyer J. Aortic dissection detected by transesophageal echocardiography. Int J Card Imaging 1986; 2: 31-35.

50. Portner PM, Oyer PE, Pennington DG, Baumgartner WA, Griffith BP, Frist WR, Magilligan DJ, Noon GP, Ramasamy N, Miller PJ, Jassawalla JS. Implantable electrical left ventricular assist system: bridge to transplantation and the future. Ann Thorac Surg 1989; 47: 142-150.

51. Reichart B, ‹berfuhr P, Welz A, Kemkes BM, Klinner W, Reble B, Funccius W, Hammer C, Ertel W, Reichenspurner H, Peters D, Gokel JM, Franke N, Land W. Heart transplantation at the University of Munich - the first one and a half years. J Heart Transplant 1983; 2: 266-269.

52. Reichenspurner H, Kemkes BM, Haberl R, Angermann CH, Lersch CH, Osterholzer G, Anthuber M, Weber M, Gokel JM. Patienten‚berwachung nach Herztransplantation an der Universit‰tsklinik M‚nchen, Groflhadern. Z Herz-, Thorax-, Gef‰flchir 1987; 1: 79.

53. Rubenson DS, Tucker CR, London E, Miller DC, Stinson EB, Popp RL. Two-dimensional echocardiographic analysis of segmental left ventricular wall motion before and after coronary artery bypass surgery. Circulation 1982; 66: 1025-1033.

54. R‚ckel A, Kasper W, Meinertz T, Bechtold H, Pop T, G‚nther R. Diagnostik thorakaler Aortenaneurysmen mittels zweidimensionaler Echografie. Dtsch med Wschr 1983; 108: 976-981.

55. Schartl M, Rutsch W, Paeprer H, M‚ller U. Stellenwert der zweidimensionalen Echokardiografie in der Diagnostik akuter transmuraler Erstinfarkte. Z Kardiol 1984; 73 (1): 56-65.

56. Schiessler A, Warnecke H, Friedel N, Hennig E, Hetzer R. Clinical use of the Berlin biventricular assist device as a bridge to transplantation. Trans Am Soc Artif Intern Organs 1990; 36: M706-708.

57. Schmidli J, Rothlin ME, Turina M, Senning A. Langzeitresultate nach Mitralklappenoperation wegen Mitralinsuffizienz 1972-1982. Schweiz med Wschr 1985; 115 (13): 430-439.

58. Sch‚tz A, Kemkes BM, Kugler C, Angermann C, Schad N, Rienm‚ller R, Fritsch S, Anthuber M, Neumaier P, Gokel M. The influence of rejection episodes on the development of coronary artery diseases after heart transplantation. Eur J Cardio-thorac Surg 1990; 4: 300-308.

59. Sch‚tz A. Die Kinetik und Dynamik der akuten Abstoflungsreaktion nach Herztransplantation im t‰glichen invasiven und nichtinvasiven Monitoring. Wolfgang Papst Verlag, Lengerich 1992.

60. Smuckler AL, Nomeir AM, Watts LE, Hackshaw BT. Aortic root dissection. Another false positive echocardiographic diagnosis. Chest 1982; 82 (4): 497-498.

61. Spielmann RP, Langkowski J, Roden K, Schuchert A, Maas R, Witte G, Heller M. Kernspintomografie der thorakalen Aortendissektion. Fortschr Rˆntgenstr 1988; 148: 121-126.

62. Trompler AT, Sold G, Vogt A, Kreuzer H. Nichtinvasive Bestimmung des Herzzeitvolumens mit spektraler Doppler-Echokardiografie. Z Kardiol 1985; 74: 322-326.

63. Van Herwerden LA, Gussenhoven WJ, Roelandt J, Bos E, Ligtvoet CM, Haalebos MM, Mochtar B, Leicher F, Witsenburg M. Intraoperative epicardial two-dimensional echocardiography. Eur Heart J 1986; 7: 386-395.

64. Vetter HO, Kaulbach HG, Reichenspurner H, Rˆll W, Schindler G, Pfeiffer M, Reichart B. ‹berbr‚ckung bis zur Herztransplantation mit dem Linksherzunterst‚tzungssystem Novacor. Herz Kreislauf 1993; 25 (6): 184-187.

65. Victor MF, Mintz GS, Kotler MN, Wilson AR, Segal BL. Two dimensional echocardiographic diagnosis of aortic dissection. Am J Cardiol 1981; 48: 1155-1159.

66. Wheat MW, Wilson JR, Bartley JD. Successful replacement of the entire ascending aorta and aortic valve. JAMA 1964; 188: 234.

67. Yacoub MH, Reid CJ, Al-Khadimi RH, Radley-Smith R. Cardiac transplantation - the London experience. Z Kardiol 1985; 74 (6): 45-50.

68. Zwischenberger JB, Shalaby TZ, Conti VR. Viable Cryopreserved Aortic Homograft for Aortic Valve Endocarditis and Annular Abscesses. Ann Thorac Surg 1989; 48: 365-370.

The role of imaging techniques in the routine diagnosis and management of critically ill patients is growing steadily, due to the great technological advances made in the past few years. Echocardiography, which is a harmless, noninvasive, readily available, and highly sensitive technique, has become a virtually indispensable tool for cardiac diagnosis.

In 10 to 20 % of all patients with heart disease, echocardiography cannot be performed from the transthoracic route, due to obesity, chest deformity, pulmonary emphysema, or intensive care measures such as artificial respiration. Transesophageal echocardiography (TEE) therefore plays a major role in cardiac intensive care and emergency medicine [6, 22, 23].

Indications for echocardiography in intensive care patients

1. Monitoring ventricular function
   ▸ Acute myocardial infarction with complications
   ▸ Congestive heart failure in myocardial heart disease
   ▸ Mechanical circulatory support

2. Diagnosis of cardiac abnormalities
   ▸ Fever of unknown origin
   ▸ Congestive heart failure in native valve disease
   ▸ Silent aortic stenosis
   ▸ Severe acute aortic insufficiency
   ▸ Differential diagnosis mitral stenosis vs. cor triatriatum sinistrum
   ▸ Severe acute mitral insufficiency
   ▸ Cardiac insufficiency due to shunts

3. Thrombo-embolism
   ▸ Atrial tumors and thrombi
   ▸ Ventricular thrombi

4. Aortic aneurysms
   ▸ Dissecting aneurysms
   ▸ Posttraumatic aneurysms
   ▸ Atherosclerotic aneurysms

5. „Upper inflow obstruction"
   ▸ Pericardial effusion
   ▸ Pericardial tamponade
   ▸ Hematoma compromising the right atrium

6. Massive pulmonary embolism
7. Acute rejection after heart transplantation

In patients with unexplained symptoms of shock, the physician must quickly determine whether circulatory failure is of cardiac origin. Cardiogenic shock is caused primarily by acute myocardial infarction. Cardiogenic shock frequently occurs in extensive myocardial infarction - with the exception of the predominantly right coronary supply type. Also, cardiogenic shock occurs more frequently in anterior than in posterior infarctions. Echocardiographic parameters to assess the pumping function of the heart include ventricular wall motion analysis, ventricular diameter and geometry, fractional shortening (FS), and left ventricular ejection fraction (LVEF). Doppler techniques can be used to measure cardiac output in the left ventricular outflow tract.

Echocardiography is often able to distinguish ischemic but vital tissue from scar tissue. A wall motion analysis can be performed to roughly quantitate the amount of ischemic muscle. Wall motion abnormality is more sensitive for detection of regional myocardial ischemia than ECG changes or pulmonary capillary wedge pressure. In this regard, echocardiography is three to four times more sensitive than ECG.

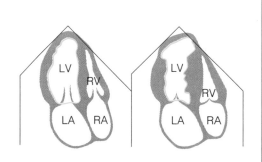

Extensive but well delimited dyskinesis of the anterior apex. Total and residual LVEF can be determined by echocardiography. This provides the surgeon additional information for surgery.

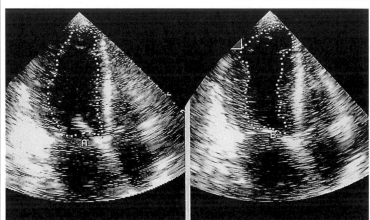

Apical four-chamber view in diastole (left) and systole (right).

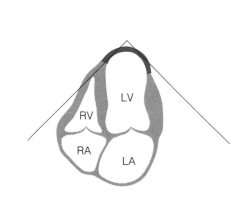

Dyskinesis of the anterior apex is highlighted, and LVEF is calculated by means of ultrasonic backscatter analysis (acoustic quantification).

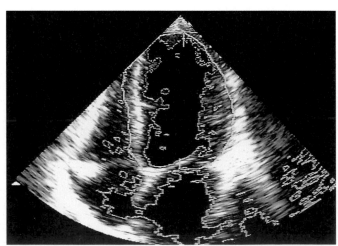

Acoustic quantification. Apical four-chamber view.

Echocardiography permits diagnosis of ventricular septal rupture, which can occur in both anterior and posterior infarctions. Echocardiography often provides direct visualization of the perforation site. Right ventricular enlargement and pulmonary artery dilation are further echocardiographic signs of right ventricular volume overload as an expression of a new ventricular septal defect. Shunts can be visualized after administration of an echo contrast agent (*e.g.* Echovist®).

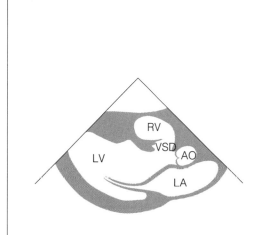

Subvalvular break in continuity of the interventricular septum, indicating postinfarction septal rupture.

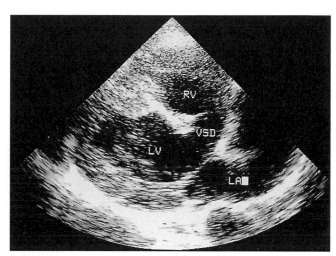

Parasternal long-axis view.

During myocardial infarction, papillary muscle dysfunction or rupture can occur, thereby causing severe acute mitral regurgitation. With echocardiography, it is possible to visualize systolic mitral regurgitation as well as the torn papillary muscle, which can be seen floating in the bloodstream.

Myocardial infarction may also induce rupture of the ventricular free wall, which is usually rapidly fatal. Echocardiography can provide evidence of hemopericardium and is sometimes able to visualize the perforation itself. Important echocardiographic signs of free wall rupture are fluid trapped between the epicardium and pericardium, a „swinging heart", and inspiratory displacement of the septum towards posterior in conjunction with an increase in right ventricular diameter and a decrease in left ventricular diameter.

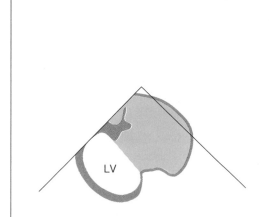

Extensive postinfarction aneurysm (inferior wall, with involvement of the posterolateral wall), and perforation of the ventricular free wall.

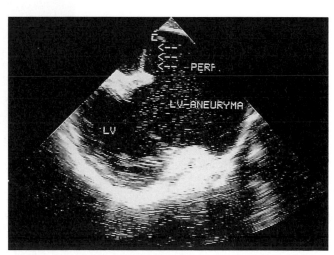

Transgastric short-axis (transverse) view.

M-mode and two-dimensional (2-D) echocardiography are important diagnostic tools for detection, differentiation, and follow-up of delated, hypertrophic or restrictive cardiomyopathies, and for assessment of treatment results. To be suitable for use in cardiac intensive care and emergency medicine, the imaging technique must be able to detect reduced global systolic pumping function in one or both ventricles in patients with dilatative cardiomyopathies, and to detect any hemodynamically significant obstruction of the left ventricular outflow tract that leads to dyspnoe or syncope. The technique must also be able to detect severe diastolic and systolic left ventricular dysfunction in patients with restrictive cardiomyopathies.

The resulting treatments range from anticoagulation to the implantation of a mechanical circulatory support system as a bridge to cardiac transplantation.

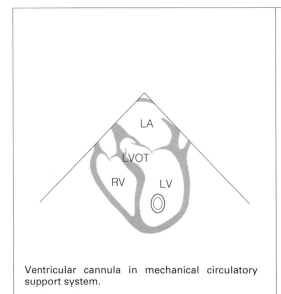

Ventricular cannula in mechanical circulatory support system.

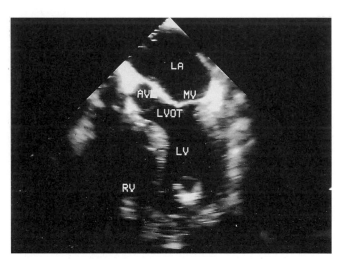

Transesophageal short-axis (transverse) view.

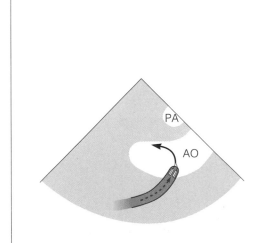

Upright position of the cannula in the ascending aorta causing increased hemolysis.

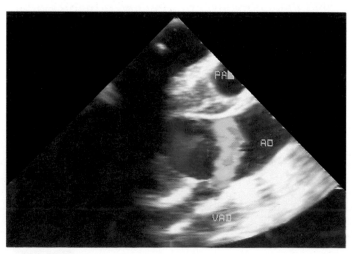

Color-encoded transesophageal long-axis echocardiogram.

Echocardiography plays an important role in patient monitoring. It provides important information for deciding whether and when to ween the patient from the circulatory support or cardiac replacement system. Echocardiography alone was able to identify the underlying cause of complications in over 10% of our patients requiring circulatory support.

The underlying causes identified by echocardiography include right atrial or ventricular hematoma causing a significant reduction in cardiac output, patent foramen ovale causing insufficient oxygenation of blood in conjunction with mechanical circulatory support, and upright position of the anastomosis causing increased hemolysis.

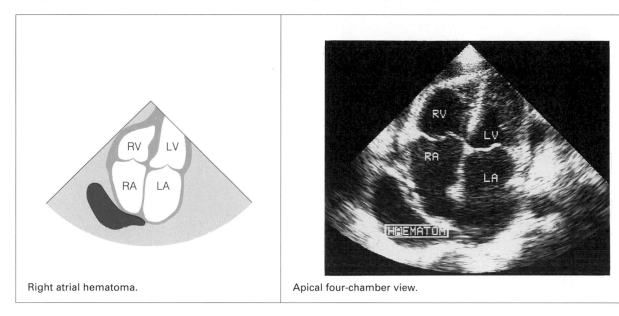

Right atrial hematoma.

Apical four-chamber view.

6. Cardiac Ultrasound Diagnosis in Intensive Care and Emergency Medicine
6.2 Diagnosis of Cardiac Abnormalities

Doppler color flow mapping is helpful in the identification of valvular insufficiency. As in Sellers' angiographic quantitation method, color Doppler permits semiquantitation of tricuspid, pulmonary, mitral, and aortic regurgitation and shunts. When used in combination with 2-D and M-mode echocardiography, color Doppler can identify the hemodynamic effects of regurgitation in the form of atrial and ventricular dilatation.

The modified Bernoulli equation can be used in Doppler sonography to determine the severity of valvular stenosis. Even in patients with reduced cardiac output, the valve orifice area, derived either by planimetry or from the continuity equation, can also be used to identify severe valvular stenosis as the underlying cause of cardiogenic shock. Without echocardiography and Doppler, silent aortic stenosis would go undiagnosed and untreated.

Echocardiography alone permits differential diagnosis of cor triatriatum sinistrum, the clinical symptoms of which resemble those of mitral stenosis. Echocardiography is able to visualize the membrane of the cor triatriatum opening. Openings smaller that 5 mm in size have a relatively poor prognosis; these patients usually die in the first 3 to 5 years of life. In comparison, patients with an opening larger than 10 mm in size usually live to an age of 38 to 70 years. The most common concomitant defects are atrial septal defect (60%) and anomalous pulmonary vein opening (15 to 25 %). The coexistence of such defects must be proven or excluded.

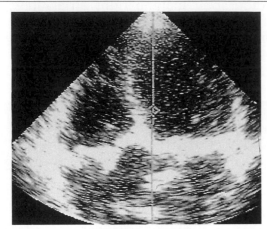

Apical four-chamber echocardiogram demonstrating „silent" aortic stenosis. Because left ventricular function is severely restricted, there is only a slight gradient. The aortic valve area calculated using the continuity equation equals 0.68 cm². The patient has severe aortic stenosis.

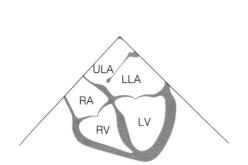

Cor triatriatum sinistrum membrane divides the left atrium in upper (ULA) and lower (LLA) segments.

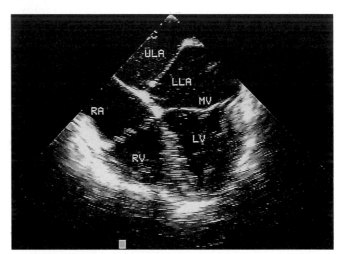

Transesophageal short-axis (transverse) view.

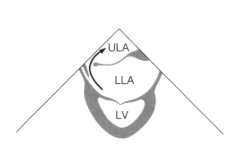

Cor tritriatum sinistrum. The membrane dividing the left atrium into upper (ULA) and lower (LLA) segments has a defect that gives rise to shunt flow.

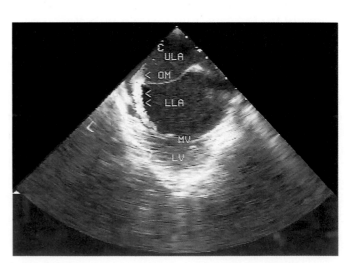

Color-encoded transesophageal short-axis (transverse) view.

Echocardiography has become the method of choice for detection and follow-up of endocarditis. Septic-embolic complications are not infrequent. 2-D echocardiography can be used to assess the size, shape, and mobility of vegetations. TEE further improves the sensitivity of echocardiographic diagnosis.

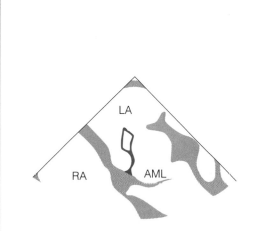

Mitral valve endocarditis. Echocardiography detects a threadlike vegetation extending from the anterior mitral leaflet (AML); it floats freely in the left atrium (LA).

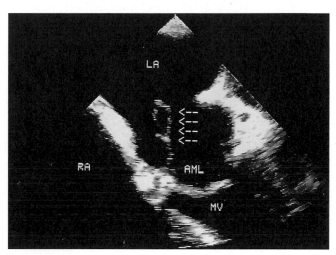

Transesophageal short-axis (transverse) echocardiogram.

6.   **Cardiac Ultrasound Diagnosis in Intensive Care and Emergency Medicine**
6.3   **Aortic Dissection**

Transesophageal echocardiography is a highly sensitive and specific method for preoperative diagnosis of aortic dissection. In urgent cases, surgery can be performed on the basis of the TEE diagnosis alone. However, the prerequisite for this is careful interrogation to precisely determine the extent of dissection and to detect the presence of possible complications. When allowed to run its natural course, acute aortic dissection has a poor prognosis: 3 to 5 % of untreated patients die immediately after the onset of aortic dissection, 20 to 40 % die within 24 hours after onset, 60 to 80 % die within two weeks, and 65 to 85 % die within one month, 70 to 90 % die within three months, and 85 to 95 % die within six months. In the Seventies, the hospital mortality rate was still 40%, despite conservative treatment and surgical intervention. The current hospital mortality rate is 10% and lower.

For clinical diagnosis of aortic dissection, the following points must be clarified and described:

- ▶ Evidence of a true and false lumen
- ▶ Extent; entry and re-entry sites
- ▶ Dissection type: communicating or non-communicating?
- ▶ Thrombus formation
- ▶ Supra-aortic vessel involvement?
- ▶ Coronary vessel involvement?
- ▶ Aortic insufficiency?
- ▶ Pericardial effusion?

The critical need for surgery is indicated when:

1. Rupture is imminent (increased pericardial effusion, enlargement of the mediastinum)
2. Regurgitation becomes increasingly severe (especially in severe aortic regurgitation)
3. Neurologic complications occur (peripheral paralytic symptoms, disturbance of consciousness)
4. Acute coronary ischemia occurs (when the dissection displaces the coronary ostia)
5. The diameter of the aneurysm is large (> 5 to 6 cm).

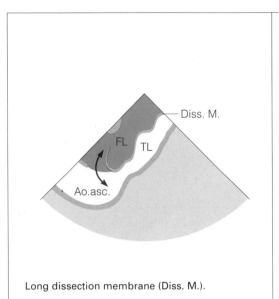

Long dissection membrane (Diss. M.).

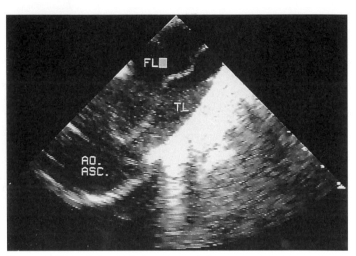

Transesophageal short-axis (transverse) view.

6. **Cardiac Ultrasound Diagnosis in Intensive Care and Emergency Medicine**
6.4 **Acute Rejection after Heart Transplantation**

The diagnosis of acute rejection after cardiac transplantation is still made on the basis of endomyocardial biopsy results [2, 18]. The introduction of cyclosporine in immunosuppressive therapy has improved the survival rate. However, cyclosporine also reduces the sensitivity of noninvasive rejection markers [19, 33]. More than 90% of all heart transplant patients experience at least one rejection episode [24]. The duration and frequency of these episodes seems to be a determining factor in the development of chronic rejection [15]. The primary role of echocardiography in following heart transplant patients is therefore monitoring rejection.

An advanced rejection episode influences systolic right and left ventricular function according to the sequence of the ischemia cascade. Diastolic ventricular function is diminished in the initial rejection phase, and reduction of systolic ventricular function occurs only in the advanced stages of rejection. Increasing left ventricular dilatation occurs in conjunction with reduced ejection fraction and decreased fiber shortening fraction. The amplitude of left ventricular posterior wall contractions is also reduced.

Doppler echocardiography is very helpful for early detection of rejection episodes [3, 9-12]. Reduced isovolumic relaxation time [1, 4, 5, 31], reduced early diastolic left ventricular area rate of change [1], increased left ventricular posterior myocardial relaxation time, and decreased early diastolic passive inflow into the left ventricle [29, 30] are relevant parameters that can be derived from Doppler mitral flow measurements [8, 14, 16, 17, 20, 25, 27-30, 32]. Various studies have shown that Doppler measurements correlate well with those of angiographic and scintigraphic methods [7, 21, 26].

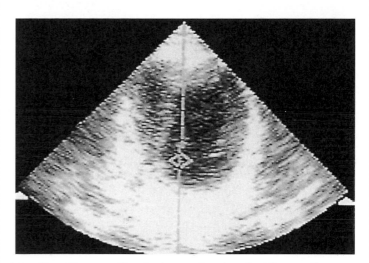

2-D echocardiogram with pulsed-wave Doppler mitral flow profile.

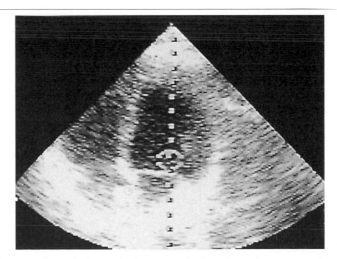

Transesophageal short-axis (transverse) view from the same patient after rejection episode. Diminished E-wave and increased A-wave indicate new contractile abnormality.

Ultrasonic backscatter analysis (acoustic quantitation) can be used to measure left ventricular areas and volumes in a user-defined region, and to calculate parameters of diastolic and systolic function. The derived cycle-to-cycle volume change curves makes it possible to distinguish between passive (E) from active (A) left ventricular inflow. The suspicion of rejection is confirmed when there is an increase in end-diastolic and end-systolic volumes and a decrease in the peak filling rate (mm/s).

Early diastolic functional abnormality is sometimes indicated by a reduction in the E/A ratio as an expression of reduced left ventricular compliance. This finding supports the suspected diagnosis of rejection.

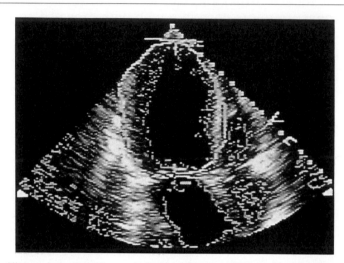

Ultrasonic backscatter analysis (acoustic quantification) is used for on-line assessment of diastolic and systolic LV function.

References

1. Angermann CE, Spes CH, Hart RJ, Kemkes BM, Gokel MJ, Theisen K. Echokardiographische Diagnose akuter Abstoßungsreaktionen bei herztransplantierten Patienten unter Cyclosporintherapie. Z Kardiol 1989; 78: 243-252.
2. Billingham ME. Diagnosis of cardiac rejection by endomyocardial biopsy. J Heart Transplant 1981; 1: 25-30.
3. Brutsaert DL, Rademakers FE, Sys SU, Gillebert TC, Housemans PR. Analysis of relaxation in the evaluation of ventricular function in the evaluation of ventricular function of the heart. Progr Cardiovasc Di 1985; 28: 143-163.
4. Dawkins KD, Oldershaw PJ, Billingham ME, Hunt S, Oyer PE, Jamieson SW, Popp RL, Stinson EB, Schumway NE. Changes in diastolic function as a noninvasive marker of cardiac allograft rejection. J Heart Trasplant 1984; 3: 286-294.
5. Desruennes M, Corcos T, Cabrol A, Gandjbakhch I, Pavie A, Leger P, Eugene M, Bors V, Cabrol C. Doppler echocardiography for the diagnosis of acute cardiac allograft rejection. J Am Coll Cardiol 1980; 12: 63-70.
6. Erbel R, Mohr-Kahali S, Drexler, Pfeiffer D, Börner D, Schuster S. Diagnostischer Stellenwert der trans-ösophagealen Echokardiopgraphie. Dtsch med Wschr 1987; 112: 23.
7. Friedman BJ, Drinkovic N, Miles H, Shih WJ, Mazzoleni A, De Maria AN. Assessment of left ventricular diastolick function: comparison of Doppler and gated blood pool scintigraphy. J Am Coll Cardiol 1986; 8: 1348-1354.
8. Fujii J, Yazaki Y, Sawada H, Aizawa T, Watanabe H, Kato H. Noninvasive assessment of left and right ventricular filling in myocardial infarction with a two-dimensional Doppler echocardiographic method. J Am Coll Cardiol 1985; 5: 1155-1160.
9. Gaasch WH, Cole JS, Quinones MA, Alexander JK. Dynamic determinants of left ventricular diastolic pressure-volume relations in man. Circulation 1975; 51: 531-535.
10. Gaasch WH, Levine JH, Quinones MA, Alexander JK. Left ventricular compliance: mechanisms and clinical implications. Am J Cardiol 1976; 38: 645-653.
11. Grossman W, McLaurin LP. Diastolic properties of the left ventricle. Ann Intern Med 1976; 84: 316-326.

12. Hammersmeister KE, Warbasse JR. The rate of change of left ventricular volume in man. II Diastolic enents in health and disease. Circulation 1974; 49: 739-747.

13. Hanrath P, Kremer P, Langenstein BA, Matsumoto M, Bleifeld W: Transösophageale Echokardiographie. Ein neues Verfahren zur dynamischen Ventrikelfunktionsanalyse. Dtsch med Wschr 1981; 106: 523.

14. Inouye I, Massie B, Loge D. Abnormal left ventricular filling: an early finding in mild to moderate systemic hypertension. Am J Cardiol 1984; 53: 120-126.

15. Kemnitz J, Cohnert T, Schäfers JH et al. A classification of cardiac allograft rejection. Am J Surg Path 1987; 11: 503-515.

16. Kitabatake A, Inoue M, Asao M, Tanouchi J, Masuyame T, Abe H, Morita H, Senda S, Matsuo H. Transmitral blood flow reflecting diastolic behavior of the left ventricle in health and disease: a study by pulsed Doppler technique. Jpn Circ J 1982; 46: 92-102.

17. Kücherer H, Ruffmann K, Schaefer E, Kübler W. Nichtinvasive Bestimmung linksvenrikulärer diastolischer Füllungsparameter mittels Dopplerechokardiographie: Klinische Anwendung bei Patienten mit KHK. Z Kardiol 1989; 77: 179-184.

18. Myerowitz PD, Gilbert E. Myocardial biopsy following heart transplantation. In: Myerowitz PD (ed). Heart Transplantation. Futura Mount Kisco, New York 1987; 219.

19. Oyer PE, Stinson EB, Jamieson SW, Hunt SA, Perlroth M, Billingham M, Shumway NE. Cyclosporine in cardiac transplantation: A 2 1/2 year follow-up. Transplant Proc 1983; 15: 2546-2552.

20. Phillips RA, Coplan NL, Krakoff LR, Yeager, Ross RS, Gorlin R, Goldman ME. Doppler echocardiographic analysis of left ventricular filling in treated hypertensive patients. J Am Coll Cardiol 1987; 9: 317-322.

21. Rokey R, Kuo L, Zoghbi WA, Limacher MC, Quinones MA. Determination of parameters of left ventricular diastolic filling with pulsed Doppler echocardiographic: comparison with cineangiography. Circulation 1985; 71: 543-550.

22. Schlüter M, Hanrath P. The clinical application of transesophageal echocardiography. Echokardiographie 1984; 1: 427.

23. Schlüter M, Thier W, Kremer P, Siglow V, Hanrath P. Klinischer Einsatz der transösophagealen Echokardiographie. Dtsch med Wschr 1984; 108: 722.

24. Schütz A, Kemkes BM, Kugler CH, Angermann CH, Schad N, Rienmüller R, Fritsch S, Anthuber M, Neumcicr P, Gokel JM. The influence of rejection episodes on the development of coronary artery disease after heart transplantation. Eur J Cardio-Thorac Surg 1990; 4; 300-308.

25. Snider AR. Doppler evaluation of left ventricular diastolic filling in children with systemic hypertension. Am J Cardiol 1985; 56: 921-926.

26. Spirito P, Maton BJ, Bonow RO. Noninvasive assessment of left ventricular diastolic function: comparative analysis of Doppler echocardiographic and radionuclide angiographic techniques. J Am Coll Cardiol 1986; 7: 518-526.

27. Störk T, Müller R, Ewert C, Piske G, Wienhold S, Hochrein H. Wirkung von Nikotin auf die linksventrikuläre Funktion bei koronarkranken Patienten: eine echokardiographische Studie. Dtsch med Wschr 1990; 116: 610-617.

28. Störk T, Müller R, Piske G, Ewert C, Hochrein H. Noninvasive measurement of left ventricular filling pressures by means of pulsed Doppler ultrasound, Am J Cardiol 1989; 64; 655-660.

29. Störk T, Walkowiak T, Müller R, Siniawski H, Hetzer R, Hochrein H. Nichtinvasive Erfassung der Abstoßungsreaktion nach Herztransplantation mittels Dopplerechokardiographie. Klin Wochenschr 1990; 68 (suppl XIX): 186.

30. Störk T, Walkowiak T, Siniawski H, Müller R, Hetzer R, Hochrein H. Nichtinvasive Erfassung der Abstoßungsreaktion nach Herztransplanttaion mittels Dopplersonographie. Z Kardiol 1990; 79 (suppl I): 74.

31. Valentine HA, Fowler MB, Hunt SA, Naasz C, Halte LK, Billingham ME, Stinson EB, Popp RL. Changes in Doppler echocardiograhic indexes of left ventricular function as potential markers of acute cardiac rejection. Circulation 1987; 76 (suppl V): 86-92.

32. Wind BE, Snider AR, Buda AJ, O'Neill WW, Popol EJ, Dilworth LR. Pulsed Doppler assessment of left ventricular diastolic filling in coronary artery disease before and immediately after coronary angioplasty. Am J Cardiol 1987; 59: 1041-1046.

33. Yacoub MH, Reid CJ, Al-Khadimi RH, Radley-Smith R. Cardiac transplantation - the London experience. Z Kardiol 1985; 74 (suppl VI): 45-40.

Cellular and molecular bonds can be loosened and broken down by high-intensity ultrasound.

A 2.5 MHz ultrasound wave travels through the body at a velocity of 1540 m/s and a wavelength of 0.616 mm. With a conventional transducer, the ultrasound intensity equals approximately 100 W/cm^2 (18 times the hearing threshold), and the sound level equals 180 dB(A). Considerable amplitude excursion of the scanned object and immediately adjacent objects occurs. In high-intensity ultrasound, this phenomenon can be applied for breakage of structural bonds. By focusing the ultrasound wave, intensities of up to 10^4 W/cm^2 and a sound level of 200 dB(A) can be achieved. This is many 10th powers higher than the sound intensity of a jet power unit.

High-intensity ultrasound already has many technological applications. For instance, focused ultrasound pressure waves can be used to remove dirt and impurities from laboratory vessels, the dispersive effect of ultrasound can be used to emulsify oil in aqueous solutions, ultrasound homogenization techniques are used in the pharmaceutical industry, and ultrasound can be used to remove odontolith in dentistry.

This obviously implies an increase in potential side effects as well as new perspectives for cardiac ultrasound. The first therapeutic application of cardiac ultrasound was in the decalcification of stenotic valves.

The preliminary results were good: a satisfactory amount of calcium was removed. However, scar tissue retraction which ultimately led to severe regurgitation was shown to develop a few weeks later. Apparently, the main problem in ultrasonic valvular decalcification efforts is learning to control the intensity and site of energy expenditure.

In addition to removing valvular calcification, another potential application of high-intensity ultrasound is removal of atherosclerotic calcific plaques. The effectiveness of ultrasound for the removal of such plaques in the systemic arteries was studied in animal experiments. High-intensity ultrasound (ca. 40 W) was shown to break down fibrotic and calcific arterial plaques by altering the pressure-volume relationship within the stenosis. Further research on ultrasonic ablation of atherosclerotic lesions may one day make it possible to perform routine ultrasound pretreatment in patients scheduled for mechanical interventions such as PTCA.

A further interesting perspective of therapeutic ultrasound is combined ultrasound and thrombolytic treatment. The efficacy of a thrombolytic agent is limited by the size of the clot, which provides only a small surface area for bonding. The potency of the thrombolytic agent is apparently increased by pre- and post-thrombolysis ultrasound treatments. By using ultrasound bursts at an intensity of 2 W/cm^2 and a duration of ca. 2 seconds, thrombus bonds were successfully loosened, which increased the number of available fibrin bonding sites.

Vegetations associated with endocarditis often do not respond to antibiotics due to the physicochemical properties of the pathogen and to the size of the vegetations. Therefore, it has been hypothesized that it may be possible to perforate, make porous, or loosen the bacterial capsule by means of focused, high-intensity ultrasound waves. As in the concept of combined ultrasound and thrombolytic treatment, the goal is to create a larger surface area for the antibiotics to react with.

In order for potential therapeutic cardiac ultrasound applications to be clinically feasible, the techniques must be noninvasive. This means that high-intensity ultrasound must be applied via the transthoracic route. Furthermore, extensive focussing problems must first be solved: absorption, reflection and scatter along the way to the target structure must be avoided. In two ultrasound transmitters currently under study, the beam is superimposed only on the target structure. When this structure is the heart, superimposition and phase extinction must be triggered in such a way that heart motion can be distinguished from chest wall motion. The use of an electronically timed window in conjunction with transducers capable of emitting ultrashort (millisecond to microsecond), focused, high-intensity bursts of ultrasound seems to be the only feasible solution.

Part Two

CLINICAL APPLICATIONS
OF CARDIAC ULTRASOUND DIAGNOSIS

Over the past few years, echocardiography has become a decisive diagnostic tool in pediatric cardiology. With only a few exceptions, currently available echocardiographic techniques make it possible to diagnose all congenital cardiac defects. Many invasive techniques have lost their former significance since the advent of cardiac ultrasound diagnosis. Echocardiography is, for example, superior to invasive angiography in the assessment of such cardiac structures as the atrioventricular valves.

This chapter is based on the European system of nomenclature and diagnosis of congenital heart disease. Its goal is to provide a systematic, segmental approach to echocardiographic diagnosis of each individual cardiac defect. Therefore, more emphasis has been placed on practical aspects of cardiac ultrasound diagnosis, rather than on the more theoretical aspects of embryology and terminology.

8.	Congenital Heart Disease
8.1	Position and Situs Anomalies

In both children and adults with congenital cardiac defects, situs anomalies of the heart and other unpaired epigastric organs can occur (*e.g.* in situs inversus and dextrocardia). To properly diagnose and evaluate malposition, the cardiologist must have a good understanding of the anatomy of the epigastric organs and the great interabdominal vessels.

In *situs solitus*, or normal configuration, the heart and the spleen are position on the left, and the liver is on the right. Dextrocardia, dextroversion, and mesocardia do not necessarily imply the absence of situs solitus. In *isolated dextrocardia*, there is mirror image reversal of the heart with normal configuration of the lung and abdominal organs. In *dextroversion*, the heart is positioned in the right hemithorax without mirror image reversal, i.e. the right and left atria are respectively right and left sided, and the cardiac apex points to the right. In *mesocardia*, the heart is located in middle of the thorax with the apex midline, and it is impossible to specify whether it is predominantly in the left or right hemithorax.

These cardiac situs anomalies with normal configuration (situs solitus) of the lung and abdominal organs must be differentiated from the following situs anomalies:

Situs anomalies
▸ Situs inversus partialis
▸ Situs inversus totalis
▸ Situs ambiguus

In *situs inversus partialis (thoracalis)*, there is mirror image reversal of all thoracic organs. The heart is positioned in the right hemithorax, the anatomic right trilobe lung is located on the left, and the anatomic left bilobe lung is located on the right.

In contrast to partial situs inversus, where the configuration of the abdominal organs is normal, there is mirror image reversal of thoracic *and* abdominal organs in *situs inversus totalis*. If the display image could be "turned around", the anatomic relationships would appear normal.

In *situs ambiguus*, on the other hand, the situs cannot be defined. The clinical diagnosis of situs ambiguus is important, because of the number of congenital cardiac defects associated with it. A good knowledge of epigastric anatomy is essential for diagnosis of situs ambiguus.

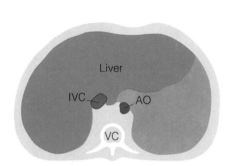

Normal epigastric anatomy. The vertebral column (VC) separates the inferior vena cava (IVC) and the aorta (AO).

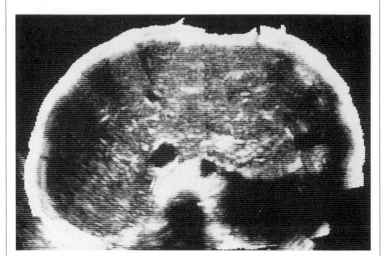

Compound sonography. Short-axis view of the liver.

In their normal configuration (situs solitus), the hepatic veins and the inferior vena cava enter the right atrium, slightly to the right of the vertebral column, and the abdominal aorta lies to the left of the vertebral column. The vertebral column therefore "separates" the abdominal aorta and the inferior vena cava. In situs inversus, the anatomic relationship is reversed, but the vertebral column still separates the aorta and the inferior vena cava. In situs ambiguus, however, this is no longer the case. The abdominal aorta and the inferior vena cava are located on the same side of the vertebral column. This is termed *juxtaposition of the great abdominal arteries*. Additionally, the liver is located in the mid-abdomen, the branches of the portal veins often extend horizontally, and the portal vein exits almost vertically.

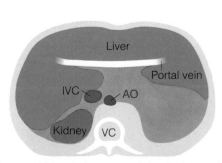

Juxtaposition of the great abdominal vessels. The portal vein (V. portae) courses horizontally through the abdomen. The aorta (AO) and inferior vena cave (IVC) are located on the same side of the vertebral column (VC). This configuration corresponds to situs ambiguus. In this case, there is right atrial isomerism, *i.e.*, asplenia.

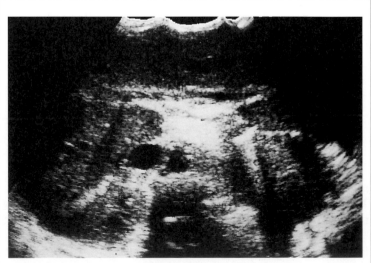

Compound sonography. Short-axis view of the liver.

The thoracic anatomy is also atypical in situs ambiguus. There may be either two anatomic right lungs and right atria on both sides, or two anatomic left lungs and left atria. The anatomic right lung is trilobular, and the upper lobe bronchus exits high. The left lung is bilobular, and the upper lobe bronchus exits low. The atria can be identified in (filtered high-voltage) chest x-rays by the anatomy of the bronchial tree.

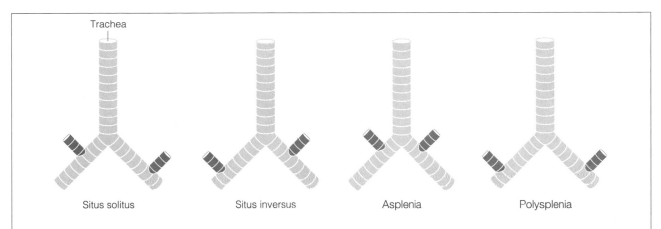

Normal morphology of the bronchial tree. The upper lobe bronchus exits high in the anatomic right lung, and low in the anatomic left lung. From left to right: situs solitus, situs inversus, asplenia (right atrial isomerism), and polysplenia (left atrial isomerism).

The right and left atria can also be distinguished on the basis of their appendages. The right atrial appendage is a broad, pyramidal structure with a broad base, whereas the left atrial appendage is long and narrow. It is difficult, and often impossible, to assess the atrial appendages from the transthoracic route. However, visualization can usually be achieved from the transesophageal route.

According to the anatomy of the bronchial tree and the atria (*i.e.* atrial appendages), situs ambiguus is classified as
1. *asplenia* (right atrial isomerism) and
2. *polysplenia* (left atrial isomerism). Both types are usually associated with dextrocardia.

Right atrial isomerism, or asplenia, is defined as bilateral "right-sidedness". Absence of the spleen (asplenia) is an important, but not the primary characteristic of right atrial isomerism. The defining features of right atrial isomerism are bilateral anatomic right atria, bilateral trilobular lungs (in most cases), and upper lobe bronchi that exit high. Juxtaposition of the great abdominal vessels is a further echocardiographic indication. A number of complex cardiac defects are associated with right atrial isomerism (asplenia). In order to detect these lesions, the anatomy must be assessed using a thorough segmental approach.

Associated cardiac defects in right atrial isomerism (asplenia)
▸ Total anomalous pulmonary venous return
▸ Transposition of the great arteries
▸ Pulmonary stenosis or atresia
▸ Atrial septal defects or monoatrium
▸ Double outlet right ventricle
▸ Double inlet left ventricle

Left atrial isomerism, or polysplenia, is characterized by bilateral "left-sidedness". Both atria resemble anatomic left atria, both lungs are (usually) bilobular, and upper lobe bronchi exit low. The primary echocardiographic findings for diagnosis are juxtaposition of the great vessels, *i.e.,* location of the abdominal aorta and inferior vena cava on the same side of the vertebral column, and azygos continuity of the inferior vena cava.

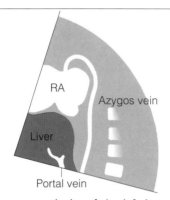

In azygos continuity of the inferior vena cava (IVC), the IVC anomalously courses directly in front of the vertebral column and drains into the azygos vein. The azygos vein then courses behind the right atrium (RA) and connects with the superior vena cava above the right atrium. Azygos continuity is common in left atrial isomerism (polysplenia).

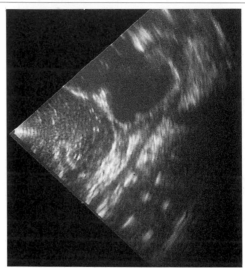

Subcostal long-axis scan.

With polysplenia the hepatic portion of the inferior vena cava is absent, and the IVC drains into the embryologically "older" azygos vein. Infrequently, the inferior vena cava drains into the hemiazygos vein, which then connects with the persistent left superior vena cava. The hepatic veins drain into the left atrium separate from the inferior vena cava. In rare cases, the right and left hepatic veins also drain separately in the right and left atria, respectively.

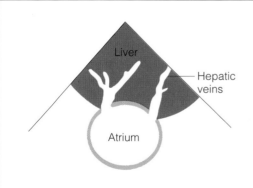

Polysplenia: The left and right hepatic veins drain separately into the same atrium, in the absence of an atrial septum. This is a common characteristic of left atrial isomerism (polysplenia).

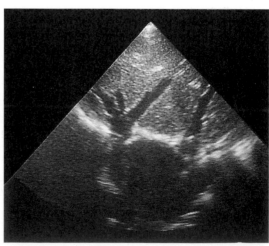

Subcostal short-axis (transverse) scan.

A number of complex cardiac defects are associated with left atrial isomerism (polysplenia). In order to detect these lesions, the anatomy must be assessed using a thorough segmental approach.

Associated cardiac lesions in left atrial isomerism (polysplenia)

▸ Complete AV canal with monoatrium
▸ Total anomalous pulmonary venous return
▸ Pulmonary stenosis or atresia
▸ Transposition of the great arteries

Summary of Position and Situs Anomalies

▸ Situs solitus (normal configuration)
Heart and spleen located on the left, liver on the right.

▸ Situs inversus totalis
Heart and spleen on the right, liver on the left.

▸ Dextrocardia
Mirror image reversal of thoracic organs, the anatomic right atrium is on the left, and the anatomic left atrium on the right.

▸ Dextroversion (dextroversio cordis)
The heart is located in the right hemithorax without mirror image reversal. The anatomic right atrium is on the right, and the anatomic left atrium is on the left.

▸ Mesocardia
The heart is in the mid-thorax, with the cardiac apex in the middle line of the thorax.

▸ Asplenia (right atrial isomerism)
Bilateral anatomic right atria, juxtaposition of the great abdominal vessels, the liver is located in the mid-abdomen, and the portal vein exits vertically.

▸ Polysplenia (left atrial isomerism)
Bilateral anatomic left atria, juxtaposition of the great abdominal vessels, azygos continuity of the inferior vena cava. The liver is located in the mid-abdominal region, and the portal vein exits vertically.

| 8. | Congenital Heart Disease |
| 8.2 | Systemic Vein Anomalies |

In addition to situs anomalies, the possibility of systemic vein anomalies must also be assessed using a thorough and systematic approach.

Defects and anomalies of the inferior vena cava are rare. The inferior vena cava is normally located on the right side of the vertebral column. Directly below the diaphragm, it extends ventrally through the liver, and connects, together with the hepatic veins, with the right atrium.

A *double inferior vena cava* is a remnant of the double inferior vena cava formed during embryological development. This explains how the inferior vena cava can "change sides". In very rare cases, the inferior vena cava fails to develop, and is replaced by a vascular plexus around the aorta (circumaortic renal collar). Anomalous return of the inferior vena cava and/or hepatic veins to the left atrium are also very rare anomalies (principle sign: cyanosis) that occur primarily in situs anomalies with complex cardiac defects.

Azygos continuity, which was discussed above under left atrial isomerism (asplenia), very rarely occurs in absence of left atrial isomerism (polysplenia). In azygos continuity, the abdominal portion of the azygos vein drains into the azygos vein, which connects with the superior vena cava.

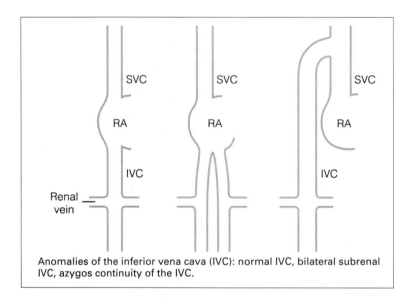

Anomalies of the inferior vena cava (IVC): normal IVC, bilateral subrenal IVC, azygos continuity of the IVC.

Additionally, such *acquired lesions* as stenosis or thrombosis of the superior vena cava can occur subsequent to surgery or central venous catheterization. In echocardiography, this can usually be identified as echo-dense material in the inferior vena cava. In some cases, however, the defect cannot be distinguished from surrounding connective tissue. Most commonly, thrombus involves the section of the inferior vena cava located below the origin of the renal veins.

Anomalies of the superior vena cava are much more common than anomalies of the inferior vena cava. Pediatric patients have a large thymus, which makes it possible to visualize the superior vena cava from the parasternal portal. The superior vena cava proximal to the heart can also be visualized from the subcostal portal. A *persistent left superior vena cava* is the most common anomaly of the systemic veins. A persistent left SVC usually drains into the coronary sinus, which is enlarged due to the increased blood volume. This can be demonstrated in parasternal long-axis scans. Total or partial anomalous pulmonary venous return to the coronary sinus must be excluded from the diagnosis by assessing the right and left pulmonary veins in apical four-chamber or subcostal scans. In total anomalous pulmonary venous return, the left ventricle is usually compromised by the right ventricle, which is always massively enlarged. A peripheral contrast study (left arm injection) may also be performed. When the coronary sinus is enlarged due to a persistent left superior vena cava, the echo contrast agent is first detected in the coronary sinus, then in the right atrium.

Contrast echocardiography is also provides indirect evidence of communication between the left and right superior vena cava. When communication exits, simultaneous contrast of the coronary sinus and the right superior vena cava occurs. Preoperative confirmation or exclusion of right and left superior vena cava communication is important for surgical planning, particularly in patients connected to a heart-lung machine. If communication exists, the left SVC can be simply ligated. Otherwise, the coronary sinus must be selectively cannulated during surgery.

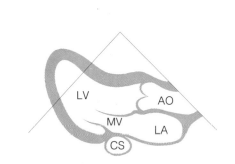

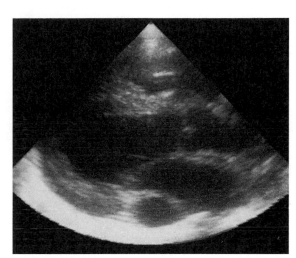

Massively enlarged coronary sinus (CS) in persistent left superior vena cava (SVC). The left ventricle (LV), mitral valve (MV), left atrium (LA), and aortic root (AO) are normal. Pathological dilatation of the coronary sinus is characteristic of total anomalous pulmonary venous return to the coronary sinus and persistent left superior vena cava.

Parasternal long-axis scan.

Infrequently, a persistent left superior vena cava can be connected directly to the left atrium (mainly in situs ambiguus). Even more infrequently, a persistent left superior vena cava may connect with an "unroofed" coronary sinus. In both cases, cyanosis may occur, and a left-to-right shunt may develop when the left atrial pressure becomes higher than the venous systemic pressure. The diagnosis may be confirmed or suggested by peripheral echo contrast studies (left arm injection).

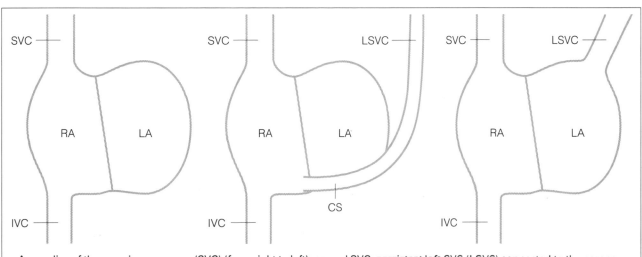

Anomalies of the superior vena cava (SVC) (from right to left): normal SVC; persistent left SVC (LSVC) connected to the coronary sinus (CS); and persistent LSVC connected to the right atrium (RA).

Dilatation of the (right) superior vena cava can occur in extremely rare cases of SVC aneurysm. Much more frequently, it is seen when there increased blood flow through the superior vena cava, which occurs when there is total anomalous pulmonary venous return to the superior vena cava or innominate vein (principle sign: massive RV enlargement), and arteriovenous fistula. When massive dilatation of the superior vena cava is detected in newborns, sonography must be performed to assess the possibility of vena cerebri magna aneurysm (intracerebral vena cerebri magna aneurysm due to arterial fistula; principle sign: systolic-diastolic head murmur; diagnosis via cerebral sonography).

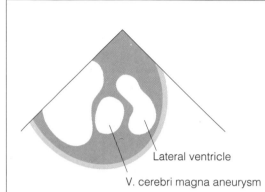

Lateral ventricle

V. cerebri magna aneurysm

The aneurysm can be seen in the echo-free space between the two (dilated) lateral ventricles. The vena cerebri magna aneurysm is located behind the third ventricle. Doppler color flow imaging permits visualization of blood flow in the aneurysm (due to the arteriovenous fistula).

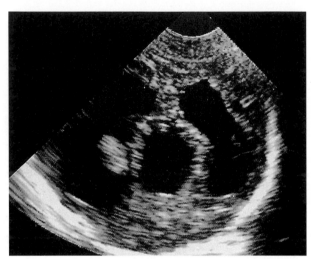

Cerebral sonography through the open fontanelle. Short-axis scan.

Persistent left superior vena cava must be differentiated from a levoatrial or levocardinal vein, which forms a connection between the left atrium and innominate vein. The levoatrial vein ascends dorsally, not ventrally, to the pulmonary artery, similar to a persistent left superior vena cava. A levoatrial vein is found predominantly in patients with mitral atresia and a constricted or obstructed atrial septum. Pulmonary venous blood therefore flows through the levoatrial vein into the innominate vein, which causes (right) superior vena cava dilatation in these patients.

| 8. | Congenital Heart Disease |
| 8.3 | Pulmonary Vein Anomalies |

The pulmonary veins develop from the primitive lung, with secondary connection to the left atrium. When this process proceeds abnormally, the pulmonary veins are not connected to the left atrium. The result is either pulmonary venous atresia, which normally has an unfavorable prognosis, or total anomalous pulmonary venous return. Echocardiography usually is not able to provide the diagnosis of pulmonary atresia. However, echocardiography is so sensitive for diagnosis of total anomalous pulmonary venous return that the echocardiographic diagnosis often obviates the need for preoperative invasive diagnosis. In pediatric patients, normal pulmonary venous return can be visualized in subcostal or apical four-chamber scans. In adults, transesophageal echocardiography is usually necessary.

There are several types of total anomalous pulmonary venous return. In all types, a confluence of pulmonary veins forms behind the left atrium, but fails to connect to the atrium.
The confluence of veins can be visualized by echocardiography. Total anomalous pulmonary
venous return is classified according to the site of pulmonary venous return (*i.e.*, supracardiac, cardiac, infradiaphragmatic).

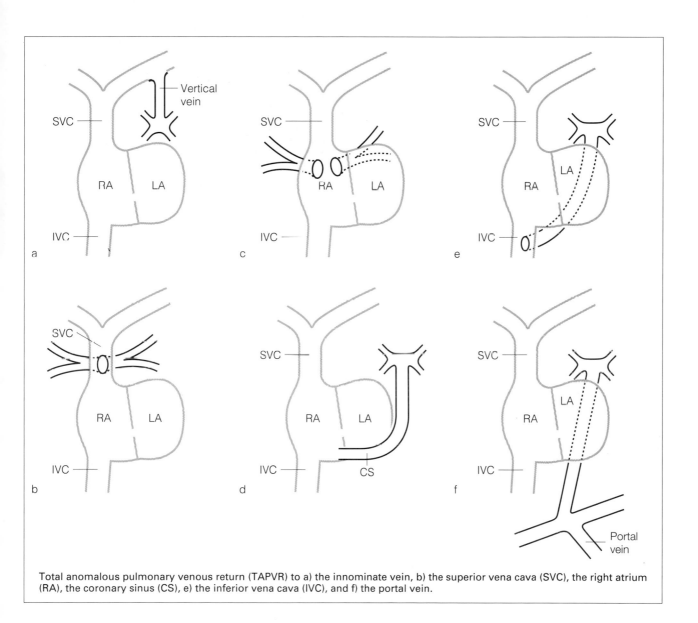

Total anomalous pulmonary venous return (TAPVR) to a) the innominate vein, b) the superior vena cava (SVC), the right atrium
(RA), the coronary sinus (CS), e) the inferior vena cava (IVC), and f) the portal vein.

Supracardiac types of total anomalous pulmonary venous return:

In supracardiac total anomalous pulmonary venous return, the confluence of pulmonary
veins drains either via a collecting vessel or directly into the superior vena cava. Most commonly, there exists a collecting vessel (vena verticalis) that enters the innominate artery.
Infrequently, the vertical vein enters the azygos or hemiazygos vein.

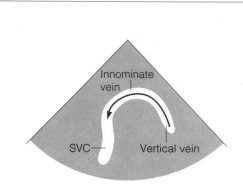

Total anomalous pulmonary venous return (supracardiac). The pulmonary veins connect via the vena verticalis to the innominate vein. Blood in the vertical vein flows towards the transducer. Blood in the dilated superior vena cava (SVC) flows away from the transducer. The innominate vein courses across the aortic arch.

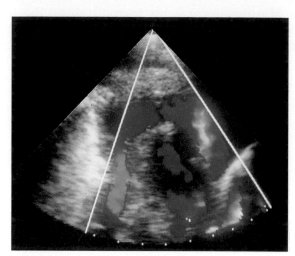

Suprasternal long-axis scan with color flow mapping.

In the other type of supracardiac total anomalous pulmonary venous return, the pulmonary veins drain directly into the (right) superior vena cava in the absence of a collecting vessel. Since pulmonary venous inflow is frequently obstructed, the site of drainage can best be identified by Doppler color flow imaging.

Cardiac total anomalous pulmonary venous return:

In cardiac total anomalous pulmonary venous return, the confluence of pulmonary veins behind the left atrium connects directly to the coronary sinus, or connects via a persistent left SVC to the coronary sinus. Direct connection between the confluence of veins and the right atrium is also possible. The site of drainage can best be identified by Doppler color flow imaging.

Infradiaphragmatic total anomalous pulmonary venous return:

For diagnosis of infradiaphragmatic total anomalous pulmonary venous return, the epigastric anatomy must be carefully assessed. In infradiaphragmatic total anomalous pulmonary venous return, the confluence of pulmonary veins connects via a collecting vessel to the dilated portal vein, or (more infrequently) to the inferior vena cava. As in supracardiac total anomalous pulmonary venous return to the innominate vein, the collecting vessel is called the vena verticalis. The presence of three vessels seen coursing through the diaphragm (i.e., the aorta, the inferior vena cava, and the vena verticalis) is an essential diagnostic indication. The vena verticalis extends behind the heart, similar to the IVC in azygos continuity, with the difference being that the inferior vena cava is normal.

An obligatory atrial septal defect (usually of the ostium secundum type) is present in all types of total anomalous pulmonary venous return. The defect provides the sole passage for blood from the right atrium to enter the left atrium and left ventricle. This results in extensive right ventricular volume overload and a decrease in left ventricular dimension. The left ventricle is also compromised by the dilated right ventricle. The ventricular septum bulges into the left ventricle and exhibits paradox septal motion.

Usually, the echocardiographic diagnosis of total anomalous pulmonary venous return must be made on the basis of indirect signs, *i.e.*, the absence of veins entering the left atrium. In newborns and young infants, Doppler color flow maps of apical or subcostal four-chamber scans are usually able to provide the diagnosis. An additional indication is an echo-free space behind the left atrium that corresponds to the confluence of pulmonary veins.

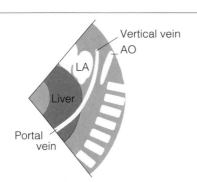

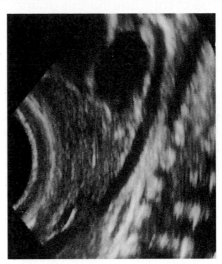

Total anomalous pulmonary venous return to the portal vein. The pulmonary veins drain via a collecting vessel (vertical vein). This vein originates behind the left atrium (LA) and courses caudad to join the portal vein. At diaphragm level, the vertical vein courses in front of the aorta (AO) and beside the inferior vena cava (IVC). The IVC can be visualized by angulating the transducer, or by scanning the ventricular short-axis.

Subcostal long-axis scan.

Particularly in parasternal long-axis scans, the aorta, which is located behind the left atrium, can simulate a confluence of pulmonary veins. However, this is almost never occurs in subcostal four-chamber scans. When in doubt, a pulsed-wave Doppler recording can be made to determine whether blood flow in the confluence is pulmonary venous or arterial flow. Furthermore, the echocardiographer can select a scanning plane that simultaneously visualizes the left atrium, the confluence, and the descending aorta. This makes it practically impossible to confuse the structures.

Besides determining the size and position of the confluence of pulmonary veins and of the left atrium, the site of abnormal connection must also be identified before performing surgical repair. Infradiaphragmatic total anomalous pulmonary venous return, usually to the portal vein, is the easiest type to diagnose. First, the confluence of pulmonary veins behind the left atrium is visualized from the subcostal four-chamber view. The transducer is then rotated until the imaging plane is parallel to the vertebral column and the descending aorta. The three vessels that pass through the aorta can be visualized by carefully sweeping the transducer back and forth. Next, the transducer is rotated 90° to obtain the short-axis view through the epigastrium. In total anomalous pulmonary venous return to the portal vein, the epigastrium is always massively enlarged, and can hardly be overlooked by a skilled echocardiographer. Doppler color flow maps can often demonstrate the continued flow of pulmonary venous blood from the portal vein through the venous duct to the right atrium.

Total anomalous pulmonary venous return to the inferior vena cava is more difficult to diagnosis. The vertical vein must then be followed up to its origin, which is usually identified in Doppler color flow images as an area of accelerated flow.

Supracardiac total anomalous pulmonary venous return is relatively simple to diagnose. After identifying the confluence of pulmonary veins, the vena verticalis is visualized from the supraclavicular portal. An indirect sign of supracardiac total anomalous pulmonary venous return is dilatation of the superior vena cava, which usually can be identified in color flow maps as an area of accelerated flow.

Total anomalous pulmonary venous return to the superior vena cava is more difficult to diagnose, because the only identifiable pathological structure is the confluence of pulmonary veins behind the left atrium. Therefore, Doppler detection of accelerated flow plays an important role in the diagnosis.

This is also true of total anomalous pulmonary venous return to the right atrium. The connection between the confluence of pulmonary veins and the right atrium must be carefully sought and identified by means of Doppler color flow imaging. In contrast, total anomalous pulmonary venous return to the pulmonary sinus is relatively simple to diagnose, because the enlarged coronary sinus is easy to detect.

Mixed forms of total anomalous pulmonary venous return with multiple anomalous connection sites are relatively difficult to diagnose. Because the velocity of abnormal pulmonary venous return is reduced, it is more difficult to identify in Doppler color flow imaging. When a vena verticalis exists, total anomalous pulmonary venous return can be diagnosed on the basis of the pathological presence of that vessel. However, it is difficult to additionally identify the connection to the right atrium or superior vena cava. Therefore, all potential anomalous connection sites must be thoroughly and systematically interrogated, especially when the blood flow velocity at the assumed sole connection site is only moderately increased.

If neither pulmonary venous return to left atrium, nor a confluence of pulmonary veins, nor entry sites of the pulmonary veins can be found, pulmonary atresia must be considered in the diagnosis. However, because pulmonary atresia is extremely rare, this diagnosis must be made with great reservation. Because total anomalous pulmonary venous return is frequently associated with situs ambiguus (left atrial isomerism), the presence of associated complex cardiac defects can also be expected.

8.3   **Pulmonary Vein Anomalies**
8.3.2   **Partial Anomalous Pulmonary Venous Return**

Partial anomalous pulmonary venous return is another possibility in which only some of the pulmonary veins connect abnormally. Partial anomalous pulmonary venous return is frequently associated with an atrial septal defect of the sinus venosus type. Indeed, partial anomalous pulmonary venous return is rarely found in absence of an atrial septal defect. The right pulmonary veins, most of which drain into the superior vena cava, right atrium, or connect to the junction of the inferior vena cava and the right atrium, are usually involved. Infrequently, the left pulmonary veins anomalously drain into a vena verticalis or a persistent left superior vena cava. The scimitar deformity is a special type of partial anomalous pulmonary venous return. The lower and middle right pulmonary veins drain into a collecting vein, which extends to the right atrium and connects to the inferior vena cava. The echocardiographic structure resembles a Turkish saber (scimitar). Although the site of drainage can be visualized in subcostal scans, it is difficult to make the actual diagnosis.

The echocardiographic diagnosis of atrial septal defect is usually made by direct visualization of the defect via two-dimensional echocardiography. Subcostal four-chamber scans are particularly effective for this purpose, because the beam is then perpendicular to the atrial septum. However, in apical four-chamber and apical short-axis scans, the beam is parallel to the atrial septum. Therefore, defects are often simulated by inadequate ultrasound reflection (echo dropout). As compared to echo dropout, the edges of a true atrial septal defect appear to be thickened.

Doppler color flow imaging can be used to identify the shunt through the defect. Again, this can be demonstrated best in subcostal four-chamber scans, because the beam is parallel to the blood flow through the defect. In contrast, the beam is perpendicular to the direction of blood flow in apical four-chamber and apical short-axis scans.

Contrast echocardiography is a very sensitive method for detection of very small defects in the atrial septum. Even in "pure" left-to-right shunts, there is a minimal right-to-left shunt that often can be demonstrated only by means of contrast echocardiography. When the possibility of persistent left superior vena cava must be assessed, scans should be made after peripheral venous (left arm) injection of echo contrast agent .

It is usually relatively easy to obtain direct visualization of atrial septal defects in pediatric patients. However, this is more difficult in adolescents and adults, because the intercostal spaces are smaller, and the distance from the transducer to the target structure is larger. Contrast echocardiography is often helpful in such cases, and transesophageal echocardiography can reliably visualize the defect. Especially when planning surgical repair of an interventricular septal defect, it is necessary to have an accurate picture of the defect. Therefore, transesophageal scans must usually be used in adolescents and adults, whereas subcostal echocardiography is the superior imaging technique in children younger than 6 to 8 years of age.

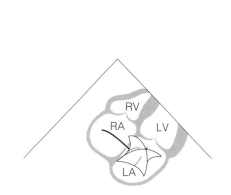

Repair of an atrial septal defect using a buttoned device. The surgical intervention is performed under echocardiographic control, which allows optimal positioning of the device. The "umbrella" is opened in the left atrium.

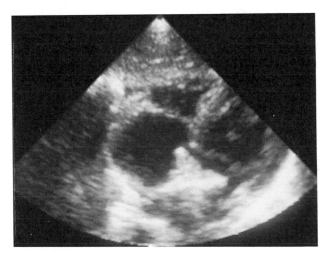

Subcostal four-chamber view.

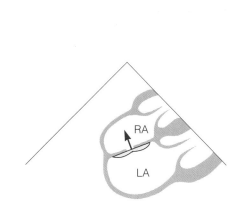

Repair of an atrial septal defect using a buttoned device. The "umbrella" is opened and positioned to cover defect (right). The results of defect repair are checked using Doppler color flow imaging.

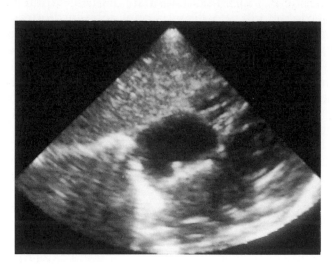

Subcostal four-chamber scan.

Patent foramen ovale, an atrial septal "defect" that conducts oxygenated blood from the placenta via the umbilical vein and venous duct to the left atrium, is also worth mentioning. A patent foramen ovale is common in the first few weeks and months of life. There is a minimal right-to-left shunt, which can be visualized by contrast echocardiography. Because the foramen ovale opening may appear relatively wide in newborns, it is sometimes mistaken for a "true" atrial septal defect. All atrial septal "defects" should be cautiously evaluated in the first few months of life, because such findings may actually be due to a patent foramen ovale. Even in older children, adolescents, and adults, the patent foramen ovale may persist and go on to cause paradox embolisms. The most reliable way to visualize right-to-left shunt through a patent foramen ovale is to record contrast echocardiographic scans while performing Valsalva's maneuver. In adults, it is usually necessary to make these scans from the transesophageal route.

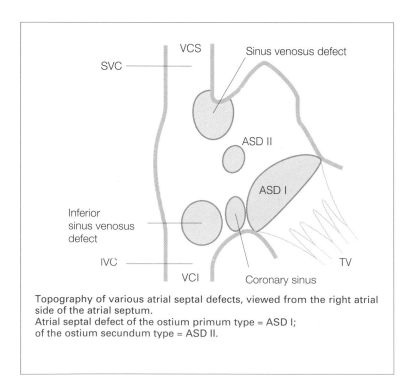

Topography of various atrial septal defects, viewed from the right atrial side of the atrial septum.
Atrial septal defect of the ostium primum type = ASD I;
of the ostium secundum type = ASD II.

Atrial septal defects are classified into five to six morphological types. The most common are atrial septal defects of the *ostium secundum type (ASD II)*, which are located in the region of the fossa ovalis. Echocardiography reveals a "halo" of atrial septal tissue around the defect. Ostium secundum defects are often associated with mitral valve prolapse, which usually is not hemodynamically significant. A variation of ostium secundum defect is "aneurysm" of the foramen ovale, in which the foramen ovale protrudes aneurysmalally into the right atrium. Patho-anatomical studies show multiple small defects in the region of the foramen ovale, giving the structure a sieve-like appearance.

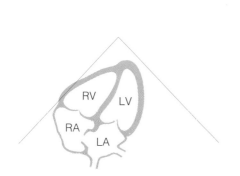

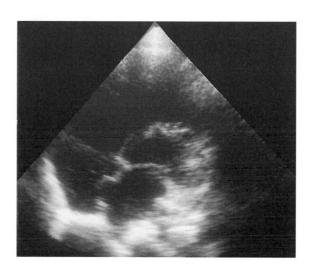

Aneurysm of the fossa ovalis. The fossa ovalis protrudes from the left atrium (LA) into the right atrium (RA). A defect is seen in the middle of this "protrusion". However, the defect cannot reliably be distinguished from echo dropout, because the beam is parallel to the target structure.

Modified (shortened) apical four-chamber scan.

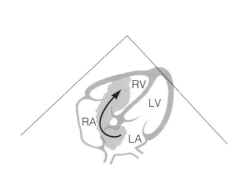

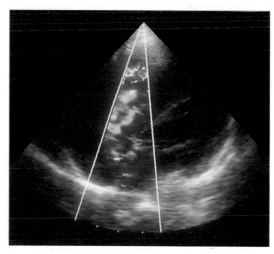

The Doppler color flow map reveals an extensive left-to-right shunt extending from the LA through the fossa ovalis aneurysm to the RA and right ventricle (RV). This corresponds to an atrial septal defect. There are multiple small perforations. They can be visualized on the Doppler color flow map of the left-to-right shunt.

Color flow map of modified (shortened) apical four-chamber scan.

Atrial septum defects of the *ostium primum type (ASD I)* are located in the basal aspect of the atrial septum at atrioventricular valve level. Ostium primum defects are sometimes mistaken for the junction of a dilated coronary sinus in persistent left superior vena cava, or for anomalous pulmonary venous return to the coronary sinus.

However, the proper diagnosis can be made from the parasternal long-axis view. The dilated coronary sinus demonstrates the typical appearance. Because the ostium primum defect also belongs to the group of atrial septal defects, the tricuspid and mitral valves insert at the same level of the ventricular septum. This cleft is always oriented towards the tricuspid valve, never towards the aortic root (see AV septal defects). Defects that extend as far as the ventricular septum are AV septal defects, which will be discussed in the following section.

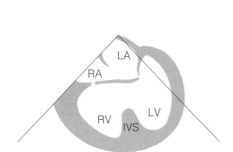

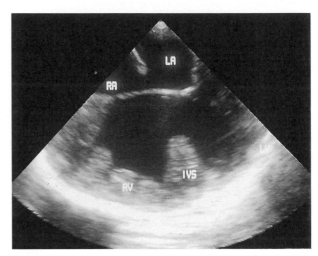

Atrial septal defect of the ostium primum type (ASD I). AV septal defect. The atrial septum (IAS) does not reach the AV valve plane. This corresponds to an atrial septal defect of the ostium primum type. Characteristically, the septal AV valve segments merge together. In addition to ASD I, there is a ventricular septal defect directly below the AV valve. IVS = interventricular septum.

Intraoperative transesophageal short-axis (transverse) scan.

Atrial septal defects of the *sinus venosus type* are located in the upper atrial septum, near the junction of the left pulmonary veins and the left atrium. They are also characterized by a total absence of atrial septal tissue between the superior vena cava and the pulmonary veins, and are usually associated with partial anomalous pulmonary venous return. Sinus venosus defects are more difficult to surgically correct. The defect must first be enlarged to ensure that blood flows freely from the superior vena cava and left pulmonary veins after the defect has been repaired.

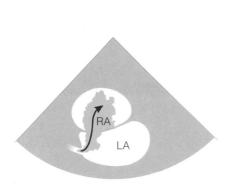

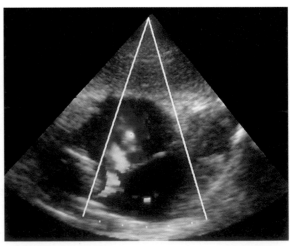

Sinus venosus defect. The defect is located in high in the septum (IAS), near the junction of the upper right pulmonary veins and the superior vena cava. Blood flows through the defect from the left atrium (LA) to the right atrium (RA).

Color flow map of a subcostal four-chamber scan.

Inferior sinus venosus defects are rare atrial septal defects located in the lower aspect of the atrial septum, near the site where the inferior vena cava enters the right atrium which, unlike the ostium primum defect, is separated from the atrioventricular valve level by atrial septal tissue. *Coronary sinus defects*, which are located near the site where the coronary sinus enters the right atrium, are also rare. Because they sometimes reach (almost) as far as atrioventricular valve, coronary sinus defects are sometimes mistaken for ostium primum defects. The difference is that, in coronary sinus defects, the insertion of the septal tricuspid leaflet is deeper than that of the mitral leaflet (in apical four-chamber scans). Hemodynamically speaking, this defect is no different from an unroofed coronary sinus, which provides communication between the two atria. Unroofed coronary sinus, which is difficult to surgically correct, is a significant tentative diagnosis. Whereas it is relatively easy to make an echocardiographic diagnosis or differential diagnosis of ostium secundum, ostium primum, and sinus venosus defects, echocardiographic differentiation of inferior sinus venosus defects and coronary sinus defects is not always possible.

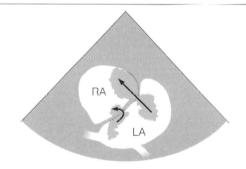

Coronary sinus defect. Deep-seated defect in the IAS, with left-to-right shunt from the LA to RA. Unlike the ostium primum defect, the coronary sinus defect is not located above the AV valve, but posterior to it. Therefore, scans must be made in the far posterior region (almost) through the fibrous ring. In addition to the coronary sinus defect, there is a small defect in the mid-IAS suggestive of a persistent foramen ovale or a very small ostium secundum defect.

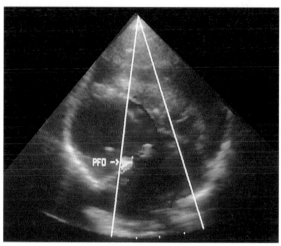

Color flow map of subcostal four-chamber scan.

Monoatrium, the final special type of atrial septal defect, is characterized by complete absence of the atrial septum. Isolated monoatrium is a very rare occurrence. It is more frequently found in patients with AV septum defects or complex defects arising from situs anomalies (particularly polysplenia). Therefore, the site of the defect must be carefully determined.

Juxtaposition of the atrial appendages, which may simulate an atrial septal defect, is of differential diagnostic significance. In juxtaposition, the atrial appendages are located on the same side of the heart, *i.e.*, one appendage extends to the contralateral side posteriorly around the great arteries. Naturally, the atrial septum is not located inside the appendage. Juxtaposition of the atrial appendages is sometimes mistakenly interpreted as an atrial septal defect.

All atrial septal defects produce similar hemodynamic effects. In the presence of the left-to-right shunt, the right ventricle is enlarged, the ventricular septum is flattened along the short axis, or it protrudes into the left ventricle. M-mode echocardiograms reveal paradox septal motion. Two-dimensional echocardiograms reveal that the ventricular septum is affected by contraction of the right ventricle, not the left. Therefore, the size of the left ventricle often appears to be reduced, although it is usually normal.

A truly hypoplastic left ventricle can occur only in newborns and in young infants. In these cases, the left ventricle fails to develop, because the pulmonary venous blood flow across the defect drains to the right.

Tricuspid insufficiency usually develops when right ventricular dilation becomes more severe. This insufficiency normally is not hemodynamically significant, but is useful when making pulsed or continuous-wave Doppler assessments of right ventricular pressure. For practical reasons, the "gradient" across the tricuspid valve is measured and added to the estimated atrial pressure (4 to 8 mmHg). This RV pressure estimate can be used to determine the presence of pulmonary hypertension, which develops via pulmonary recirculation (Eisenmenger's reaction). Eisenmenger's reaction leads to massive enlargement of the right ventricle, left ventricular compression and inversion of the curvature of the ventricular septum. Tricuspid insufficiency then becomes hemodynamically significant. Ebstein's anomaly of the tricuspid valve, which is usually associated with an atrial septal defect, must be considered in the differential diagnosis. In Ebstein's anomaly, the tricuspid valve is displaced into the right ventricle, and is incompetent. Pulmonary hypertension is almost never found in Ebsteins's anomaly of the tricuspid valve, because a predominant right-to-left shunt develops due to tricuspid regurgitation through the atrial septal defect. This is aggravated by pulmonary stenosis, which often coexists.

Mitral valve lesions are more rare. Different investigators report different rates of occurrence of mitral valve prolapse, which is only very seldom hemodynamically significant. When mitral regurgitation exists, ostium primum defect must be excluded from the diagnosis. When ostium primum defect exists, there is a cleft in the mitral valve, which must be sought.

Associated partial anomalous pulmonary venous return must be excluded from the diagnosis, especially when there is a sinus venosus defect. This is done by following the right and left pulmonary veins to their origins. If no atrial septal defect can be found, but the right ventricle is enlarged without any other abnormality, the possibility of partial anomalous pulmonary venous return without atrial septal defect must be considered. In this case, there is usually partial anomalous pulmonary venous return to the superior vena cava (supracardiac), to the right atrium or coronary sinus (cardiac) or, more infrequently, to the innominate vein. Infradiaphragmatic partial anomalous pulmonary venous return, which occurs in the scimitar deformity, is rare.

| 8. | Congenital Heart Disease |
| 8.5 | Atrioventricular Septal Defects (AV Canal Defects) |

The group of atrioventricular septal defects includes a variety of congenital cardiac malformations that have similar embryological origins. Because of the central location of the atrioventricular septum, involvement of the lower portions the atrial septum (septum primum), the atrioventricular valves and their connection to the ventricles and the ventricular septum (inlet septum) below the AV valves can occur. AV septal defects are relatively common in patients with trisomy 21 syndrome (Down's syndrome).

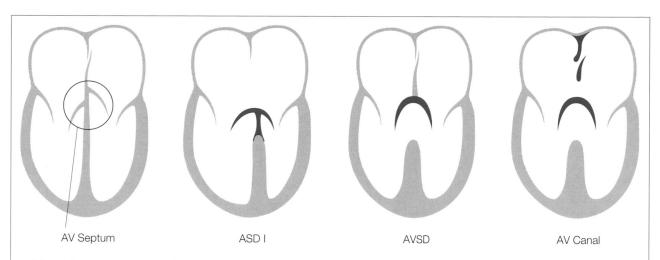

Schematic representation of the characteristic changes observed in AV septal defects. The AV valves normally insert at different levels of the ventricular septum. However, in atrioventricular septal defects (AVSD), the septal leaflet segments merge (four-chamber view).

The AV valves are normally separated by the aortic root, which is positioned between them. If significant amounts of the AV septum are missing, the aortic root develops in front of the AV valves, not between them. When the AV valve plane is viewed from above, the AV valves no longer look like a pair of "glasses", but form a single oval structure. The orientation of the papillary muscles is also changed: These are no longer appear "twisted", as though the aortic root had pushed them apart, but are situated vis-a-vis.

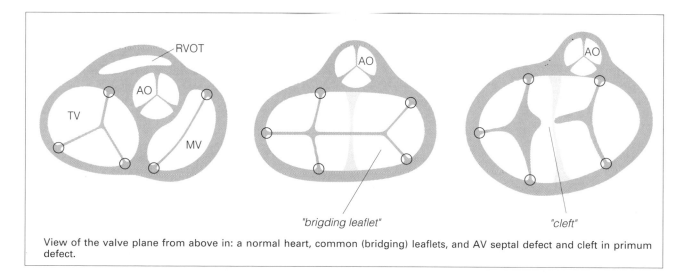

View of the valve plane from above in: a normal heart, common (bridging) leaflets, and AV septal defect and cleft in primum defect.

The principle anomaly is found in the AV valves. Instead of forming two separate structures, common atrioventricular valve connection develops. This common atrioventricular valve connection typically has five leaflets: two "true" tricuspid leaflets, one "true" mitral leaflet, and common anterior and common posterior AV valve leaflets (bridging leaflets). In one extreme, the common valve rudiment can develop to form a common AV valve with prominent bridging leaflets. In the other extreme, it can form two divided atrioventricular ostia with a cleft mitral valve.

This defect is usually falsely classified as a cleft anterior leaflet of the mitral valve. In AV septal defects, the cleft usually points towards the other (right) ostium - never towards the aortic root. This fact is not simply of theoretical interest, because there actually exists a type of congenital cleft anterior mitral leaflet that points towards the aortic root. The latter type does not belong to the group of atrioventricular septal defects (see mitral valve anomalies).

Atrioventricular septal defects can usually be easily diagnosed by echocardiography on the basis of their characteristic appearance. The septal portions of the atrioventricular valve typically insert at the same level of the ventricular septum. In normal subjects, the septal tricuspid valve leaflet inserts (2 to 4 mm) deeper than the mitral valve. The abnormal location of the aortic root, which does not appear between the atrioventricular valves, but in front of the common AV valve leaflets, can be identified indirectly. This is done by demonstrating that it is not possible to visualize the aorta and the atrioventricular valves together in the same plane, even with careful angulation of the transducer from the apical four-chamber position.

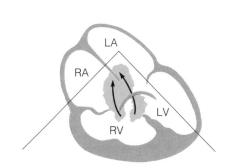

AV septal defect. There is an ostium primum atrial septal defect and a ventricular septal defect directly below the AV valves. Septal leaflet segments are located at the same level and merge (bridging leaflets). The color flow map reveals a jet in the right or left atrium, corresponding to mitral or tricuspid regurgitation, respectively.

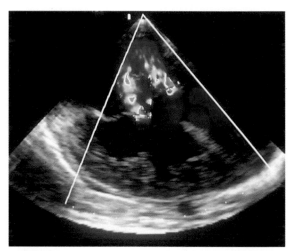

Color flow map of a transesophageal short-axis echocardiogram.

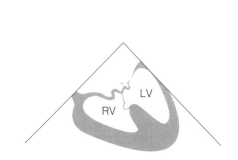

AV septal defect with common AV valve. The dysplastic AV valve leaflets are irregular. Chordae tendineae reach to the edge of the ventricular septal defect. The IAS cannot be visualized because of a large primum defect.

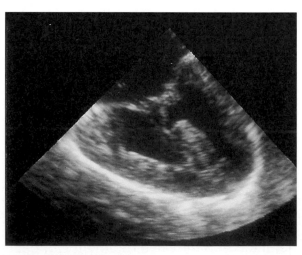

Transesophageal short-axis view.

Evaluation of the common AV valve is the most time-consuming part of echocardiographic assessment of AV septal defects. Initial two-dimensional scans from the four-chamber view reveals that the septal segments of both AV valves insert at the same level of the ventricular septum and merge together. The decisive questions to be clarified are whether there are two separate valves or one common valve, and where the corresponding chordae insert. When the ventricular defect is small, the two valve segments are usually extensively divided. In primum defects with an intact ventricular septum, there are two separate valves, and the AV valve anomaly is limited to the cleft mitral valve. It is easiest to visualize the cleft in the mitral valve from the short-axis view. The cleft always points towards the AV ostium, never towards the aortic root.

In the other extreme, when there is a large primum defect and a large ventricular defect, the common (bridging) leaflets are usually prominent, whereas the others are hypoplastic. Some of the left atrial chordae then extend through the ventricular septal defect to the right ventricle (straddling). There is a broad spectrum of AV valve anomalies between the extremes. Several classification of severity of AV septal defects have been proposed. However, an individualized description of the anatomy of the atrioventricular valves appears to be always superior to such rigid classifications.

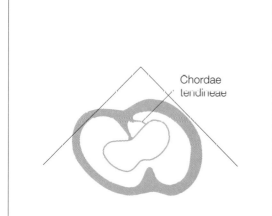

Common AV valve in AV septal defect. The bridging leaflets of the common AV valve extend through a large defect in the IAS. The chordae insert at the edge of the ventricular septal defect.

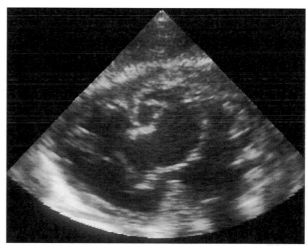

Subcostal short-axis frame in diastole.

After visualizing the papillary muscles and the AV valve in the short-axis view (from the subcostal or parasternal position), the transducer is then adjusted to the four-chamber view. From the four-chamber view, the scanning plane is rotated towards posterior in order to assess the size of the anterior common leaflet, the anatomy of the respective chordae, and their insertion sites. In order to decide whether two separate valves or one common valve exist, it is helpful to determine whether the medial aspect of the bridging leaflet is attached to bridging tissue, or whether it moves freely. Then, by carefully angulating the transducer in the plane of the chordae tendineae, the chordae can be tracked up to their insertions. It is important to determine whether the chordae pass through the ventricular defect into the opposite ventricle when considering surgery. If this is the case, the ventricular septal defect cannot be surgically corrected without altering the valvular apparatus.

Chordae tendineae that insert at the upper edge of the ventricular septal defect pose no surgical problems. The anterior bridging leaflet can also be assessed by angulating the scanning plane ventrally.

In addition to describing the features of AV valve morphology, two-dimensional echocardiography is also helpful in assessing functional competence, *i.e.*, the presence and extent of right or left atrial AV valve regurgitation. AV valve incompetence tends to be an unfavorable prognostic factor for surgical outcome, and may be an indication of dysplastic valvular tissue. Doppler echocardiography is helpful in assessing pressure relationships. Right and left ventricular pressure is always at equilibrium in the presence of large ventricular defects.

When there is a common AV valve, ventricular dominance or an unbalanced AV septal defect often exists. This implies an imbalance in ventricular development, whereby the left ventricle is usually underdeveloped or hypoplastic, but the right ventricle seldom is.

The abnormal spatial relationship of the atrioventricular valves and the aortic root only infrequently causes constriction of the left ventricular outflow tract. Residual defects in the atrial septum or ventricular septum and AV valve dysfunction, *i.e.* mitral or tricuspid valve incompetence or stenosis, is found after surgical correction.

| 8. | Congenital Heart Disease |
| 8.6 | Ventricular Septal Defects |

Ventricular septal defects can be isolated or may occur in association with other congenital cardiac defects. An ventricular septal defect is often found as an integral part of other cardiac anomalies, such as tetralogy of Fallot, double outlet right ventricle, and pulmonary atresia, which will be discussed later. An isolated ventricular septal defect can result in left-to-right shunt across the defect and, thus, to left atrial and left ventricular enlargement. The hemodynamic consequences of the ventricular septal defect depend on its size. When the ventricular septal defect is relatively small, the pressure in the right ventricle is normal or only slightly elevated. When the ventricular septal defect is relatively large, equalization of systolic pressures in the two ventricles may result. The pressure gradient across the defect can be determined by cardiac Doppler. The right ventricular pressure can then be derived from the right and left ventricular pressure gradient and the systolic blood pressure. However, the pressure gradients cannot be used in the presence of lesions such as aortic stenosis, in which the left ventricular pressure differs from the systolic blood pressure.

An increase in RV pressure, *i.e.* low pressure gradient across the defect, occurs in large defects with pressure equalization. Eisenmenger's reaction may develop in older left-to-right shunts. The left-to-right shunt decreases as pulmonary resistance increases, and shunt reversal may occur. Right-to-left shunt and cyanosis result when pulmonary resistance becomes higher than systemic resistance. Left ventricular volume overload decreases in this process, *i.e.*, the left atrium and left ventricle are no longer enlarged, but there are signs of right ventricular volume overload. The right ventricle then becomes enlarged, and the ventricular septum protrudes into the left ventricle.

Ventricular septal defects can be divided into four different types according to their morphology:

> ▸ Atrioventricular septal defects
> ▸ Muscular ventricular septal defects
> ▸ Perimembranous ventricular septal defects, and
> ▸ Doubly committed (juxta-arterial) ventricular septal defects.

This classification is based on the "texture" of the defect margin. By definition, a muscular ventricular septal defect is completely surrounded by muscular tissue, an AV septal defect borders on the common atrioventricular valve plane, a perimembranous ventricular septal defect borders with the aortic valve and its fibrous connection to the tricuspid valve, and a doubly committed ventricular septal defect borders on the continuous aortic and pulmonic valves. This classification was devised by morphologists, and tends to be impractical for clinical use. However, it is currently the only available morphological classification for ventricular septal defects.

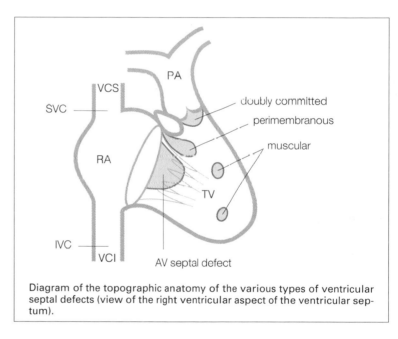

Diagram of the topographic anatomy of the various types of ventricular septal defects (view of the right ventricular aspect of the ventricular septum).

8.6 Ventricular Septal Defects
8.6.1 Atrioventricular Septal Defects

Atrioventricular septal defects were discussed in the previous section. Due to the moderate to extensive absence of the AV septum, defects occur in the lower aspect of the atrial septum (septum primum), atrioventricular valves, and the ventricular septum. In extremely rare cases, the atrial septum is closed, and there is a "pure" ventricular septal defect. When scanning from the four-chamber view, the echocardiographic diagnosis of atrioventricular septal defects can be made by the fact that the septal aspects of the two AV valves anomalously insert at the same level of the ventricular septum and merge, *i.e.*, the septal tricuspid valve leaflet does not insert below the level of the mitral valve.

The upper margin of a ventricular septal defect is formed by the merging AV valvular tissue. It has no visible relationship to the aortic root, which is not located between the two AV valves, but in front of the common valve. Very large defects that reach the free walls of the two ventricles may also extend as far as the aorta in the parasternal long axis.

8.6   **Ventricular Septal Defects**
8.6.2   **Muscular Ventricular Septal Defect**

Muscular ventricular septal defects are, by definition, completely surrounded by muscular tissue, and can occur in all sections of the ventricular septum. Commonly, multiple muscular defects occur and, in extreme cases, the ventricular septum may be so filled with "holes" that it resembles "Swiss cheese". Muscular ventricular septal defects can also occur in combination with non-muscular ventricular septal defects.

The diagnosis of muscular defects still is relatively simple, because the majority of these defects arise in trabecular components of the septum. This also makes them easy to distinguish from all other defects. Echocardiographic visualization is best achieved in apical four-chamber scans. However, muscular defects located in the extreme apical aspect lie in the near field and may be easily overlooked. Therefore, addition scans should also be made from the subcostal position. Muscular defects may occur throughout the entire ventricular septum, and they may occur in combination with other defect types. Therefore, the entire septum must be carefully and systematically interrogated. Muscular defects get smaller in systole and become "invisible" for two-dimensional echocardiography. In this case, Doppler color flow imaging can usually demonstrate the jet through the defect.

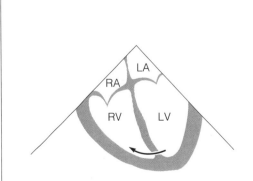

Small muscular ventricular septal defect located in the extreme apical IVS. The color flow map shows the jet passing through the defect, from the LV to the RV. In apical four-chamber scans, apically located defects lie in the near field of the transducer and may therefore be overlooked.

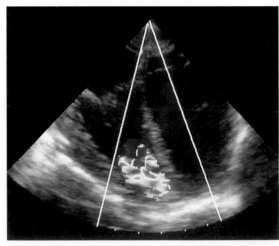

Transesophageal short-axis (transverse) scan with color flow mapping.

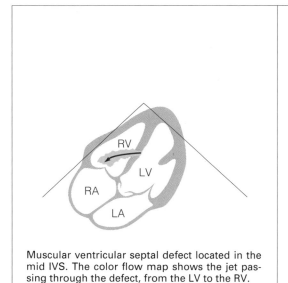

Muscular ventricular septal defect located in the mid IVS. The color flow map shows the jet passing through the defect, from the LV to the RV.

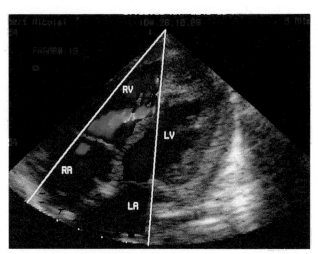

Apical four-chamber scan with color flow mapping.

When there is only a minimal residual halo of myocardium around the muscular ventricular septal defect, it can be difficult to impossible to differentiate it from other defect types. However, such differentiation is only of theoretical interest and has no practical relevance.

| 8.6 | Ventricular Septal Defects |
| 8.6.3 | Perimembranous Ventricular Septal Defects |

Perimembranous defects are the most common type of ventricular septal defects. The upper margin of the defect is usually formed by the fibrous continuity between the aortic valve and the tricuspid valve ring. Viewed from the right ventricular aspect, perimembranous defects can usually be found below the septal tricuspid leaflet. They are often covered with tricuspid valvular tissue.

Spontaneous closure of perimembranous defects occurs in cases where tricuspid valvular tissue adheres to the defect. In the course of this spontaneous closure, a "pocket" of tricuspid valvular tissue develops. This pocket of tissue, resembling a sail, protrudes from the left ventricular outflow tract into the right ventricle. Because of its "aneurysmal" appearance, such pocket formations are sometimes classified as "septum membranaceum aneurysm", although it is not a true aneurysm.

Echocardiography can visualize most perimembranous defects located in the parasternal long axis and in subaortic regions. Viewed from the right ventricle, perimembranous defects can extend in three directions: to the AV septum, to the apical septum, or to the right ventricular outflow tract. The linear extent of perimembranous defects is best appreciated in the parasternal long-axis view.

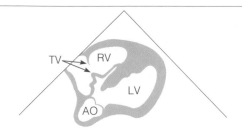

Perimembranous ventricular septal defect located below the aortic valve (AO) in the IVS. The septal leaflet of the tricuspid valve (TV) borders on the defect and partially covers the defect. In motion, parts of this leaflet are immobile, and are joined to the IVS. This covering and adhesion of tricuspid valvular tissue commonly leads to spontaneous closure of the ventricular septal defect. Tricuspid valvular tissue protruding from the LA into the RA is classified as a septum membranaceum aneurysm, although it is not a true aneurysm.

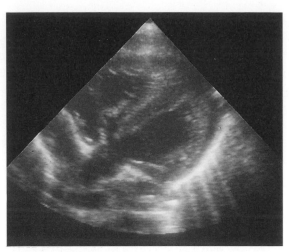

Apical four-chamber scan.

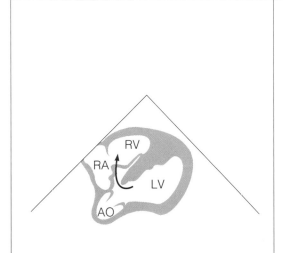

The color flow map reveals a left-to-right shunt through the ventricular septal defect.

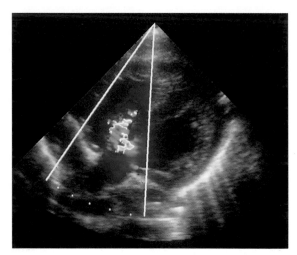

Color flow map of apical four-chamber scan.

Since the noncoronary aortic valve cusp is immediately adjacent to the upper margin of the perimembranous ventricular septal defect, the cusp may prolapse into the defect. Therefore, the possibility of aortic insufficiency due to a prolapsing aortic valve cusp must always be evaluated during echocardiographic diagnosis of perimembranous ventricular septal defects. Doppler color flow imaging and PW Doppler are used for this purpose. Two-dimensional echocardiography can often demonstrate the increased mobility of the prolapsing aortic valve cusp.

A special type of ventricular septal defect is the *doubly committed defect*. The upper margin of this defect is formed by the juxtaposition of the pulmonary and aortic valves. Doubly committed defects are possible only in cases where the aortic and pulmonic valves lie directly adjacent to one another. In other words, both great arteries must arise from a single (double outlet) ventricle. Straddling of semilunar valves is also common, *i.e.*, the respective vessel overrides the ventricular septal defect. Theoretically, the ventricular septal defect in truncus arteriosus (communis) is also a doubly committed ventricular defect, because the truncus valve corresponds to both the aortic and pulmonic valves.

As was stated before, the above described morphological classification of ventricular septal defects is impractical for use in routine echocardiographic diagnosis. Therefore, a topographic classification for practical use is hereby presented. The ventricular septum is thereby divided into inlet, trabecular, and outlet segments.

Inlet septum defects that extend as far as the AV valve plane are usually classified as AV septal defects. Characteristically, the septal parts of the two AV valves insert at the same level and merge. Muscular ventricular septal defects can also be located in the inlet septum. These defects are clearly separated from the AV valve plane and the aortic valve by muscular tissue. If the defect extends as far as the tricuspid and aortic valves, and if the tricuspid valve inserts below the level of the mitral valve, the defect is a perimembranous ventricular septal defect that extends into the inlet septum.

Trabecular septum defects must, by definition, be surrounded on all sides by muscular septal tissue. Therefore, these defects are exclusively muscular ventricular septal defects. However, one must keep in mind that these defects commonly occur in combination with other defect types. Extremely large AV septal defects or perimembranous ventricular septal defects can also extend to the trabecular septum. However, they are neither limited to the trabecular septum nor easy to differentiate.

Outlet defects in the right ventricular outflow tract can be muscular, perimembranous, or doubly committed (juxta-arterial) defects. A muscular outlet defect exists when there is evidence of septal muscular tissue between the aortic and pulmonic valves and the defect. In perimembranous defects, the defect reaches as far as the aortic valve, but not the pulmonary valve. In contrast, juxta-arterial ventricular septal defects extend to reach both the pulmonary and aortic valves.

The aorta overriding a "subaortic" ventricular septal defect is not a morphological entity. In echocardiography, however, this is such a typical and diagnostically relevant finding, that it will be discussed separately.

Normally, the anterior wall of the aorta and the ventricular septum appear to merge and form a straight line when scanned from the parasternal long-axis view. When a subaortic ventricular septal defect exists, however, there is a "step" between the upper margin of the ventricular septum and the aortic anterior wall, and the aorta overrides the ventricular septal defect. Therefore, it no longer arises exclusively from the left ventricle. The extent of overriding, which is quantified as a percentage of the aortic diameter, varies.

This defect is a guiding sign in the diagnosis of tetralogy of Fallot, pulmonary atresia with ventricular septal defect, truncus arteriosus communis, and double outlet right ventricle (DORV). When transposition of the great arteries exists, the pulmonary artery may also override the ventricular septal defect (Taussig-Bing syndrome, DORV). From a purely morphological point of view, the majority of these defects (with the exception of most DORV / juxta-arterial defects) are perimembranous defects that extend in to the outlet septum.

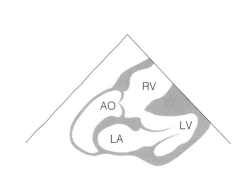

"Subaortic" ventricular septal defect (VSD) over-ridden by the aorta (AO). The defect is directly below the AO, which extends across and over-rides the defect. This clinically significant finding is a guiding sign in the diagnosis of tetralogy of Fallot, pulmonary atresia with ventricular septal defect, truncus arteriosus communis, and double outlet ventricles.

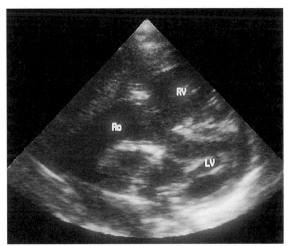

Subcostal four-chamber scan.

Gerbode's defect is a defect in the membranous atrioventricular septum. Because the tricuspid valve normally inserts below the mitral valve (except in AV septal defects), a potential communication between the left ventricle and right atrium exists between the insertions of the two AV valves. Due to the small size of the membranous septum, Gerbode's defects are usually small. However, an extensive left-to-right shunt still exists due to the great difference in pressures in the left ventricle and the right atrium. The diagnosis is made using Doppler color flow imaging. The jet passing from the left ventricle to the right atrium must be differentiated from tricuspid insufficiency.

Last to be discussed are ventricular septal defects that occur in a *"univentricular" heart* in which only one ventricle has developed normally. In addition to one main, or dominant, ventricle, there usually is also a rudimentary ventricle lacking connection to the atria. The rudimentary ventricle is almost always filled via a defect in the ventricular septum. This defect, which provides the only means of diastolic filling of the rudimentary ventricle, is not comparable to a defect between two normal ventricles. Therefore, it is not classified as a ventricular septal defect, but as an interventricular foramen. Univentricular heart will be discussed in detail in Section 8.8.

As was described above, AV septal defects are commonly associated with anomalies of the atrioventricular valve and atrial septum, whereas doubly committed (juxta-arterial) ventricular septal defects occur almost exclusively in double outlet left and right ventricles (DORV and DOLV). Septum membranaceum aneurysm and aortic insufficiency caused by a prolapsing aortic valve cusp secondary to a perimembranous ventricular septal defect have also been discussed.

Additional accompanying anomalies include right ventricular hypertrophy secondary to infundibular, muscular outflow tract obstruction. Usually, such RVOT obstructions recede after surgical or spontaneous closure of the defect. Surgery is indicated when RVOT obstruction persists after spontaneous defect closure.

Isolated ventricular septal defects, particularly AV septal defects and trisomy 21, are commonly associated with a patent ductus arteriosus. Muscular ventricular septal defects are commonly associated with coarctation of the aorta. Juxta-arterial ventricular septal defects are commonly associated with discontinuity of the aortic arch.

| 8.7 | Anomalous Origin of the Great Arteries |
| 8.7.1 | Transposition of the Great Arteries |

Instead of discussing the various theories on the embryology and classification of transposition of the great arteries, we will concentrate on the original, simple definition of the term: In transposition of the great arteries, the positions of the aorta and pulmonary artery have been "switched" in absence of any further anatomical cardiac abnormalities. The aorta arises from the right ventricle, and the pulmonary artery arises from the left ventricle. In almost all cases, the aorta lies in front of the pulmonary artery.

Dextrotransposition (D-transposition) of the great arteries exists when the aorta lies in front of and to the right of the pulmonary artery. *Corrected transposition* (mixed levocardia) exists when the aorta lies to the left of the pulmonary artery.

Echocardiographic diagnosis of transposition of the great arteries is relatively simple. First, it must be demonstrated that the aorta arises from the right ventricle instead of from the left ventricle, in the presence of otherwise normal cardiac anatomy. Secondly, it must be demonstrated that the pulmonary artery arises from the left ventricle instead of from the right ventricle. These findings fulfil the criteria for diagnosis of corrected transposition (L-transposition) and D-transposition.

In D-transposition of the great arteries, the lack of communication between the pulmonary and systemic circulatory systems results in cyanosis. The echocardiographic diagnosis is made by identifying the switched position of the great arteries. In normal individuals, the pulmonary aorta arises on the right and in front of the aorta, and extends towards the left in front of the aorta. In transposition of the great arteries, a bifurcation in the artery that arises posteriorly can be visualized well from a subcostal or parasternal view. This bifurcation is the morphological identifier of the pulmonary artery. This therefore proves that the artery that arises posteriorly and from the left ventricle is the pulmonary artery.

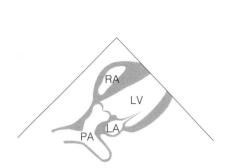

D-transposition of the great arteries. The pulmonary artery (PA) arises from the left ventricle (LV). The LV is characterized by a continuity between the semilunar and AV valves. The PA can be identified by its bifurcation.

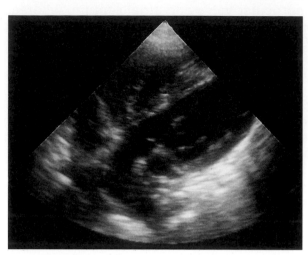

Subcostal four-chamber scan.

The aortic and pulmonic valves can often be visualized together in the parasternal short-axis plane; the anterior semilunar valve is located somewhat to the right of the posterior semilunar valve. The posterior semilunar valve has a typically star-shaped configuration in D-transposition, in contrast with the Y-shaped configuration in normal individuals. The aortic arch can best be visualized from the supraclavicular position. The vessels arising from the aortic arch are an unmistakable feature of the aortic arch. The aorta is located in front of the pulmonary artery and arises from the right ventricle. In newborns, Botallo's duct extends from the pulmonary artery and connects directly to the descending aorta. Therefore, this "Botallo's arch" may be mistaken for the aortic arch. In order to avoid this mistake, identification of the aortic arch should always be made by visualization of the aortic arch vessels.

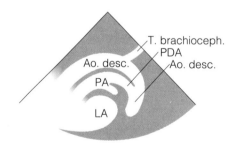

Transposition of the great arteries. The position of the aorta typically in front of the pulmonary artery (PA) is characteristic of D-transposition, corrected transposition, and "malposition". The aortic arch can be unequivocally identified by the aortic origin of the brachiocephalic trunk and thereby differentiated from a patent ductus arteriosus (PDA). A PDA is located between the PA and the descending aorta.

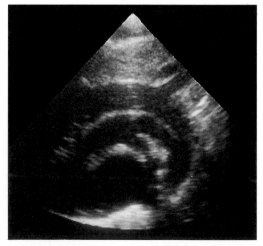

Suprasternal long-axis scan.

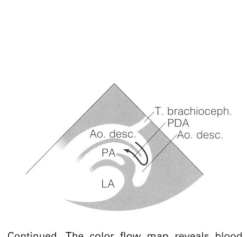

Continued. The color flow map reveals blood flow through the PDA, which proceeds from the AO into the PA.

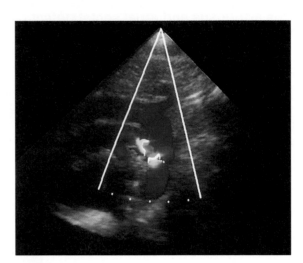

Color flow map of suprasternal long-axis scan.

After echocardiographically identifying the transposition of the great arteries, both arteries must be followed to their origins in order to visualized their connection to the ventricle. The anterior vessel (which was identified as the aorta) arises from the anterior ventricle. The posterior vessel (which was identified as the pulmonary artery) arises from the posterior ventricle. Although, in normal individuals, the posterior ventricle is the anatomical right ventricle, and the posterior ventricle is the anatomical left ventricle, the anatomical relationships are switched in transposition of the great vessels. Therefore, it must be demonstrated that the anterior ventricle is actually the anatomical right ventricle, and that the posterior ventricle is the anatomical left ventricle.

An anatomical left ventricle is characterized by continuity between the anterior mitral leaflet and the posterior wall of the artery arising from the left ventricle. In other words, there is no muscular tissue between the artery and the mitral valve, i.e., there is continuity between the two structures. A right ventricle, in contrast, is characterized by the presence of muscular tissue between the tricuspid valve and the artery arising from the right ventricle. The two structures are thereby separated, i.e., there is discontinuity. This muscular tissue separates the right ventricular inflow and outflow tracts, and it can be visualized echocardiography by adjusting the view for simultaneous visualization of the right ventricular inflow and outflow tracts. An additional characteristic identifier of the right ventricle is the moderator band, which can be appreciated in the four-chamber view.

The main reason for early diagnosis of D-transposition of the great arteries is not merely to start early treatment, but to perform corrective surgery as soon as possible. Preferably, corrective surgery should be performed within the first two weeks of life. The great arteries are transsected and "switched", and the coronary ostia from the anterior vessels are transferred to the posterior vessel. In order for surgical repair to be successful, the patient must have a suitable coronary anatomy, and the left ventricle must be capable of supplying the systemic circulatory system. The left ventricle supplies the pulmonary artery, which rapidly loses pressure after birth. Therefore, the postnatal left ventricle quickly loses its ability to the supply systemic circulation. In echocardiography, this is appreciated as increasing protrusion of the ventricular septum from the right ventricle into the left ventricle.

Simple D-transposition exists when there is no associated cardiac anomaly. In this case, patent ductus arteriosus and atrial septal defect do not count as associated anomalies, because survival is possible only if such a defect provides a mixing site for venous and atrial blood. Infusions of prostaglandin E1 can be administered to maintain patency of the ductus arteriosus.

If the atrial septal defect is too small, it can be enlarged during the neonatal period by means of balloon atrioseptostomy. Balloon atrioseptostomy is usually successful and effective when the atrial septal defect is one-third the length of the atrial septum, as visualized in the subcostal four-chamber view.

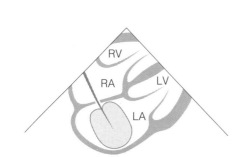

Balloon atrioseptostomy (BAS) performed under echocardiographic control. In some cardiac defects (D-transposition, mitral atresia, etc.), BAS is performed to improve mixing of atrial and venous blood, or to provide an drainage out of the LA. At most hospitals today, BAS is usually performed under echocardiographic control instead of in the cardiac catheterization laboratory.

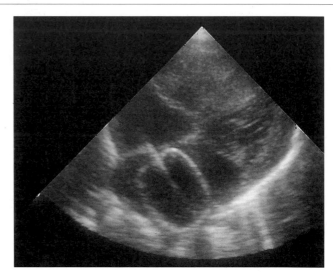

Subcostal four-chamber scan.

Complex D-transposition exists when associated anomalies other than patent ductus arteriosus or atrial septal defect occur. Most commonly, there are one or more ventricular septal defects, particularly muscular defects. These defects are significant when planning anatomic correction, because they provide mixing sites for venous and atrial blood and increase the pressure in the left ventricle, thereby keeping it "fit". Surgical repair of associated ventricular septal defects can be performed after the second week of life. The pressure gradient across the defect can be measured by cardiac Doppler. The gradient can then be used to estimate the left ventricular pressure, which should more than 70% higher than the pressure in the right ventricle.

Subpulmonary stenoses (stenoses in the left ventricular outflow tract) are of great significance, because they often make surgical repair difficult or impossible to perform. Subpulmonary stenoses are often muscular in nature, and are caused solely by protrusion of the ventricular septum into the left ventricle. They therefore revert after surgery. However, fibrous or fibromuscular stenoses are found in some patients. These stenoses must be resected during surgery.

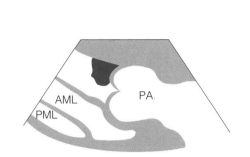

Left ventricular outflow tract obstruction in D-transposition. A fibromuscular "bulge" located immediately below the pulmonary valve causes localized subpulmonary stenosis and left ventricular tract obstruction.

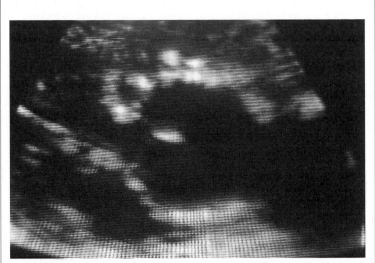

Parasternal long-axis scan.

Anatomic correction is not possible in stenosis of the pulmonary valve, which postoperatively becomes the aortic valve. If there is an associated ventricular septal defect in addition to pulmonary stenosis, the Rastelli procedure can be performed for surgical repair. In this procedure, the ventricular septal defect is closed in such a manner as to restore left ventricular and aortic continuity. The pulmonary artery is transsected, and a conduit is inserted between the distal main pulmonary artery and the right ventricle, so as to restore right ventricular and pulmonary artery continuity.

In corrected transposition of the great arteries, the aorta is located to the left and in front of the pulmonary artery. As in D-transposition, the aorta arises from the anatomical right ventricle, and the pulmonary artery arises from the morphological left ventricle. In corrected transposition, however, the ventricles are "switched": the right ventricle is connected to the left atrium (via a tricuspid valve), and the left ventricle is connected to the right atrium via a mitral valve. Therefore, the pulmonary artery receives venous blood, even though it arises from the left ventricle, and the aorta receives arterial blood from the left atrium even through it arises from the right ventricle. The transposition is therefore said to be "corrected". Atrioventricular and ventriculo-arterial discordance exists in corrected transposition of the great arteries.

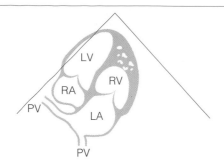

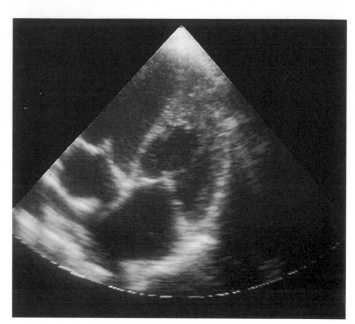

Ventricular inversion in corrected transposition. The atria are located normally, but the ventricles are inverted. The right ventricle (RV) is located below the left atrium LA, which can be identified by the openings of the pulmonary veins (PV). The RV can be identified by the mitral valve, which inserts lower, and the apical moderator band. Additionally, discontinuity between the aortic valve and semilunar valve can be visualized in the parasternal long-axis view. The RA can be identified by the openings of the venae cavae and hepatic veins, which are not visualized here. They can be visualized by slightly angulating the int transducer. The RA opens into the LV. The LV can be identified by the mitral valve, which inserts higher, by the absence of a moderator band, and by the continuity between the AV and semilunar valve (viewed from the long axis).

Apical four-chamber scan.

As in D-transposition, echocardiography reveals that the aorta is in front of the pulmonary artery, but arises to the left and in front of the pulmonary artery. In corrected transposition, however, the anatomical left atrium is connected to the right ventricle. The pulmonary veins drain into the atrium on the left, which opens into the anatomical right ventricle. The superior and inferior venae cavae drain into the right atrium, which opens into an anatomical left ventricle. The anatomical right ventricle can be identified by the visualization of a moderator band and by inflow and outflow tract discontinuity. The anatomical left ventricle is identified by continuity between the posterior wall of the pulmonary artery and the anterior mitral leaflet. The abnormal position and abnormal hemodynamic stresses on the two ventricles makes it difficult to visualize the ventricular septum. Frequently, it is not possible to visualize the ventricular septum in the parasternal long-axis view.

Valvular pulmonary stenosis is a common associated anomaly. CW Doppler is helpful in determining the pressure gradient. Because the pulmonary artery is the posterior vessel, pulmonary stenosis can be mistaken for aortic stenosis when the echocardiographer is unaware that corrected transposition exists. Ventricular septal defects, which are most frequently located in the subpulmonary region, may also occur. Tricuspid valve dysplasia (TVD) is another possible associated anomaly. In TVD the septal or inferior leaflet of the tricuspid valve displaces into the right ventricle (Ebstein's malformation), which can lead to extensive tricuspid insufficiency. When the diagnosis of corrected transposition is not known, the resulting tricuspid insufficiency can easily be mistaken for mitral insufficiency.

Malposition of the great arteries exists when the anatomy of the great arteries corresponds to the position observed in transposition, but the connections of the great arteries to the ventricles do not meet the definition of transposition. In other words, the aorta lies in front of the pulmonary artery. However, the aorta does not arise from the right ventricle, or the pulmonary artery does not arise from the left ventricle. Malposition of the great arteries also exists when both arteries arise side-by-side from the anterior (double outlet) ventricle.

This distinction is important, not only with regard to nomenclature. Communication between the great arteries and the ventricles is of decisive hemodynamic significance. Malposition is observed in complex cardiac anomalies such as double outlet right or left ventricle or "uni-ventricular" heart (only one ventricle is normal, while the other is only rudimentary).

8.7	Anomalous Origin of the Great Arteries
8.7.2	Double Outlet Ventricles (DORV, DOLV),
	and Overriding of a Great Artery

In contrast with transposition of the great arteries, where both arteries arise from the "wrong" ventricle, both arteries arise from the same ventricle in double outlet ventricles. In double outlet ventricles, the orientation of the great arteries may be normal, or they may demonstrate dextro- or corrected transposition.

Double outlet right ventricle (DORV) is common, whereas double outlet left ventricle (DOLV) is extremely rare. The two types are differentiated on the basis of the anatomy of the ventricle.

Echocardiography is often superior to angiography for demonstration of double outlet right ventricle, because of its better ability to demonstrate the spatial relationship of the semilunar valves and the ventricular septum. The origins of the two arteries can usually be visualized in the parasternal short-axis view, whereby the semilunar valves are seen in front of the ventricular septum.

In double outlet right ventricle, the semilunar valve are usually located adjacently and at the same level. There is commonly an associated ventricular septal defect, which is usually of the juxta-arterial type. Because both arteries arise from the right ventricle, the ventricular septal defect provides the sole "outlet" for the left ventricle. Blood flow through the defect can be visualized using Doppler color flow imaging. By slightly angulating the transducer, the spatial relationship of the defect and the arteries can be studied from both parasternal and apical four-chamber views.

In the past, arterial and mitral valve discontinuity was interpreted as an sign of double outlet right ventricle. Although this is a very helpful indication, it alone is not diagnostic of DORV. The more essential indication is proof that both arteries arise from a single ventricle, which means following both arteries down to their origins. In almost all cases, it is possible to demonstrate the exact origin of the two arteries and to visualize one of the arteries overriding the ventricular septal defect. An overriding great vessel is defined as one whose origin straddles the ventricular septal defect. Overriding can be specified in terms of percentage of vessel diameter. The parasternal long-axis view is well suited for this purpose. The artery is always classified according to the ventricle that is predominantly arises from.

8.7   **Anomalous Origin of the Great Arteries**
8.7.2   **Double Outlet Ventricles (DORV, DOLV),**
and Overriding of a Great Artery

344

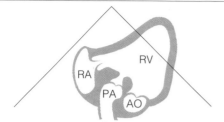

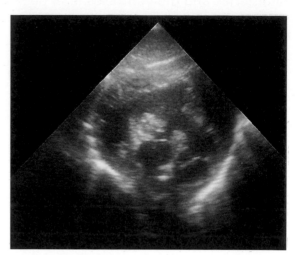

Double outlet right ventricle (DORV). Both the aorta (AO) and pulmonary artery (PA) arise from the right ventricle (RV). Under both semilunar valves, there is muscular tissue corresponding to an infundibulum (bilateral infundibulum). A teardrop shaped mass of muscular tissue from between the two arteries protrudes into the RV. This "teardrop" is a classical angiographic indication of DORV. The AO arises in front of the PA, *i.e.*, there is malposition. The origin and spatial relationship of the two arteries must be assessed in another scanning plane, *i.e.*, by rotating the transducer 90° along its axis from the parasternal or suprasternal position.

Subcostal four-chamber scan.

Subcostal scanning is very helpful in assessing the spatial relationships of the two ventricles, the great arteries, and the ventricular septal defect. However, many errors are made by inexperiences echocardiographers. The majority of false echocardiographic diagnoses occur due to misinterpretation of the spatial relationship between the ventricle and artery seen in subcostal scans.

Although the position of the vessels can, theoretically, be normal in double outlet right ventricle, malposition usually exists. Frequently, the large arteries are not located one in front of the other, but side-by-side. An infundibulum is commonly found under the two great arteries. In this case, a fibromuscular structure can be identified between the arteries. This structure protrudes into the right ventricle and separates the two infundibula. In angiography, this is called a "teardrop" structure, because of its characteristic appearance. In most cases where both arteries arises side by side, their origins can be visualized only from the subcostal position. Subcostal studies often are also the only means of visualizing the infundibulum underneath the two arteries (Doppler "cone").

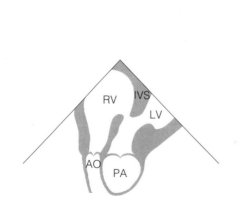

Double outlet right ventricle. Both the AO and PA arise from the RV. A ventricular septal defect provides the sole outlet for the LV.

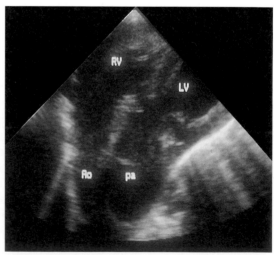

Subcostal four-chamber scan.

Echocardiography is an excellent technique for studying the spatial relationship of a ventricular septal defect to the great arteries. When planning anatomical correction, it is essential to know whether the ventricular septal defect is in direct communication with the pulmonary artery, the aorta, or both vessels. The size of the defect is also a decisive factor for the success of surgical correction. Not only must the defect must have a close relationship to the aorta, it must also be large enough to later function as the left ventricular outflow tract.

A large variety of associated lesions may coexist with DORV. The most common are pulmonary stenosis and pulmonary atresia. The degree of pulmonary stenosis should be quantitated in a continuous Doppler study, in order to obtain an estimate of pulmonary arterial pressure. In the absence of pulmonary stenosis, pulmonary hypertension tends to develop at an early age. Therefore, pulmonary stenosis "protects" the pulmonary circulation in patients with double outlet right ventricle. Atrioventricular valve dysplasia with abnormal inserting chordae tendineae in the ventricular septal defect are not uncommon.

The characteristic feature of *truncus arteriosus (communis)* is the lack of separation of the aorta and pulmonary artery. Thus, the aorta, pulmonary arteries, and coronary arteries originate from one great artery. Pulmonary atresia, another malformation in which only one vessel arises from the heart, must be excluded from the diagnosis. In contrast to truncus arteriosus, pulmonary atresia is characterized by absence of the pulmonary arteries.

There are four types of truncus arteriosus:

Type I   A single pulmonary artery arises from the truncus
Type II The right and left pulmonary arteries arise close together but independently from the truncus
Type III The right and left pulmonary arteries arise independently from opposite sides of the truncus
Type IV Absence of pulmonary arteries; today type IV is no longer considered to be a form of truncus arteriosus, but rather is a type of pulmonary atresia with ventricular septal defect.

In truncus arteriosus, the truncus "overrides" an obligatory ventricular septal defect. The overriding truncus can be visualized best in the parasternal long-axis view. The common origin of the aorta and pulmonary arteries from the truncus can also be visualized well in parasternal long and short-axis views. Additionally, the truncus can also be visualized in suprasternal notch or (in newborns and infants) subcostal scans.

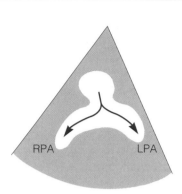

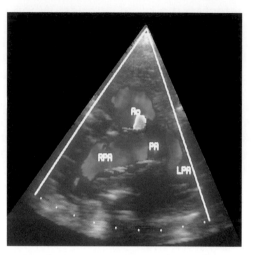

Truncus arteriosus communis. The left (LPA) and right (RPA) pulmonary arteries arise together from the aorta (AO), *i.e.*, truncus arteriosus. The AO and PA are not separate, but form a common vessels, the truncus arteriosus communis.

Parasternal short-axis scan with color flow mapping.

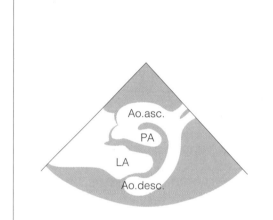

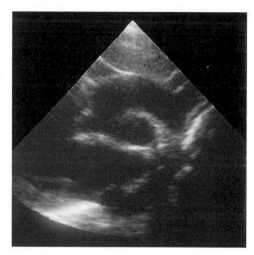

Truncus arteriosus communis. Division of the truncus into the ascending aorta (Ao. asc.) and PA, immediately superior to the truncus valve.

Suprasternal long-axis scan.

Truncus arteriosus can be unequivocally differentiated from pulmonary atresia by demonstrating the truncal origin of the pulmonary arteries. A typical feature of truncus arteriosus is a quadricuspid semilunar valve, but this is neither obligatory, nor is it diagnostic of truncus arteriosus. The valve is commonly incompetent.

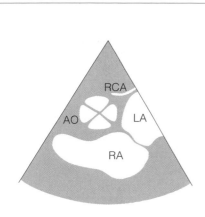

Quadricuspid truncus valve. Truncus arteriosus is virtually the only cardiac anomaly in which a quadricuspid valve occurs. Quadricuspid valves are often incompetent. RCA = right coronary

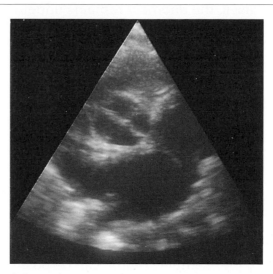

Parasternal short-axis scan.

Associated lesions: A patent ductus arteriosus is present in around 50% of all patients with truncus arteriosus. Pulmonary atresia is a rare associated lesion with patent ductus arteriosus. Interruption of the aortic arch is a relatively common associated lesion (10-19 %).

Pulmonary hypertension develops early (within the first months of life) in patients with truncus arteriosus. In patients without hypertension, Doppler reveals systolic-diastolic flow in the pulmonary arteries. However, when pulmonary hypertension occurs, only systolic flow occurs.

8.7   **Anomalous Origin of the Great Arteries**
8.7.4   **Aortopulmonary Window**

An *aortopulmonary window* is characterized by incomplete separation of the aorta and pulmonary artery, *i.e.,* direct communication between the two arteries exists. This communication is best demonstrated in the parasternal short-axis view. Doppler color flow imaging reveals a color jet extending from the aorta to the pulmonary artery. A bidirectional shunt develops when pulmonary hypertension occurs. However, this is difficult to visualize, even with the help of Doppler color flow imaging.

8.7   **Anomalous Origin of the Great Arteries**
8.7.5   **Patent Ductus Arteriosus**

Patent ductus arteriosus (PDA) is not a cardiac anomaly, but a patent, normal fetal vessel. In many cardiac anomalies, survival would not be possible if the ductus arteriosus were to close. In other words, these anomalies are compatible with life only in the presence of a patent ductus arteriosus.

In many cases, the anomaly remains undetected until the ductus arteriosus starts to close in the first days to weeks of life. Examples include D-transposition of the great arteries (early closure of the PDA within 2 to 3 days), pulmonary atresia, tetralogy of Fallot (closure of PDA within 1 to 2 weeks), coarctation of the aorta, and aortic stenosis (closure of PDA within 5 to 10 days).

Patent ductus arteriosus is best studied from suprasternal notch and supraclavicular positions, whereby the aortic arch and pulmonary artery serve as orientational structures. The two vessels are usually connected by the ductus arteriosus in such a way that the ductus arteriosus forms a direct extension of the pulmonary artery. The PDA extends like a second aortic arch and connects to the descending aorta. This "ductus arch" is sometimes mistaken for the aortic arch (differential diagnosis of D-transposition). The aortic arch is distinguished from the PDA by the vessels that exit the aortic arch. Doppler color flow imaging reveals systolic-diastolic flow through the PDA. In any case, this typical flow profile should be verified using pulsed Doppler. When it is not possible to directly visualize the ductus arteriosus, color Doppler can usually reveal the typical flow profile in the pulmonary artery. Alternatively, the pulsed Doppler sample volume can be positioned at the site where the left pulmonary artery exits from the main pulmonary trunk. In patients with pulmonary hypertension, the flow profile changes from systolic-diastolic to purely systolic flow.

In newborns and infants the patent ductus arteriosus can usually be visualized from the subcostal position. In ventilated patients, overdistension of the lungs obstructs scanning from the supraclavicular and parasternal routes. Then, the subcostal position is often the available portal for visualizing the ductus arteriosus.

A patent ductus arteriosus (PDA) is essential for survival in a number of congenital heart defects, which are listed below.

Group 1   Coarctation of the aorta, interrupted aortic arch, hypoplastic left ventricle
In coarctation of the aorta and interrupted aortic arch, the descending aorta is located posterior to the stenosis or interruption, or it is insufficiently perfused. The PDA ensures perfusion of the aorta posterior to the stenosis or interruption. In hypoplastic left ventricle, the PDA provides the means of perfusion of the entire systemic circulatory system.

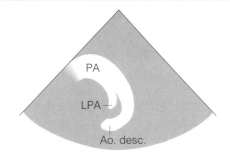

Persistent ductus arteriosus (PDA) in a hypoplastic left ventricle. The PDA forms a direct continuation of the PA. The origin of the ductus is identified by the exit of the LPA. The aortic arch lies outside of this scan plane. The PA, PDA, and descending aorta for an "arch" that can be easily mistaken for the aortic arch, especially with lesser quality images, as in this case. Therefore, the origins of vessels exiting the aortic arch must be visualized to identify the aortic arch and the PDA.

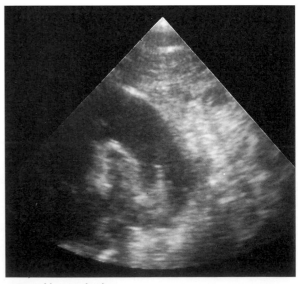

Suprasternal long-axis view.

Group 2 D-transposition of the great arteries

In D-transposition of the great arteries, the systemic and pulmonary circulatory systems do not communicate. Therefore, a patent ductus arteriosus or a patent foramen ovale provide the only site for mixing of arterial and venous blood.

Group 3 Pulmonary atresia, tetralogy of Fallot

A patent ductus arteriosus provides the only means of pulmonary artery perfusion in pulmonary atresia with ventricular septal defect, and it provides the primary means of perfusion in tetralogy of Fallot. In this group, atypical origin and course of the ductus is common. The ductus usually arises from the aortic arch rather than in the region of the isthmus. Then it proceeds caudad to the pulmonary artery. In this case, it does not resemble a continuation of the pulmonary artery. However, pulmonary atresia with an intact ventricular septum and in critical pulmonary stenosis, the ductus extends as described in group 1.

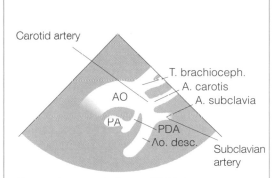

Patent ductus arteriosus (PDA) in pulmonary atresia. In pulmonary atresia or tetralogy of Fallot, the PDA often arises prematurely from the aortic arch (AO). Then, it does not continue parallel to the AO as a continuation of the pulmonary artery (PA), but runs almost perpendicular to the AO and parallel to the descending aorta.

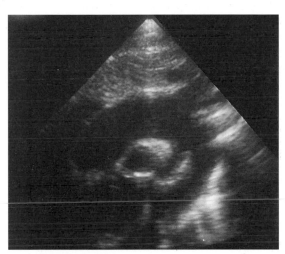

Suprasternal long-axis scan.

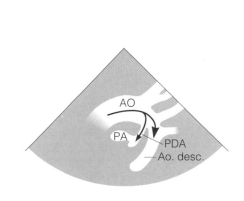

Continued. The Doppler color flow map reveals turbulent flow in the PDA. In addition to pulmonary atresia, there is malposition of the great arteries.

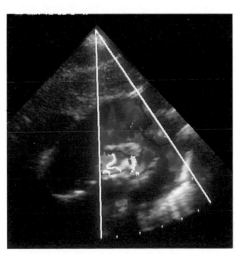

Color flow map of the suprasternal long-axis scan.

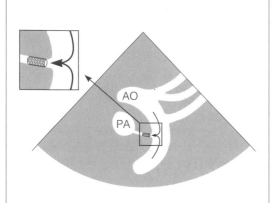

Palmaz stent in patent ductus arteriosus (PDA) in pulmonary atresia. The metallic Palmaz stent appears on the color flow map as a highly echo reflective region around the PDA. This disturbance makes it impossible to assess the scan.

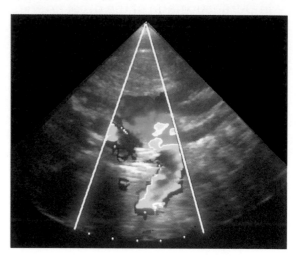

Suprasternal long-axis scan with color flow mapping.

Another special type of PDA is bilateral Botallo's duct. Embryologically, Botallo's duct arises from the sixth pharyngeal arch artery. Because the arch arteries arise in pairs, the right-sided ductus usually recedes when a left descending aorta is formed. In the presence of a left descending aorta, the left Botallo's duct arises from the region of the aortic isthmus, and the right Botallo's duct arises from the right subclavian artery. However, in the presence of a right descending aorta, the right Botallo's duct arises from the region of the aortic isthmus, and the left Botallo's duct arises from the left subclavian artery.

| 8.7 | Anomalous Origin of the Great Arteries |
| 8.7.6 | Coarctation of the Aorta and Interrupted Aortic Arch |

Coarctation of the aorta is defined as a narrowing in the region of the distal aortic arch, *i.e.*, the aortic isthmus. Coarctation is usually congenital, but may also occur postnatally, due to a contracture of ductus tissue. Coarctation may also worsen postnatally after ductus tissue contracture.

The region of the aortic isthmus can be visualized by in suprasternal notch or supraclavicular echocardiograms. It can also be visualized from the parasternal position in newborns and young infants, who have a large imaging window created by the thymus. Echocardiographic visualization of the isthmus from the subcostal position is also possible in these patients and in ventilated patients with restricted windows. Usually, narrowing of the isthmus can be visualized only in two-dimensional echocardiograms. However, because closely positioned, air-filled structures such as the trachea, bifurcation, and esophagus often create artifacts, a diagnosis based on 2-D echocardiography alone must be made with caution. Coarctation of the aorta can be identified by the pressure gradient across the isthmus region, which is demonstrated as flow acceleration in pulsed or continuous-wave Doppler studies. A low flow amplitude in the abdominal aorta is an indirect sign of coarctation of the aorta.

Coarctation of the aorta causes reduced perfusion of poststenotic regions, which may result in underperfusion of the liver. In newborns perfusion of the poststenotic region is almost maintained by a patent ductus arteriosus. This function is assumed by the collateral vessels after the ductus closes. The collateral vessels thus "bypass" the coarctation of the aorta, but they cannot be visualized by echocardiography.

Coarctation of the aorta may be either tubular or circumscript. In good quality echocardiograms, both types can be distinguished. In some cases, the aortic isthmus is so severely stenotic that it is functionally occluded (atresia). The pressure gradient cannot be detected in these patients, because of the lack of blood flow across the aortic isthmus. The following types of coarctation of the aorta are classified according to location:

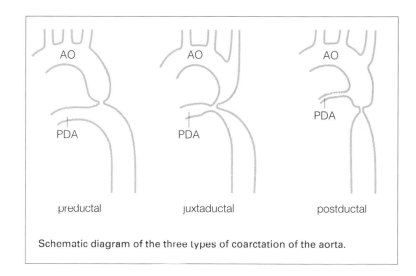

Schematic diagram of the three types of coarctation of the aorta.

1. **Preductal coarctation of the aorta**
   The majority of coarctations are preductal, *i.e.*, the coarctation is located above the origin of the ductus arteriosus. Preductal coarctations are most common in newborns. Perfusion for the lower half of the body is maintained by means of a patent ductus arteriosus.

2. **Juxtaductal coarctation of the aorta**
   The aortic isthmus is located opposite from the origin of the ductus arteriosus. This duct has basically the same hemodynamic effects as a preductal coarctation. However, closure of the ductus increases the degree of stenosis.

3. **Postductal coarctation of the aorta**
   Postductal coarctation is rare. In this case, coarctation is located distal to the origin of the ductus arteriosus. Because the ductus enters the proximal to the constriction, the lower body must be supplied by means of collateral circulation. This used to be defined as "adult" coarctation, as compared with "infantile" coarctation. However, this classification is questionable, mainly because it usually is not possible to detect the origin of the ductus in adults. Postductal coarctation of the aorta is very rare in newborns. These infants usually already have extensive collateral vessels to bypass the constriction of the coarctation of the aorta.

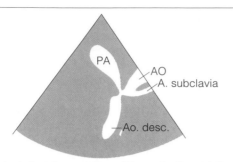

Juxtaductal coarctation of the aorta. Constriction of the aortic isthmus directly across from the PDA, which also narrows distally. The posterior segment of the aortic arch (AO) and the subclavian artery (A. subclavia) are positioned above the constriction. The descending aorta (Ao. desc.) is positioned underneath the constriction. Overshadowing caused by air in the esophagus and tracheal bifurcation often makes it difficult to visualize the isthmus region, which can be identified better in moving imaging than in static images.

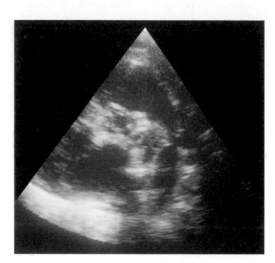

Parasternal long-axis scan.

In newborns, coarctation of the aorta is frequently associated with tubular hypoplasia of the aortic arch, which is hypoplastic from the origin of the innominate artery to the constriction of the aortic isthmus. Tubular hypoplasia of the aortic arch causes additional constriction and, thus, to flow acceleration prior to the original constriction. In this case, the Bernoulli equation can no longer be used to determine the gradient across the isthmus.

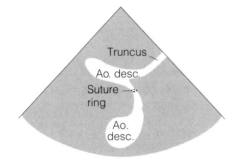

Tubular hypoplasia of the aortic arch after surgical correction of coarctation of the aorta (COA). In tubular hypoplasia, a constriction similar to that of COA develops. In this case, the preexisting COA was surgically corrected by resection and end-to-end anastomosis. The dotted line represents the suture ring.

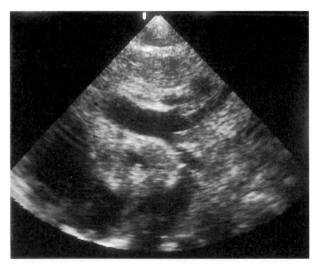

Suprasternal long-axis scan.

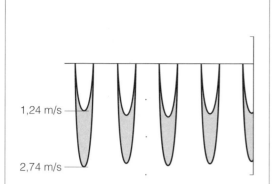

1,24 m/s

2,74 m/s

A CW Doppler recording was made at the suture site. The pressure gradient in the region of tubular hypoplasia appears as a second curve (1.24 m/s) on the Doppler spectral curve (2.74 m/s). The pressure gradient across the suture site is equal to the difference of the two velocities, in accordance with the complete Bernoulli equation.

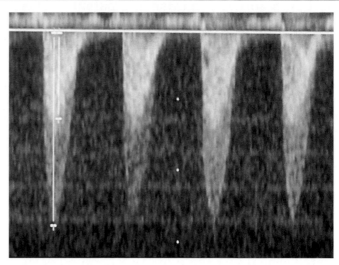

CW Doppler recording.

Although two-dimensional echocardiography provides the evidence suggestive of coarctation of the aorta, definitive proof is the demonstration of the pressure gradient or of flow acceleration across the suspected constriction. The following factors must be taken into consideration when measuring the pressure gradient across the isthmus.

1. Tubular hypoplasia of the aortic creates a gradient prior to the actual constriction of the isthmus. Flow velocity therefore is already increased prior to the isthmus constriction. The increased prestenotic velocity must, therefore, be taken into consideration when determining the pressure gradient across the isthmus. The complete Bernoulli equation, not the simplified version, must therefore be used for calculations.
2. When extensive collateral circulation has developed, the pressure in the lower extremities can be almost normal. Therefore, the pressure gradient across the constriction may be only slight.
3. The same effect may occur in conjunction with a very wide ductus arteriosus and increased pulmonary arterial pressure, which is normal in the postnatal phase. When the pressures in the aorta and pulmonary artery are equal, there is no pressure gradient across the constriction. In this case, contrast echocardiography may be helpful in demonstrating the leakage of contrast agent into the descending aorta. Doppler color flow imaging is usually able to demonstrate the flow of blood from the pulmonary artery to the descending aorta.
4. If the ductus arteriosus closes, a pressure gradient across the stenotic duct develops. This gradient can be mistaken for the gradient across the aortic isthmus. In order to avoid this mistake, the direction of flow must also be taken into consideration.
5. When there is no constriction, but rather atresia of the aortic isthmus, there is absolutely no flow across the isthmus. Therefore, no gradient can be detected.

Because of the number of sources of interpretational error, echocardiographic diagnosis of coarctation of the aorta must be performed very cautiously and critically. However, when the diagnosis has been made using a careful and systematic technique, corrective surgery of coarctation of the aorta can be performed without the need for further invasive diagnosis.

The hemodynamic effects of coarctation of the aorta vary greatly between newborns, young infants, and adults. In older children and adults, the ductus arteriosus is closed, and collateral vessels usually maintain perfusion of the lower body. Blood pressure prior to the constriction of the aortic isthmus is compensatorily increased in order to achieve adequate perfusion of the lower body. Extensive hypertrophy therefore results from the extreme pressure overload of the left ventricle.

In newborns and young infants, a patent ductus arteriosus ensures perfusion of the lower body, which causes pressure and volume overload occur in the right ventricle. Right ventricular pressure increases in order to increase the pulmonary arterial pressure. The RV volume increases to ensure perfusion of the lungs and the lower body.

Associated lesions commonly occur in coarctation of the aorta. Bicuspid aortic valve or aortic stenosis is common. Ventricular septal defects are also relatively common. Another associated lesion is Shone's complex, which is a combination of coarctation of the aorta and parachute mitral valve.

Aortic atresia is a severe form of left ventricular outflow tract obstruction. Anatomically, aortic atresia resembles coarctation of the aorta with primary or secondary closure of the residual lumen. Aortic atresia can be distinguished from coarctation of the aorta by the absence of all pressure gradients, as measured in PW and CW Doppler.

A difference in the flow profile of the aortic arch and the descending aorta can also be demonstrated. The flow profile in the ascending aorta and in the aortic arch are normal, whereas the profile in the descending aorta is flattened and has a marked portion of diastolic flow.

Interruption of the aortic arch is another severe form of LVOT obstruction. A patent ductus arteriosus provides perfusion of the aorta distal to the interruption. Interruption of the aortic arch is classified according to the location of the interruption. Type A - in the region of the aortic isthmus; type B - between the left common carotid artery and the left subclavian; type C - between the innominate artery and the left common carotid artery. The right subclavian artery or the innominate artery can be aberrant (*i.e.* it arises as last branch distal to the interruption) in all three types. Isolation of the right subclavian or innominate arteries is rare, but possible. Blood is supplied to the isolated vessel by means of the pulmonary artery and a persistent right ductus arteriosus.

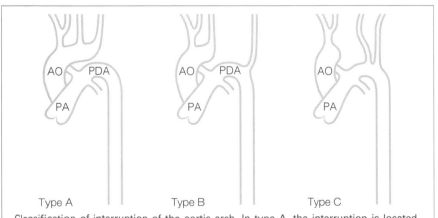

Type A Type B Type C

Classification of interruption of the aortic arch. In type A, the interruption is located behind the exit of the left subclavian artery in the region of the aortic isthmus. In type B, it is located between the left common carotid artery and the left subclavian artery. In type C, it is located between the innominate artery and the left common carotid artery.

In an interrupted aorta, echocardiography reveals a descending aorta perfused by a patent ductus arteriosus. Part of the aortic arch, corresponding to the site of interruption, cannot be visualized. Doppler color flow imaging provides visualization of the interruption of flow in the aortic arch. However, it sometimes is not possible to visualize a part of the aortic arch because of poor imaging conditions. Evidence of retrograde flow in the distal aorta (which occurs in types B and C), *i.e.*, behind the interruption, is strongly suggestive of interruption. With good quality images, the interruption of the aortic arch and the anatomy of the vessels of the aortic arch can be unequivocally assessed by echocardiography, which can then supplement or replace angiographic diagnosis.

Ventricular septal defects of the juxta-arterial type are also common associated cardiac anomalies. An interrupted aorta is commonly observed in conjunction with complex cardiac defects. Other associated cardiac anomalies include univentricular heart and double outlet right ventricle.

Ring and loop formations around the trachea and/or esophagus are clinically diagnosed (radiologically or angiographically) as congenital stridor. Echocardiography is suggestive, but not diagnostic of congenital stridor, except in a few examples such as double aortic arch.

8.   **Congenital Heart Disease**
8.8   **Univentricular Heart and Atresia**

The use of the term "univentricular heart" has varied greatly in the literature, which has led to some confusion. In this chapter, we will use the term to describe the morphological ventricular anomaly for which it is characteristic, and not as the disease entity, *per se.* A typical "univentricular" heart has a large, dominant ventricle, which is the only functional ventricle, and an easily overlooked, rudimentary ventricle, which is functionally insignificant. Therefore, although one ventricle is abnormally developed, two ventricles still exist. The term "univentricular heart" is therefore a misnomer.

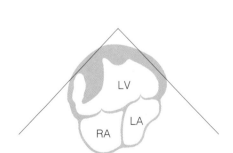

In "univentricular heart" with a double inlet left ventricle. There are two normal atria and AV valves, but only one "dominant" ventricle that corresponds to the left ventricle (LV). Upon close scrutiny, the "rudimentary" right ventricle (RV) can be found. Both AV valves connect to the dominant ventricle (double inlet ventricle). A defect in the IVS (bulboventricular foramen) forms the only inlet into the rudimentary ventricle.

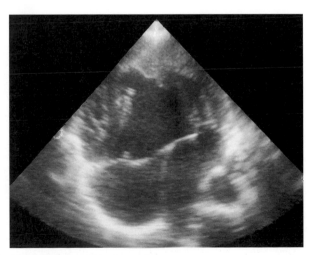

Apical four-chamber 2-D echocardiogram.

In *double inlet ventricle*, both atrioventricular valves arise from one ventricle, which means that both atrioventricular valves and, thus, both atria are connected to one dominant ventricle. In addition to the dominant ventricle, there is also a rudimentary ventricle without direct connection to the atrioventricular valves. The rudimentary ventricle receives blood from the dominant ventricle solely across a ventricular septal defect. One of the large arteries usually arises from this ventricle which, accordingly, is named the subaortic or subpulmonary ventricle. Only in rare cases is the rudimentary ventricle not connected to one of the great arteries, *i.e.*, it has neither an inlet nor an outlet. In this case, the dominant ventricle is a double outlet - double inlet ventricle.

The dominant ventricle is classified as either a *double inlet left ventricle* or a *double inlet right ventricle*, according to its anatomy. The morphology of the atrioventricular valves is determined by the ventricle located below the valves, *e.g.*, there are two mitral valves in a double inlet left ventricle, and two tricuspid valves in a double inlet right ventricle. Double inlet right and left ventricles can be differentiated by echocardiography. In double inlet left ventricle, the dominant valve is situated behind the rudimentary valve; in double inlet right ventricle (exception: ventricular inversion), it is in front of the rudimentary valve. In very rare cases, no rudimentary ventricle can be found, and one cannot determine whether the dominant ventricle is a right ventricle or a left ventricle *(undetermined ventricle)*. When one suspects that there is an undetermined ventricle, the possibility of a large ventricular septal defect and a complete atrioventricular canal with "absence" of the ventricular septum must be excluded from the diagnosis.

Echocardiographic diagnosis of double inlet ventricle is superior to angiographic diagnosis. Echocardiography provides better visualization of the atrioventricular valves and of their spatial relationship to the dominant ventricle. The diagnosis is made by demonstrating the two separate atrioventricular valves that drain into one dominant ventricle, from an apical or subcostal four-chamber view. Infrequently, transthoracic scan quality is not sufficient, and transesophageal scans must be made to secure the diagnosis. Regurgitation in one or both of the atrioventricular valves can be detected by Doppler color flow imaging.

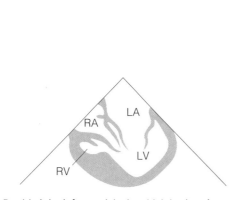

Double inlet left ventricle, in which both atrioventricular (AV) valves drain into one "dominant" left ventricle (LV). The rudimentary right ventricle (RV) does not communicate with either AV valve. Only the bulboventricular foramen supplies the RV with blood from the "dominant" ventricle.

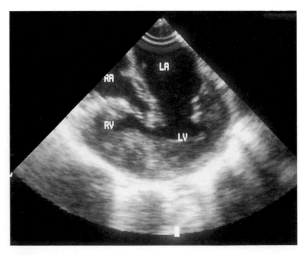

Transesophageal short-axis 2-D echocardiogram.

The rudimentary ventricle, which often is not immediately apparent, can be identified best in subcostal or parasternal short-axis scans. It is often helpful to interrogate region below the two great arteries, because one of the arteries usually arises from the rudimentary ventricle. The rudimentary ventricle can frequently be visualized in apical scans by rotating the transducer from the four-chamber view into the long axis. The rudimentary ventricle then is usually found below the origin of one of the great arteries.

After identifying the rudimentary ventricle, the next task is to determine whether the communication between the two ventricles, *i.e.* the interventricular foramen, is large enough or not. When the interventricular foramen is restrictive, stenosis will develop between the dominant ventricle and the great artery that arises from the rudimentary ventricle. This is defined as aortic occurs when the vessel is the aorta, and as pulmonary stenosis when the vessel is the pulmonary artery. A gradient across this interventricular communication can easily be detected using continuous-wave Doppler.

In double inlet left ventricle, malposition of the great arteries commonly occurs, whereby the aorta may lie to the left (*L*-malposition) or to the right (*D*-malposition) of the aortic artery. Usually, the aorta arises from the right, rudimentary ventricle and the interventricular foramen is restrictive, which causes pulmonary stenosis. Frequently, valvular pulmonary stenosis, which can be quantitated with CW Doppler, also exists. Pulmonary stenosis is a significant factor, because it protects the pulmonary circulatory system against pulmonary hypertension (Eisenmenger's reaction). The pulmonary artery pressure (systolic pressure - gradient) must be estimated using the arterial blood pressure and the gradient across the pulmonary valve. The systolic pulmonary artery pressure should not be higher than 20 to 30 mmHg.

In double inlet right ventricle, the aorta almost always arises from the dominant ventricle. A double inlet / double outlet right ventricle exists in cases where the pulmonary artery arises from the dominant ventricle. In other words, both atrioventricular valves drain into the dominant ventricle, and both great arteries arise from it. In that case, the rudimentary ventricle has no communication with the atria or the great arteries. This constellation is seen virtually only in double inlet right ventricle, and never in double inlet left ventricle. Pulmonary atresia is common in double inlet right ventricle. In that case, the origin of the pulmonary artery cannot be identified, because there is usually muscular atresia in the absence of a pulmonary trunk.

Situs anomalies are commonly associated with double inlet right or left ventricle. Then, the double inlet ventricle is accompanied by additional anomalies, such as total anomalous pulmonary venous return or atrioventricular canal-like defects of the atrioventricular valves.

8.8 **Univentricular Heart and Atresia**
8.8.2 **Straddling and Overriding of the Atrioventricular Valves**

There are transitional types of double inlet ventricle, which is defined as the connection of both atrioventricular valves to a single dominant ventricle. In transitional types, one of the two atrioventricular valves partially communicates with the rudimentary ventricle. Because the rudimentary ventricle then (at least partially) communicate with an AV valve, it develops better than ventricles totally lacking communication. Purely descriptive terminology is used to describe this type of "partial" communication. This is done by evaluating the anatomy and other relationships of the valve ring as well as the insertions of the chordae tendineae.

Straddling is said to occur when chordae tendineae of one AV valve cross a ventricular septal defect or interventricular foramen and insert into the opposite ventricle, *i.e.,* the chordae of one AV valve insert into both ventricles. Straddling is relatively common in AV septal defects.

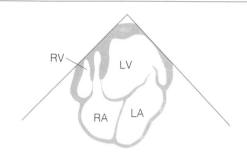

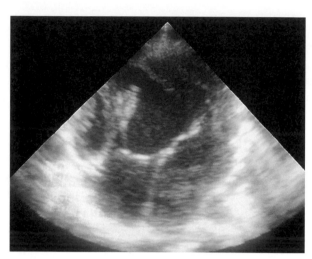

Overriding AV valve and straddling in double inlet left ventricle. The right AV valve drains predominantly in the dominant left ventricle (LV), but overrides part of the rudimentary right ventricle (RV). Because of the overriding AV valve, the rudimentary ventricle is relatively well developed. Straddling also exists. The chordae tendineae of the right AV valve insert in the IVS and, to some extent, in the rudimentary RV.

Apical four-chamber 2-D echocardiogram.

In *overriding*, the AV valve ring lies across the ventricular septum. The extent of overriding is given as a percentage of the valve ring. The AV valve is designated as part of the ventricle with the largest percentage of valve ring area.

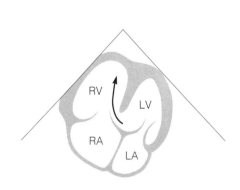

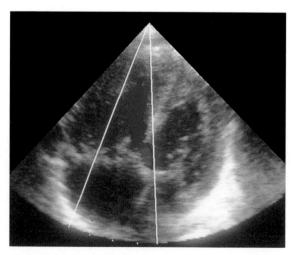

Overriding tricuspid valve. Both ventricles are developed. A ventricular septal defect is located below atrioventricular (AV) valve level. The right (tricuspid) AV valve "overrides" the defect. The tricuspid valve extends across both the enlarged right ventricle and the smaller left ventricle.

Color flow map of apical four-chamber 2-D echocardiogram.

An ventricular septal defect or an interventricular foramen is a prerequisite for straddling or overriding. The possibility of straddling and overriding should always be considered when one of the ventricles is underdeveloped or appears too small. Straddling is particularly common in atrioventricular septal defects, corrected transposition (*L*-transposition), and univentricular heart. Echocardiography is clearly superior to angiography for the assessment of straddling and overriding.

| 8.8 | Univentricular Heart and Atresia |
| 8.8.3 | Atrioventricular Valve Atresia (Tricuspid, Mitral) |

In this group of cardiac anomalies, one of the two atrioventricular valves is atretic. Therefore, one of the two atria does not communicate with the AV valve or its respective ventricle. The sole outlet for the involved atrium is an atrial septal defect. Tricuspid atresia exists when the morphological right atrium is involved, regardless of whether the left atrium drains into the left ventricle via an anatomical mitral valve, or drains into the right ventricle via an anatomical tricuspid valve.

The terminology tends to get somewhat confusing, especially when tricuspid atresia occurs when a tricuspid valve exists. The hemodynamically decisive factor is the fact that the right atrium has no direct communication with the ventricles, and that it drains solely through a atrial septal defect. On the other hand, the anatomy of the ventricle under the non-atretic valves is less significant, but it determines the anatomy of its respective valve. Confusion could be avoided by classifying tricuspid atresia as "atresia of the right atrioventricular communication", and by classifying mitral atresia as "atresia of the left atrioventricular communication". Even though this terminology is less confusing, it has not gained wide acceptance. The simpler and older established terms, "tricuspid atresia" and "mitral atresia", are still preferred.

Tricuspid atresia occurs in the absence of a right-sided atrioventricular communication, *i.e.*, agenesis of the AV valve between the right atrium and the ventricle below it. In tricuspid atresia, the AV valve of the right atrium is atretic. Tricuspid atresia can be classified into two anatomical types:
1. *classical tricuspid atresia* and
2. *tricuspid atresia with an atretic (imperforate) valve*.

Classical tricuspid atresia is the much more common type in which the embryonic rudiment of the right AV valve is completely absent. In tricuspid atresia with an atretic valve, a valve rudiment exists, but it has an imperforate (atretic) membrane.

Classical tricuspid atresia is characterized by the complete absence of a valve rudiment between the right atrium and one of the two ventricles. From a patho-anatomical point of view, the deepest site of the right atrium (where the valve rudiment should be) borders with the left ventricle. Classical tricuspid atresia has a characteristic echocardiographic appearance. Similar to the double inlet ventricle, only one dominant ventricle is found in apical or subcostal four-chamber views. In contrast with double inlet ventricle, only one AV valve connects to the dominant ventricle. This valve connects the left atrium to the dominant ventricle. In addition to the dominant ventricle, a rudimentary right can also be found in front and to the right.

The rudimentary right ventricle does not communicate with both atria, it only communicates with the left ventricle via an interventricular foramen. The interventricular foramen usually is in the upper portion of the ventricular septum, and there is often an additional defect in the apical portion of the septum. In tricuspid atresia, the foramen often is or becomes restrictive. In terms of hemodynamics, this causes subvalvular stenosis of the artery arising from the rudimentary ventricle.

As in double inlet (left or right) ventricle (DILV, DIRV), it is essential to measure the gradient at the interventricular foramen between the left and right ventricles by means of pulsed or continuous-wave Doppler. In rare cases the interventricular foramen closes completely. This is possible only when the pulmonary artery arises from the rudimentary ventricle.

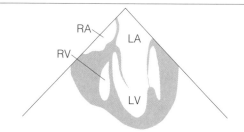

"Classical" tricuspid atresia with the ventricular anatomy of a "univentricular heart", *i.e.*, a dominant left (LV) and a rudimentary right ventricle (RV). An AV valve opens into the dominant ventricle, but there is no normal "inlet" into the rudimentary ventricle. There is also no right valve to provide an "outlet" for the right atrium (RA). The highly echo reflective material between the right atrium and the rudimentary ventricle corresponds to epicardial fat and connective tissue. The only "outlet" out of the RA is an atrial septal defect (not shown), and the only "inlet" into the rudimentary right ventricle is a bulboventricular foramen.

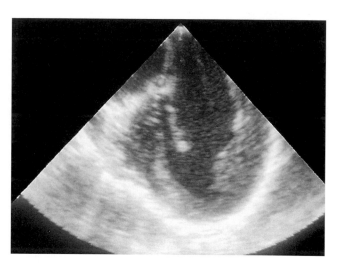

Transesophageal short-axis 2-D echocardiogram.

After evaluating the ventricular anatomy (apical and subcostal four-chamber views), the position and origin of the great arteries are then assessed. The position of the great arteries may be normal, *i.e.*, the aorta lies in back and to the right, and the pulmonary artery lies in front and to the left. However, malposition of the great arteries (*D*-malposition or *L*-malposition) is also possible. Three different types are differentiated according to position of the great arteries, as described below.

Type I   Normal position of the great arteries
Type II   *D*-malposition of the great arteries
Type III   *L*-malposition of the great arteries

Pulmonary stenosis or even pulmonary atresia are common associated lesions. In normal position of the great arteries, these lesions may be aggravated by a restrictive communication between the dominant and the rudimentary ventricle. Assessment of the pulmonary artery is important when considering surgical management, *i.e.*, the Fontan procedure. The Fontan procedure can be performed only when pulmonary artery pressure is low. Because of the importance of pulmonary artery pressure in treatment decision-making, tricuspid atresia is grouped into three types according to the extent of pulmonary stenosis:

Type A   Pulmonary atresia
Type B   Pulmonary stenosis
Type C   Normal pulmonary circulation

In type A, pulmonary circulation occurs across a patent ductus arteriosus, and enhancement of pulmonary blood flow is indicated (aortopulmonary shunt). In type C, pulmonary blood flow is increased, and banding of the pulmonary artery is indicated.

In contrast with the pulmonary valve, the aortic valve is almost never stenotic. Aortic stenosis occurs only in malposition (types II and III) with restrictive communication between the right and left ventricles.

The communication between the two atria is of hemodynamic importance, because it represents the only outlet out of the right atrium. In most cases, the defect is located in the fossa ovalis. Sinus venosus defects and primum defects are less common. Venous inflow may be limited when the defect is small and restrictive. A pressure gradient across the atrial septal defect can easily be detected using PW Doppler. Today, a gradient across the atrial septal defect is considered unfavorable, because right atrial overextension is believed to be associated with later arrhythmias. Therefore, the gradient at the atrial septum should not exceed 8 mmHg. When considering the Fontan procedure, insufficiency of the (only) AV valve, the cause of reduced pulmonary venous flow, must first be excluded.

Tricuspid atresia with an atretic valve is a rare form of tricuspid atresia that became diagnosable only after the advent of echocardiography. Four-chamber scans show a normal or enlarged left ventricle and a small, hypoplastic right ventricle. As compared with "classical" tricuspid atresia, a highly echo reflective membrane is situated between the right atrium and right ventricle. This corresponds to the atretic rudiment of the tricuspid valve. Commonly, a (rudimentary) valve apparatus can also be demonstrated beneath the atretic membrane, *i.e.*, valve. Diagnosis of this type of tricuspid atresia is clinically important, because the membrane can be opened and replaced by a valve, whereas this is not possible in "classical" tricuspid atresia, which is characterized by complete valve agenesis. Dysplasia of the atretic tricuspid valve, which is often displaced into the right ventricle (Ebstein's malformation), is not uncommon. Cor triatriatum dextrum may simulate tricuspid atresia with an atretic valve. In cor triatriatum dextrum, an enlarged Eustachian valve rides over and obstructs the tricuspid valve.

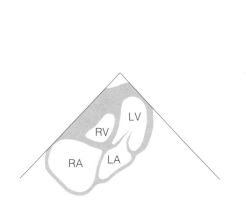

Tricuspid atresia with atretic valve. A highly echo reflective membrane, corresponding to the atretic tricuspid valve, is located between the small right ventricle (RV) and the dilated right atrium (RA).

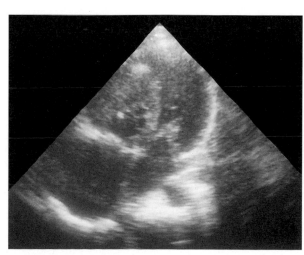

Apical four-chamber 2-D echocardiogram.

In *mitral atresia*, there is no communication between the left atrium and the left ventricle. Although the anatomy of the valve is determined by the respective ventricle, the term "mitral atresia" is still used despite the morphology of the atretic valve, because the AV valve of the left atrium is atretic. In contrast to tricuspid atresia, the presence of a primitive, but atretic communication between the left atrium and left ventricle (imperforate valve) is much more common than complete absence of the communication between the structures.

There are two fundamental types of mitral atresia, namely:

1. mitral atresia with ventricular septal defect, and
2. hypoplastic left heart syndrome.

In *hypoplastic left heart syndrome*, the ventricular septum is intact, and the left ventricle does not develop due to mitral atresia. Hypoplastic left heart syndrome is almost always associated with aortic atresia. However, in *mitral atresia with ventricular septal defect*, the ventricle can develop because it can receive blood and drain via the defect.

Mitral atresia with ventricular septal defect is morphologically and anatomically similar to tricuspid atresia. However, in mitral atresia with ventricular septal defect, the AV valve of the left atrium is atretic, not the AV valve of the right atrium. In contrast to tricuspid atresia, the existence of an atretic communication between the left atrium and the left ventricle (imperforate valve) is more common. The origin of the great arteries may vary. Tricuspid atresia is frequently accompanied by pulmonary stenosis and pulmonary atresia.

In addition to assessing the ventricular anatomy, position and origin of the great arteries, and gradients across the pulmonary valve, the echocardiographic examination must also determine whether or not the communication between the two atria is restrictive. Because pulmonary venous blood must drain via a defect in the atrial septum, a restrictive atrial septal defect can obstruct pulmonary venous blood flow and, thus, lead to "passive" hypertension. In this case, interventional or surgical enlargement of the atrial septal defect is indicated to relieve the condition.

In mitral atresia with a developed, but atretic (imperforate) valve, apical four-chamber scans reveal a normal or enlarged right ventricle and a smaller left ventricle. If the valvular apparatus can be identified below the imperforate membrane, cor triatriatum sinistrum and supravalvular mitral stenosis must be excluded from the diagnosis.

The term *hypoplastic left heart syndrome* is used to describe a number of aortic and mitral valve anomalies in which both valves may be stenotic or atretic. A rudimentary valve is, in any case, present. In some cases, atresia is so severe that the left ventricle can neither fill nor drain. Usually, the aortic valve is atretic, and the mitral valve is extremely stenotic, thickened, and dysplastic. Left ventricular filling may be impaired, but contraction is isovolumic due to the aortic stenosis. Independent of this anatomical variation, the left ventricle is hypoplastic and there is usually endocardial fibroelastosis in hypoplastic left heart syndrome. Perfusion of the systemic circulatory system does not occur via the left ventricle, but rather via the right ventricle by means of a patent ductus arteriosus. The descending aorta is hypoplastic. Retrograde perfusion from the ductus supplies the aorta which, in turn, supplies the coronary vessels. In almost all cases, there is an atrial septal defect across which pulmonary venous blood can flow.

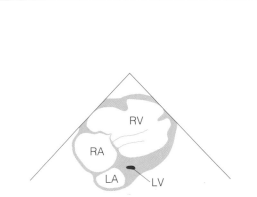

Hypoplastic left heart syndrome. The right ventricle (RV) is massively enlarged and extremely trabeculated; the right atrium (RA) is also dilated. The left atrium (LA) is small; an atrial septal defect of the secundum type is found. The LV is so small that it can easily be overlooked. The aortic (not shown) and mitral valves are atretic.

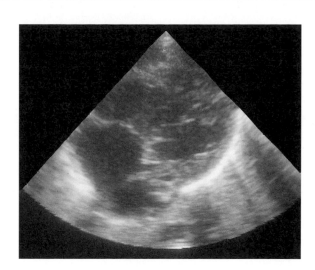

Subcostal four-chamber 2-D echocardiogram.

The first abnormality noticed in the echocardiographic examination is massive enlargement of the right ventricle, which is responsible for perfusion of the lungs as well as for systemic circulation. In contrast, it often takes a long time to find the (hypoplastic) left ventricle, even though it is always situated at the back and to the left. The hypoplastic left ventricle can often be identified by increased echogenicity, which is attributable to the highly echo reflective structures of endocardial fibroelastosis. The mitral valve is identified as a membranous structure; sometimes, a small opening in the membrane can be detected. Because atretic membranes also move, motion of the membrane should not be mistakenly interpreted as motion of the true valve. Frequently, the valvular apparatus is completely absent; otherwise, individual plump chordae tendineae without papillary muscles can be found.

In addition to the massively enlarged right ventricle, the next identifiable abnormality is the dilated pulmonary artery. A wide, patent ductus arteriosus is always present. The ductus, which looks like an extension of the pulmonary artery, drains into the descending aorta. The right ventricle and the pulmonary artery can easily be demonstrated in parasternal and subcostal scans. The ductus arteriosus and its relationships to the pulmonary artery and the aorta are best visualized in supraclavicular scans. Doppler color flow imaging or PW Doppler can demonstrate that blood moving across the patent ductus arteriosus flows exclusively from the pulmonary artery to the aorta.

Another abnormality found when assessing the pulmonary artery and the ductus arteriosus is that, even though the aortic arch and the vessels exiting from it can be visualized, the ascending aorta appears to be "absent" or is hypoplastic. Doppler studies reveal retrograde flow in the aortic arch. The direction of flow, which should normally be anterior-posterior (*i.e.* away from the transducer), is towards the transducer. This retrograde perfusion of the aortic arch is practically diagnostic of severe obstruction of the aortic valve, *i.e.*, hypoplastic left heart syndrome. With careful scanning, the ascending aorta can always be visualized. The aorta is variably hypoplastic and is usually only 2 to 3 mm in diameter. There is also retrograde perfusion of the ascending aorta. However, it is not always easy to demonstrate because of the small diameter of the ascending aorta, and because of the possibility of error due to the closely adjacent, wide pulmonary artery. Usually, it is easier to demonstrate the ascending aorta from suprasternal or supraclavicular positions than from the parasternal position.

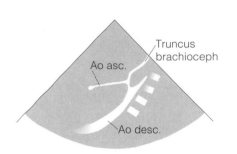

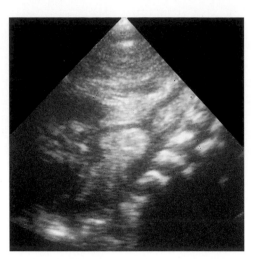

Hypoplastic left heart syndrome. The caliber of the descending aorta (Ao. desc.) is normal, but the ascending aorta (Ao. asc.) is extremely hypoplastic (narrower than the brachiocephalic trunk). The Ao. asc. ends in a dilatation that corresponds to the aortic root (bulbus) and the origins of the coronary vessels. The aortic valve is atretic. There occurs retrograde perfusion across the hypoplastic Ao. asc. The sole function of the Ao. asc. is to supply blood to the coronary vessels.

Suprasternal long-axis scan.

In the last step, the communication between the two atria should be analyzed in subcostal scans, and the pressure gradient should be measured using PW Doppler. A restrictive communication leads to restricted flow out of the pulmonary veins and, thus, to pulmonary edema. Little can be done to treat newborns with hypoplastic left heart syndrome. Two possibilities are heart transplantation and palliation by means of the Norwood techniques. In many hospitals, these patients are classified as untreatable, so the echocardiographic diagnosis of hypoplastic left heart syndrome is virtually a death sentence for these patients.

Some authors classify other, in some cases treatable, anomalies as "hypoplastic left heart syndrome". Therefore, these anomalies should not be classified as "hypoplastic left heart syndrome". Instead, a detailed description of the anomaly should be made. In aortic atresia with ventricular septal defect, the left ventricle can be normally developed, and the mitral valve is usually normal. Surgical "correction" is usually possible in these cases. The left ventricle is hypoplastic in unbalanced AV septal defects. However, hypoplasia of the left ventricle is the only similarity with hypoplastic left heart syndrome.

Another point should be stressed again: Especially in echocardiographic diagnosis, it is of utmost importance to strictly differentiate between "classical" hypoplastic left heart syndrome and other cardiac anomalies with a hypoplastic left ventricle. Some examples of correctable cardiac anomalies with, in some cases, a seemingly extremely „hypoplastic" left ventricle are total anomalous pulmonary venous return and persistent fetal circulation. The latter is not a cardiac anomaly, but a postnatal adaptation defect.

In *pulmonary atresia with an intact ventricular septum*, the pulmonary artery is closed and the right ventricle cannot eject any blood. Atresia is usually of the membranous type, *i.e.*, an atretic rudimentary valve exists. Muscular atresia is more uncommon. In pulmonary atresia with an intact ventricular septum, an incompetent tricuspid valve provides the only outlet out of the right ventricle. There is commonly dysplasia of the tricuspid valve corresponding to Ebstein's malformation, *i.e.*, the tricuspid valve is displaced into the right ventricle.

Because tricuspid incompetence provides the only possibility for the right ventricle to eject blood, the right ventricle develops abnormally and becomes hypoplastic. A rule of thumb is: the more severe the tricuspid incompetence, the larger the right ventricle. The size of the right ventricle can vary greatly.

The right ventricle can be as small as a hardly detectable residual lumen (similar to hypoplastic left heart syndrome), or almost as large as a normal ventricle (as in normal hearts). Venous blood reaches the left atrium by means of an atrial septal defect. Perfusion of the pulmonary circulation is ductus-dependent.

Anomalies of the coronary vessels, particularly myocardial sinusoids, are common. Myocardial sinusoids are embryonic communications between the right ventricle and the coronary vascular system. Because right ventricular pressure is regularly suprasystemic, venous blood from the right ventricle is ejected into the coronary venous system. Often in addition to coronary perfusion with undersaturated blood, stenoses are found in the communications between the myocardial sinusoids and coronary vessels, which can lead to myocardial ischemia. Also, coronary vascular occlusions may be as severe as atresia of both coronary ostia, with retrograde perfusion of the coronary vascular system via the myocardial sinusoids with venous blood from the right ventricle. In pulmonary atresia with an intact ventricular septum, echocardiography reveals a normal to slightly enlarged left ventricle and a hypoplastic right ventricle. Tricuspid incompetence is always present. Continuous-wave Doppler can be used to measure the pressure gradient across the tricuspid valve and, thus, to derive the pressure in the right ventricle. Frequently, the tricuspid valve appears to be dysplastic, the valve leaflets appear plump and are often displaced to the right ventricle, and the chordae tendineae are thickened and rarefied.

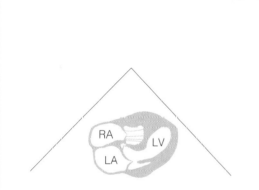

Pulmonary atresia with an intact ventricular septum (IVS). In pulmonary atresia with intact IVS, there is always more or less extensive hypoplasia of the RV and hypertrophy of the right ventricular myocardium. Additionally, there is dysplasia and hypoplasia of the tricuspid valve, the leaflets and chordae of which are plump in appearance.

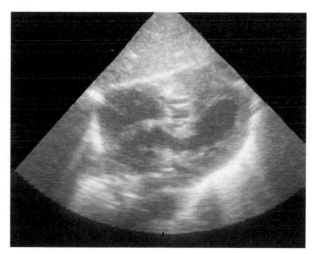

Subcostal four-chamber 2-D echocardiogram.

An additional finding is that the right ventricular outflow tract is atretic. Usually, one finds a fused valve lacking any opening whatsoever. Infrequently, the infundibulum is also atretic. It is almost always possible to visualize the pulmonary artery trunk. Blood circulation in the pulmonary trunk is maintained by a patent ductus arteriosus. Therefore, retrograde flow in the pulmonary trunk is a typical sign of pulmonary atresia. In Doppler color flow imaging, predominantly retrograde flow is often seen in addition to antegrade flow (at least for a brief duration). The ductus flushes the atretic pulmonary trunk, which resembles a closed sac.

The ductus arteriosus and flow in the pulmonary trunk are visualized best in supraclavicular and suprasternal scans. The ventricular anatomy, the tricuspid valve, and the right ventricular outflow tract can be visualized in parasternal and subcostal scans. The atrial septal defect can also be visualized best in subcostal scans. Only rarely can myocardial sinusoids be demonstrated by echocardiography.

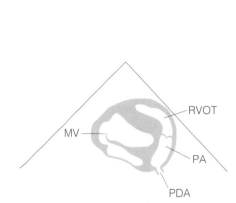

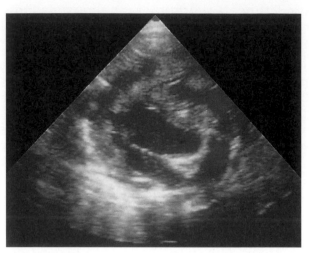

Pulmonary atresia. Between the right ventricular outflow tract (RVOT) and the pulmonary artery (PA) is an echo reflective membrane that corresponds to an atretic valve. The patent ductus arteriosus (PDA) drains into the PA.

Subcostal short-axis scan.

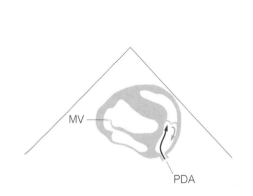

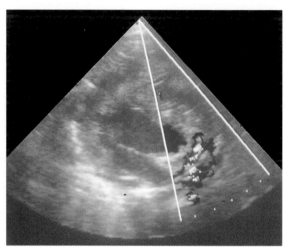

Continued. The color flow map demonstrates the blood flow across the PDA to the PA. Then, it bounces off the atretic membrane and reverses direction. In contrast with the PA, no blood flow is found in the RVOT. In other words, blood flow in the PA is completely dependent on the PDA.

Subcostal short-axis 2-D echocardiogram with color flow mapping.

---

8.   Congenital Heart Disease
8.9   Tetralogy of Fallot and Pulmonary Atresia with Ventricular Septal Defect

Tetralogy of Fallot and pulmonary atresia with ventricular septal defect are similar cardiac anomalies. Therefore, both anomalies will be discussed together in this section. Both anomalies have a ventricular septal defect, pulmonary stenosis or atresia, an abnormal right ventricular outflow tract, and an aorta that overrides the ventricular septal defect.

Tetralogy of Fallot is characterized by the combination of pulmonary stenosis, a subaortic ventricular septal defect, and an overriding aorta. Of hemodynamic significance is the fact that pulmonary stenosis and the overriding aorta lead to leakage of venous blood into the aorta and, thus, to cyanosis.

The more severe the stenosis, the more severe the cyanosis. When both pulmonary stenosis and overriding are slight, cyanosis is minimal ("pink Fallot").

The aorta overriding the subaortic ventricular septal defect (overriding indicated in %) can be visualized in parasternal long-axis scans. When overriding exceeds 50%, many authors classify the anomaly as "double outlet right ventricle". In the first few years of life, the overriding aorta can also be visualized from the subcostal portal, or it can be visualized by angulating the transducer anteriorly from the apical four-chamber position, until the aorta comes into view.

Although an overriding aorta is a key diagnostic sign, an overriding aorta can also be found in such anomalies as truncus arteriosus (communis), pulmonary atresia with ventricular septal defect, and double outlet (right and left) ventricles. These anomalies can be differentiated from tetralogy of Fallot by evaluating the pulmonary arteries. A pulmonary artery arising from the right ventricle excludes truncus arteriosus from the diagnosis. The demonstration of antegrade flow in the pulmonary trunk excludes pulmonary atresia. The pulmonary artery can be assessed especially well using Doppler color flow imaging. Pulmonary stenosis, which is usually associated with tetralogy of Fallot, leads to aliasing and increased variance. Thus, a narrowed pulmonary artery is "colorfully" and markedly demonstrated in color flow maps. The gradients in the pulmonary artery and right ventricular outflow tract can be determined using CW Doppler. In tetralogy of Fallot, the gradient is usually ca. 50 mmHg in newborns, and 70 to 90 mmHg in older patients. Right and left ventricular pressures are equal. Therefore, there can be no gradient across the ventricular septal defect. Two-dimensional echocardiography often permits direct visualization of the infundibular stenosis. A high-frequency (7.5 MHz) transducer with a short near field and a low depth of penetration should be used for this purpose. The bifurcation of the pulmonary arteries can often be visualized in parasternal scans. The pulmonary arteries are usually small, and special attention should be given to stenoses in the region of the bifurcation. Frequently, the ductus arteriosus remains patent throughout the first year of life; there is then sufficient perfusion of the lungs. The ductus can usually be visualized best from the suprasternal notch. Patency of the ductus arteriosus is of clinical significance, because a life-threatening reduction in lung perfusion can develop if the ductus closes.

In very rare cases of tetralogy of Fallot, the pulmonary valve is completely absent. Then, the pulmonary artery trunk and the proximal main branches of the pulmonary artery are massively dilated, thereby restricting the trachea and the main bronchi. One main branch of the pulmonary artery (usually the left branch) may also be atretic. Usually, the branch is then perfused by a patent ductus arteriosus.

Atrial septal defect, *i.e.* a patent foramen ovale, is a common associated anomaly. This combination used to be termed "pentalogy of Fallot", but today this terminology is seldom used. In the "pentalogy" of Fallot, the aortic arch lies on the right and, in elderly patients, there is mild aortic insufficiency. Typically, there is also a subaortic ventricular septal defect over which the aorta "rides", and a muscular ventricular septal defect, which can be visualized best in the apical four-chamber view. When looking for additional ventricular septal defects, one must remember that right and left ventricular pressures are usually equal. Therefore, color Doppler will be an unreliable method of detection. Two-dimensional echocardiography should preferably be used in this case.

Especially in patients with trisomy 21, tetralogy of Fallot can occur with an AV canal defect. Echocardiography reveals the typical AV valve defect (the septal leaflets insert at the same level) and an AV septal defect.

Morphologically, pulmonary atresia with ventricular septal defect is very similar to tetralogy of Fallot, but the pulmonary artery is atretic. Blood travels to and from the lungs either via a patent ductus arteriosus or aortopulmonary collaterals. The latter are abnormal vessels that arise from the descending aorta, aortic arch, or coronary arteries and perfuse the pulmonary circulatory tract. In pulmonary atresia with ventricular septal defect, parasternal long-axis echocardiograms reveal the aorta riding over a ventricular septal defect. By rotating the transducer laterally and slightly clockwise, the right ventricular outflow tract and the pulmonary arteries can usually be seen. Often, it is not possible to visualize the pulmonary artery, and the right ventricular outflow tract may also be "absent". In tetralogy of Fallot, Doppler color flow imaging can easily demonstrate severe pulmonary stenosis despite hypoplasia of the pulmonary vessels. In pulmonary atresia with ventricular septal defect, however, no blood flow whatsoever can be detected. Only when the pulmonary vessels are well developed can the pulmonary trunk be found, and its relationship to the right ventricle can be analyzed. From parasternal and supraclavicular portals, it is often possible to visualize and measure the right pulmonary artery behind the ascending aorta and in front of the superior vena cava in cross section, and it is sometimes possible to visualize the hypoplastic pulmonary artery trunk, which cannot be visualized from the suprasternal position due to air artifacts.

It is difficult to make the diagnosis when no pulmonary artery can be visualized. Truncus arteriosus can be excluded only when the truncal origin of the pulmonary artery has been demonstrated. In truncus arteriosus, the main branches of the pulmonary artery are usually dilated, whereas they are usually hypoplastic in pulmonary atresia. A chest x-ray may be very helpful: in pulmonary atresia, the pulmonary vascular markings are decreased; in truncus arteriosus, they are increased.

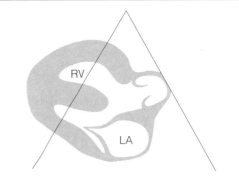

Pulmonary atresia with ventricular septal defect (VSD). In pulmonary atresia with VSD, there is typically a subaortic VSD over which the aorta "rides". In contrast to tetralogy of Fallot, none of the vessel structures in front of the ascending aorta corresponds to a pulmonary artery. The left ventricle is relatively small; the IVS and the right ventricular myocardium are excessively thickened.

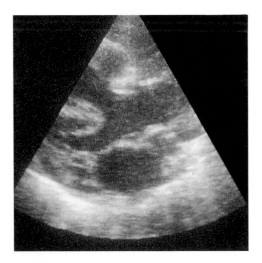

Subcostal long-axis 2-D echocardiogram.

Aortopulmonary collaterals usually cannot be visualized by echocardiography, because of their intrapulmonary course after they emerge from the descending aorta. In the auscultatory examination, however, to-and-fro murmurs can be heard in the paravertebral region of the back. A surgically implanted aortopulmonary shunt can usually be detected in the suprasternal region.

On the whole, anomalies of the mitral valve are rare, but they are hemodynamically very significant. It is difficult to make an angiographic assessment of mitral valve deformities. In echocardiography, the mitral valve is examined in three planes: the apical or subcostal four-chamber view, the parasternal long-axis view, and the parasternal short-axis view. In adolescents and adults, transesophageal echocardiography significantly improves the imaging of the mitral valve, whereas in newborns and infants, it is of limited diagnostic value because the mitral valve often lies in the near field of the transducer, rendering at least Doppler echocardiography impossible.

Assessment of the mitral valve involves the assessment of the valve leaflets, the chordae tendineae, and the papillary muscles.

AV Septal Defect

AV septal defects were discussed in depth in the section on septal defects. The four-chamber view reveals that the septal sections of both atrioventricular valves insert or join at the same level on the ventricular septum. The septal tricuspid valve leaflet does not insert lower (2 to 4↑mm) than the mitral valve, as it normally does. Attempting to angulate the imaging plane from the apical four-chamber view so as to show the aorta together with atrioventricular valves will not be successful, because the root of the aorta does not lie between the two atrioventricular valves, but in front of the common atrioventricular connection. A cleft in the mitral valve appears in the short axis, which in an AV septal defect is always is aligned in the direction of the right AV ostium and never toward the root of the aorta. The involvement of the atrioventricular valves ranges from a cleft mitral valve to a common valve. The decisive question in echocardiography diagnostics is whether the two separate valves appear in the image or one single one. In extreme cases, only the bridging leaflets are discernible, and the greater part of the chordae tendineae passes through the defective section of the ventricle into the right ventricle. In the four-chamber view, the imaging plane is inclined posteriorly to reveal the size of the common posterior leaflet, the anatomy of the appropriate chordae tendineae, and their insertion at the ventricular septum in one or both ventricles. Finally, it must be determined whether the center section of the bridging leaflet appears to be attached to a tissue bridge or moves completely freely. If the bridging leaflet appears to be attached, then this would indicate that, to a certain extent, two separate valve sections have formed, whereas completely free motion at the site of the AV defect would indicate that there is no separation between two valve sections. The anterior bridging leaflet is analyzed accordingly after inclining the imaging plane ventrally. It is often possible to visualize the anatomy of the atrioventricular valve sections in the short axis, but not the chordae tendineae.

Isolated Anterior Cleft Mitral Valve

In addition to the cleft mitral valve observed in the AV defect, there is also a rare "isolated" mitral cleft that occurs independently of an AV defect. In contrast to the cleft observed in the AV defect, this "isolated" cleft lies in the anterior mitral leaflet and is aligned in the direction of the root of the aorta, whereas the cleft AV defect is always aligned in the direction of the ventricular septum. The fact that the septal sections of both atrioventricular valves insert or join at the same level in the case of the AV septal defect aids in differential diagnosis. In the case of the isolated mitral cleft, the septal tricuspid valve leaflet inserts 2 to 4 mm lower than the mitral valve (in the four-chamber view).

Hypoplasia and Dysplasia of the Mitral Valve

Often the mitral valve can only be categorized as hypoplastic or dysplastic. Hypoplasia means that the mitral valve is too small. Viewing the tricuspid valve and the mitral valve in the short axis (from a parasternal or subcostal view) will produce a particularly distinct echocardiographic image of hypoplasia of the mitral valve.

Dysplasia of the mitral valve describes the condition in which the mitral valve appears abnormal, the mitral leaflets are thickened and limited in their range of motion, and the chordae tendineae are rarefied and plump. Dysplasia is generally accompanied by hypoplasia of the mitral valve. The papillary muscles are often abnormally short or missing entirely so that the plump chordae tendineae begin at the free wall of the left ventricle or the ventricular septum without papillary muscles.

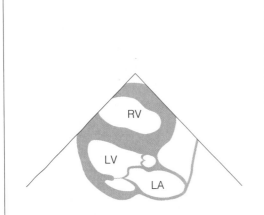

Congenital mitral stenosis. Thickened (dysplastic) mitral valve. There is doming of the mitral leaflets into the left ventricle; a short papillary muscle can be seen.

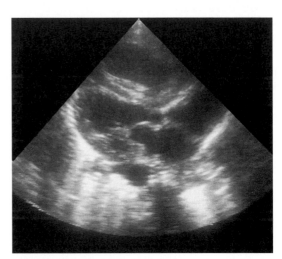

Parasternal long-axis 2-D echocardiogram.

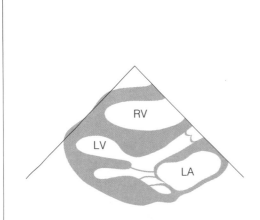

Dysplastic mitral valve. The chordae tendineae are shortened and plump. The mitral valve appears to have shifted into the hypoplastic left ventricle. A papillary muscle is not visible.

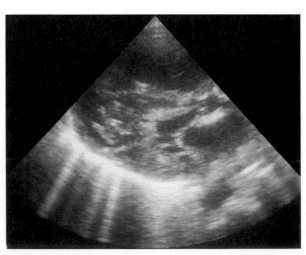

Parasternal long-axis 2-D echocardiogram.

Mitral Atresia

Mitral atresia was discussed in depth in the section on atresia. Either there is total agenesis of the mitral valve, or, more frequently, there will be an imperforate membrane between the left atrium and ventricle.

Double Orifice Mitral Valve

Double orifice mitral valve is extremely rare and generally can be visualized more distinctly in the short-axis view than in the four-chamber view. Two adjacent mitral ostia in the short-axis view are impressive findings.

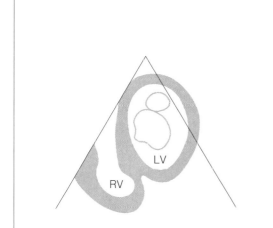

Double orifice mitral valve. Instead of a mitral ostium there are two mitral ostia. The two orifices appear on the echocardiogram like two separate valves.

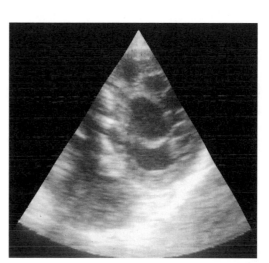

Subcostal short-axis 2-D echocardiogram.

Mitral Valve "Arcade" Formation

In mitral valve "arcade" formation, the chordae tendineae are shortened and the papillary muscles extend to the edges of the mitral leaflets.

Parachute Mitral Valve

This malformation of the mitral valve is a typical finding in Shone's anomaly. The malformation of the mitral valve is accompanied by coarctation of the aorta and aortic (subvalvular) stenosis. The malformation of the mitral valve is characterized by a single papillary muscle on which the chordae tendineae of both mitral leaflets are attached. The structure resembles a parachute. In short-axis echocardiograms, one can demonstrate the presence of a single papillary muscle onto which all chordae tendineae of the mitral valve are attached.

Floppy Mitral Valve

Floppy mitral valve is comparatively rare in children as opposed to adults. A pronounced prolapse of the mitral valve should always be regarded as a possible indication of Marfan's syndrome or homocystinuria. Slight prolapsing of the mitral valve is seen relatively often in atrial septal defects of the secundum type, but this is almost never of any clinical significance.

Atrioventricular Discordance

Atrioventricular discordance refers to the condition in which the left atrium is joined with the right ventricle and the right atrium is joined with the left ventricle such as in a corrected (L) transposition. Since the atrioventricular valves develop from the ventricle, the mitral valve always belongs to the left ventricle and the tricuspid valve belongs to the right ventricle. This can lead to confusion when analyzing the echocardiogram if the clinician fails to notice that the ventricles have been "switched", as is the case with the corrected transposition.

Supravalvular Ring

Above the mitral valve there is a fibrous ring that has, at least partially, fused with the mitral valve, and which obstructs flow out of the left atrium. This membrane often is not discernible on the echocardiogram when the mitral valve is closed, because the mitral leaflets are in direct contact with the ring. If the membrane has fused together with the mitral leaflets or adheres to them, then the echocardiogram will not reveal this defect.

Cor Triatriatum Sinistrum

In this rare malformation the left atrium is subdivided into proximal and distal chambers by a fibromuscular membrane. Whereas the veins of the lung empty into the proximal chamber of the atrium, the distal chamber includes the atrial appendage and the opening of the mitral valve into the left ventricle. There are always one or more defects in this fibromuscular membrane that almost always obstruct the flow of blood from the pulmonary veins into the left ventricle (restrictive membrane). Extremely rarely, there will be nonrestrictive communication between the two atrial chambers.

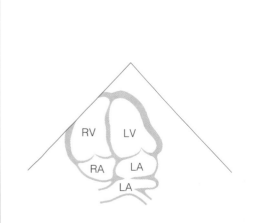

Cor triatriatum sinistrum. A membrane which divides the atrium into two chambers, thereby impeding the flow of blood from the pulmonary veins, appears in the left atrium.

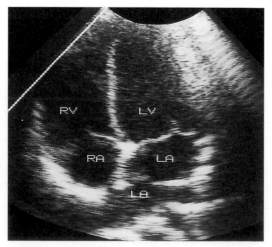

Apical four-chamber 2-D echocardiogram.

In about 50% of patients with cor triatriatum sinistrum, the atrial septum is closed. In the other patients there is an atrial septal defect which is almost always in the fossa ovalis and which generally (in about 75% of all cases) communicates with the distal atrial chamber. Echocardiographic diagnosis of cor triatriatum sinistrum is simple: The left atrium is divided into two parts by a membranous structure. This membrane is most distinct in the apical or subcostal four-chamber 2-D echocardiogram. Often a membrane in the left atrium can also be seen in the parasternal long-axis 2-D echocardiogram. Here, however, care must be taken to avoid making a false diagnosis, because the wall of the left atrium often protrudes into the left atrium and simulates a membrane.

In addition to clearly visualizing a membrane in the left atrium, echocardiography must also determine the extent of the restriction caused by this membrane and the location of a possible atrial septal defect. Doppler echocardiography can be used to estimate the degree of obstruction of pulmonary venous drainage. The greater the obstruction, the better it will show up in color Doppler echocardiography. An atrial septal defect is best localized by visualizing the shunt in color Doppler flow maps.

| 8.10 | **Congenital Valve Defects** |
| 8.10.2 | **Tricuspid Valve Anomalies** |

Ebstein's Malformation of the Tricuspid Valve

Ebstein's malformation is characterized by displacement of the attachment of some or all of the tricuspid valve leaflets into the right ventricle. The leaflets are also dysplastic. Ebstein's malformation can appear in a variety of forms; mild cases can be completely free of symptoms. In mild cases, only the septal leaflet of the tricuspid valve is displaced into the ventricle. In moderately severe cases, the posterior leaflet is also involved. In severe cases, the septal and posterior leaflets are displaced as far as the right ventricular apex, and are attached to the free wall or the ventricular septum. Then, only a small amount of leaflet tissue in the apical region can move. Involvement of the anterosuperior leaflet is evidenced by abnormal insertion at a muscle bundle, which prevents this leaflet from moving freely and thus impedes the function of the valve.

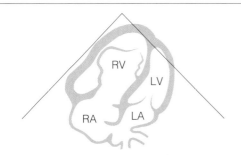

Ebstein's malformation of the tricuspid valve. The right atrium and right ventricle are enlarged, whereas the left atrium and the left ventricle appear comparatively small. The tricuspid valve leaflets are fused with the myocardium, so that the tricuspid valve is functionally displaced into the apex of the right ventricle. Tricuspid insufficiency. There is an additional interatrial septal defect, which can result in right-to-left shunt and cyanosis, due to the increased pressure in the right atrium.

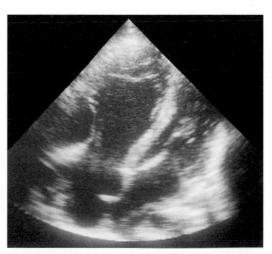

Apical four-chamber 2-D echocardiogram.

From a functional point of view, Ebstein's malformation leads to tricuspid insufficiency of a magnitude corresponding to the severity of the displacement of the posterior and septal leaflets. The displacement of the tricuspid valve into the right ventricle "atrializes" the right ventricle, *i.e.* the parts proximal to the displaced tricuspid valve form a functional part of the right atrium. Coupled with the tricuspid insufficiency, this leads to a reduction in the size of the right ventricle and, thus, to right ventricular incompetence.

Delayed closing of the tricuspid valve 0.065 seconds after the mitral valve is an established M-mode criterion of Ebstein's malformation. Today two-dimensional echocardiography is used to directly visualize displacement of the septal and posterior leaflets. The apical four-chamber 2-D echocardiogram is particularly suited for this purpose. Only the displacement of the septal tricuspid leaflet can generally be visualized in the parasternal long-axis 2-D echocardiogram. Usually the abnormal attachment of the anterosuperior leaflet can also be visualized in four-chamber 2-D echocardiograms. No normal opening or closing motion is noticeable in the leaflet, which appears as a sail-like structure stretched tightly between the atrioventricular passage and the apex of the right ventricle. Since the right ventricle (both the atrialized and ventricular parts) is dilated, the valve apparatus is generally well discernible from the apical position. Difficulties can arise only in the case of extremely severe forms in which the septal and posterior leaflets are displaced so far apically that the leaflets can only be found if the transducer is placed as far apically as possible. Displacement of the tricuspid valve can be overlooked if the transducer is placed farther parasternally. Subcostal scanning is helpful in this case, because it offers a better view of apical sections of the right ventricle. The functional effects are best analyzed using color Doppler and PW Doppler echocardiography (to determine the orifice area of the valve).

Associated malformations regularly include an atrial septal defect of the secundum type and pulmonary stenosis, which gives rise to a right-to-left shunt, due to the increased pressure in the right atrium. Every patient suffering from Ebstein's malformation should specifically be examined for an atrial septal defect and pulmonary stenosis. Ebstein's malformation is common in patients with pulmonary atresia and an intact ventricular septum, but in most of these cases, pulmonary atresia is the primary disorder. Finally, Ebstein's malformation also occurs with atrioventricular discordance or corrected transposition of the great arteries. Since the aorta arises from the right ventricle in this case, tricuspid insufficiency is of particular clinical significance, because it has the same hemodynamic effects as mitral insufficiency.

Hypoplasia and Dysplasia of the Tricuspid Valve

In some patients, the tricuspid valve can only be categorized as hypoplastic or dysplastic. Although the leaflets are attached normally, indicating the absence of Ebstein's malformation, the tricuspid valve is hypoplastic, *i.e.*, too small. The simultaneous view of the tricuspid valve and the mitral valve in the short axis (from the parasternal or subcostal position) is especially helpful in revealing hypoplasia of the tricuspid valve. Dysplasia of the tricuspid valve is a condition in which the valve leaflets are thickened and limited in their range of motion, and the chordae tendineae are rarefied and plump. Hemodynamically, tricuspid stenosis is generally the primary disorder. Often an atrial or ventricular septal defect will accompany this condition.

Uhl's Anomaly of the Right Ventricle

This extremely rare anomaly is characterized by the complete absence of the right ventricular myocardium. The right ventricle is a massively dilated fibrous sack without any muscle tissue.

Right Ventricular Dysplasia

This disorder is characterized by fatty infiltration of the right ventricular myocardium, while the left ventricle remains unaffected. Symptoms (arrhythmias) only begin to appear in adolescence or young adulthood. The right ventricle is dilated. Generally there is paradoxical septal motion and impairment of global right ventricular function.

Cleft Tricuspid Valve

In the setting of AV septal defects a cleft can be observed, not only in the mitral valve, but also in the tricuspid valve as well. This can lead to tricuspid insufficiency. In rare cases, cleft tricuspid valve occurs independently of an underlying AV septal defect. In echocardiography, this cleft cannot always be shown directly in the short-axis view, but tricuspid insufficiency can easily be demonstrated near the AV septum using color flow imaging.

Eustachian Valve and Cor Triatriatum Dextrum

The Eustachian valve is a normal structure at the origin of the inferior vena cava in the right atrium. It is particularly prominent in newborns and young infants. This is due to the significance of the Eustachian valve in the fetus: Arterialized blood that flows through the ductus venosus and reaches the right atrium at the origin of the inferior vena cava is diverted by the Eustachian valve to the foramen ovale and, thus, to the left atrium. The Eustachian valve can persist into adults in varying size and then often causes confusion. A genuine cor triatriatum dextrum is extremely rare, occurring either as a result a genuine membrane formation in the right atrium, as in cor triatriatum sinistrum, or as a result of an extremely large Eustachian valve that overrides the tricuspid orifice. The hemodynamic result is tricuspid atresia.

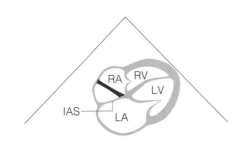

Eustachian valve. In the right atrium there is a membrane that appears to divide the right atrium. This Eustachian valve is a normal structure that extends from the origin of the inferior vena cava far into the atrium; it does not cause any obstruction. In the fetus, the Eustachian valve conducts blood from the inferior vena cava and the umbilical vein through the foramen ovale. Obstruction caused by an extremely large Eustachian valve is extremely rare.

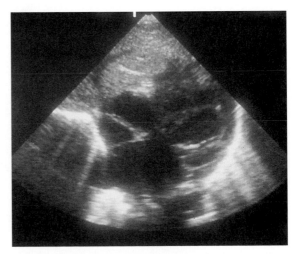

Subcostal four-chamber 2-D echocardiogram.

Valvular Aortic Stenosis

Valvular aortic stenosis is the most frequent cause of a stenosis of the left ventricular outflow tract during childhood. The aortic valve is thickened and the commissures are fused together. The aortic valve often has a primarily bicuspid form, However, tricuspid forms also occur where one leaflet is hypoplastic and fused to the adjacent leaflet so that the valve, although tricuspid, opens like a bicuspid valve. In congenital aortic stenosis the valve ring is almost always hypoplastic. Since surgical valve replacement is only possible if the annulus is sufficiently wide, measuring the valve ring by means of echocardiography plays an integral part in the examination of these children. Relatively low-risk valve replacement is possible only with a valve ring measuring at least 15 to 16 mm.

The morphology of the aortic valve and its opening can be observed in a parasternal short-axis echocardiogram. An apical or suprasternal CW Doppler recording is used to determine the gradient across the aortic valve. While the Doppler gradient at the aortic stenosis is a reliable indication of the severity of the aortic stenosis after the first few months of life, during these first few months it can be an unsuitable parameter for severity. This is because in this critical aortic stenosis in a newborn the function of the left ventricle is so greatly restricted that no pressure gradient can occur.

The echocardiogram shows a dilated left ventricle with restricted function and a thickened aortic valve. The ductus arteriosus is patent and shows an antegrade flow of blood to the aorta, *i.e.*, the right ventricle has assumed part of the systemic perfusion (as is the case in coarctation of the aorta or hypoplastic left heart syndrome). If the ductus arteriosus is open and there is increased pressure in the pulmonary artery, the pressure in the aorta will no longer be able to fall below the pressure in the pulmonary artery, thus causing a further decrease in the pressure gradient across the aortic valve.

Some newborns with critical aortic stenosis develop endocardial fibroelastosis of the left ventricle, which then does not dilate but can be small. In this case, there is almost always a patent ductus arteriosus, through which the right ventricle supplies at least part of the systemic circulation. This form of critical aortic stenosis represents a link to hypoplastic left heart syndrome with a dilated right ventricle and hypoplastic left ventricle.

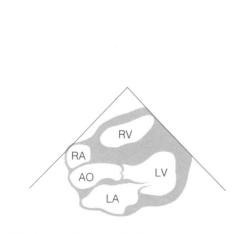

Valvular aortic stenosis in a newborn. The markedly thickened aortic valve is accompanied by endocardial fibroelastosis of the left ventricle.

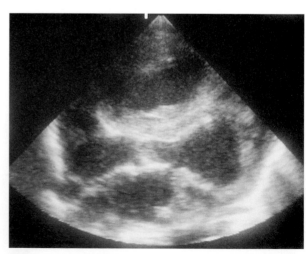

Subcostal long-axis 2-D echocardiogram.

8.10   **Congenital Valve Defects**   **377**
8.10.3   **Obstruction of the Left Ventricular Outflow Tract**
              and Defects of the Aortic Valve

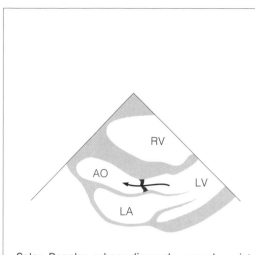

Color Doppler echocardiography reveals a jet behind the stenotic aortic valve (aliasing due to the high flow velocity).

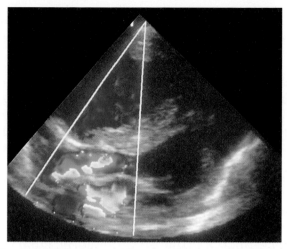

Color flow map of the subcostal four-chamber 2-D echocardiogram.

In older children the right ventricle is of normal size, while the left ventricle exhibits myocardial hypertrophy, the extent of which reflects the severity of aortic stenosis. The valvular aortic stenosis is generally accompanied by at least mild aortic insufficiency.

On the whole, the clinical syndrome of aortic stenosis in older children is similar to that in adults. Yet in contrast to adults, calcification is extremely rare before the age of eighteen.

Associated malformations are seldom found in children. However, coarctation of the aorta often appears as an associated disease in newborns and young infants. This is difficult to diagnose, because there is generally no gradient at the aortic isthmus. Additional pathological conditions include anomalies of the mitral valve and ventricular septal defects.

Subvalvular Aortic Stenosis

Subvalvular aortic stenosis is characterized by a fibrous ridge a few millimeters below the valve in the left ventricular outflow tract. This fibrous ridge appears as an echo-producing structure primarily in parasternal and apical long-axis views. It can be visualized best from the subcostal position in newborns and young infants. This fibrous ridge can be fused with the aorta, in which case it will hardly be discernible in the echocardiogram. Generally it will lie close to the aortic valve and can be distinguished from a valvular aortic stenosis by means of color Doppler echocardiography.

Subvalvular aortic stenosis may be isolated, or it can occur in conjunction with a valvular aortic stenosis, an interrupted aortic arch, or coarctation of the aorta.

Supravalvular Aortic Stenosis

Supravalvular aortic stenosis occurs almost exclusively in Williams-Beuren syndrome. Typically, the ascending aorta will be constricted just above the aortic root. Associated malformations include peripheral pulmonary stenosis, stenosis of the origins of the vessels of the aortic arch, and progressive hypoplasia of the aortic arch and the descending aorta.

8.10   **Congenital Valve Defects**   378
8.10.3   **Obstruction of the Left Ventricular Outflow Tract**
                     and Defects of the Aortic Valve

Aortic Insufficiency

Isolated congenital aortic insufficiency is extremely rare. However, aortic insufficiency frequently occurs following surgical correction of valvular aortic stenoses and ventricular septal defects, and in Marfan's syndrome.

Postoperative aortic insufficiency regularly occurs following commissurotomy of a valvular aortic stenosis and after balloon dilation of a valvular aortic stenosis. The fused dysplastic cusps will almost always fail to close properly after surgery as well as after cardiological intervention. Slight aortic insufficiency is even desirable, because experience has shown that it leads to enhanced growth of the hypoplastic valve ring.

Aortic insufficiency with a ventricular septal defect is a rarer cause of aortic insufficiency during childhood. This is seen primarily in conjunction with a perimembranous ventricular septal defect, in which the non-coronary or right coronary aortic cusp is immediately adjacent to the upper edge of the ventricular septal defect. In this condition, in the cusp can prolapse into the defect. Such a prolapse of an aortic cusp can often be directly visualized in two-dimensional echocardiograms. Simultaneous detection of aortic insufficiency and a perimembranous ventricular septal defect by means of color Doppler echocardiography makes this a probable diagnosis. In addition to this "classic" cause of aortic insufficiency during childhood, aortic insufficiency also occurs in older patients with tetralogy of Fallot and in the truncus arteriosus (communis). In the latter case, this is due to insufficiency of the truncus valve.

A common cause of isolated aortic insufficiency is Marfan's syndrome. In addition to constitutional symptoms and iridodonesis, there are also cardiological findings. These include an expanded ascending aorta and aortic insufficiency due to the massively dilated root of the aorta. This is frequently accompanied by a prolapse of the mitral valve. In its outward appearance, Marfan's syndrome can be mistaken for homocystinuria.

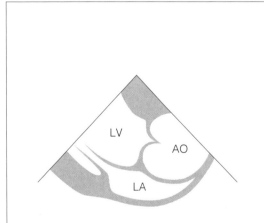

Marfan's syndrome with dilated root of the aorta. Massively dilated root of the aorta (AO) in a patient with Marfan's syndrome. The left ventricle is greatly rounded and expanded due to aortic insufficiency (not visible here).

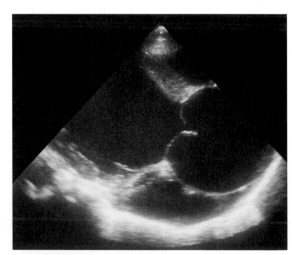

Parasternal long-axis 2-D echocardiogram.

Aortic insufficiency must be differentiated from two rare anomalies, namely, perforated sinus of Valsalva aneurysm and left ventricular atrioventricular tunnel.

Ruptured Aneurysm of the sinus of Valsalva

An aneurysm of the sinus of Valsalva can be either congenital or acquired (endocarditis). Generally the right aortic sinus is affected, less frequently the non-coronary or left aortic sinus. Symptoms only begin to appear when a perforation of the aneurysm of sinus of Valsalva occurs. In most cases, a communicating passage between the aortic sinus and the right ventricle, right atrium, or pulmonary artery will appear. The two-dimensional echocardiogram will show the aneurysmally expanded sinus of Valsalva. Unlike the aneurysmal dilation of the entire root of the aorta in Marfan's syndrome, only one sinus is affected. Color Doppler echocardiography reveals the communicating passage to the right ventricle, right atrium, or pulmonary artery. With a perforation into the right ventricle, a differential diagnosis must eliminate the possibility of a ventricular septal defect; with a perforation into the right atrium, a coronary fistula and Gerbode's defect; and with a perforation into the pulmonary artery, an aortopulmonary window must be excluded.

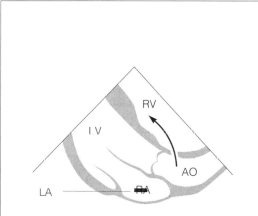

Perforated aneurysm of sinus of Valsalva above the right coronary cusp communicating with the right ventricle. Color Doppler echocardiography reveals a jet with aliasing from the root of the aorta to the right ventricle.

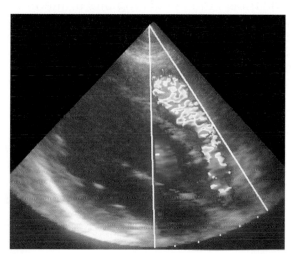

Color flow map of the parasternal long-axis 2-D echocardiogram.

Tunnel Between the Aorta and the Left Ventricle

This is a congenital defect between the right aortic sinus and its aortic cusp. The tunnel between the aorta and the left ventricle creates a direct hemodynamic connection between these two structures. The echocardiogram reveals the right aortic sinus to be massively dilated, and color echocardiography shows regurgitation next to the aortic valve.

Since such a tunnel between the aorta and the left ventricle represents the most common cause of aortic insufficiency beginning as early as in newborns, the examination should specifically search for this phenomenon in cases of isolated aortic insufficiency occurring before the second year of life.

8.10	Congenital Valve Defects	380
8.10.4	Obstruction of the Right Ventricular Outflow Tract and	
	Defects of the Pulmonary Valve	

Valvular Pulmonary Stenosis

In valvular pulmonary stenosis, the cusps are thickened and are fused together. The valve can have a primarily bicuspid, tricuspid, or quadricuspid form. Generally fusion of the commissures is the primary disorder, but this fusion can become less important. In such a case stenosis is caused by a mucoid thickening of the cusps (dysplastic valve). This is of therapeutic significance, because opening the commissures will have no significant effect on the stenosis.

In the case of an isolated pulmonary stenosis, myocardial hypertrophy is present and the ventricle tends to be small. The pulmonary artery is often extremely distended due to the dilation downstream of the stenosis, and this dilation often causes the valve ring to appear narrow. The pulmonary valve itself lies in the near field, which means that it generally cannot be visualized as clearly as the aortic valve. However, systolic doming of the valve leaflets is often visible, and a central jet will appear in the color Doppler echocardiogram. A parasternal CW Doppler recording is used to determine the pressure gradient.

In aortic stenosis the thickening and limited range of motion of the aortic cusps can be easily diagnosed in the 2-D echocardiogram, but this is not the case with the pulmonary valve. The valve can appear thickened and abnormal without any stenosis. Caution is required particularly in the case of newborns, because pulmonary valves that exhibit this type of thickening can revert to normal.

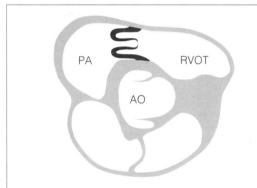

Valvular pulmonary stenosis. Thickened pulmonary valve with doming of the cusps. Since the pulmonary valves lies in the near field, the cusps generally cannot be visualized as clearly as in aortic stenosis. Particularly in the case of newborns, a normal pulmonary valve can appear thickened, making it essential to measure the pressure gradient across the valve.

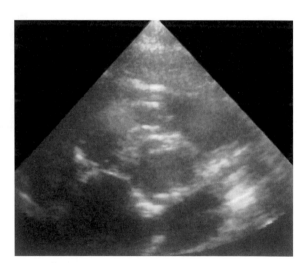

Subcostal short-axis 2-D echocardiogram.

Genuine pulmonary stenosis must be distinguished from a flow-induced stenosis. In the case of recirculation defects (ventricular septal defect, atrial septal defect, complex defects without pulmonary stenosis) the flow through the pulmonary artery is several times greater than normal. The velocity of flow through the pulmonary valve rises accordingly. Measuring the flow velocity upstream of the suspected stenosis in the Doppler analysis will reveal that there is already an increased flow velocity before the stenosis. In this case, the velocity upstream of the stenosis must be taken into account, *i.e.* use of the simplified Bernoulli equation is no longer acceptable.

Often a valvular pulmonary stenosis will appear as part of another anomaly. Complex heart defects in (tricuspid atresia, univentricular heart, etc.) are often associated with valvular pulmonary stenosis.

8.10   **Congenital Valve Defects**
8.10.4   **Obstruction of the Right Ventricular Outflow Tract and**
               Defects of the Pulmonary Valve

381

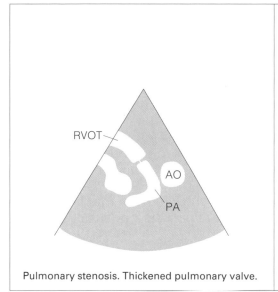

Pulmonary stenosis. Thickened pulmonary valve.

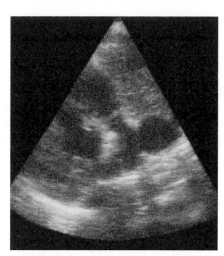

Parasternal short-axis 2-D echocardiogram.

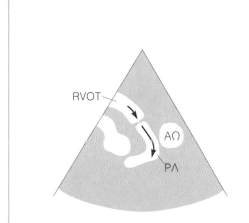

Color Doppler echocardiography reveals a jet with aliasing behind the pulmonary stenosis, indicating the presence of a pressure gradient.

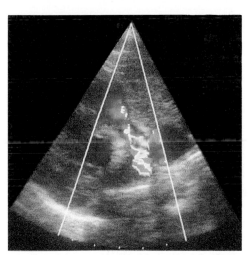

Color flow map of the parasternal short-axis 2-D echocardiogram.

Infundibular Pulmonary Stenosis

Here the pulmonary valve is normal, but the infundibulum of the right ventricle is narrowed. Infundibular stenosis will can often be visualized in the parasternal or apical view when high-frequency transducers and a short near field are used. PW Doppler echocardiography can be used to show that the pressure gradient lies upstream of the pulmonary valve.

Infundibular pulmonary stenosis often appear in conjunction with a valvular pulmonary stenosis; it is rarely isolated. One relevant cause of an isolated infundibular stenosis is found in patients with a ventricular septal defect: The pulmonary recirculation causes infundibular hypertrophy and, ultimately, infundibular pulmonary stenosis. If the ventricular septal defect closes spontaneously, "isolated" infundibular pulmonary stenosis will remain.

8.10	Congenital Valve Defects	382
8.10.4	Obstruction of the Right Ventricular Outflow Tract and	
	Defects of the Pulmonary Valve	

Rare Causes of Pulmonary Stenosis

Other causes of obstruction of the right ventricular outflow tract are rare.

Hypertrophy of the muscles below the infundibulum can produce intraventricular stenosis and divide the right ventricle in two (two-chambered right ventricle). This generally occurs in conjunction with a ventricular septal defect, and can best visualized in the subcostal or apical view. Even when the echocardiogram appears to show an intraventricular obstruction, the possibility of an infundibular and valvular pulmonary stenosis must always be excluded, because secondary myocardial hypertrophy can cause the stenosis to produce an echocardiographic image that looks like intraventricular obstruction.

In rare cases, a large aneurysm of the septum membranaceum ventriculorum that bulges into the right ventricular outflow tract can obstruct the tract. Tumors can also obstruct the right ventricular outflow tract.

Supravalvular pulmonary stenoses occur primarily in conjunction with valvular pulmonary stenoses or tetralogy of Fallot. "Isolated" supravalvular pulmonary stenoses occur in patients who have had banding of the pulmonary artery during childhood.

Peripheral Pulmonary Stenoses

Only central pulmonary vessel stenoses, *i.e.*, stenoses at the bifurcation, can be detected on echocardiograms. They seldom appear in isolation and are generally observed in conjunction with other defects (tetralogy of Fallot, transposition, pulmonary atresia with ventricular septal defect) Even in Williams-Beuren syndrome, peripheral pulmonary stenoses occur. Here, they generally lie far in the periphery (*i.e.*, in the intrapulmonary region) and therefore cannot be visualized on an echocardiogram.

Pulmonary Insufficiency

Pulmonary insufficiency rarely occurs as an isolated lesion. Mild pulmonary insufficiency, generally hemodynamically insignificant, occurs with defects that cause dilation of the pulmonary artery as well as with increased pressure within the pulmonary artery. More extensive pulmonary insufficiency can occur following surgery or balloon dilation of the pulmonary valve, since the pathologically deformed valve is no longer capable of closing after the commissures have been opened.

Agenesis of the pulmonary valve, a special form of tetralogy of Fallot, represents the only congenital type of pulmonary insufficiency. The pulmonary valve fails to develop, and narrowing of the valve ring occurs. The regurgitation and the stenotic effect of the narrow valve ring combine to produce a grotesque dilation of the central pulmonary arteries, so that stridor resulting from compression of the bronchial tree appears as the cardinal symptom.

| 8.11 | Tumors and Myocardial Heart Disease |
| 8.11.1 | Anomalies and Diseases of the Coronary Arteries |

Anomalies and acquired changes in the coronary arteries are very rare in childhood. The predominant symptom is myocardial ischemia and, thus, regional wall motion abnormality.

Regional wall motion disturbances are extremely rare in children, so the symptom is virtually pathognomic. An exception, however, is paradox septal motion in right ventricular volume overload.

Causes of regional wall motion in the absence of echocardiographic signs of coronary changes include coronary stenoses subsequent to surgery of the coronary vessels (anatomical correction of transposition), compression of the left coronary artery after pulmonary artery banding due to transposition of the great arteries, familial hyperlipidemia, and infantile polyarteritis nodosa. None of these diseases can be directly diagnosed by echocardiography. The diagnosis of pulmonary atresia with intact ventricular septal defect and myocardial sinusoids can, at least, be suggested by echocardiography. Atresia of the coronary ostia also cannot be visualized. Coronary artery changes that can be diagnosed by echocardiography are described below.

Origin of the Coronary Arteries From the Pulmonary Artery (Bland-White-Garland Syndrome)

In Bland-White-Garland syndrome, the left coronary artery arises from the pulmonary artery. The hemodynamic effects of this are determined by the extent of collateralization. When there is sufficient collateralization, the right coronary artery "shares" with the left coronary artery, and there is retrograde perfusion of the left coronary artery. Myocardial ischemia does not occur, but there left-to-right shunting from the aorta through the coronaries into the pulmonary artery occurs. In echocardiography, this shunt can be identified as a diastolic jet in the pulmonary artery at the origin of the left coronary artery.

When collateralization is insufficient, myocardial ischemia or infarction occurs. Then, left ventricular dysfunction becomes the central problem. Echocardiography reveals a dilated, dysfunctional left ventricle. Regional contractility is abnormal, particularly in the region of the left ventricular posterior wall. Usually, there is mitral insufficiency due to left ventricular dilatation or papillary muscle enlargement. The echogeneity of the papillary muscles is often increased due to fibrosis. Left ventricular thrombus is an infrequent finding. The diagnosis is suggested when the left coronary artery cannot be visualized. However, a diastolic jet in the pulmonary artery is a sure sign.

Coronary Fistula

With coronary fistula, the origin of the coronary arteries is normal, but there is "short-circuit" communication with the low pressure system. Coronary fistula may drain into the right atrium, right ventricle, left ventricle, or pulmonary artery. Due to the difference in pressure between the origin of the fistula and the aorta, systolic-diastolic flow or purely diastolic flow occurs through the fistula. Echocardiography is often able to directly visualize the massively dilated coronary artery of the fistula itself. The origin of the fistula can often be identified by the jet in Doppler color flow imaging. Anomalies that must be considered in the differential diagnosis are: Gerbode's defect when the fistula drains into the right atrium, ventricular septal defect and a perforated sinus of Valsalva aneurysm when the fistula drains into the right ventricle, mitral insufficiency when the fistula drains into the left atrium, aortic insufficiency or an aortic left ventricular tunnel when the fistula drains into the left ventricle, and patent ductus arteriosus and Bland-White-Garland syndrome when the fistula drains into the pulmonary artery.

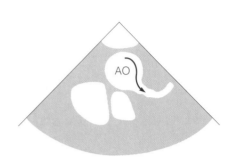

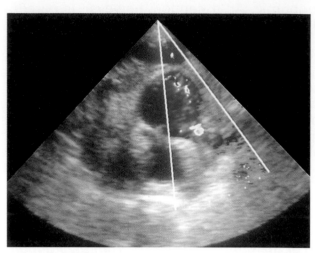

Coronary fistula. Dilated coronary artery in which Doppler color flow imaging clearly revealed diastolic blood flow. In contrast to coronary aneurysms of Kawasaki's syndrome, there is no local dilatation corresponding to aneurysm. Instead, the vascular contours are smooth in appearance. This case corresponds to a coronary fistula to the right atrium.

Parasternal short-axis 2-D echocardiogram with color flow mapping.

Kawasaki's Syndrome

In Kawasaki's syndrome, *i.e.*, mucotaneous lymph node syndrome, dilated coronary arteries have a typical aneurysmal appearance. The diagnosis of proximal aneurysms can be made in cross-sectional scans with a high degree of accuracy. When the aneurysm is located in peripheral locations, it may be difficult to impossible to visualize.

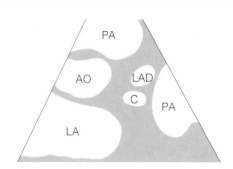

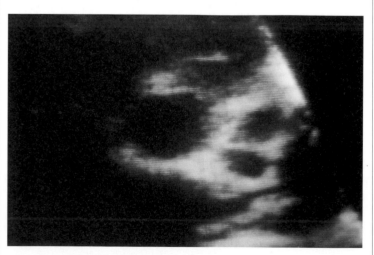

Coronary aneurysm in Kawasaki's syndrome. This parasternal short-axis scan visualizes the area between the aorta (AO) and pulmonary artery (PA), through which the left coronary artery courses. There are two circular, echo-free areas that correspond to aneurysms of the circumflex artery (C) and the left anterior descending (LAD) coronary artery. The PA appears twice, because it courses in an arch.

Parasternal short-axis 2-D echocardiogram.

Primary disease of the myocardium is rare in children. The causes are the same as in adults, *i.e.* dilated, restrictive, and hypertrophic cardiomyopathies. Congenital diseases that produce the same symptoms must be excluded from the diagnosis. For example, in order to diagnose dilated cardiomyopathy, left ventricular pressure overload and myocardial ischemia (*e.g.*, Bland-White-Garland syndrome) must be excluded from the diagnosis. In hypertrophic cardiomyopathy, secondary myocardial hypertrophy due to chronic pressure overload must be excluded from the diagnosis (*e.g.*, aortic stenosis, coarctation of the aorta).

Primary *endocardial fibroelastosis (EFE) and myocardial storage diseases* are characteristic types of primary myocardial disease that may occur in pediatric patients. Endocardial fibroelastosis affects newborns: massive thickening of the endocardium leads to systolic contractile dysfunction and impaired diastolic filling. The left ventricle is usually dilated, but can also be small (as in restrictive cardiomyopathy). Echocardiography demonstrates the thickened endocardium as a highly echo reflective lining of the left ventricle. Secondary thickening of the endocardium occurs in other lesions (*e.g.*, critical aortic stenosis in newborns).

As in adults, myocardial storage disease in children can simulate hypertrophic cardiomyopathy. In some cases, thickening of the myocardium (which often causes increased echodensity) is much more severe than that observed in adults. Naturally, secondary myocardial hypertrophy due to chronic left ventricular pressure overload must be excluded from the diagnosis.

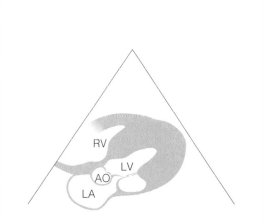

Pompe's disease (glycogen storage disease). Severe myocardial thickening, the echodensity of the myocardium is greatly increased. The lumen of the left ventricle is hardly visible, even in diastole.

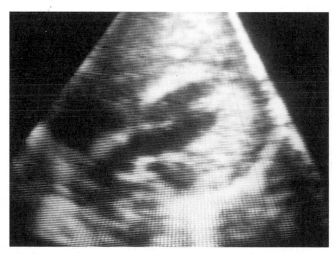

Subcostal four-chamber 2-D echocardiogram.

| 8.11 | Tumors and Myocardial Heart Disease |
| 8.11.3 | Tumors |

In pediatric patients, cardiac tumors are rare, but usually treatable. Therefore, it is important to diagnose these tumors. Echocardiography is clearly superior to angiography in the diagnosis of cardiac tumors. The tumors appear on the echocardiogram as an echo reflective mass. Because of their movement in the bloodstream, pediculate tumors are hard to overlook. Intramyocardial tumors, however, can be detected only from sizes of ca. 0.5 to 1.0 cm and up. Thrombus and endocarditic vegetations must be considered in the differential diagnosis.

A *rhabdomyoma* is an intramyocardial tumor that protrudes into the right or left ventricular cavity only as a secondary phenomenon. Rhabdomyomas are usually multiple. They are associated with tuberous cerebral sclerosis, and occur primarily in the first years of life. Frequently, these tumors spontaneously disappear. Echocardiography usually reveals a broad-based tumor connected to the myocardium; the echodensity of the tumor often is slightly increased.

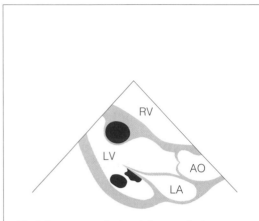

Rhabdomyoma of the left ventricular myocardium. Multiple echo reflective tumors are present in the myocardium. Multiple rhabdomyomas are common in patients with Pringle's disease (tuberous sclerosis), and they usually have a good prognosis.

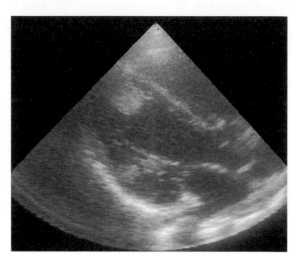

Apical long-axis 2-D echocardiogram.

Fibromas are fibrous tumors that arise in the myocardium as pediculate tumors on the cardiac valves. Usually, the echodensity of the fibromas is clearly increased.

Myxomas can occur in adolescents, but are much more common in adults.

Tetromas contain components of all three germ layers; their location is usually intrapericardial; calcification is common.

Hemangiomas are rare masses that occur primarily in the atrial and epicardial regions.

Malignant cardiac tumors are extremely rare. They usually lead to myocardial infiltration and (hemorrhagic) pericardial effusion.

Cardiac metastases are extremely rare in pediatric patients. Like malignant tumors, they also commonly lead to (hemorrhagic) pericardial effusion.

| 8. | Congenital Heart Disease |
| 8.12 | Analysis of Complex Congenital Heart Anomalies: The Segmental Approach |

The diagnosis and assessment of congenital heart anomalies, particularly situs anomalies, requires a systematic analysis of the anatomy of the heart and vessels. Although this may be difficult at first, and because echocardiography tempts the observer to make *prima vista* diagnoses, it is necessary to abide by a systematic approach with every patient.

Otherwise, associated lesions that are not immediately visible could easily be overlooked. The segmental, systematic approach to the evaluation of congenital cardiac anomalies was developed by the "English School". Although it may seem complicated at first, the use of such a systematic approach has definite advantages. It permits diagnosis and classification of even complex congenital heart defects. The systematic approach described below is an excellent method for cardiac ultrasound diagnosis of congenital heart defects.

Step One:
Definition of Situs

The situs, *i.e.* atrial anatomy, is sonographically determined by examining the epigastric anatomy. The following types are distinguished: normal situs (situs solitus), mirror-image situs (situs inversus), right isomerism (asplenia syndrome), and left isomerism (polysplenia syndrome).

Step Two:
Definition of Ventricular Anatomy

The left ventricle is characterized by slight trabecularization and continuity between the semilunar and atrioventricular valves. The right ventricle is characterized by a moderator band, discontinuity, and rough trabecularization.

Step Three:
Definition of Atrioventricular Communication

The type and manner of communication must be defined.

Type of communication:
Communication between the atria and the ventricles can be *concordant* (communication between left atrium and left ventricle, and right atrium and right ventricle, resp.), *discordant* (*e.g.*, right atrium connected to left ventricle), or *ambiguous* (*e.g.* two left atria).

Manner of communication:
As in a normal heart, communication can consist of two valves that each communicate with one respective ventricle, or with one common ventricle. In other cases, the valve may ride over a ventricular septal defect, etc. *(overriding)*, or its chordae tendineae may insert in the contralateral side of the ventricular septum *(straddling)*. Only one atrioventricular valve may be developed due to a variety of factors, namely: failure of the atrioventricular valves to divide (AV septal defect); agenesis of an atrioventricular valve (*e.g.*, "classical" tricuspid atresia with no communication to the right atrium); the valve exists, but is imperforate (atretic).

Step Four:
Definition of the Ventriculo-arterial Communication

Type of communication:
Again, the communication may be concordant (the aorta arises from a left ventricle, and the pulmonary artery from a right ventricle), discordant (*e.g.* transposition), both great arteries can arise from a single ventricle (double outlet ventricle), or there may be only one great artery (*e.g.* truncus communis).

Manner of communication:
The manner of communication can consist in an imperforate valve (*i.e.*, and atretic membrane) or overriding (as in tetralogy of Fallot or truncus arteriosus).

Step Five:
Identification of Specific Cardiac Anomalies
Isolated cardiac anomalies provide details required to systematically describe the "building plan" of the heart.

▸ **Anomalies of the systemic veins:**
Azygos continuity of the inferior vena cava, persistent left superior vena cava with drainage in the coronary venous sinus, etc.

▸ **Anomalies of the pulmonary veins:**
Partial and total anomalous pulmonary venous return.

▸ **Atrial septal defects:**
Ostium primum and secundum defects, sinus venosus defects, aneurysms of the fossa ovalis, etc.

▸ **Assessment of the atria:**
Cor triatriatum, Eustachian valve, atrial tumors, etc.

▸ **Anomalies of the atrioventricular valves:**
Ebstein's malformation, atresia, hypoplasia, dysplasia, insufficiency, cleft, AV septal defects, prolapse, etc.

▸ **Anomalies of the semilunar valves:**
Atresia, stenosis, insufficiency, etc.

▸ **Assessment of the ventricular septum:**
Defects, asymmetrical septum hypertrophy, tumors, etc.

▸ **Assessment of the ventricle:**
Hypoplasia, cardiomyopathies, tumors, etc.

▸ **Assessment of the great arteries:**
Aortopulmonary window, patent ductus arteriosus, coarctation of the aorta.

▸ **Assessment of the coronary arteries:**
Kawasaki's syndrome (mucotaneous lymph node syndrome), Bland-White-Garland syndrome, coronary fistula, etc.

The following tables list various normal values for echocardiographic measurements in children in terms of body surface area. In contrast to graphic representations, the disadvantage of tables is the need to interpolate between the different ranges. However, in clinical practice, tables are much easier to use. We, therefore, decided to list the data in table form. The tables give the most important normal values for M-mode echocardiography and Doppler, plus the standard deviation. The data was not compiled from the literature, but was measured in healthy young children and adolescents. Therefore, all of the data were obtained from a single normal collective, were measured using a single echocardiograph, and were obtained (mostly) by a single observer (Dr. Kampmann).

Table 1. Echocardiographic normal values for children (n = 124)

		LVEDD	LVESD	RVEDD	IVS-EDD	IVS-ESD	LVPW-EDD	LVPW-ESD	LVFS	LVEF	Mean Vcf	Mean Vcfc
		cm	cm	cm	cm	cm	cm	cm	%	%	circ/s	circ/s
BSA ≤ 0.5 m²	mean	2.33	1.43	0.97	0.39	0.52	0.43	0.63	38	71	1.6	0.85
	SD	0.24	0.19	0.17	0.06	0.07	0.04	0.08	3.5	4.1	0.3	0.1
	10th perc.	1.92	1.2	0.7	0.3	0.41	0.37	0.52	35	66	1.25	0.73
	90th perc.	2.6	1.68	1.2	0.49	0.61	0.5	0.75	45	78	2.24	1
BSA 0.51 - 0.75 m²	mean	3.16	1.95	1.18	0.45	0.68	0.49	0.79	38	69	1.3	0.84
	SD	0.36	0.26	0.23	0.05	0.11	0.05	0.08	4.6	5.9	0.2	0.09
	10th perc.	2.6	1.6	0.9	0.4	0.55	0.4	0.66	32	61	0.97	0.69
	90th perc.	3.6	2.36	1.5	0.5	0.9	0.6	0.9	44	77	1.59	0.96
BSA 0.76 - 1.0 m²	mean	3.64	2.39	1.53	0.58	0.77	0.59	0.87	34	64	1.07	0.75
	SD	0.24	0.18	0.25	0.09	0.13	0.08	0.09	3.4	4.6	0.13	0.08
	10th perc.	3.3	2.1	1.24	0.42	0.45	0.5	0.76	30	58	0.93	0.65
	90th perc.	4	2.65	2.04	0.7	0.94	0.7	1.05	40	71	1.32	0.89
BSA 1.01 - 1.25 m²	mean	4	2.59	1.79	0.63	0.87	0.66	1.05	35	65	1.15	0.81
	SD	0.27	0.22	0.21	0.12	0.14	0.09	0.13	3.1	4.3	0.19	0.1
	10th perc.	3.7	2.31	1.51	0.49	0.65	0.53	0.89	32	60	0.92	0.71
	90th perc.	4.4	2.9	2.03	0.8	1.1	0.8	1.2	39	70	1.39	1.01
BSA > 1.25 m²	mean	4.48	2.88	2.01	0.69	0.92	0.77	1.12	35	65	1.1	0.79
	SD	0.32	0.34	0.39	0.09	0.16	0.09	0.14	4.1	5.3	0.16	0.1
	10th perc.	4	2.43	1.34	0.54	0.69	0.6	0.9	32	60	0.88	0.64
	90th perc.	4.99	3.4	2.5	0.84	1.12	0.9	1.3	40	71	1.41	0.98
Total	mean	3.66	2.33	1.56	0.57	0.78	0.61	0.93	36	67	1.23	0.81
	SD	0.76	0.54	0.46	0.14	0.19	0.14	0.2	4	5.5	0.26	0.1
	10th perc.	2.5	1.6	0.93	0.39	0.53	0.43	0.68	32	60	0.94	0.67
	90th perc.	4.6	2.9	2.1	0.79	1	0.8	1.24	42	74	1.56	0.96

Table 2. Echocardiographic normal values for children by body surface area (BSA) (n = 124)

		LVEDD/m²	LVESD/m²	RVEDD/m²	IVS-EDD/m²	IVS-ESD/m²	LVPW-EDD/m²	LVPW-ESD/m²
		cm/m²	cm/m²	cm/m²	cm/m²	cm/m²	cm/m²	cm/m²
BSA ≤ 0.5 m²	mean	6.53	4.01	2.7	1.1	1.49	1.2	1.8
	SD	1.03	0.69	0.6	0.29	0.39	0.18	0.32
	10th perc.	4.92	2.84	1.64	0.77	1	0.88	1.22
	90th perc.	8	5.1	3.69	1.67	2.2	1.5	2.24
BSA 0.51 - 0.75 m²	mean	5.03	3.09	1.89	0.71	1.09	0.78	1.27
	SD	0.5	0.35	0.45	0.12	0.23	0.1	0.18
	10th perc.	4.26	2.5	1.4	0.54	0.86	0.66	0.98
	90th perc.	5.8	3.5	2.34	0.89	1.52	0.96	1.55

Table 2. Echocardiographic normal values for children by body surface area (BSA) (n = 124) (continued)

		LVEDD/ m² cm/m²	LVESD/ m² cm/m²	RVEDD/ m² cm/m²	IVS-EDD/ m² cm/m²	IVS-ESD/ m² cm/m²	LVPW-EDD/ m² cm/m²	LVPW-ESD/ m² cm/m²
BSA 0.76 - 1.0 m²	mean	4.23	2.78	1.78	0.67	0.89	0.68	1.02
	SD	0.31	0.28	0.25	0.13	0.14	0.1	0.08
	10th perc.	3.68	2.3	1.47	0.52	0.67	0.56	0.89
	90th perc.	4.6	3.1	2.2	0.91	1.09	0.84	1.12
BSA 1.01 - 1.25 m²	mean	3.5	2.27	1.56	0.55	0.76	0.58	0.91
	SD	0.24	0.2	0.15	0.09	0.12	0.08	0.11
	10th perc.	3.2	2.04	1.3	0.44	0.6	0.47	0.73
	90th perc.	3.8	2.48	1.74	0.7	0.96	0.69	1.06
BSA > 1.25 m²	mean	3.03	1.96	1.35	0.47	0.62	0.51	0.76
	SD	0.25	0.24	0.25	0.06	0.09	0.06	0.99
	10th perc.	2.64	1.62	0.98	0.4	0.49	0.45	0.65
	90th perc.	3.4	2.21	1.77	0.54	0.75	0.6	0.88
Total	mean	4.24	2.68	1.77	0.66	0.92	0.71	1.09
	SD	1.26	0.76	0.55	0.24	0.34	0.24	0.37
	10th perc.	2.93	1.87	1.28	0.43	0.59	0.47	0.72
	90th perc.	6.05	3.75	2.48	0.95	1.47	1.12	1.6

Table 3. Doppler normal values for children (n = 124)

				mean	SD
Tricuspid valve					
	E wave		m/s	0.82	0.15
	A wave		m/s	0.52	0.1
	E/A ratio			1.60	
Pulmonary valve			m/s	0.98	0.15
	RVFVT		cm	19.77	2.45
	RVET		ms	317.0	48.45
	RVETc		ms	401.0	35.5
	RVAT		ms	121.5	23.13
	RVAT/ET			0.387	0.05
Mitral valve					
	E wave		m/s	0.93	0.17
	A wave		m/s	0.52	0.12
	E/A ratio			1.78	
Aortic valve			m/s	1.14	0.18
	LVFVT		cm	20.31	2.797
	LVET		ms	304.4	40.5
	LVETc		ms	456.4	36.4
	LVAT		ms	92.8	14.97
	LVAT/ET			0.305	0.04
Ascending aorta			m/s	0.9	
Descending aorta			m/s	0.88	
Vena cava			m/s	0.5 to 1.5	

Key to Abbreviations	
BSA	Body surface area
IVS-EDD	Interventricular septal end-diastolic diameter
IVS-ESD	Interventricular septal end-systolic diameter
LVAT	Left ventricular acceleration time
LVEDD	Left ventricular end-diastolic diameter
LVEF	Left ventricular ejection fraction
LVESD	Left ventricular end-systolic diameter
LVET	Left ventricular ejection time
LVETc	Left ventricular ejection time, corrected
LVFS	Left ventricular fractional shortening
LVFVT	Left ventricular flow velocity integral
LVPW-EDD	Left ventricular posterior wall end-diastolic diameter
LVPW-ESD	Left ventricular posterior wall end-systolic diameter
Mean Vcf	Mean velocity of circumferential fiber shortening
Mean Vcfc	Mean velocity of circumferential fiber shortening, corrected
RVAT	Right ventricular acceleration time
RVEDD	Right ventricular end-diastolic diameter
RVET	Right ventricular ejection time
RVFVT	Right ventricular flow velocity integral

There are two main problems associated with the diagnosis of myocarditis. On the one hand, myocarditis is commonly misdiagnosed, as autopsy studies have shown. On the other hand, a variety of heart muscle diseases of otherwise unknown origin are classified as "myocarditis" unjustified in the everyday clinical setting. The diagnosis of myocarditis is currently based on histological evidence. However, the accuracy of the diagnosis depends on removal of the biopsy material from a "representative" site, and on the skill and experience of the pathologist. Furthermore, all of the clinical and pieces of the diagnostic mosaic are unspecific. Echocardiographic signs of acute, inflammatory heart disease are left ventricular enlargement, impaired left ventricular function, and pericardial effusion.

The following tests provide supplementary evidence of recent infection:
1. positive ^{67}gallium myocardial scintigraphy,
2. isolation of the virus (seldom successful) from lavages, blood, or stools during the first few days after onset, and
3. a four-fold titer increase in serological tests during the second week after onset.

Therefore, the primary role of cardiac ultrasound diagnosis is to provide additional indications to support the evidence of endomyocardial biopsy and to follow the course of the disease. The significance of raw data analysis for tissue characterization, primarily in cellular and pericellular edema, remains unclear.

9.	**Myocardial Disease**
9.2	**Cardiomyopathies**
	(Irmtraut Kruck)

According to the recommendations of the World Health Organization (WHO), cardiomyopathies are classified into three types, according to the observed patho-anatomical and pathophysiological changes. The three types are:

1. dilated cardiomyopathy
2. hypertrophic cardiomyopathy, and
3. restrictive (infiltrative) cardiomyopathy.

| 9.2 | **Cardiomyopathies** |
| 9.2.1 | **Dilated Cardiomyopathy** |

Dilated cardiomyopathy is described according to etiology as follows [55]:

▸ Cryptogenic ("Idiopathic")
▸ Inflammatory ▸ Metabolic ▸ Toxic ▸ Familial - Hereditary

A positive family history is found in only 5 to 10 percent of all patients with cardiomegaly [44]. The most common cause of dilated cardiomyopathy is myocarditis, which may be either infectious or noninfectious and acute, subacute, or chronic. Histologically, lymphocytic infiltration and myocardial cell necrosis can be observed [2]. These changes may be caused by infectious organisms and/or toxins or other autoimmune processes and allergies. They may occur either peri or post partum. Predominant right ventricular dilated cardiomyopathy, in which ventricular tachycardia and sudden cardiac death frequently occur, is rare.

Dilated cardiomyopathy is characterized by left and right ventricular enlargement with increased systolic and diastolic ventricular volumes and a reduced ejection fraction. Usually, the ventricles become globular in shape [29]. The left and right atria commonly become dilated in the later course of the disease.

Cardiac Ultrasound Diagnosis

The enlarged ventricles provide good conditions for echocardiograpy. Multiple views from the usual portals are required for diagnosis and assessment (parasternal long and short-axis views, apical two and four-chamber views, and subcostal views).

Conventional Echocardiography

Two-dimensional echocardiography:
(dilated cardiomyopathy)

* Enlarged left ventricle with impaired contractility.

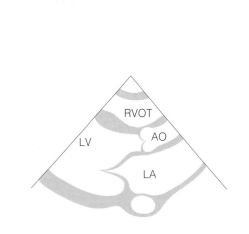

The left ventricle (LV) and left atrium (LA) are enlarged compared with the aorta (AO) and right ventricular outflow tract (RVOT).

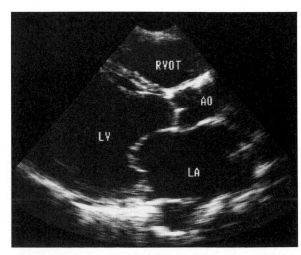

Parasternal long-axis 2-D echocardiogram.

Left ventricular *contraction abnormalities* can be demonstrated especially well in the ventricular short axis and in both apical planes [1]. The *stroke volume* and the *ejection fraction* can be quantitated by planimetry of the diastolic and systolic endocardial contours of the left ventricle in apical four and two-chamber scans.

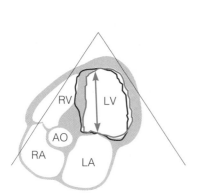

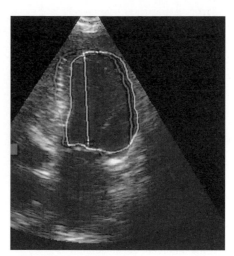

Calculation of end-diastolic and end-systolic volumes, ejection fraction, and stroke volumes by planimetry of the left ventricle in systole (green) and in diastole (red), according to the area-length method.

Apical four-chamber 2-D echocardiogram.

In dilated cardiomyopathy, regional and diffuse wall motion abnormalities may occur. Therefore, echocardiography is unable to differentiate between dilated cardiomyopathy and diffuse coronary artery disease [36, 64, 66]. Enlargement of the left ventricle is also found in the advanced stages of severe aortic and mitral insufficiency [3, 7]. In this case, the existence of valvular changes facilitates the differential diagnosis.

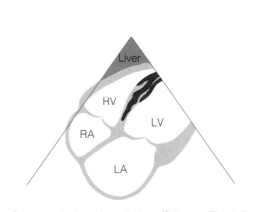

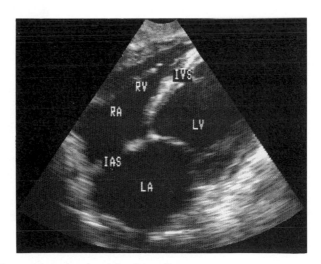

Severe mitral and aortic insufficiency. The left ventricle (LV) and left atrium (LA) are enlarged compared to the other right heart cavities. The interventricular septum (IVS) exhibits a striated echo pattern, and it appears to have increased overall echo density.

Subcostal four-chamber 2-D echocardiogram.

Characteristic signs of dilated cardiomyopathy are *echo dense myocardial areas*, which probably occur due to fibrotic changes in the myocardium [6].

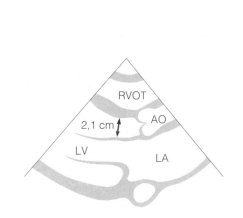

The distance of the maximally opened anterior mitral leaflet to the interventricular septum is enlarged (2.1 cm).

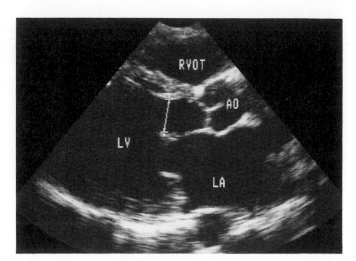

Parasternal long-axis 2-D echocardiogram.

Decreased mitral valve opening and such complications as *thrombus, pericardial effusion,* and *pleural effusion* can be identified in moving images [22, 23]. *Spontaneous echocardiographic contrast* in the left ventricle and left atrium are a common finding in dilated cardiomyopathy; they are considered to be thrombogenic factors [16, 45].

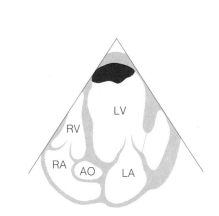

Relatively weakly marked echo-dense structures (arrows) that project into the enlarged left ventricle can be seen in the region of the apical septum. This corresponds to apical thrombus.

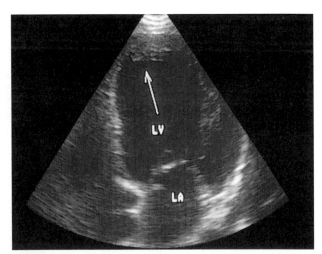

Apical four-chamber 2-D echocardiogram.

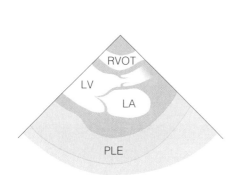

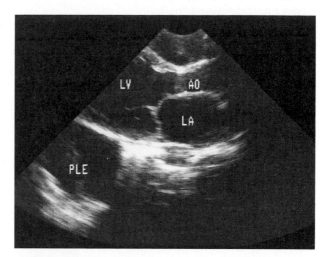

The left atrium and left ventricle are enlarged. An echo-free space (PLE) is located behind the posterior wall of the left ventricle. This corresponds to large, left-sided pleural effusion.

Parasternal long-axis 2-D echocardiogram.

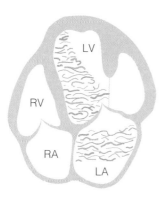

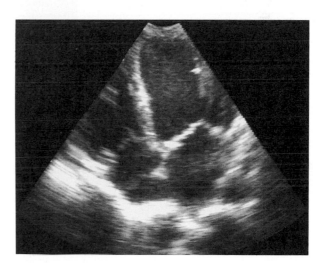

Fine echo-dense structures are found in the left atrial and ventricular cavities. Because these are not scatter artifacts, the movement of these "schlieren" in the bloodstream can be detected in real-time images.

Apical four-chamber 2-D echocardiogram.

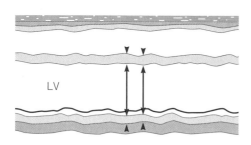

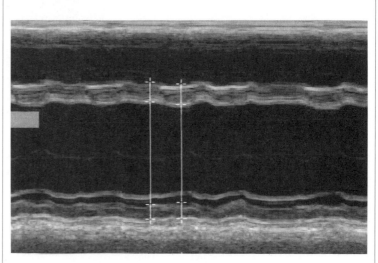

Dilated left ventricle with end-diastolic and end-systolic dimensions of 64 and 61 mm, respectively. The regional fractional shortening of 0.05 is highly pathological. The septum and anterior wall are almost akinetic. The ejection fraction is only 0.14.

M-mode parasternal long-axis recording.

M-mode echocardiography:
(dilated cardiomyopathy)

- In manifest dilated cardiomyopathy, the left ventricle is enlarged to more than 60 mm. The right ventricle may also be enlarged, but quantification of the right ventricle is difficult, due to its irregular geometry [4, 14, 18, 19]. The left atrium is also enlarged in symptomatic patients. Wall thicknesses may be normal or thin, and contractility (systolic contractile motion) may be regionally or globally impaired to varying degrees.

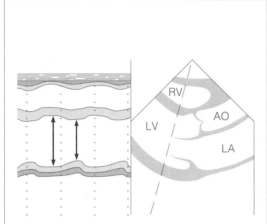

Calculation of regional fractional shortening (FS) from the left ventricular end-diastolic and end-systolic dimensions. In this case, the FS is pathologically reduced (0.18).

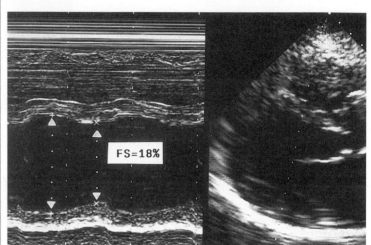

Parasternal long-axis M-mode and 2-D echocardiograms.

Regional *fractional shortening* and the *ejection fraction* are pathologically reduced.

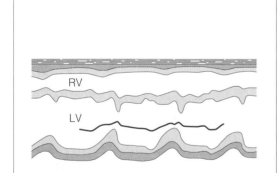

The inwards motion of the interventricular septum (top arrow) is slower than that of the posterior wall (bottom arrow) in impaired left ventricular relaxation.

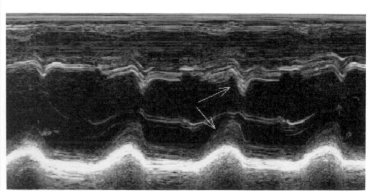

M-mode parasternal long-axis recording.

The motion of the interventricular septum can also be *biphasic*. This is an indication of impaired or paradox relaxation with a coexistent left bundle-branch block.

9.2   **Cardiomyopathies**
9.2.1   **Dilated Cardiomyopathy**
         399

The mitral valve apparatus is displaced dorsally due to dilation. The *mitral septum distance* (MDS or ES distance) increases. A mitral septum distance greater than 6 mm is interpreted as pathological. However, this sign is unspecific, because it may occur in other diseases with left heart insufficiency. The mitral valve may also exhibit rapid, protodiastolic closure.

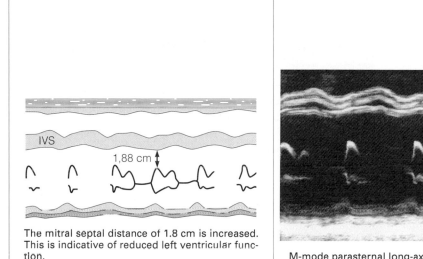

The mitral septal distance of 1.8 cm is increased. This is indicative of reduced left ventricular function.

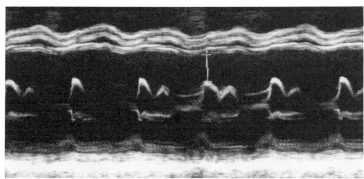

M-mode parasternal long-axis recording.

Mitral valve closure is premature and incomplete. This produces a "shoulder" at the end of the A-C slope.

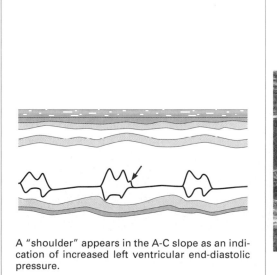

A "shoulder" appears in the A-C slope as an indication of increased left ventricular end-diastolic pressure.

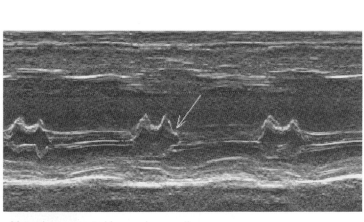

M-mode parasternal long-axis recording.

Increased end-diastolic pressure is characterized by absence of the A wave. The left atrium becomes larger. When the stroke volume is reduced, the excursion of the aortic root becomes markedly reduced, and the aortic valve cusps often exhibit early or meso-systolic closure.

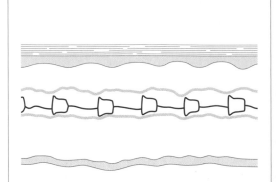

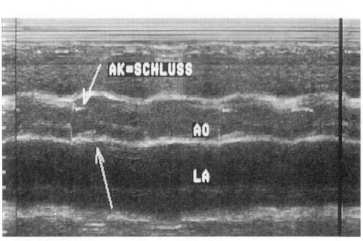

The left atrium is dilated. The excursion amplitude of the aortic root (bottom arrow) is reduced, and the right coronary aortic valve cusp causes early systolic closure (top arrow), which indicates impaired left ventricular function.

M-mode parasternal long-axis recording.

In the ventricular short axis, the mitral valve orifice area is clearly reduced.

Particularly in cytostatic therapy, M-mode follow-up examinations are especially important for determining, for example, the need to increase the dosage or to repeat the therapy. M-mode-derived parameters are also of prognostic importance [59].

Conventional Doppler Echocardiography

Pulsed-wave Doppler (CW Doppler)

- In patients with dilated cardiomyopathy, the *peak systolic flow velocity* in the aorta or pulmonary artery is often significantly lower than in healthy subjects.

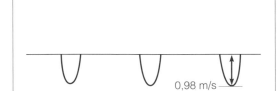

Reduced peak instantaneous flow velocity across the aorta (ca. 1 m/s).

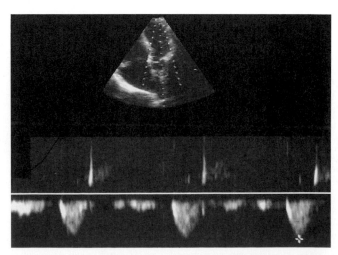

Apical five-chamber 2-D echocardiogram and CW Doppler recording.

Stroke volumes and cardiac output measurements from the suprasternal position were shown to correlate well with invasively obtained data. The *acceleration time, i.e.,* the time to peak flow velocity, and the *left ventricular ejection time* are reduced. As the degree of diastolic dysfunction increases, the *isovolumic relaxation time* may also increase. Transmitral and transtricuspid inflow may be altered due to altered relaxation and ventricular compliance. This, in turn, alters the *E/A ratio, i.e.,* the ratio of E to A wave velocity.

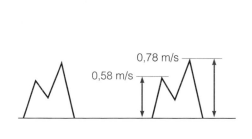

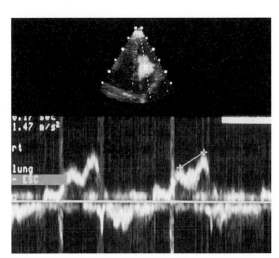

Transmitral flow. The early diastolic flow velocity of 0.58 m/s is clearly lower than the end-diastolic flow velocity of 0.78 m/s.

Apical four-chamber view (top). PW Doppler (bottom).

In that case, the quotient is less than one. However, when concomitant mitral insufficiency is present (which is commonly the case in dilated cardiomyopathy), the early diastolic velocity increases again. This leads to pseudonormalization of the E/A ratio. Coexistent mitral or tricuspid regurgitation can be detected and semiquantitated by PW Doppler. Pulmonary hypertension can also be detected using PW Doppler.

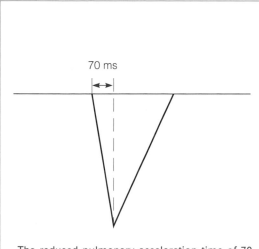

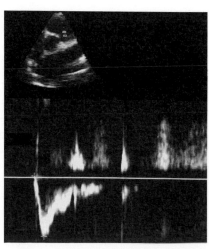

The reduced pulmonary acceleration time of 70 ms is an indication of increased mean pulmonary artery pressure (> 20 mmHg).

Parasternal short-axis view (top). PW Doppler (bottom).

Continuous-wave Doppler (CW Doppler)

- CW Doppler is used primarily to detect associated mitral and tricuspid insufficiency. The peak systolic right ventricular pressure and pulmonary artery pressure can be derived from the peak tricuspid flow velocity.

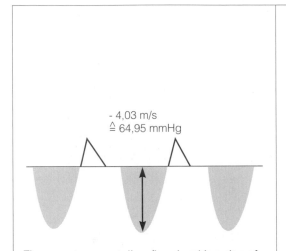

- 4,03 m/s
≙ 64,95 mmHg

The very strong systolic reflux signal is a sign of severe mitral insufficiency. The systolic pressure in the left ventricle is reduced.

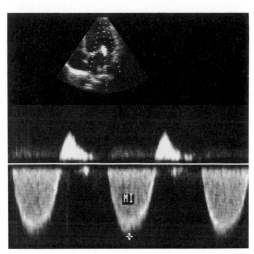

Apical four-chamber 2-D echocardiogram and CW Doppler recording.

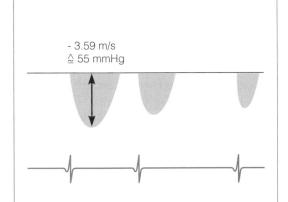

- 3.59 m/s
≙ 55 mmHg

The strong reflux signal is a sign of severe tricuspid insufficiency. Right ventricular systolic pressure is increased (ca. 55 mmHg in this measurement). Very different pressure values are measured when atrial fibrillation exists.

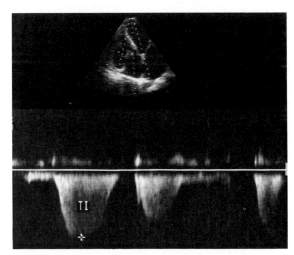

Apical four-chamber 2-D echocardiogram and CW Doppler recording.

Doppler color flow imaging (2-D and M-mode)

- Graphic visualization of associated tricuspid and mitral regurgitation.

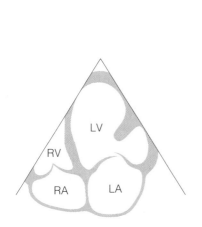

Enlargement of the left ventricle and left atrium in dilated cardiomyopathy.

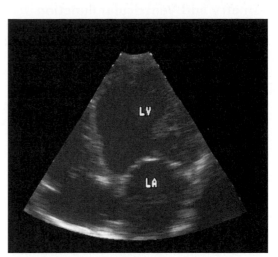

Apical four-chamber 2-D echocardiogram.

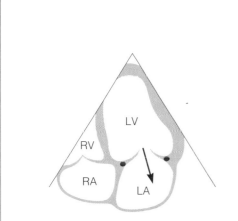

Continued. "Relative" mitral insufficiency in dilated cardiomyopathy.

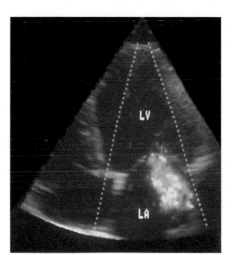

Apical four-chamber 2-D echocardiogram with color flow mapping.

Transesophageal echocardiography (single and multiplane)

- Visualization of thrombus in left atrial appendage, atrium, or ventricle, and visualization of spontaneous contrast, which indicates the risk of thrombus formation.

Morphometry and Ventricular Function

RVEDD	_____	mm	Right ventricular end-diastolic diameter
LADmax	_____	mm	Maximum diameter of the left atrium
LVEDD	_____	mm	Left ventricular end-diastolic diameter
LVESD	_____	mm	Left ventricular end-systolic diameter
LVFS	_____		Fractional shortening
LVEF	_____		Left ventricular ejection fraction
Wall motion analysis			

Valve Morphology and Dynamics

- ▸ Reduced aortic root excursion
- ▸ Premature mitral valve closure
- ▸ Reduced mitral and aortic valve opening amplitude
- ▸ "Shoulder" in the A-C slope
- ▸ Proto-mesosystolic closure of the aortic valve?

Ventricular Function and Pressure-Flow Relationships (Doppler)

- ▸ *Regurgitations:*
  Qualitative visual proof and semiquantitation
    - detection, velocity measurement, and mapping of regurgitaions
    - follow-up of mitral and tricuspid regurgitation
    - graphic display of regurgitations
- ▸ Determination of mean pulmonary artery pressure
- ▸ Determination of cardiac output

Transesophageal Echocardiography

- ▸ Detection of intracardiac thrombi
- ▸ Image quality superior to that of transthoracic echocardiography

9.2	Cardiomyopathies
9.2.2	Hypertrophic Cardiomyopathy

There are two main types of hypertrophic cardiomyopathy:
1. *obstructed* and
2. *non-obstructed* hypertrophic cardiomyopathy.

Obstructed hypertrophic cardiomyopathy still is commonly called "idiopathic hypertrophic subaortic stenosis" in the U.S.A.

Hypertrophic cardiomyopathy is a congenital disease, the transmission of which is probably autosomal-dominant. Hypertrophic cardiomyopathy is characterized by either symmetrical or asymmetrical ventricular hypertrophy with a normal-sized or abnormally small ventricular cavity. By definition, systemic hypertension, aortic stenosis, and other diseases that cause hypertrophy must be absent.

The left heart muscle is commonly involved; involvement of the right heart muscle is less common. Because of the variable distribution of hypertrophy, hypertrophic cardiomyopathy can be further classified as follows:

Left ventricular hypertrophy

▶ Asymmetric hypertrophy
  - ventricular septum hypertrophy
  - mid-ventricular hypertrophy
  - apical hypertrophy
  - posteroseptal and/or lateral wall hypertrophy
▶ Symmetric (concentric) hypertrophy

Right ventricular hypertrophy

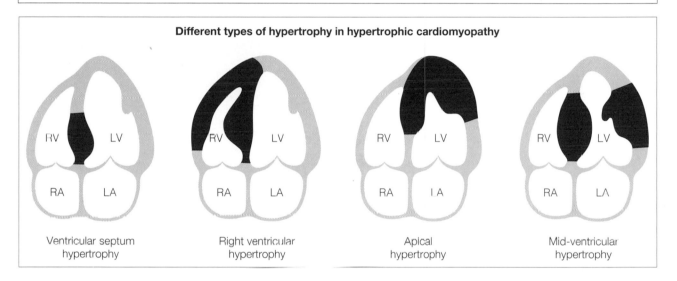

Different types of hypertrophy in hypertrophic cardiomyopathy

| Ventricular septum hypertrophy | Right ventricular hypertrophy | Apical hypertrophy | Mid-ventricular hypertrophy |

Cardiac Ultrasound Diagnosis

In order to detect and assess hypertrophy, images must be obtained from multiple views, *i.e.*, parasternal long and short-axis views, apical two and four-chamber views, and subcostal four-chamber view.

| 9.2.2 | Hypertrophic Cardiomyopathy |
| 9.2.2.1 | Obstructed hypertrophic Cardiomyopathy (HOCM) |

Conventional Echocardiography

Two-dimensional echocardiography (2DE):
(obstructed hypertrophic cardiomyopathy)

2DE can be used to detect and/or assess:
  • the extent of hypertrophy

- the distribution of hypertrophy
- the geometry of the ventricle
- left ventricular systolic and diastolic function
- the size of the atria
- morphological changes in the mitral valve
- morphological changes in the papillary muscles
- mitral and papillary muscle motion

In the majority of cases (90%), there is asymmetrical septum hypertrophy of the left ventricle.

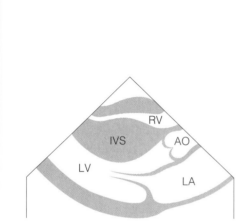

In systole it is hard to detect the ventricular cavities. Because of massive septum hypertrophy, the septum and posterior wall appear to come in contact.

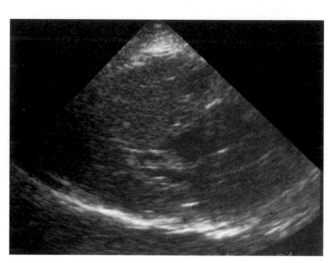

Parasternal long-axis 2-D echocardiogram.

First and foremost, the proximal and distal portions of the septum are involved. Involvement of the anterolateral wall or of the right ventricular septum also is commonly found.

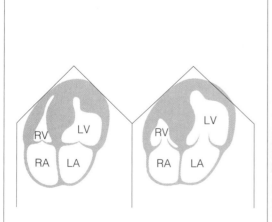

Systole (left) and diastole (right). Marked hypertrophy of the septum, including the right ventricular septum. The lateral wall is not affected by hypertrophy.

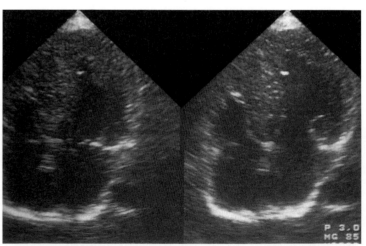

Apical four-chamber 2-D echocardiogram.

From an apical view, the septum often appears to be significantly thinner than in the long-axis, due to the tangential angle of the beam. Obstructed hypertrophic cardiomyopathy is suggested when the left outflow tract is markedly narrow, or when complete obstruction of the distal intracavitary lumen occurs during systole.

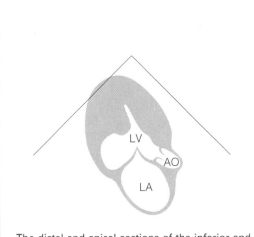

The distal and apical sections of the inferior and anteroseptal walls are hypertrophied. In systole, the two walls appear to touch.

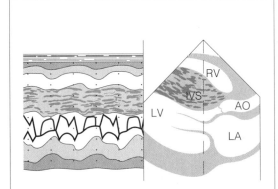

Apical long-axis 2-D echocardiogram.

Systolic anterior movement of the anterior and/or posterior mitral leaflet (SAM phenomenon) can be visualized by real-time two-dimensional echocardiography (2DE). Frame-by-frame analysis in multiple imaging planes has contributed to the better understanding of mechanism of systolic anterior movement.

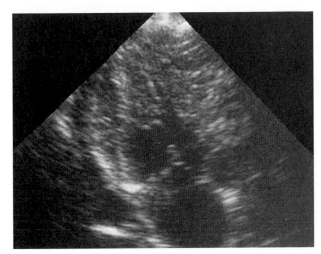

The septum is massively thickened compared to the posterior wall. The left atrium is dilated. The M-mode recording reveals a striated structural pattern in the septum, and systolic anterior motion (SAM) of the mitral valve apparatus. In 2DE, SAM can be visualized only in real-time

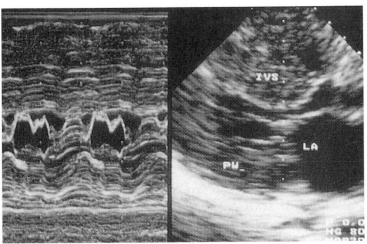

Parasternal long-axis M-mode and 2-D echocardiograms.

It was shown that obstruction can be caused, not only by displacement of the mitral valve apparatus, but also by the altered motion of the hypertrophied papillary muscles in conjunction with the altered geometry of the left ventricle and, therefore, altered left ventricular contractility.

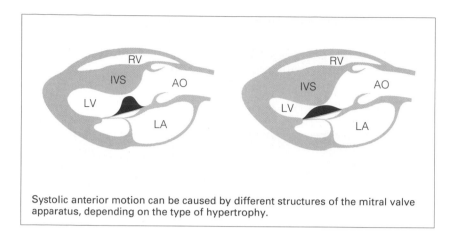

Systolic anterior motion can be caused by different structures of the mitral valve apparatus, depending on the type of hypertrophy.

On the other hand, the absence of systolic anterior motion can be expected in apical hypertrophy which, itself, is relatively uncommon (3%). In hypertrophic cardiomyopathy the overall contractility of the involved wall segment is reduced. The acoustic characteristics of the involved portion of the myocardium are also altered. The myocardium then appears more echodense and commonly inhomogeneous due to the increase in reflected echo impulses.

M-mode echocardiography:
(obstructed hypertrophic cardiomyopathy)

- *Asymmetric septum hypertrophy:*
  The typical M-mode sign of hypertrophic cardiomyopathy is extensive septal hypertrophy (up to 40 mm), usually with normal thickness of the left posterior wall. A septum to posterior wall ratio (IVS-EDD to LVPW-EDD) of >1.3 [29, 55] is considered suggestive, but not diagnostic of HOCM, because this may also occur in patients with aortic stenosis, arterial hypertension, in athletes, and in storage diseases. The thickness of the septum may be over- or underestimated in tangential scans. When the boundaries of the right ventricular endocardium cannot be distinguished, wall thicknesses cannot be measured. In the follow-up of asymmetric septum hypertrophy, septal thickness plays an important role in the progression of the disease and in treatment success. However, one should keep in mind that considerable measurement differences can result when measurements are made from a more oblique angle or from a different intercostal space. The ratio should not be pathological in apical and lateral hypertrophy.
- *Systolic anterior motion (SAM):*
  Early or mesosystolic anterior motion of the mitral valve apparatus is a classical echocardiographic sign of obstructed hypertrophic cardiomyopathy. When SAM occurs, convex arch-shaped or box-shaped anterior movement of the mitral valve apparatus can be observed. This movement is attributable to the Venturi (suction) effect, which can be explained, in part, by the pressure gradient between the left ventricle and the aorta and, in part, by altered contractile function. As the severity of obstruction increases, longer and closer contact between the mitral valve and interventricular septum can often be observed.

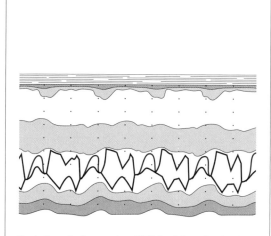

Systolic anterior motion (SAM) of the mitral valve apparatus.

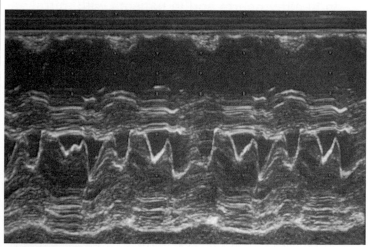

Parasternal long-axis 2-D echocardiogram.

Attempts have been made to quantitate the severity of obstruction, but these methods have not yet gain acceptance, due to the lack of systolic anterior motion (SAM) in the distal or apical third of the left ventricle in obstructed hypertrophic cardiomyopathy. SAM is not a suitable index for follow up or for evaluation of treatment results. SAM can be provoked by the Valsalva maneuver, nitrate, amyl nitrate, or other sympathomimetic agents.

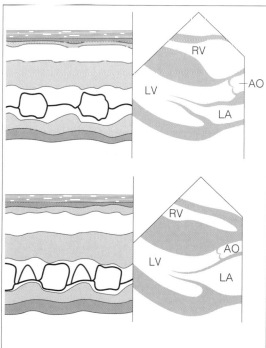

In the upper panel, no SAM is detected. After administration of glycerol nitrate (lower panel), marked SAM is provoked. Obstruction can also be induced by administration of nitrate.

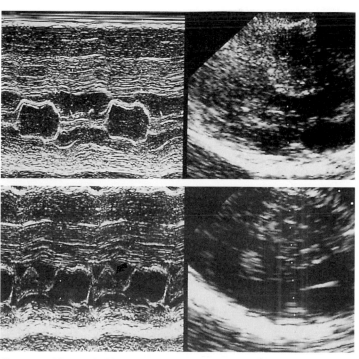

Parasternal long-axis M-mode and 2-D echocardiograms.

However, it must be stressed that systolic anterior motion (SAM) can also be observed in healthy hearts and in patients with mitral valve prolapse, inferior myocardial infarction, left ventricular aneurysm, secondary left ventricular hypertrophy, congenital heart defects, and (infrequently) pericardial effusion.

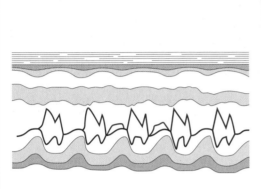

Discrete systolic anterior motion (SAM) of the mitral valve apparatus (arrow) in concentric hypertrophy due to hypertension.

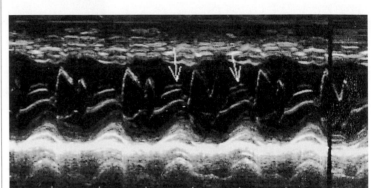

M-mode parasternal long-axis recording.

- *Early or mesosystolic closure of the aortic valve:*
  Early or mesosystolic closure of the aortic valve is another classical sign of obstructed hypertrophic cardiomyopathy.

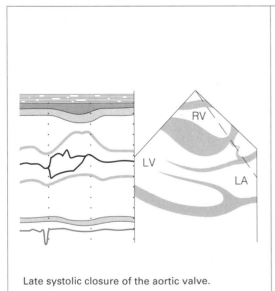

Late systolic closure of the aortic valve.

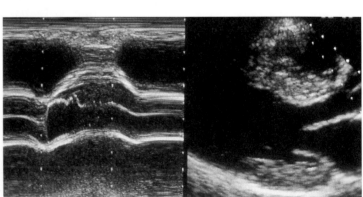

Parasternal long-axis M-mode and 2-D echocardiograms.

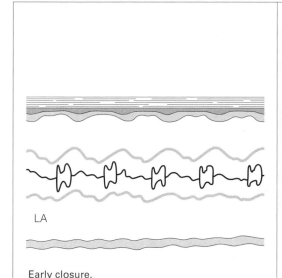

Early closure.

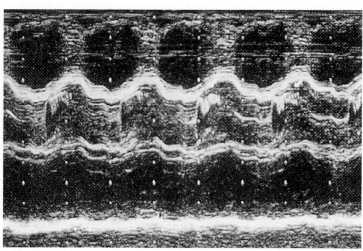

M-mode parasternal long-axis recording.

Early or mesosystolic closure also occurs in subvalvular aortic stenosis (due to membranous or fibromuscular structures), and in patients with dilated cardiomyopathy and impaired ventricular function. Closure is then followed by late systolic opening. However, the absence of this echocardiographic sign does not exclude the possibility of obstruction.

- *Reduced E-F slope:*
  A reduced E-F slope (< 36 mm/s) of the anterior mitral leaflet is an nonspecific M-mode criterion which can also occur in other hypertrophic diseases due to reduced compliance.

- *Ventricular function:*
  In hypertrophic cardiomyopathy, the end-diastolic diameter of the left ventricle is usually normal, whereas the end-systolic diameter is reduced. Therefore, regional fractional shortening and the ejection fraction are usually in the upper limits of normal.

- *Dilatation of the left atrium:*
  Atrial dilatation occurs due to increased left ventricular end-diastolic filling pressure and reduced compliance. Commonly, associated mitral incompetence is present. This can cause additional atrial enlargement.

Conventional Doppler Echocardiography

Continuous-wave Doppler (CW Doppler):

- *CW Doppler can be used to detect high-velocity turbulent or laminar flow in the left ventricular outflow tract, and to identify the presence and site of obstruction. CW Doppler can also detect coexistent mitral insufficiency. The diastolic inflow signal can be analyzed to assess left ventricular relaxation and compliance abnormalities.*

The CW Doppler cursor is placed in the left ventricular outflow tract. Obstructed cardiomyopathy has a characteristic saber-shaped flow profile with a late systolic peak, due to the gradual increase in velocity during early systole. In conjunction with obstruction, acceleration again occurs in late systole.

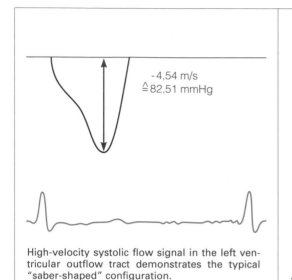

-4,54 m/s
≙ 82,51 mmHg

High-velocity systolic flow signal in the left ventricular outflow tract demonstrates the typical "saber-shaped" configuration.

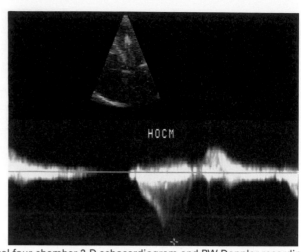

HOCM

Apical four-chamber 2-D echocardiogram and PW Doppler recording.

The signal intensity usually decreases at the end of systole. Therefore, the detection and measurement of peak velocity may be difficult. Probably, only relatively few blood particles are accelerated, and the peak velocity signal is therefore weak. Flow velocities in the left ventricular outflow tract can be as high as 2 to 5 m/s. As in aortic stenosis, the modified Bernoulli equation can be used to compute the intraventricular pressure gradient from the maximum flow velocity.

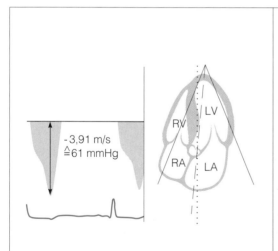

-3,91 m/s
≙ 61 mmHg

LV
RV
RA
LA

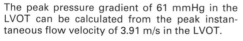

The peak pressure gradient of 61 mmHg in the LVOT can be calculated from the peak instantaneous flow velocity of 3.91 m/s in the LVOT.

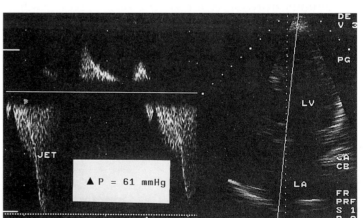

JET

▲ P = 61 mmHg

DE
V 3
PG
LV
CA
CB
LA
FR
PRF
S 1
P O

CW Doppler recording and apical four-chamber 2-D echocardiogram.

It is sometimes difficult to distinguish a mitral regurgitant signal from a obstruction jet, because both move in the same direction. Usually, mitral regurgitant jets are directed towards the lateral wall, and obstruction jets are directed towards the septum. Therefore, with careful mapping, it is possible to differentiate between the two. The severity of mitral insufficiency can vary greatly; regurgitation is almost always present.

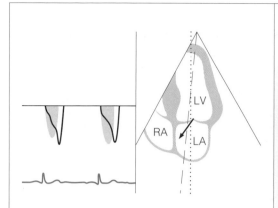

Intracavitary obstruction jets and associated mitral regurgitation are detected along the CW Doppler beam. It is sometimes possible to differentiate between the two signals. In this case, there is a weaker mitral regurgitant signal (left arrow) and a saber-shaped obstruction jet (right arrow).

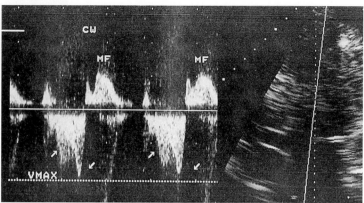

CW Doppler recording and apical four-chamber 2-D echocardiogram.

Pulsed-wave Doppler (PW Doppler):

- *PW Doppler can be used to detect turbulent or laminar flow in the left ventricular outflow tract (LVOT) in order to prove or exclude the presence of obstruction and to locate the site of obstruction. PW Doppler can detect turbulent flow in the left atrium to provide evidence of coexistent mitral insufficiency. Analysis of the diastolic inflow signal provides a means for assessment of relaxation and compliance abnormalities of the left ventricle. PW Doppler also permits measurement of isovolumic relaxation and left ventricular ejection times.*

Pulsed-wave Doppler studies are performed mainly from the apical long-axis (RAO equivalent) view and apical four and five-chamber views. PW Doppler findings: In obstructed hypertrophic cardiomyopathy, one usually finds flow acceleration that begins relatively deep in the left ventricular outflow tract. There, flow is still laminar, but it becomes turbulent in the region of the obstruction.

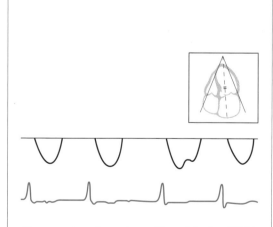

The sample volume is positioned in the LVOT. There, the flow velocity is relatively low, and flow is laminar.

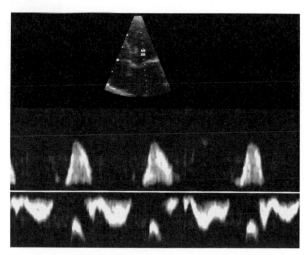

Apical four-chamber 2-D echocardiogram and PW Doppler recording.

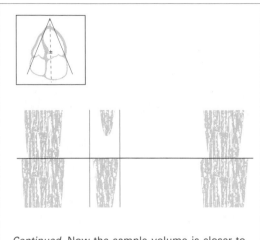

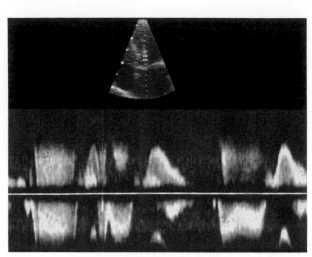

Continued. Now the sample volume is closer to the aortic valve. Turbulent flow, which is recorded on both sides of the baseline, corresponds to obstruction.

Apical four-chamber 2-D echocardiogram and PW Doppler recording.

By placing the sample volume in the region of the mitral valve or above the mitral valve plane, associated mitral insufficiency and additional systolic turbulent flow signals can be detected.

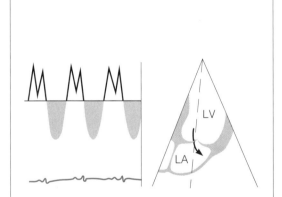

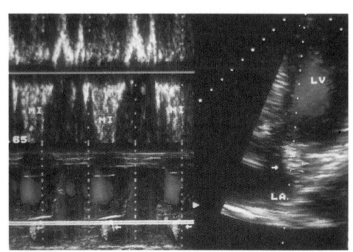

The sample volume is now located in the left atrium near the mitral valve. The mitral regurgitant jet can be easily identified in the color flow map. There is also a turbulent signal below the baseline (mitral insufficiency).

PW Doppler, apical four-chamber view, with color flow mapping.

Therefore, pulsed-wave Doppler permits differentiation and localization of systolic turbulent flow signals. In obstructed hypertrophic cardiomyopathy the systolic ejection time is also increased. This can be easily measured using PW Doppler (from the onset of the aortic flow signal to the aortic valve closure signal).

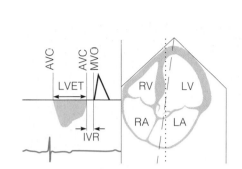

The left ventricular ejection time (LVET) can be calculated from the time from aortic valve opening (AVO) to closure (AVC). The LVET is longer in obstructed hypertrophic cardiomyopathy (HOCM). The isovolumic relaxation time (IVR) is defined as the time from aortic valve closure (AVC) to mitral valve opening (MVO). IVR is also increased in HC (> 80 ms).

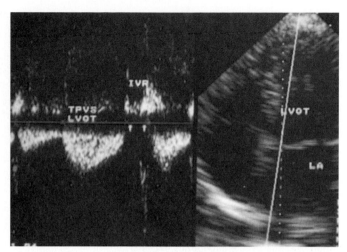

CW Doppler recording and apical four-chamber 2-D echocardiogram.

PW Doppler studies have demonstrated that flow in the descending aorta is abruptly reduced at the onset of obstruction, *i.e.*, early closure of the aortic valve. Then, low flow velocities are detected in early systole [20, 26, 31, 42, 46]. When the site of obstruction is in the apical ventricle, it can be very difficult to distinguish the turbulent PW Doppler signal from systolic wall motion artifacts.

As compared with conventional M-mode and 2-D echocardiography, it is easier to assess the diastolic function of the left ventricle and, if necessary, right ventricle by PW Doppler [17, 21, 24, 41, 52]. A pathological E/A ratio is a very common finding. Therefore, this cannot be taken as a specific sign of impaired diastolic function. The E/A ratio changes when left ventricular compliance and relaxation are impaired, and is also affected by pressure and compliance of the left atrium and pulmonary capillary bed [17, 38, 52]. Frequently, the early diastolic drop in velocity is delayed, and the isovolumic relaxation time is increased [15]. Antegrade and retrograde flow signals from low velocities during the isovolumic relaxation time are not uncommon. This is caused by changes in energy-dependent relaxation [39, 56-58]. The parameters of diastolic function can vary greatly, depending on the extent and location of hypertrophy. Unfortunately, they also are unspecific, because they also occur in all secondary forms of hypertrophy [52]. However, parameters of diastolic function are suitable for follow-up and assessment of treatment results.

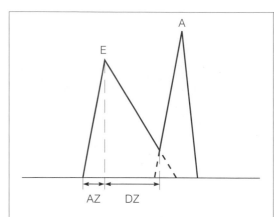

The end-diastolic flow velocity (A) is higher than the early diastolic velocity (E). Normally, the E/A ratio is reversed. Increased early diastolic acceleration (AZ) and deceleration times (DZ) indicate impaired left ventricular compliance.

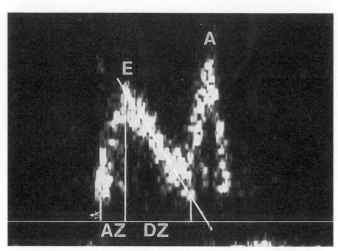

PW Doppler recording (apical four-chamber 2-D echocardiogram).

Doppler color flow imaging (2-D and M-mode)

- *Doppler color flow imaging can be used to graphically display turbulent obstruction jets in the left ventricular outflow tract and to detect and semiquantitate associated mitral insufficiency.*

  With Doppler color flow imaging, it is possible to distinguish between hypertrophic non-obstructed and hypertrophic obstructed cardiomyopathies [28, 48, 65]. When obstruction is present, a color mosaic flow signal pattern is observed.

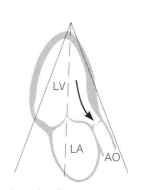

With Doppler color flow imaging, systolic flow acceleration in the left ventricular outflow tract (LVOT) can be identified as color reversal from blue to red. This is followed by a turbulent flow signal that extends to the aortic valve, which is a sign of obstruction.

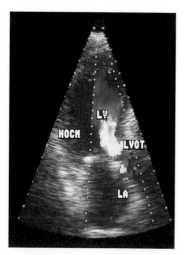

Color flow map of apical long-axis 2-D echocardiogram

Flow acceleration, which begins prior to the obstruction, can be identified as a red-encoded signal in the left ventricular outflow tract. In order to thoroughly detect and record areas of turbulence, Doppler color flow maps should be made of all the usual views, and of atypical views. Furthermore, associated mitral insufficiency in the left atrium should be identified immediately.

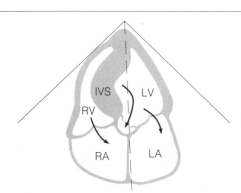

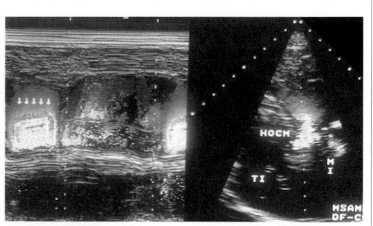

Turbulent obstructed flow in the left ventricular outflow tract (right). Turbulence in the left atrium (LA) indicates the presence of concomitant mitral insufficiency. The few color signals detected in the right atrium during systole are a sign of tricuspid insufficiency. The increase in turbulence in late systole (arrows) is clearly visible in the M-mode echocardiogram.

M-mode and 2-D apical four-chamber view. Color flow mapping.

Color M-mode echocardiography, with its superior temporal resolution, can demonstrate the coincidence of occurrence of systolic anterior motion (SAM) and turbulence in the outflow tract. At the onset of systole, blue laminar flow with a low flow velocity is usually still present. Then, flow acceleration, usually with aliasing, and turbulence develop in late systole. Color M-mode is helpful for temporal identification of turbulence, especially in combined lesions. For example, it is able to differentiate the diastolic turbulence of aortic insufficiency from the systolic turbulence in the left ventricular outflow tract in obstructed hypertrophic cardiomyopathy.

Transesophageal Echocardiography (Single and Multiplane)

- *Transesophageal echocardiography (TEE) can be used to visualize obstructions and associated mitral insufficiency in patients unsuitable for transthoracic scanning or when there are eccentric obstruction jets or associated diseases of the ventricle or valves.*

9.2.2   **Hypertrophic Cardiomyopathy**
9.2.2.2   **Hypertrophic Non-obstructed Cardiomyopathy**

Cardiac Ultrasound Diagnosis

Conventional Echocardiography

Two-dimensional echocardiography:
(hypertrophic non-obstructed cardiomyopathy)

- Two-dimensional echocardiographic findings in hypertrophic non-obstructed cardiomyopathy can vary greatly, depending on the location of hypertrophy [37].

As in obstructed hypertrophic cardiomyopathy, hypertrophy must therefore be visualized from parasternal and apical scanning positions. Frequently, the papillary muscles are also massively hypertrophied and may be displaced towards anterior.

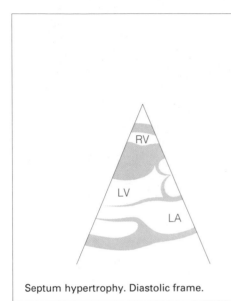

Septum hypertrophy. Diastolic frame.

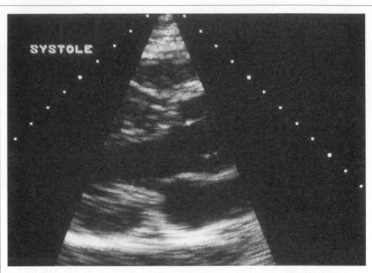

Parasternal long-axis 2-D echocardiogram.

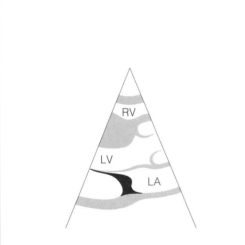

Systolic frame. The subvalvular mitral apparatus is thickened without obstruction.

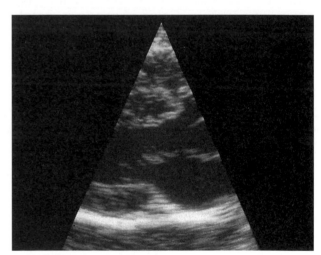

Parasternal long-axis 2-D echocardiogram.

M-mode echocardiography:
(hypertrophic non-obstructed cardiomyopathy)

- Depending on the type of hypertrophy (particularly in apical hypertrophy), wall thicknesses may be normal. Systolic anterior motion (SAM) may occur in hypertrophic non-obstructed cardiomyopathy, but is usually minimal. Proto- or mesosystolic closure of the aortic valve does not occur. When the diastolic pressure is increased, the left atrium may be enlarged.

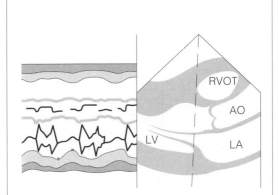
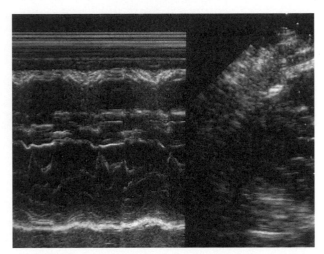

Hypertrophy of the septum, with inhomogeneous echo texture. Systolic anterior motion (SAM) is not detected.

Parasternal long-axis M-mode and 2-D echocardiograms.

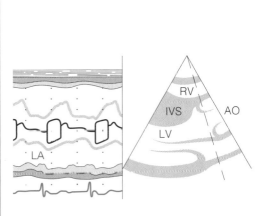
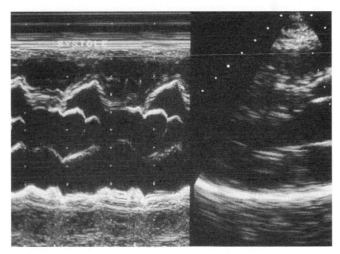

Same patient. The M-mode recording of the aortic valve is normal. No closure occurs in either early nor late systole.

Parasternal long-axis M-mode and 2-D echocardiograms.

Conventional Doppler Echocardiography

Continuous-wave Doppler (CW Doppler):

- CW Doppler studies reveal increased flow velocities with an additional late systolic increase in velocity. However, the velocities are not as high as those measured in hypertrophic obstructed cardiomyopathy. In the non-obstructed type, peak velocities are usually less than 2 m/s.

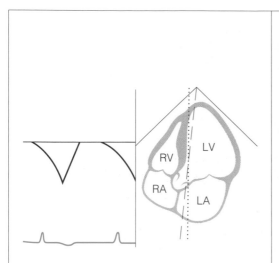

Peak velocity occurs only in late systole, and is only 1.1 m/s.

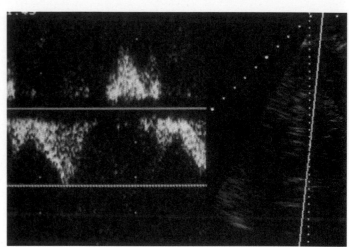

CW Doppler recording. Apical four-chamber view, with color flow mapping.

Pulsed-wave Doppler (PW Doppler):

- In hypertrophic non-obstructed cardiomyopathy, PW Doppler signals with aliasing are recorded relatively far into the left ventricle, but there is no turbulent flow. In conventional PW Doppler, the diastolic flow profile can be changed, as in hypertrophic cardiomyopathy. Long ejection times can also occur. Additionally, systolic flow signals corresponding to associated mitral insufficiency can also be observed.

Doppler color flow imaging (2-D and M-mode)

In Doppler color flow imaging, accelerated flow signals, *i.e.*, aliasing, in the left ventricular outflow tract can be easily identified. Color reversal from blue to red occurs deep in the left ventricle. Turbulent flow signals do not occur. Accordingly, only laminar red and blue flow patterns are observed in color M-mode studies.

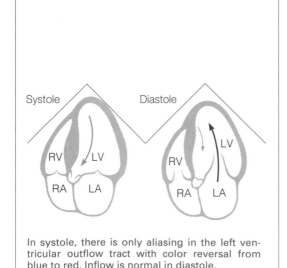

In systole, there is only aliasing in the left ventricular outflow tract with color reversal from blue to red. Inflow is normal in diastole.

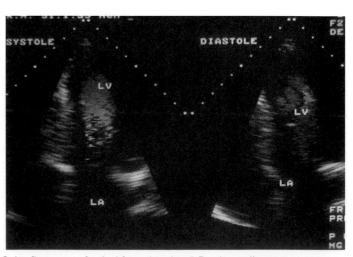

Color flow map of apical four-chamber 2-D echocardiogram.

Transesophageal Echocardiography (Single and Multiplane)

Transesophageal echocardiography (TEE) is indicated only when transthoracic visualization or measurement is of insufficient quality.

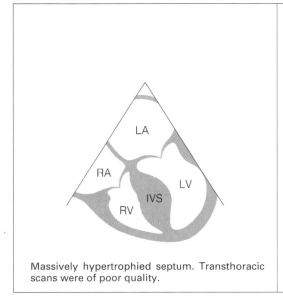

Massively hypertrophied septum. Transthoracic scans were of poor quality.

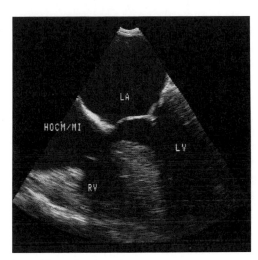

Transesophageal four-chamber view.

9.2.2   **Hypertrophic Cardiomyopathy**
9.2.2.3   **Special Measurement Program and Quick Reference**

Morphometry and Ventricular Function

IVS-EDD	_____	mm	End-diastolic diameter of the interventricular septum
LVPW-EDD	_____	mm	End-diastolic diameter of the left ventricular posterior wall
LADmax	_____	mm	Maximum diameter of the left atrium
LVEDD	_____	mm	Left ventricular end-diastolic diameter
LVESD	_____	mm	Left ventricular end-systolic diameter
LVFS	_____		Fractional shortening
LVEF	_____		Left ventricular ejection fraction

Parameters of diastolic function
E wave
A wave
E/A ratio
E-DT

Assessment of the various types of hypertrophic cardiomyopathy in two-dimensional images

Valve Morphology and Dynamics
▸ Systolic anterior motion (SAM) phenomena
▸ Proto-mesosystolic closure of the aortic valve?

Ventricular Function and Pressure-Flow Relationships (Doppler Echocardiography)
▸ Regurgitation:
  Qualitative visual proof and semiquantitation of regurgitation
  (detection, velocity measurement, mapping, and
  follow-up of mitral and tricuspid regurgitation;
  graphic display of regurgitation)
▸ Determination of mean pulmonary artery pressure
▸ Determination of cardiac output

▸ Turbulent or laminar flow signal in the LVOT? (PW and CW Doppler)
▸ Measurement of intracavitary pressure gradients (CW Doppler)
▸ Measurement of left ventricular ejection time (PW and CW Doppler)
▸ Measurement of isovolumic relaxation time (PW and CW Doppler)

9.2   **Cardiomyopathies**
9.2.3   **Restrictive (and infiltrative) Cardiomyopathy**

Infiltrative diseases of the myocardium can be divided into two subgroups: infiltrative and storage diseases. Infiltrative cardiomyopathies are is characterized by infiltration of the interstitium. In storage diseases, iron, glycogen, or lipids is deposited in the cells [10, 51, 60]. Infiltrative cardiomyopathy most commonly occurs in sarcoidosis and amyloidosis. In storage diseases, cardiac involvement is most common in hemochromatosis. Restriction develops in the advanced stages of disease [27]. The anatomical, physiological, and clinical spectrum of these diseases can vary greatly, and is dependent, primarily, on the duration and severity of disease.

Cardiac Ultrasound Diagnosis

Echocardiographic scans should be obtained from the usual planes (parasternal long and short-axis views, apical two and four-chamber views, and subcostal four-chamber view).

Conventional Echocardiography

Two-dimensional echocardiography:
B-model Restrictive (infiltrative) cardiomyopathy)
• The ventricle is usually normal-sized or small, with marked wall thickening of the left and right ventricles.

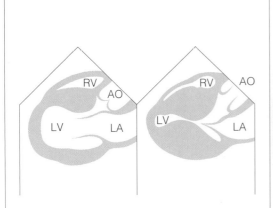

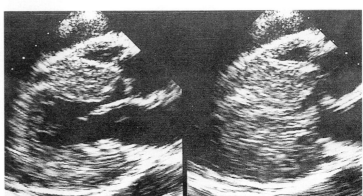

Left ventricle (LV) exhibits massive, concentric hypertrophy. During systole (right) the left ventricle is displaced. The aortic valve cusps are thickened, but open satisfactorily.

Parasternal long-axis 2-D echocardiogram.

The interatrial septum, interventricular septum, papillary muscles, and the cardiac valves can also be involved.

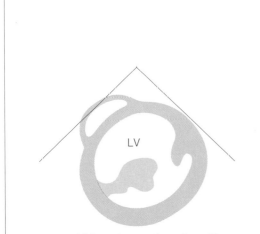

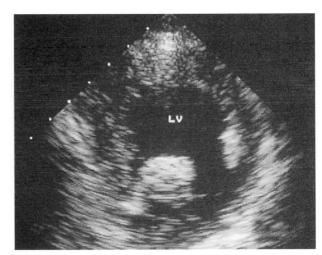

Massively thickened anterolateral papillary muscle. The posteromedial papillary muscle was normal.

Parasternal short-axis 2-D echocardiogram.

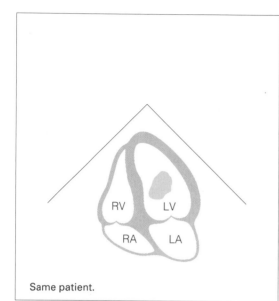

Same patient.

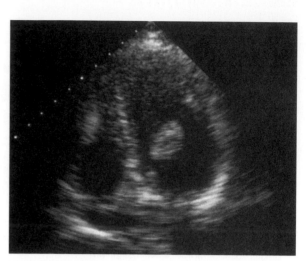

Apical four-chamber 2-D echocardiogram.

As in hypertrophic cardiomyopathy, hypertrophy can be asymmetrical [47, 49, 53]. In advanced stages of disease, the systolic function may be impaired. The atria are usually dilated, and slight to moderate amounts of pericardial effusion may develop.

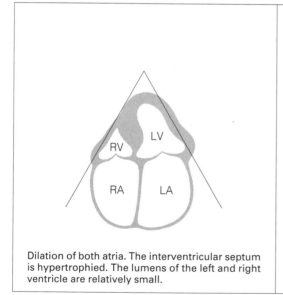

Dilation of both atria. The interventricular septum is hypertrophied. The lumens of the left and right ventricle are relatively small.

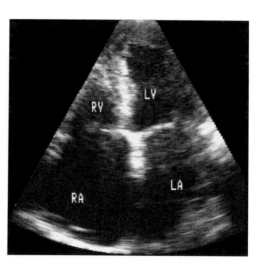

Apical four-chamber 2-D echocardiogram.

Regional wall motion abnormalities have also been reported to occur in infiltrative cardiomyopathy [61]. Inhomogeneous, sometimes very bright echo textures are very commonly in amyloidosis. This phenomenon can be attributed to differences in acoustic properties of normal and pathological tissue, i.e., amyloid deposits are much more echo reflective than normal tissue. Amyloid deposits can be found in different locations [61]. However, these findings are nonspecific, and they also occur in chronic renal insufficiency. Sarcoidosis hearts are characterized primarily by the occurrence of variable contraction patterns [11]. Regional wall thickening and thinning can occur side-by-side. Diastolic parameters can be altered is sarcoidosis as well as in amyloidosis.

M-mode echocardiography:
B-mode (Restrictive (infiltrative) cardiomyopathy)

- As in 2-D echo, the left ventricle may be normal-sized, small, or enlarged. The walls may display inhomogeneous, thin, or normal thicknesses, or they may be hypertrophied [12, 63]. In advanced stages of disease, regional fractional shortening is pathologically reduced, and the left atrium is enlarged. In rare cases, systolic anterior motion (SAM) may also be observed. In M-mode studies, impaired diastolic function is identified on the basis of increased isovolumic relaxation time and decreased diastolic filling time [30].

Conventional Doppler Echocardiography

Continuous and pulsed-wave Doppler (CW and PW Doppler)

- In infiltrative-restrictive cardiomyopathy, PW Doppler, CW Doppler and Doppler color flow imaging techniques are used to detect and/or assess valvular insufficiency and to assess diastolic function.

  PW Doppler is particular well suited for detection of impaired diastolic function. Typical signs of restriction are increased early diastolic flow velocity (E), reduced late systolic flow velocity (A) across the mitral valve and, thus, an increased E/A ratio [25, 34, 35, 62]. However, the E/A ratio can also be inverted. In restrictive cardiomyopathy, the deceleration rate is reduced due to the abrupt increase in diastolic left ventricular pressure.

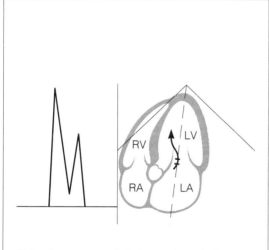

Following a normal increase in velocity, the deceleration rate is reduced. The end-diastolic velocity is clearly reduced.

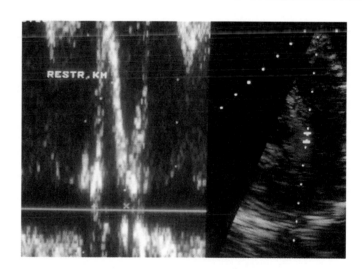

PW Doppler. Apical four-chamber view with color flow mapping.

The isovolumic relaxation time is commonly reduced. The flow profiles of the superior vena cava and the hepatic vein are also altered. Whereas the systolic flow velocity increases and the diastolic flow velocity decreases, there is flow reversal in the pulmonary veins with an increase in diastolic flow velocity and a decrease in systolic flow velocity. Deep inspiration can additionally accentuate this signal variation [34, 54].

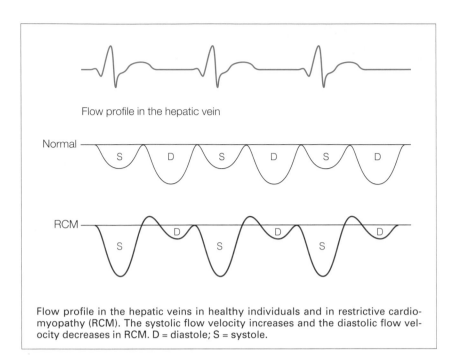

Flow profile in the hepatic vein

Flow profile in the hepatic veins in healthy individuals and in restrictive cardiomyopathy (RCM). The systolic flow velocity increases and the diastolic flow velocity decreases in RCM. D = diastole; S = systole.

The extent of these flow velocity variations may vary greatly, depending on the severity
of the primary disease.

Amyloidosis	
Doppler echocardiographic criteria in different stages of cardiac amyloidosis	
Early Stage	**Advanced stage**
v_{max} E, mitral valve ↓ v_{max} A, mitral valve ↑ E/A ratio ↓ Deceleration time ↑ (>240 ms) Isovolumic relaxation ↑ (>80 ms) v_{max} systolic, hepatic vein ↑ v_{max} diastolic, hepatic vein ↓ Mild valvular incompetence possible	v_{max} E, mitral valve ↔ ↑ v_{max} A, mitral valve ↓ E/A ratio ↑ Deceleration time ↓ (<160 ms) Isovolumic relaxation ↔ (↓) v_{max} systolic, hepatic vein ↓ v_{max} diastolic, hepatic vein ↑ Mild valvular incompetence possible

Doppler color flow imaging (2-D and M-mode)

- In infiltrative-restrictive cardiomyopathy, Doppler color flow imaging is of only limited
  importance for demonstration of existing regurgitation and, when applicable, obstruction [32, 35, 50].

1. Abasi AS, Chahine RA, Macalpin RN. Ultrasound in the diagnosis of primary congestive cardiomyopthy. Chest 1973; 63: 937-942.
2. Aretz HT, Billingham NE, Edwards ED. Myocarditis: a histopathologic definition and classification. Am J Cardiovasc Pathol 1986; 1: 3-11.
3. Balleseter M, Jajoo J, Rees S et al. The mechanism of mitral regurgitation in dilated left ventricle. Clin Cardiol 1983; 3: 333-338.
4. Baran A, Nanda NC, Falkoff S, Barold S, Gallagher JJ. Two-dimensional echocardiographic detection of arrhythmogenic right ventricular dysplasia. Am Heart J 1982; 103: 1066-1077.
5. Betocchi S, Cannon RO, Watson RM. Effects of sublingual nifedipine on hemodynamics and systolic and diastolic function in patients with hypertrophic cardiomyopathy. Circulation 1985; 72: 1001-1007.
6. Bhandari AK, Nanda NC. Two dimensional echocardiographic recognition of abnormal changes in the myocardium. Ultrasound in Med & Biol 1983; 8: 663-671.
7. Boltwood CM, Tei C, Wong M et al. Quantitative echocardiography of the mitral complex in dilated cardiomyopathy: the mechanism of functional regurgitation. Circulation 1983; 68: 498-508.
8. Bonow RO, Dilizian V, Rosing DR, Maron BJ, Bacharaw SI, Green MV. Verapamil-induced improvement in left ventricular diastolic filling and increased exercise tolerance in patients with hypertrophic cardiomyopathy; short- and longterm effects. Circulation 1985; 72: 853-864.
9. Bonow, RO, Rosing DR, Bacharach, SL, Green MV, Kent KM, Lipson LC, Maron BJ, Leon MB, Epstein SE. Effects of verapamil on left ventricular sytolic function and diastolic filling in patients with hypertrophic cardiomyopathy. Circulation 1981; 64: 787-796.
10. Borer J, Henry WL, Epstein SE. Echocardiographic observations on patients with systemic infiltrative disease involving the heart. Am J Cardiol 39 1977; 39: 184-189.
11. Burstow DJ, Tajik AJ, Bailey KR, DeRemee RA, Taliercio CP. Two-dimensional echocardiography findings in systemic sarcoidosis. Am J Cardiol 1989; 63: 478-485.
12. Child JS, Levisman JA, Abbasi AS, Mac Alpin RN. Echocardiographic manifestations of infiltrative cardiomyopathy. A report of seven cases due to amyloid. Chest 1976; 70: 726-731.
13. Cooper M, Shaddy R, Silverman N, Enderlein M. Usefullness of Doppler echocardiography for determining hemodynamic improvement with intravenous verapamil in hypertrophic cardiomyopathy. Am J Cardiol 1985; 56: 210-202.
14. Corya B, Feigenbaum H, Rasmussen S et al. Echocardiographic features of congestive cardiomyopathy compared with normal subjects and patients with coronary artery disease. Circulation 1974; 49: 1153-1159.
15. Curtius JM, Neumeier WM, Loogen F. Dopplerechocardiographische Analyse des linsventrikulären Einflußverhaltens bei hypertrophischer obstruktiver Kardiomyopathie prä- und postoperativ. 7 Kardiol 1988; 77: 271-277.
16. Doud DN, Jacobs WR, Moran JF, Scanlon PJ. The natural history of spontaneous contrast. J Am Soc Echo 1990; 3: 465-470.
17. Downes TR, Nomeir AM, Smith KM, Steward KP, Little WC. Mechanism of altered pattern of left ventricular filling in aging in subjects without cardiac disease. Am J Cardiol 1989; 64: 523-527.
18. Dyczynski J, Schweitzer L. Neue echokardiographische paraapikale Technik zur Bestimmung der Masse und der Dicke der Wand des rechten Ventrikels bei Probanden und Patienten mit dilatativer Kardiomyopathie. Z Kardiol 1987; 76: 751-760.
19. Fitchett DH, Sugrue DD, MacArthur J, Oakley CM. Right ventricular dilated cardiomyopathy. Br Med J 1984; 51: 25-29.
20. Gardin JM, Debastani A, Glasgow GA, Butman S, Burn CS, Henry WL. Echocardiographic and Doppler flow observation in obstructed and nonobstructed hypertrophic cardiomyopathy. Am J Cardiol 1985; 56: 614-621.
21. Gidding,SS, Snider AR, Rocchini AP, Peters J, Farnstworth R. Left ventricular diastolic filling in children with hypertrophic cardiomyopathy; assessment with pulsed Doppler echocardiography. J Am Coll Cardiol 1986; 8: 310-316.
22. Gottdiener JS, Van Voorhees L, Gay J et al. Incidence and embolic potential of left ventricular thrombus in cardiomyopathy: assessment by two-dimensional echocardiography. Am J Cardiol 1982; 49: 1029.
23. Hangland JM, Asinger RW, Mikell FL et al. Embolic potential of left ventricular thrombi detected by two dimensional echocardiography. Circulation 1984; 70: 588-598.
24. Hanrath P, Manthey DG, Siegert R, Bleifeld W. Left ventricular relaxation patterns in different forms of left ventricular hypertophy: an echocardiographic study. Am J Cardiol 1980; 45: 15-20.
25. Hatle L, Appleton CP, Popp RL. Constrictive pericarditis and restrictive cardiomyopathy differentiation by Doppler according to atrioventricular flow velocities. Am J Coll Cardiol 1987; 9: 178.
26. Hatle L. Noninvasive assessment and differentiation of left ventricular outflow obstruction with Doppler ultrasound. Circulation 1981; 64: 381-387.
27. Hirota Y, Shimizu G, Kita Y, Nakayama Y, Suwa MM Kawamura K, Nagata S, Sekiguchi M. Spectrum of restrictive cardiomyopathy; report of the national survey in Japan. Am Heart J 1990; 120: 188-191.
28. Hoit BD, Penonen E, Dalton N Sahn DJ. Doppler color flow mapping studies of jet formation and spatial orientation in obstructive hypertrophic cardiomypathy. Am Heart J 1989; 117: 1119-1125.
29. Hutchins GM, Bukley BH, Moore GW, Piasio MA, Lohr FT. Shape of the human cardiac ventricles. Am J Cardiol 1978; 41: 646-671.

30. Increased right ventricular wall thickness on echocardiography in amyloid infiltrative cardiomyopathy. Am J Cardiol 1979; 44: 1391-1395.
31. Jenni RK, Ruffmann K, Vieli A, Anliker M, Krayenbuehl HP. Dynamics of aortic flow in hypertrophic cariomyopathy. Eur Heart J 1985; 6: 391-398.
32. Keren G, Sherez J, Megidish R, Levitt B, Laniado S. Pulmonary venous flow pattern - its relationship to cardiac dynamics; a pulsed Doppler echocardiographic study. Circulation 1985; 71: 1105-1112.
33. Kinoshita O, Hongo M, Yamada H, Misawa T, Kono J, Okubo S, Ikeda S. Impaired left ventricular diastolic filling in patients with familial amyloid polyneuropathy; a pulsed Doppler echocardiographic study. Br Heart J 1989; 61: 198-206.
34. Klein AL, Tajik AJ. Doppler assessment of diastolic function in cardiac amyloidosis. Echocardiography 1991; 8: 233-239.
35. Klein AL, Oh JK, Fletcher A, Miller A, Seward JB, Tajik J. Two-dimensional and Doppler echocardiographic assessment of infiltrative cardiomyopathy. J Am Soc Echo 1988; 1: 48-59.
36. Kronik GH, Mˆsslacher R, Schmoliner R. Differentialdiagnose zwischen diffusen Myokarderkrankungen und koronarer Herzkrankheit mit Hilfe der zweidimensionalen Echokardiographie. Herz/Kreisl 1981; 13: 113-187.
37. Kuhn H, Thelen U, Koehler E, Loesse B. Die hypertrophe nicht obstruktive Kardiomyopathie (HNCM) - klinische, haemodynamische, elektro-, echo- und angiographische Untersuchungen. Z Kardiol 1980; 69: 457-469.
38. Kuo LC, Quinones MA, Rokey R, Sartori M, Abinader EG, Zoghbi WA. Quantification of atrial contribution to left ventricular filling by pulsed Doppler echocardiography and the effect of age in normal and diseased hearts. Am J Cardiol 1987; 59: 1174-1178.
39. Maire R, Jenni R, Krayenbuehl HP. Retrograde left ventricular flow during early relaxation. J Am Coll Cardiol 1988; 11: 672-673.
40. Marcus FI, Fontaine GH, Giraudon G et al. Right ventricular dysplasia: a report of 24 adult cases. Circulation 1982; 65: 384-385.
41. Maron BJ, Spirito P, Green KJ, Wesley YE, Bonow RO, Arce J. Noninvasive assessment of diastolic function by pulsed Doppler echocardiography in patients with hypertrophic cardiomyopathy. J Am Coll Cardiol 1987; 10: 733-742.
42. Maron BJ. Hypertrophic cardiomyopathy with ventricular septal hypertrophy localized to the apical region of the left ventricle (apical hypertrophic cardiomyopathy) Am J Cardiol 1982; 49: 1838-1849.
43. Masuyama T, Nellesen M, Stinson EB, Popp RL. Improvement in left ventricular diastolic filling by septal myectomy in hypertrophic cardiomyopathy. J Am Soc Echo 1990; 3: 196-204.
44. Michels VV, Driscoll DJ, Miller FA. Familial aggregation of idiopathic dilated cardiomyopathy. Am J Cardiol 1985, 55: 1232-1239.
45. Mikell F, Asinger S, Elsperger K, Anderson W, Hodges M. Regional stasis of blood in the dysfunctional left ventricle: echocardiographic detection and differentiation from early thrombosis. Circulation 1982; 66: 755-763.
46. Murgo JP, Alter BR, Dorethy FJ. Dynamics of left ventricular ejection in obstructive and non-obstructive hypertrophic cardiomyopathy. J Clin Invest 1980; 66: 1369-1377.
47. Nicolosi GL, Pava D, Lestuzzi C, Burelli C, Zardo F, Zanuttini D. Prospective identification of patients with amyloid heart disease by two-dimensional echocardiography. Circulation 1984; 70: 432-432.
48. Nishimura RA, Tajik AJ, Reeder GS, Seward JB. Evaluation of hypertrophic cardiomyopathy by Doppler color flow imaging: initial observations. Mayo Clin Proc 1986; 61: 631-639.
49. Noma S, Askaishi M, Murayama A, Akiyama H, Ogawa S, Handa S, Nakamura Y, Sohma Y, Hosada Y, Gotoh M. Echocardiographic findings of a patient with cardiac amyloidosis and ventricular outflow obstruction. J Cardiogr 1982; 12: 267-268.
50. Oh JK, Tajik AJ, Kyle RA. Incidence of valvular regurgitation in patients with cardiac amyloidosis. Circulation 1985; 72 (suppl III): III-479.
51. Patton JN, Tajik AJ, Reeder GS, Edwards WD, Seward JB. Echocardiographic nondilated non-hypertrophic (restrictive) cardiomyopathy; clinical profle and natural history. J Am Coll Cardiol 1983; I-738.
52. Pearsons AC, Labovitz AJ, Mrosek D, Williams GA, Kennedy HL. Assessment of diastolic function in normal and hypertrophied hearts: Comparison of Doppler echocardiography and M-mode echocardiography. Am Heart J 1987; 113: 1417-1427.
53. Pierard L, Verhaught FW, Meltzer RS, Roelandt J. Echocardiographic aspects of cardiac amyloidosis. Acta Cardiol 1981; 36: 455-459.
54. Presti C, Ryan T, Armstrong WF. Two-dimensional and Doppler echocardiographic findings in hypereosinophilic syndrome. Am Heart J 1987; 114: 172-178.
55. Report of the WHO/IFSC task force on the definition and classification of cardiomyopathies. Br Heart J 1980; 44: 672-673.
56. Sasson Z, Hatle L, Appleton CP, Jewett M, Aldermann EL, Popp RL. Intraventricular flow during isovolumetric relaxation: description and characterisation by Doppler echocardiography. Am J Cardiol 1987; 10: 539-546.
57. Sasson Z, Hatle L, Rakowsky H, Wigle ED, Popp RL. Patterns of left ventricular iisovolumetric relaxation and diastolic filling in apical hypertrophy. Circulation 1988; 75 (suppl IV): IV-429.
58. Seiler CH, Jenni R, Krayenbuehl. Intraventricular blood flow during isovolumetric relaxation and diastole in hypertrophic cardiomyopathy. J Am Soc Echo 1991; 4: 247-257.

59. Shah PM, Gramiak R, Kramer DH. Ultrasound localization of left ventricular outflow obstruction in hypertrophic obstructive cardiomyopathy. Circulation 1969; 40: 3.
60. Siegel RJ, Shah PK, Fishbein MC. Idiopathic restrictive cardiomyopathy. Circulation 1984; 70: 165-169.
61. Siqueira-Filho AG, Cunha CLP, Tajik AJ, Seward JB, Schattenberg TT, Giuliani ER. M-mode and two-dimensional echocardiographic features in cardiac amyloidosis. Circulation 1981; 63: 188-196.
62. Spirito P, Lupi G, Melvendi C, Vecchio C. Restrictive diastolic abnormalities identified by Doppler echocardiography in patients with thalassemia major. Circulation 1990; 82: 88-97.
63. St.John-Sutton MJ, Reichek N, Kastor JA, Giuliani ER. Computerized m-mode echocardiographic analysis of left ventricular dysfunction in cardiac amyloid. Circulation 1982; 66: 709-199.
64. Takashashi M, Fujisawa A, Nakamura M. Localized disorders of left ventricular wall motion in congestive cardiomyopathy. J Cardiogr 1981; 11: 1241-1251.
65. Tencate FJ, Mayalla PG, Vletter WB, Roelandt J. Color-coded Doppler imaging of systolic flow patterns in hypertrophic cardiomyopathy. Int J Card Imag 1985; 1: 217-223.
66. Wallis DE, O'Connell JB, Henkin RE. Segmental wall motion abnormalities in dilated cardiomyopathies: a common finding and good prognostic sign. J Am Coll Cardiol 1984, 4: 674-679.

Isolated organic tricuspid insufficiency is rare and most commonly arises secondary to infective endocarditis [5].

Althoug genuine and isolated forms occur, the most common cause of tricuspid insufficiency is right ventricular dysfunction. This is typically associated with dilation of the right ventricle and tricuspid annulus. Such regurgitation defined as "relative" or, in case of increasing or intermittent worsening of right ventricular dysfunction, it is termed "dynamic."

Etiology of Functional and Isolated Tricuspid Insufficiency

Cardiopulmonary or pulmonary vascular disease

- ▸ Perinatal asphyxia
- ▸ Congenital heart disease
  (Ebstein's anomaly, Eisenmenger's complex, endomyocardial fibrosis, pulmonary stenosis, tricuspid valve prolapse with myxomatous leaflet degeneration (Marfan's syndrome))
- ▸ "Primary" pulmonary hypertension
- ▸ Mitral valve diseases
- ▸ Infective endocarditis
- ▸ Right ventricular myocardial infarction with ischemic tricuspid insufficiency
- ▸ Carcinoid tumor
- ▸ Cardiac tumors
- ▸ Constrictive pericarditis
- ▸ Cor pulmonale
- ▸ Traumatic tricuspid insufficiency
  (especially due to blunt chest trauma from traffic accidents and resuscitation efforts)

Echocardiography is often helpful in visualizing the anatomic abnormalities that cause tricuspid insufficiency.

Underlying anatomic causes of tricuspid insufficiency

- ▸ Tricuspid valve dysplasia
- ▸ Congenital anomalies in the form of atrioventricular canal defects
- ▸ Ebstein's anomaly
- ▸ Congenital corrected transposition of the great arteries
- ▸ Abnormal development, malalignment, dysfunction, or rupture of the papillary muscles
- ▸ Thickened, elongated, ruptured or misplaced chordae tendineae
- ▸ Rheumatic thickening and contracture of leaflets;
- ▸ Vegetations, thrombi or tumors
- ▸ Akinesia or dyskinesia of right ventricular wall sections at the base of the papillary muscles
- ▸ Dilation of tricuspid annulus

Cardiac Ultrasound Diagnosis

All echocardiographic techniques should preferably be performed using left parasternal, apical four-chamber, and subcostal four-chamber views. Additional transesophageal scans are sometimes necessary.

Conventional Echocardiography

Visualization of anatomic causes:

Two-dimensional and M-mode echocardiography:

- *Dilation of the fibrous ring;*
- *Thickened, elongated, ruptured, or abnormally positioned chordae tendineae;*
- *Papillary muscle rupture or dysfunction;*
- *Akinesia or dyskinesia of right ventricular wall sections at the base of the papillary muscles.*

Nonspecific features and possible hemodynamic effects of tricuspid insufficiency:

Two-dimensional and M-mode echocardiography:

- *Enlargement of right atrium and/or ventricle*
  (as compared with left atrium and ventricle seen from apical/subcostal view).
- *Abnormal interventricular septal motion* representing right ventricular volume overload.
- Leftward bulging of the interatrial septum (in subcostal M-mode recordings).

Contrast Echocardiography

Contrast agents for right heart contrast:

- *Extended retention time of echocontrastography agent in right heart cavities and visualization of contrast agent in inferior vena cava and hepatic veins (2-D and M-mode).*

Conventional Doppler Echocardiography

Pulsed-wave Doppler (PW Doppler):

- *To detect, map, and measure the velocity of systolic regurgitant jets in the right atrium.*

Continuous-wave Doppler (CW Doppler):

- *To detect and measure the velocity of systolic regurgitant jets at tricuspid valve level.*

Tricuspid regurgitation can usually be detected in continuous or pulsed-wave Doppler recordings from the apical four-chamber view. In CW Doppler, the beam is focused on the base of transtricuspid forward flow in the right ventricle, whereas the PW Doppler sample volume is placed immediately proximal to the tricuspid valve orifice or at the leading edge of the regurgitant jet. Doppler detection of tricuspid regurgitation appears to be slightly superior to auscultation by an experienced examiner. Although the regurgitant jet size, configuration, and direction do not affect the results of auscultation, an increase in inspiratory intensity in case of loud systolic murmurs originating from other valves may render auscultatory diagnosis more difficult.

Doppler Color Flow Imaging (2-D and M-mode)

- *Graphic display of turbulent transtricuspid regurgitant jets.*
- *Doppler color-encoding can be enhanced by contrast agents.*

Transesophageal Echocardiography (Single and Multiplane)

In transesophageal echocardiography, the posterior, septal, and anterior tricuspid valve leaflets can be visualized from the transgastric short-axis view, the long-axis views through the tricuspid valve ring, and in multiplane transesophageal images. It is difficult to make a detailed assessment of tricuspid valve morphology, as would be needed to understand the mechanism of leakage, because it is impossible to simultaneously visualize all three tricuspid valve leaflets in a single scan plane.

10.1.1   Tricuspid Insufficiency
10.1.1.1   Detection, Semiquantitation and Quantitation

In contrast to mitral regurgitation, the severity of tricuspid insufficiency needs only to be defined as "severe" or "mild", *i.e.*, requiring surgery or not. In patients undergoing left-side valve surgery, the cardiologist must determine whether tricuspid valvuloplasty is indicated. The clinically marked dichotomy usually means that a decision has to be made based on the impression of color flow images and verifiable hemodynamic consequences such as right atrial enlargement. One must decide whether to perform additional tricuspid valve reconstruction during mitral valve surgery.

In general one can assume that when tricuspid regurgitation is assessed according to the visual impression made in Doppler color flow images, severity will be overestimated as compared with hemodynamic and cine-angiocardiography determined severity. In Doppler echocardiography, all valvular regurgitations, including tricuspid regurgitation, are divided into four classes of severity according to regurgitant fraction range and cine-cardioangiographic contrast medium effects, as shown in the table below.

Tricuspid Insufficiency. Grading Scheme		
	Contrast Medium Effects	Regurgitant fraction
Mild	1+	RF $\leq$ 0.20
Moderate	2+	0.20 < RF $\leq$ 0.40
Moderately severe	3+	0.40 < RF $\leq$ 0.60
Severe	4+	0.60 < RF

In clinical practice, it is acceptable to dichotomize the lesions into those that require surgery and those that do not.

Doppler Echocardiographic Parameters for Detection and Assessment of Tricuspid Insufficiency

▸ Jet width and/or length
  (conventional Doppler or color-encoded PW Doppler).
▸ Regurgitant jet area
  (Doppler color flow imaging),
▸ Regurgitant jet width/length/area relative to right atrial length/width/area.

▸ Time-velocity integrals for tricuspid flow or for tricuspid and pulmonary flow

▸ Doppler signal intensity
  (signal amplitude, audio signal, densitometry)

▸ Regurgitant fraction

The most common method of estimating the severity of tricuspid insufficiency is relating severity to the maximum visualized color jet length and/or width and/or area. It still remains unclear whether relating the regurgitant jet length/width/area to the right atrial length/width/area actually improves the validity of this technique.

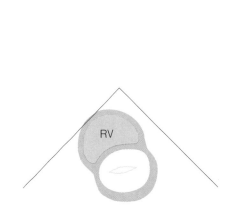

Dilatation of the right ventricle and tricuspid annulus in patient with "functional" tricuspid insufficiency.

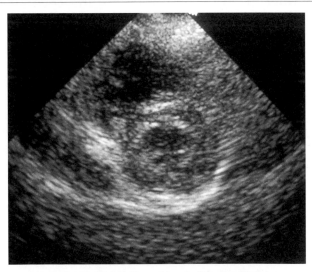

2-D parasternal short-axis 2-D view at level of the ventricle.

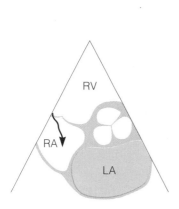

Mild "functional" tricuspid insufficiency in patient with coexistent mitral lesion and left atrial dilatation.

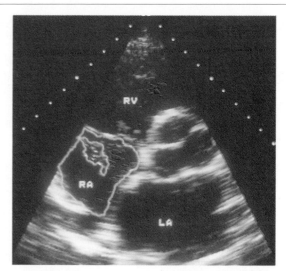

Color flow map of 2-D parasternal short-axis view at level of the aorta.

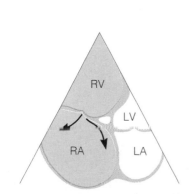

Moderate tricuspid insufficiency in setting of cor pulmonale. Note dilated right atrium. Visualization of regurgitation in color Doppler image less impressive than angiographically determined severity (2+).

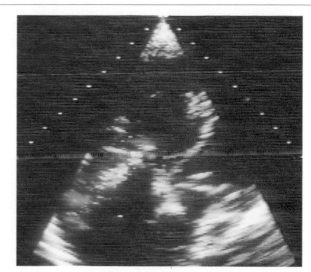

Color flow map of apical four-chamber 2-D echocardiogram.

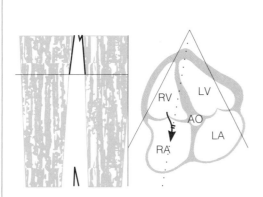

PW Doppler detection of tricuspid insufficiency; aliasing. Color flow mapping only slightly enhances visualization of regurgitant jet, but makes it easier to place the sample volume.

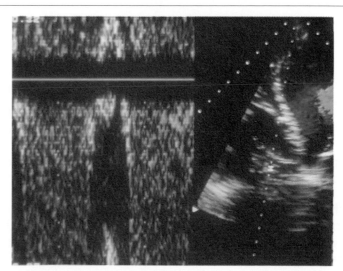

PW Doppler and apical four-chamber 2-D scans; color flow mapping.

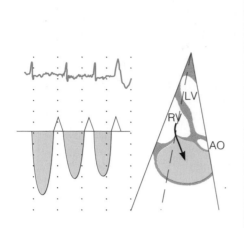

Moderate tricuspid insufficiency with severe primary mitral regurgitation, pulmonary hypertension and atrial fibrillation.

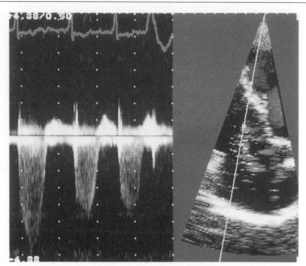

Color-encoded CW Doppler and apical four-chamber 2-D echocardiograms.

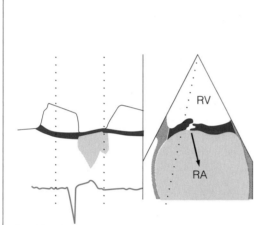

Combined tricuspid valve defect (note dark orange flow on both sides of the tricuspid valve echo) is delineated by color M-mode. Highly turbulent orthograde and retrograde flow.

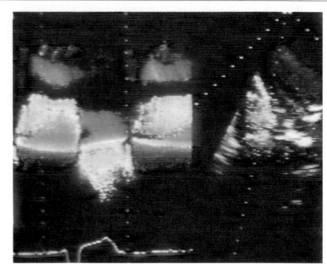

Color M-mode and 2DE images, apical four-chamber view.

10.1.1   Tricuspid Insufficiency
10.1.1.2   Sources of Error

Certain sources of error must be taken into consideration in echocardiographic detection of tricuspid insufficiency, assessment of its severity, and determination of its underlying causes.

In the short-axis view through the tricuspid valve, a localized dense area is often seen just below or adjacent to the lateral wall of the tricuspid annulus. This frequently corresponds to fatty tissue in the atrioventricular furrow and should not be misinterpreted as tumor or thrombus.

When imaging from conventional scan planes, tricuspid regurgitant jets often are not in good alignment with the ultrasound beam, because they flow in the direction of the interatrial septum. When this is the case, variable scan planes must be utilized for proper visualization of the jet.

In addition to echocardiographic findings, decisions regarding surgical timing and planning must be based on classical findings such as right atrial size, right ventricular function, concomitant peripheral edema, increased jugular vein pressure, elevated V-wave on the RA curve, auscultatory findings and, when applicable, cine-angiocardiographic findings.

Attempts to detect morphological changes in the tricuspid valve often yield false-negative findings. Echocardiographic detection of tricuspid valve prolapse is subject to the same problems as mitral valve prolapse, because most echocardiographers interrogate for tricuspid valve prolapse in the apical four-chamber view only, while failing to make M-mode recordings from the subcostal position.

10.1.1   Tricuspid Insufficiency
10.1.1.3   Ventricular Function

Right ventricular function is a critical factor in tricuspid insufficiency, because it is the most common pathomechanism for the development and aggravation of tricuspid insufficiency. Operationalized ejection phase parameters (*e.g.* right ventricular diastolic-systolic area change, measured from the apical four-chamber view) will be overestimated, because the right ventricle functions as a double outlet chamber against reduced impedance.

10.1.1   Tricuspid Insufficiency
10.1.1.4   Follow-up and Treatment Considerations

The decision to use either echocardiography or cardiac catheterization to follow up tricuspid insufficiency and to decide whether and when surgical intervention is indicated is based on the following factors.

- Primary disease (*e.g.* mitral lesion, ischemic heart disease, or primary bronchopulmonary disease);
- Severity of tricuspid insufficiency, and possible overestimation of it by Doppler echocardiography.

When following up tricuspid insufficiency by echocardiography, the general rule is: The poorer the right ventricular function and the more severe the primary disease, the shorter the time between follow-up examinations.

When tricuspid insufficiency requires surgery, two procedures may be considered: valve replacement or valve reconstruction. Prosthetic valves have proven to be a significant cause of stenosis within the regulatory low-pressure tricuspid valve system. Reconstructive techniques have been widely tried and tested. Tricuspid valve reconstruction has proven to be an exemplary method for preservation of the valve and has become the standard surgical procedure.

Doppler echocardiography is a highly specific technique for detecting tricuspid insufficiency. Besides auscultation, the only comparable complementary techniques are invasive techniques using manometry and cine-angiocardiography.

An unsolved dilemma in Doppler echocardiography, especially in color flow Doppler, is the visualization of trivial regurgitation that does not correspond to auscultatory and angiographic findings. Relying heavily on the sensitivity of Doppler echocardiography, this could be interpreted as "physiologic" regurgitation [1]. On the other hand, one could also assume it reflects hemodynamically insignificant regurgitation due to yet unexplained standardization problems in the color flow technique. However, the accuracy of these assumptions remains unclear.

This becomes especially problematic in transesophageal echocardiography, where trivial "regurgitant volumes" (due to leaflet closure motion that causes a shift in or acceleration of blood in the immediate vicinity of the tips of the leaflets) as well as other problems (*e.g.* regurgitant jets that extend to the top of the atrium) must be dealt with.

The sheer number of proposed methods for assessing the severity of tricuspid insufficiency using cardiac ultrasound techniques makes it clear that this subject has come to an impasse. The only solution is to restrict grading to only two classes of severity, namely "mild" and "severe" - as is justifiable in clinical practice.

A method that unreliably differentiates only seemingly objectivizes auscultatory findings and indications for surgery. Since the regurgitant volume cannot be determined, at least not precisely and reliably, supplementary techniques must be used to quantitate the severity of tricuspid insufficiency.

Morphometry and ventricular function

RA volume	_____	ml
RVEDD	_____	mm
RVEDV	_____	ml
LADmax	_____	mm
LA volume	_____	ml

Ventricular function. Signs of concomitant ischemic heart disease?
RV wall motion analysis.

Morphology and dynamics of tricuspid valve and subvalvular apparatus

▶ Valvular tissue defects?
▶ High DE amplitude, steep drop in EF slope, reduced rapid filling phase?

Indirect indicators of hemodynamic complications

▶ Paradoxical motion of interventricular septum?
▶ Leftward protrusion of interatrial septum?

Ventricular function and pressure-flow relationships
(contrast and conventional Doppler echocardiography)

▶ Extended contrast medium retention in right heart cavity
▶ Echocontrastography agent detected in inferior vena cava
▶ Velocity measurements (m/s)
  – maximum instantaneous velocity
  – mean transtricuspid velocity
▶ Regurgitant jets
  – qualitative visual assessment
  – semiquantitative assessment as needed
▶ Intracardiac pressure (mmHg)
  – $PA_{systolic}$
  – $PA_{diastolic}$ in patients with coexistent pulmonary insufficiency

Transesophageal Echocardiography (TEE)

▶ Detection of thrombus in right atrium
▶ Valve morphology and dynamics
▶ Detection and classification of lesions in tricuspid valve support apparatus

10.1.1   **Tricuspid Insufficiency**
10.1.1.7   **Tricuspid Insufficiency Flow Chart**
    440

SYMPTOMATOLOGY / AUSCULTATION

ECHOCARDIOGRAPHY
Conventional echocardiography: Morphometry (RA, RVEDD, RVEDV, LADmax) Ventricular function (RV wall motion analysis) Visualization of anatomic causes and hemodynamic effects Valve morphology and dynamics Detection of concomitant heart and valve disease.
Contrast, Doppler and transesophageal echocardiography Qualitative visual assessment; semiquantitative and/or quantitative assessment Visualization of underlying anatomic causes

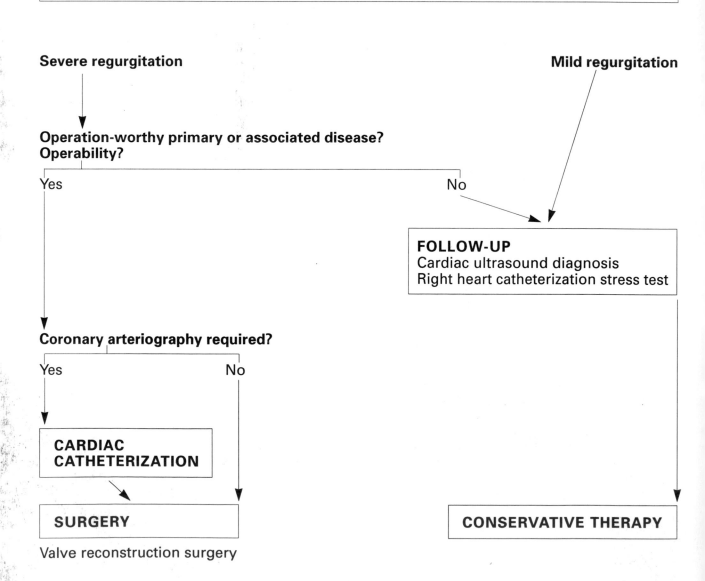

Severe regurgitation
                                    Mild regurgitation

Operation-worthy primary or associated disease?
Operability?

Yes   No

FOLLOW-UP
Cardiac ultrasound diagnosis
Right heart catheterization stress test

Coronary arteriography required?

Yes   No

CARDIAC
CATHETERIZATION

SURGERY   **CONSERVATIVE THERAPY**

Valve reconstruction surgery

The normal tricuspid valve orifice area (TVA) is approximately 7 cm². Obstruction is hemodynamically significant when the TVA is 1.5 cm² or smaller, and is critical when the TVA is smaller than 1 cm². The maximum normal transtricuspid pressure gradient is 1 mmHg (circumscribing the range of error in all methods). A pressure gradient of 2 mmHg is considered diagnostic of tricuspid stenosis. The critical effects of increased pressure gradient include increased right atrial pressure and peripheral edema formation in cases where the mean diastolic pressure gradient exceeds 5 to 10 mmHg.

Tricuspid stenosis most commonly has a rheumatic pathogenesis, usually with secondary involvement of the mitral valve [2, 7, 9, 10, 12, 13]. Tricuspid stenosis is mainly due to fibrotic tissue transformation, which may lead to commissural fusion, scar tissue formation, and consecutive contracture of leaflet tissue [3]. More unusual etiologies include tricuspid atresia, endocardial fibroelastosis, Loeffler's endomyocardial fibrosis, systemic lupus erythematosus, constrictive pericarditis, and metastasizing carcinoids. Approximately 10% of all metastasizing carcinoid tumors involve both the tricuspid and pulmonary valves [8, 11], which may additionally contain fibrous plaques. Right atrial tumors can displace the tricuspid valve orifice, thereby creating a hemodynamic situation similar to tricuspid stenosis. The underlying mechanism resembles that of valve vegetations and extracardiac tumor-related obstruction.

10.1.2 **Tricuspid Stenosis**
10.1.2.1 **Detection, Semiquantitation and Quantitation**

Cardiac Ultrasound Diagnosis

The preferred scan planes are the left parasternal short-axis view and the apical and subcostal four-chamber views.

Conventional Echocardiography

Visualization of anatomic causes:

Two-dimensional and M-mode echocardiography:
- *Abnormally thickened and/or calcified tricuspid leaflets* as demonstrated from orthogonal orientation at maximum opening; parallel multiple echos are common.

Nonspecific features and possible hemodynamic effects of tricuspid stenosis:

Two-dimensional echocardiography:
- *Diastolic doming of tricuspid leaflet into right ventricle, particularly in anterior leaflet.* Dome-like broadening of the bodies of the tricuspid leaflets occurs during blood flow, because the free edges do not allow it to open completely. Decreased separation of tips of leaflets;
- *Right atrial dilatation;*
- *Leftward protrusion of interatrial septum.*

M-mode echocardiography:
- *Flat EF slope* with absence of "A" wave in anterior and posterior leaflets [6],
- Reduced leaflet motility.

Conventional Doppler Echocardiography

Pulsed-wave Doppler (PW Doppler):

- *To detect and measure the velocity of diastolic stenotic flow jets at tricuspid valve level.*

Continuous-wave Doppler (CW Doppler):

- *To detect and measure the velocity of diastolic stenotic flow jets at tricuspid valve level.*

Tricuspid stenosis can usually be detected in pulsed or continuous-wave Doppler recordings obtained from the apical four-chamber view. The CW Doppler beam is focused on the base of transtricuspid forward flow in the right ventricle. The PW Doppler sample volume is placed in the right ventricle immediately upstream from the tricuspid valve orifice. Since transvalvular pressure gradients are very low, the probability of error is higher than in mitral valve stenosis. Therefore, only well-defined images where the stenotic flow jet is perfectly parallel to the Doppler cursor should be used for evaluation purposes.

Doppler Color Flow Imaging (2-D and M-mode)

- *Graphic display of transtricuspid turbulent stenotic flow jets.*

Transesophageal Echocardiography (Single and Multiplane)

Transesophageal echocardiography (TEE) has some slight advantages with respect to detection and quantification of severity.

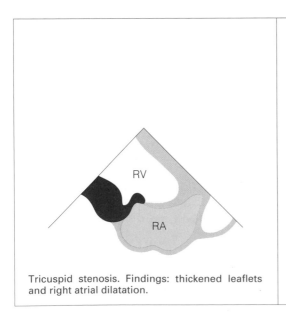

Tricuspid stenosis. Findings: thickened leaflets and right atrial dilatation.

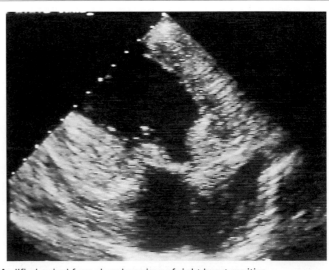

Modified apical four-chamber view of right heart cavities.

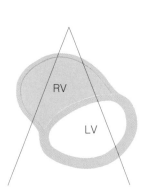

Tricuspid stenosis. Findings: turbulent stenotic flow jet in right ventricle.

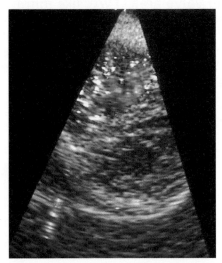

Color-encoded parasternal short-axis view from level of the ventricle.

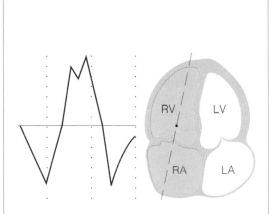

Hemodynamically significant tricuspid stenosis: instantaneous peak pressure gradient = ca. 12 mmHg; mean = 5.5 mmHg.

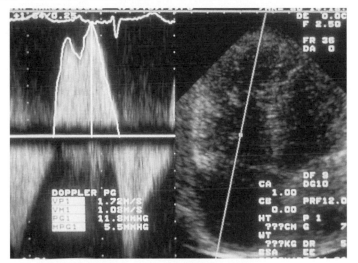

Color-encoded CW Doppler recording and apical four-chamber 2-D scan.

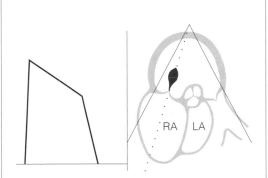

Severe tricuspid stenosis: Note small lancet-shaped stenotic flow jet near sample volume. The TVA derived from pressure half-time (387 ms) equals 0.56 cm². Despite the good envelope, quantification difficulties arose due to discrepancy between blood flow velocity and pressure half-time.

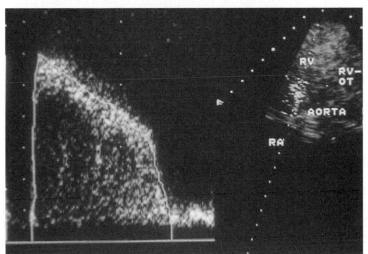

Color-encoded CW Doppler and parasternal short-axis view.

The tricuspid valve area (TVA), like mitral valve area, can be derived from the pressure half-time, *i.e.* the time in which the early diastolic peak velocity drops to $1/\sqrt{2}$ that value. TVA is obtained as the quotient of an empirical constant (220) and the pressure half-time. The pressure half-time is 39 ± 12 ms   (30 to 50 ms) in normals and 140 ± 70 ms (60 to 257 ms) in patients with tricuspid stenosis. The corresponding tricuspid valve areas are 1.96 ± 0.91 cm² (1.01 to 3.28 cm²) [4].

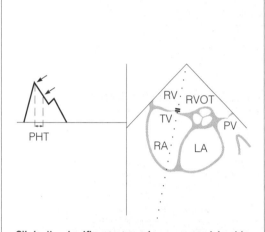

Clinically significant stenosis was noted in this patient with combined tricuspid lesions, even though the tricuspid valve area derived from the pressure half-time is larger than 2 cm².

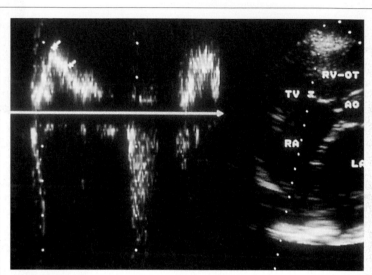

PW Doppler recording and parasternal short-axis 2-D scan.

10.1.2   Tricuspid Stenosis
10.1.2.2   Sources of Error

All echocardiographic techniques have a certain potential for error in estimation of the severity of tricuspid stenosis, particularly when the angle between the ultrasound beam and the stenotic flow jet becomes too wide. Because flow velocities in tricuspid stenosis are relatively low, pressure gradients are often underestimated, which can lead to clinically significant misinterpretations. Patients with significant coexisting tricuspid regurgitation have a high prestenotic flow velocity. The severity of tricuspid stenosis will inevitably be overestimated if this factor is disregarded, as is the case when using the simplified Bernoulli equation. Additional method-related errors arise in patients with large orifice areas and short pressure half-times. The relationship of these two values is hyperbolic. Short pressure half-times generate a steep curve. The resulting measurement inaccuracies lead to a relatively broad range of error in derived tricuspid valve area measurements.

It would therefore be advisable to adhere to the following recommendations:
1. use only perfect spectral curves with a well defined envelope area for computation purposes;
2. do not disregard the prestenotic flow velocity when using the Bernoulli equation; and
3. accelerate the paper feed in these cases (100 mm/s).

Morphometry and ventricular function

RA volume	_____	ml
RVEDD	_____	mm
RVEDV	_____	ml
LADmax	_____	mm
LA volume	_____	ml

RVEF   _____

Signs of pulmonary hypertension?
Leftward protrusion of the interatrial septum in the subcostal four-chamber view?
RVOT-EDD   _____   mm

Valve morphology and dynamics

▶ Thickening and/or calcification of tricuspid leaflets?
   Degree and extent of calcification.
▶ Reduced EF slope?
▶ Reduced leaflet motility or doming of leaflets?
▶ Involvement of subvalvular apparatus?

Ventricular function and pressure-flow relationships (Doppler echocardiography)

▶ Velocity measurements (m/s)
   – maximum instantaneous velocity
   – mean transtricuspid velocity
▶ Pressure gradients (mmHg)
   – maximum instantaneous pressure gradient
   – mean transtricuspid pressure gradient
▶ Tricuspid valve area (TVA; cm^2) and tricuspid valve area index (TVA-I; cm^2/m^2) derived
   from pressure half-time
▶ Regurgitant jet
   - qualitative visual assessment
▶ Intracardiac pressure (mmHg)
   – $PA_{systolic}$ with concomitant tricuspid regurgitation
   – $PA_{diastolic}$ with concomitant pulmonary regurgitation

---

Transesophageal echocardiography

▶ Valve morphology and dynamics

SYMPTOMATOLOGY / AUSCULTATION

ECHOCARDIOGRAPHY

Conventional echocardiography:

Morphometry (RA, RVEDD, RVEDV, LADmax)
Ventricular function (RV wall motion analysis)
Detection of underlying anatomic causes and hemodynamic effects
Valve morphology and dynamics
Detection of concomitant cardiac or valvular heart disease.

Doppler and transesophageal echocardiography:

Tricuspid valve area (TVA), tricuspid valve area index (TVA-I)
computed via pressure half-time method

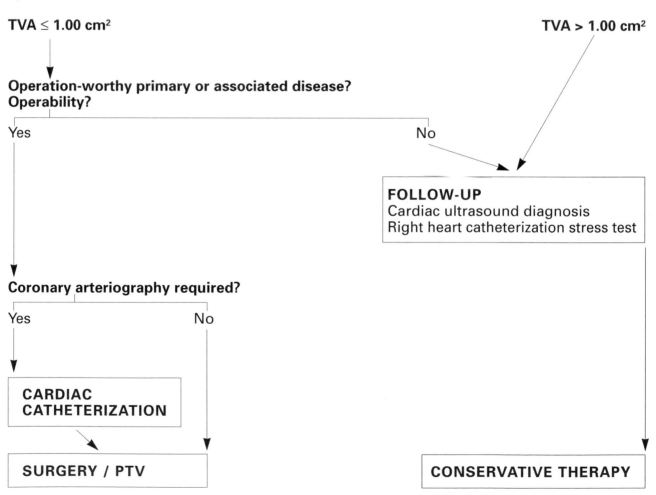

TVA $\leq$ 1.00 cm²   **TVA > 1.00 cm²**

Operation-worthy primary or associated disease?
Operability?

Yes   No

FOLLOW-UP
Cardiac ultrasound diagnosis
Right heart catheterization stress test

Coronary arteriography required?

Yes   No

**CARDIAC
CATHETERIZATION**

SURGERY / PTV   **CONSERVATIVE THERAPY**

Percutaneous transluminal valvuloplasty
Tricuspid valve reconstruction
Open or closed commissurotomy
Valve replacement surgery

1. Akamatsu S, Kagawa K, Terazawa E, Takeda T, Arakawa M, Dohi S. Physiological tricuspidal regurgitation: A study with transesophageal Doppler echocardiography. Circulation 1990: 82 (suppl III): 0178.
2. Clawson BJ. Rheumatic heart disease. An analysis of 796 cases. Am Heart J 1940; 20: 454.
3. Davies MJ. Pathology of cardiac valves. London: Butterworths, 1980.
4. Dennig K, Kraus F, Rudolph W. Doppler-echokardiographische Bestimmung des Schweregrades der Trikuspidalstenose. Herz 1986; 11: 332-336.
5. Glancy DL, Marcus FI, Cuadra M, Ewy GA, Roberts WC. Isolated organic tricuspid valvular regurgitation. Causes and consequences. Am J Med 1969; 46: 989-996.
6. Joyner CR, Hey BE Jr, Johnson J, Reid RM. Reflected ultrasound in the diagnosis of tricuspid stenosis. Am J Cardiol 1967; 19: 66-73.
7. Killip T, Lukas DS. Tricuspid stenosis. Am J Med 1958; 24: 836.
8. Ludwig J. Cardiac vein involvement in carcinoid syndrome. Possible evidence of retrograde blood flow in cardiac veins in tricuspid insufficiency. Am J Clin Path 1971; 55: 617-623.
9. Morgan JR, Forker AD, Coates JR, Myers WS. Isolated tricuspid stenosis. Circulation 1971; 44: 729-732.
10. Perloff JK, Harvey WP. The clinical recognition of tricuspid stenosis. Circulation 1960; 22: 346.
11. Ross EM, Roberts WC. The carcinoid syndrome. Am J Med 1985; 79: 339-354.
12. Smith JA, Levine SA. Clinical features of tricuspid stenosis. Am Heart J 1942; 23: 739.
13. Waller BF. Morphological aspects of valvular heart disease: Part two. Curr Prob Card 1984; 9: 1-74.

10.2	**Pulmonary Valvular Disease**
10.2.1	**Pulmonary Insufficiency**
	(Kurt J.G. Schmailzl)

In the overwhelming majority of cases, pulmonary valvular disease manifests as trivial pulmonary regurgitation secondary to pulmonary hypertension or congenital pulmonary valve stenosis. Pulmonary insufficiency is the most common manifestation of acquired pulmonary valvular disease [3, 11, 12, 13]. In rare cases neoplastic and inflammatory processes (*e.g.* rheumatic fever, infective endocarditis, syphilis, tuberculosis) have been reported to cause combined pulmonary valve lesions. In patients with severe pulmonary hypertension, high-velocity regurgitant jets develop due to dilatation of the valve ring when the pulmonary artery systolic pressure exceeds 70 mmHg. The corresponding Graham Steell murmur can be heard upon auscultation. Pulmonary regurgitations of this kind are common in chronic bronchopulmonary disease, pulmonary embolism, and severe mitral stenosis. Intracardiac and mediastinal masses, carcinoid tumors, and constrictive pericarditis can also involve the pulmonary valve or simulate valvular obstruction.

Cardiac Ultrasound Diagnosis

The preferred scan planes are the left parasternal and subcostal short-axis views. Individual cases may require additional multiplane transesophageal imaging.

Conventional Echocardiography

Visualization of anatomic causes:

2-D and M-mode echocardiography:
- *Dilatation of the fibrous ring*

Nonspecific features and possible hemodynamic effects of pulmonary insufficiency:

2-D and M-mode echocardiography:

- *Right atrial and/or right ventricular dilatation*
- *High-amplitude motion of the interventricular septum or paradoxical septal motion indicative of right ventricular volume overload*
- *Low-frequency diastolic oscillation of tricuspid valve.*

Conventional Doppler Echocardiography

Pulsed-wave Doppler (PW Doppler):

- *Detection, velocity measurement and mapping of systolic regurgitation in the right atrium.*

Continuous-wave Doppler (CW Doppler):

- *Detection and velocity measurement of systolic regurgitation jet at the pulmonary valve level.*

Pulmonary insufficiency can usually be detected in continuous or pulsed-wave Doppler recordings obtained from the parasternal or subcostal short-axis view. The CW Doppler beam should be focused on the base of transpulmonary forward flow in the right ventricle. The PW Doppler sample volume should be placed proximal to the pulmonary valve orifice or at the leading edge of the regurgitant jet.

Doppler echocardiographic detection of pulmonary valvular regurgitation and assessment of its severity does not appear to provide substantial advantages over auscultation by an experienced examiner. The high sensitivity of Doppler echocardiography is offset by false positive findings associated with "physiological" regurgitation, whereas the results of auscultation remain unaffected by the size, configuration and direction of the regurgitant jet.

Doppler Color Flow Imaging (2-D and M-mode)

- *Provides graphic display of turbulent transpulmonary regurgitant jets.*
- *Enhancing color-encoded images by contrast agents for right heart contrast.*

Transesophageal Echocardiography (Single and Multiplane)

It is difficult to make a detailed analysis of pulmonary valve morphology, as is required to understand the mechanism of leakage, because it is impossible to simultaneously visualize all three pulmonary valve cusps in a single transthoracic scan plane. In single plane TEE, it is difficult to visualize the pulmonary valve at all, except in anteflected, deep transgastric scans. Usually, scans obtained from the long-axis view through the right ventricular outflow tract are required for this purpose.

In contrast to tricuspid and mitral regurgitation, even moderately severe pulmonary insufficiency does not normally require surgical management. Clinical practice has shown that isolated pulmonary insufficiency is well tolerated in almost all patients [4]. The systolic pressure
gradient is an important tool for assessing diastolic pulmonary artery pressure. In patients
with concomitant tricuspid regurgitation, systolic and diastolic pressure gradients can be used
to quantitate both the pulmonary artery pressure and the severity of pulmonary hypertension.
These are key pieces of information for deciding whether surgery is possible in patients with
other primary diseases and for predicting their postoperative functional prognosis.

In Doppler echocardiography all regurgitations, including pulmonary regurgitation, are
divided into four grades of severity on the basis of the regurgitant fraction and cine-cardioangiographic contrast medium effects, as is shown in the table below.

Severity of Pulmonary Insufficiency. Grading System		
	Contrast medium effects	Regurgitant fraction
Mild	1+	$RF \leq 0.20$
Moderate	2+	$0.20 < RF < 0.40$
Moderately severe	3+	$0.40 < RF \leq 0.60$
Severe	4+	$0.60 \leq RF$

For practical purposes, the regurgitant fraction is not as important as the systolic pressure
gradient.

Doppler parameters for detection and assessment of pulmonary insufficiency
▸ Regurgitant jet width and/or length (conventional Doppler or color PW Doppler)   ▸ Regurgitant jet area (Doppler color flow imaging)
▸ Time-velocity integrals for flow across pulmonary valve or across pulmonary and aortic valves
▸ Doppler signal intensity   (signal amplitude, audio signal, densitometry)
▸ Regurgitant fraction
▸ Systolic pressure gradient

The most common method of estimating the severity of pulmonary insufficiency is based on
an assessment of the maximum visualized color jet length or area in conjunction with diastolic pressure gradients.

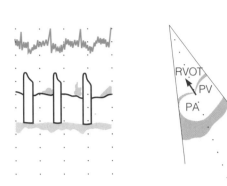

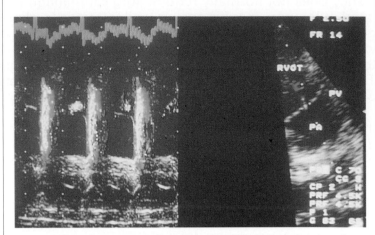

Mild pulmonary insufficiency in patient with pulmonary hypertension secondary to a mitral lesion. Small area of red encoded reflux transforms to blue due to aliasing. Color M-mode image shows bright orange reflux from severe turbulence in systole.

2-D and M-mode; parasternal cross-sectional view of aortic valve plane (long-axis view through RV); color flow imaging.

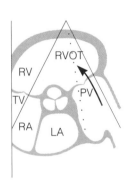

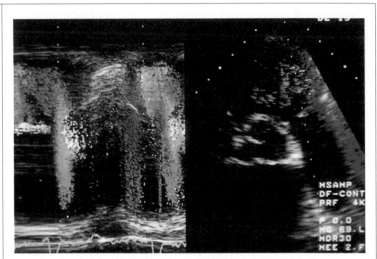

Mild pulmonary insufficiency; unequivocally detectable only in color M-mode recordings.

2-D and M-mode; parasternal cross-sectional view of aortic valve plane (long-axis view through RV); color flow imaging.

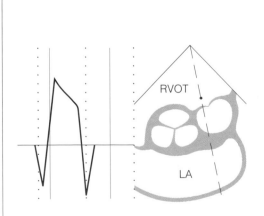

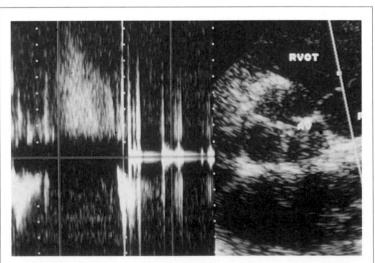

Mild pulmonary insufficiency in patient with pulmonary hypertension secondary to mitral lesion. Dilated right ventricular outflow tract.

CW Doppler recording and parasternal cross-sectional view of aortic valve plane (long-axis view through RV).

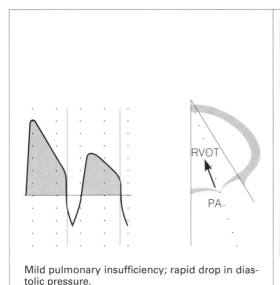

| Mild pulmonary insufficiency; rapid drop in diastolic pressure. | CW Doppler and parasternal cross-sectional view of aortic valve plane (long-axis view through RV). |

10.2.1   Pulmonary Insufficiency
10.2.1.2   Sources of Error

Error may arise in echocardiographic detection of pulmonary insufficiency and in the gross assessment of its severity.

When making decisions relevant to treatment and/or surgery, classical findings like right ventricular size and function, increased A wave in jugular vein pulses, RV curve findings, and cine-cardioangiographic classification data must also be taken into consideration.

10.2.1   Pulmonary Insufficiency
10.2.1.3   Critical Evaluation of Results and Comparison With Those of Complementary Diagnostic Techniques

Doppler echocardiography is highly sensitive for detecting pulmonary insufficiency. Besides auscultation, only invasive techniques provide comparable results.

An unsolved dilemma in Doppler echocardiography, especially in color flow Doppler, is the visualization of mostly trivial regurgitation that does not correspond with auscultatory and angiographic findings. Relying heavily on the reliability of Doppler echocardiography, this could be interpreted as "physiological" regurgitation [1]. On the other hand, one could also assume this reflects hemodynamically insignificant regurgitation due to yet unexplained standardization problems in the color flow technique. However, the accuracy of these assumptions remains unclear.

10.2.1   **Pulmonary Insufficiency**
10.2.1.4   **Special Measurement Program and**
           Quick Reference

452

Morphometry and ventricular function

RA volume	_____	ml
RVEDD	_____	mm
RVEDV	_____	ml
LADmax	_____	mm
LA volume	_____	ml

Ventricular function. Signs of concomitant ischemic heart disease? RV wall motion analysis.

Morphology and dynamics of pulmonary valve and pulmonary valve support apparatus

▸ Valvular tissue defects?

Indirect indicators of abnormal hemodynamic situation

▸ High motion amplitude in interventricular septum?
▸ Premature, gradual closure movement of pulmonary valve in systole?

Ventricular function and pressure-flow relationships (Doppler echocardiography)

▸ Velocity measurements (m/s)
 - maximum instantaneous velocity
 - mean transpulmonary velocity
▸ Regurgitation
 - qualitative visual assessment
▸ Intracardiac pressure (mmHg)
 - $PA_{systolic}$
 - $PA_{diastolic}$ with concomitant tricuspid regurgitation

Transesophageal Echocardiography

▸ Valve morphology and dynamics

SYMPTOMATOLOGY / AUSCULTATION

ECHOCARDIOGRAPHY

Conventional echocardiography:

Morphometry (RA, RVEDD, LADmax),
Ventricular function (RV wall motion analysis);
Visualization of underlying anatomic causes and hemodynamic effects,
Valve morphology and dynamics as well as
Detection of concomitant cardiac and valvular heart disease.

Doppler and transesophageal echocardiography:

Qualitative visual assessment

Visualization of underlying lesions

Detection and semiquantitation of
concomitant tricuspid regurgitation
($PA_{systolic}$)

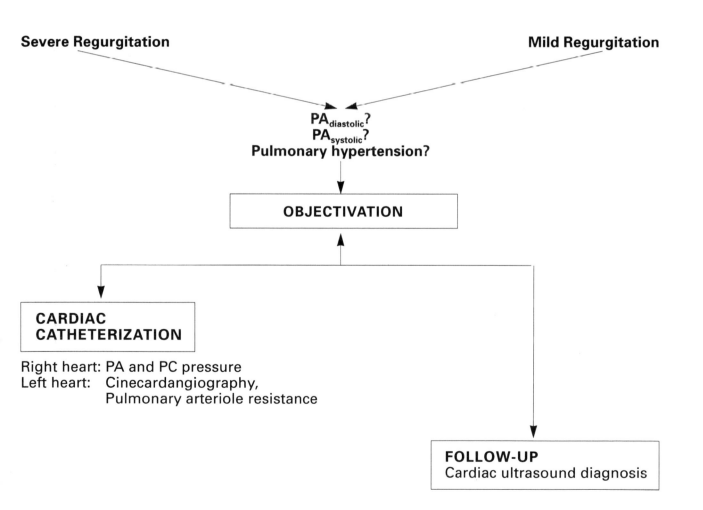

Severe Regurgitation   **Mild Regurgitation**

$PA_{diastolic}$?
$PA_{systolic}$?
Pulmonary hypertension?

OBJECTIVATION

**CARDIAC
CATHETERIZATION**

Right heart: PA and PC pressure
Left heart: Cinecardangiography,
                    Pulmonary arteriole resistance

FOLLOW-UP
Cardiac ultrasound diagnosis

Isolated (congenital) pulmonary valvular stenosis is the most common form of the right ventricular outflow tract obstruction.

Right ventricular outflow tract obstruction

- ▶ Valvular pulmonary stenosis

- ▶ Subvalvular pulmonary stenosis
  - – Infundibular stenosis
  - – Subinfundibular stenosis

- ▶ Supravalvular pulmonary stenosis
  - – Central stenosis (coarctation of the pulmonary trunk)
  - – Peripheral stenosis (pulmonary artery stenosis)

Most congenital forms of pulmonary stenosis arise from commissural fusion and adhesion or, more infrequently, from dysplastic and thickened valve cusps. Acquired forms on the other hand are mainly due to rheumatic processes, carcinoid tumors [6], or external compression by tumors and aneurysms.

10.2.2 Pulmonary Stenosis
10.2.2.1 Detection, Semiquantitation and Quantitation

Cardiac Ultrasound Diagnosis

The preferred scan plane is the left parasternal short-axis view.

If subvalvular pulmonary stenosis is suspected, the echocardiographer should look for right ventricular hypertrophy and systolic valve fluttering, a nonspecific criterion. Suspected hypoplastic defects of supravalvular branches is assessed by comparing the right pulmonary artery diameter with that of the aorta as visualized from the suprasternal notch.

Conventional Echocardiography

Visualization of anatomic causes:

Two-dimensional echocardiography:
- *Thickening and/or calcification of the pulmonary valve leaflets.* Both occur infrequently, since the overwhelming majority of pulmonary stenoses arise from commissural fusion, not cusp lesion.
- *Doming* of the pulmonary valve. When doming occurs, the valve cusps protrude into the lumen and can be delineated from the arterial wall during maximum opening.

Nonspecific features and possible hemodynamic effects of pulmonary stenosis:

Two-dimensional echocardiography:
- *Poststenotic dilatation of pulmonary trunk,*
- *Right ventricular hypertrophy.*

M-mode echocardiography:

- *"A" wave > 6 mm* [14] with presystolic opening of the valve due to increased right ventricular end-diastolic pressure. An analogous "dip" in the A wave can be seen in normals during deep inspiration as well as in patients with bradycardia and large stroke volumes.

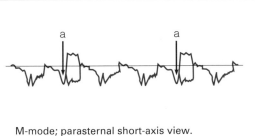

M-mode; parasternal short-axis view.

- *Increased right ventricular ejection time [9];*
- *Right ventricular hypertrophy (RVAW-EDD > 5 mm; IVS-EDD > 11 mm).*

Conventional Doppler Echocardiography

Pulsed-wave Doppler (PW Doppler):

- *Detection and measurement of velocity of stenotic flow jet at pulmonary valve level.*

Continuous-wave Doppler (CW Doppler):

- *Detection and measurement of velocity of stenotic flow jet at pulmonary valve level.*

Pulmonary stenosis can usually be detected in continuous or pulsed-wave Doppler recordings obtained from parasternal or subcostal scans of the short axis (short-axis view through the root of the aorta or long-axis view through the right ventricle).

Doppler Color Flow Imaging (2-D and M-mode)

- *Provides graphic display of turbulent transpulmonary stenotic flow jet.*

Contrast Color Doppler Flow Imaging (2-D and M-mode)

- *Enhancement of color-encoded display of turbulent transpulmonary stenotic flow jets by using echocontrastography agents.*

Transesophageal Echocardiography (Single and Multiplane)

Usually only the posterior cusp can be visualized from a transthoracic approach, but it is sometimes possible to visualize the anterior cusp as well. Anteflected, deep transgastric scans in the short-axis plane, and transesophageal scans of the right ventricular long-axis plane are the standard views for imaging the pulmonary valve. These views are superior all

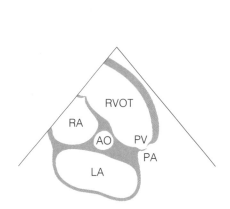

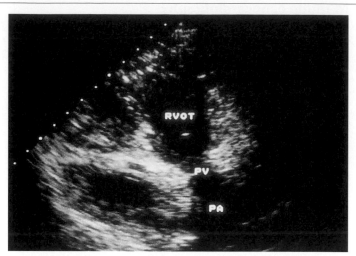

Severe pulmonary stenosis. Right ventricular hypertrophy. Dilatation of both the right ventricular outflow tract and the pulmonary trunk. Normal pulmonary valve morphology.

Parasternal cross-sectional view of aortic valve plane (long-axis view through RV).

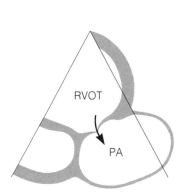

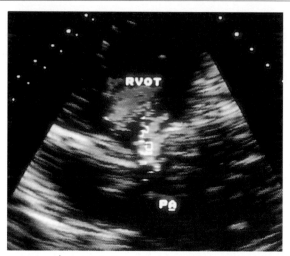

Same patient. Severe pulmonary stenosis. Systolic echocardiogram. Turbulent transvalvular flow.

Parasternal cross-sectional view of aortic valve plane (long-axis view through RV); color flow mapping.

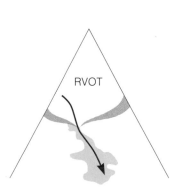

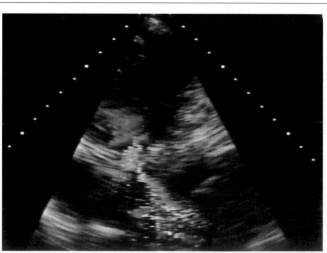

Same patient with severe pulmonary stenosis. Mid-systolic echocardiogram. Narrowing of transvalvular flow. Aliasing.

Parasternal cross-sectional view of aortic valve plane (long-axis view through RV); color flow mapping.

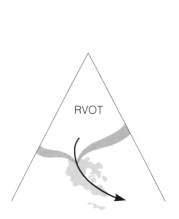

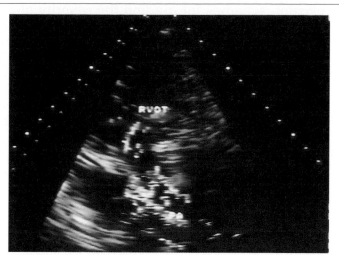

Same patient. Severe pulmonary stenosis. Highly turbulent, poststenotic flow in end-systole.

Parasternal cross-sectional view of aortic valve plane (long-axis view through RV); color flow mapping.

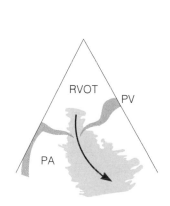

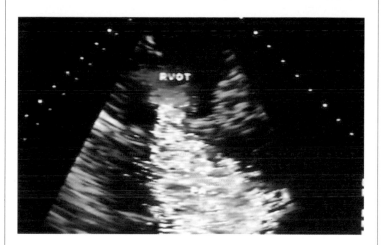

Same patient. Severe pulmonary stenosis. There is a massive stenotic flow jet in dilated pulmonary trunk in poststenotic region in end-systole.

Contrast-enhanced (D-galactose) color flow map of parasternal cross-section view of aortic valve plane (long-axis view through RV).

The pressure gradient between the right ventricle and the pulmonary trunk is considered normal as long as it does not exceed 5 to 10 mmHg [7], which frequently occurs in patients with increased pulmonary flow [5]. A pressure gradient > 15 mmHg and right ventricular systolic pressure > 30 mmHg [2] are diagnostic of pulmonary stenosis.

The existing schemes for grading the severity of pulmonary stenosis vary greatly, as can be seen below.

Pulmonary stenosis. Grading Scheme

Severity	Pressure gradient (mmHg)	Valve orifice area (cm^2)	**Valve orifice area index (cm^2/m^2)**
Mild		>2.0	**>1.2**
Moderate		2.0-1.5	**1.2-0.9**
Mod. severe		1.5-1.0	**0.9-0.6**
Severe		<1.0	**<0.6**

Grading scheme recommended by [8]

Severity	Pressure gradient (mmHg)	Valve orifice area (cm^2)	**Valve orifice area index (cm^2/m^2)**
Trivial	<25		**2.0-1.0**
Mild	25-50		**1.0-0.5**
Moderate	50-80		**0.5-0.25**
Severe	>80		**<0.25**

Grading scheme recommended by [8]

Severity	$RV_{systolic}$ (mmHg)	Valve orifice area (cm^2)	**Valve orifice area index (cm^2/m^2)**
Mild	<50		
Moderate	50-100	0,5-1,0	
Severe	>100	<0,5	

10.2.2 Pulmonary Stenosis
10.2.2.2 Sources of Error

Error in the detection and quantification of pulmonary stenosis may arise due to the difficulty in imaging the pulmonary valve itself and due to the frequent overlap of subvalvular and supravalvular pulmonary stenoses in transthoracic sections. The main sources of error are as follows:

First, anatomic changes in the pulmonary valve cusps are much more infrequent than commissural fusion. Second, echos from the posterior and anterior pulmonary valve cusps obtained via parasternal and subcostal 2-D echocardiography usually merge with arterial wall echos in systole. Third, all M-mode images are obtained with the transducer at an undefined angle with respect to the pulmonary valve. The result is that the echomorphology of the pulmonary valve can seldom be properly assessed. Finally, almost all diagnostic criteria for pulmonary stenosis are nonspecific.

Another source of error is the fact that the stenotic flow jet is often only vaguely identifiable in color Doppler images. A possible solution to this problem is the use of echocontrastography agents to enhance the vividness of color encoding.

10.2.2	**Pulmonary Stenosis**
10.2.2.3	**Special Measurement Program and**
	Quick Reference

Morphometry and ventricular function

RVAW-EDD	_____	mm
RVEDD	_____	mm
RVEDV	_____	ml
RVESV	_____	ml
RVOT-EDD	_____	mm
PVA-ESD	_____	mm
TPEDD	_____	mm
RPAESD	_____	mm

RVEF   _____

Valve morphology and dynamics

▸ Thickening and/or calcification of pulmonary valve cusps?
▸ Doming of pulmonary valve cusps?

Ventricular function and pressure-flow relationships (Doppler echocardiography)

▸ Velocity measurements (m/s)
  - maximum instantaneous velocity;
  - mean transmitral velocity
▸ Pressure gradients (mmHg)
  - maximum instantaneous pressure;
  - mean transmitral pressure gradient
▸ Pulmonary valve area (cm^2), pulmonary valve area index (cm^2/m^2)
▸ Regurgitant jet
  - qualitative visual assessment
▸ Intracardiac pressure (mmHg)
  - $PA_{systolic}$
  - $PA_{diastolic}$ with concomitant pulmonary insufficiency

---

Transesophageal echocardiography

▸ Valve morphology and dynamics

SYMPTOMATOLOGY / AUSCULTATION

ECHOCARDIOGRAPHY

Conventional echocardiography:

Morphometry
(RVAW-EDD, RVEDD, RVEDV, RVESV, RVOT-EDD, PVA-ESD, TPEDD, RPA-ESD)
Ventricular function (RVFS)
Visualization of anatomic causes and hemodynamic effects

Doppler and transesophageal echocardiography:

Pulmonary valve area (PVA), valve area index (PVA-I)

Transesophageal echocardiography:

Visualization of underlying anatomic causes and hemodynamic effects

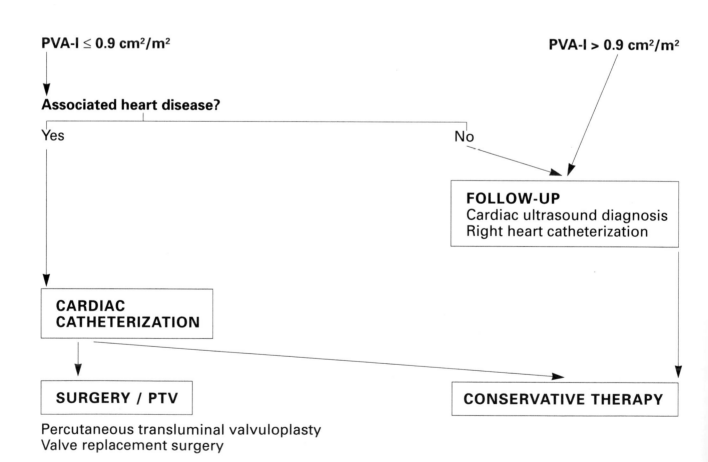

PVA-I $\leq$ 0.9 cm^2/m^2

PVA-I > 0.9 cm^2/m^2

Associated heart disease?

Yes

No

FOLLOW-UP
Cardiac ultrasound diagnosis
Right heart catheterization

**CARDIAC
CATHETERIZATION**

SURGERY / PTV

CONSERVATIVE THERAPY

Percutaneous transluminal valvuloplasty
Valve replacement surgery

1. Akamatsu S, Kagawa K, Terazawa E, Takeda T, Arakawa M, Dohi S. Physiological tricuspidal regurgitation: A study with transesophageal Doppler echocardiography. Circulation 1990: 82 (suppl III): 0178.
2. Deshmukh M, Guvenc S, Bentivoglio L et al. Idiopathic dilatation of the pulmonary artery. Circulation 1960; 21: 710.
3. Espino Vela J, Contreros R, Rustrian Sosa F. Rheumatic pulmonary valve disease. Am J Cardiol 1969; 23: 12.
4. Holmes JC, Fowler NO, Kaplan S. Pulmonary valvular insufficiency. Am J Med 1968; 44: 851-862.
5. Kjellberg SR, Mannheimer E, Rudhe U et al. Diagnosis of congenital heart disease. Chicago: Year Book Medical Publishers, 1955.
6. Ludwig J. Cardiac vein involvement in carcinoid syndrome. Possible evidence of retrograde blood flow in cardiac veins in tricuspid insufficiency. Am J Clin Path 1971; 55: 617-623.
7. Marshall RJ, Shepherd JT. Cardiac function in health and disease. Philadelphia: WB Saunders, 1968.
8. Miller G. Invasive investigation of the heart. Oxford: Blackwell Scietific Publications, 1989.
9. Nanda NC, Lombardi A, Gramiak R. Assessment of severity of pulmonary valve stenosis by echocardiography. Clin Res 1976; 24: A232.
10. Nugent EW, Freedom RM, Nora JJ, Ellison RC, Rowe RD, Nadas AS. Clinical course in pulmonary stenosis. In: Nadas AS, ed. Pulmonary stenosis, aortic stenosis, ventricular septal defect: Clinical course and indirect assessment. Report from the joint study on the natural history of congenital heart defects. Circulation 1977; 55 (suppl I):I 138-147.
11. O'Toole JD, Wurtzbacher JJ, Wearner NE, Jain AC. Pulmonary-valve injury and insufficiency during pulmonary-artery catheterization. N Engl J Med 1979; 301: 1167-1168.
12. Roberts WC, Buchbinder NA. Right-sided valvular infective endocarditis. A clinicopathologic study of twelve necropsy patients. Am J Med 1972; 53: 7 19.
13. Roberts WC, Dangel JC, Bulkley BH. Nonrheumatic valvular cardiac disease. In: Likow W, ed. Cardiovascular clinics, Vol. 5, No. 2, Valvular heart disease. Philadelphia: FA Davis, 1973, 334.
14. Weyman AE, Dillon JC, Feigenbaum H, Chang S. Echocardiographic patterns of pulmonic valve motion with pulmonary hypertension. Circulation 1974; 50: 905-910.

10.3	**Mitral Valve Disease**
10.3.1	**Mitral Insufficiency**
	(Kurt J.G. Schmailzl)

In the Western world the two most common pathogenetic types of mitral insufficiency are mitral insufficiency secondary to mitral valve prolapse syndrome and ischemic mitral insufficiency [59].

Echocardiography is sometimes in parts helpful in visualizing some of the anatomic abnormalities that cause mitral insufficiency.

Underlying Anatomic Causes of Mitral Insufficiency

▶ Incomplete or abnormal development of the mitral valve, loss or reduced integrity of valve tissue, connective tissue disorders;
▶ Calcification, destruction or dilation of the mitral annulus;
▶ Thickening, elongation, rupture or malposition of chordae tendineae;
▶ Defective development, displacement, dysfunction or rupture of papillary muscles;
▶ Akinesia or dyskinesia of left ventricular wall sections at the base of the papillary muscles.

Cardiac Ultrasound Diagnosis

The preferred scan planes for all echocardiographic techniques are the left parasternal long and short-axis views, apical two and four-chamber views, and the subcostal four-chamber view. Supplementary transesophageal imaging must be performed in some cases.

Conventional Echocardiography

Visualization of anatomic causes:

2-D and M-mode echocardiography:

- *Calcification, destruction or dilation of the mitral annulus;*
- *Thickening, elongation, rupture or malposition of chordae tendineae;*
- *Dysfunction or rupture of papillary muscles;*
- *Akinesia or dyskinesia of left ventricular wall sections at the base of the papillary muscles.*

Nonspecific features and possible hemodynamic effects of mitral insufficiency:

2-D and M-mode echocardiography:

- *Regurgitant orifice identifiable in systole* (left parasternal short-axis 2-D echocardiograms).
- *Separation of leaflets during systole,* particularly when turbulent systolic flow is found in color flow imaging (M-mode, left parasternal long-axis view).
- *Dilation of left atrium and/or left ventricle.*
- *High motion amplitude of interventricular septum,* which is suggestive of left ventricular volume overload.
- *Systolic outward movement of posterior left atrial wall.*
- *Premature, gradual closing motion of aortic valve during systole.*

M-mode echocardiography:

- *High D-E amplitude* with large transmitral stroke volume;
- *Steep EF slope;*
- *Diminished rapid filling phase.*

Conventional Doppler Echocardiography

Pulsed-wave Doppler (PW Doppler):

- *Detection, velocity measurement, and mapping of systolic regurgitant jets in the left atrium.*

Continuous-wave Doppler (CW Doppler):

- *Detection and velocity measurement of systolic regurgitant jets at mitral valve level.*

Mitral regurgitation can be usually visualized in continuous or pulsed-wave Doppler recordings obtained from the apical transducer position. The CW Doppler beam is focused in the left ventricle at the base of transmitral forward flow, whereas the PW Doppler sample volume is positioned in the left atrium proximal to the mitral orifice or at the forward edge of the regurgitant jet. It is sometimes necessary to slightly rotate the transducer in the direction of the axilla or the sternum to visualize regurgitations located further septal or lateral and/or anterior or posterior; a poor 2-D image quality must be accepted [32]. As compared with auscultation by an experienced examiner, Doppler appears to provide no advantages with regard to detection and quantitation of mitral insufficiency. The auscultatory diagnosis, is not affected by the size, configuration or direction of the regurgitant jet [31].

Doppler Color Flow Imaging (2-D and M-Mode)

- *Provides graphic representation of turbulent transmitral regurgitant jets.*
- *Transpulmonary echocontrastography agents can enhance color-encoded images [5].*

Transesophageal Echocardiography (Single and Multiplane)

A detailed analysis of mitral valve morphology is needed to understand the mechanism of leakage and to determine which patients are suitable candidates for reconstructive valve surgery. However, the nonplanar geometry of the mitral annulus and the nonlinear course of the mitral commissures make it more difficult to achieve such an analysis. A comparison of postmortem findings and epicardial and biplane transesophageal echocardiograms of the mitral valve revealed the following limitations and potentials of transesophageal echocardiography [25]: Transverse scans are able to bring the anterolateral mitral commissure and adjacent leaflet areas into view, but fail to demonstrate the posteromedial commissure. In patients with a prolapsed anterior mitral leaflet, transverse scans proximal to the posteromedial commissure frequently result in error. Longitudinal scans are ideal for studying the posteromedial commissure and the middle third of the mitral leaflet, but they poorly visualize the lateral third of the leaflet. Biplane techniques can be helpful in these cases [101].

| 10.3.1 | Mitral Insufficiency |
| 10.3.1.1 | Acute Mitral Insufficiency |

The most common causes of acute mitral insufficiency are ruptures of the chordae tendineae or papillary muscles secondary to mitral valve prolapse, acute ischemia or necrosis in the supply region of the mitral valve apparatus and its left ventricular insertions, and leaflet perforation arising from infective endocarditis. The most important echocardiographic features to be considered in the diagnosis of acute mitral insufficiency are listed below.

Nonspecific features suggestive of acute mitral insufficiency:

2-D and M-mode echocardiography:

- *Abnormal echos at mitral valve level* reflecting fluttering in the mitral valve apparatus.
- *Redundant systolic echos near the mitral valve.*
- *Detection of systolic echos from the mitral valve or mitral valve apparatus in left atrial cavity.*
- *Wall motion anomalies at the insertions of both papillary muscles,* particularly in inferior, lateral and/or posterior myocardial infarction.
- *Vegetations* on the mitral valve.

10.3.1.1   **Acute Mitral Insufficiency**
10.3.1.1.1 **Chordal Rupture and Papillary Muscle Rupture**

The sensitivity and specificity of transesophageal echocardiography (100% and 87%, resp.) for detection of chordal rupture (and papillary muscle rupture) is higher than that of transthoracic echocardiography (20% and 100%, resp.) [16, 33]. Transesophageal echocardiography makes use of the same diagnostic indicators as transthoracic color flow imaging: eccentric, peripheral, arch-shaped regurgitant jets frequently found near one of the atrial walls (anterior mitral leaflet involved = posterolateral atrial wall; posterior mitral leaflet involved = posterior aortic wall and anterior atrial wall) [66]. TEE, too, has difficulties in identifying chordae of commissures *(strut chordae)*, which are of strategic importance in surgical planning [16].

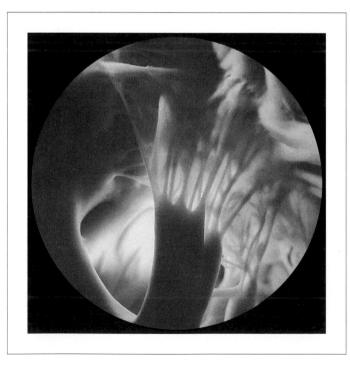

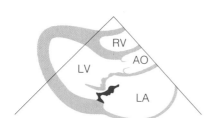

Moderately severe mitral insufficiency in chordal rupture involving the posterior leaflet; parts of the leaflet are visible in the left atrium in systole.

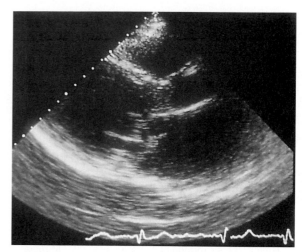

2-D left parasternal long-axis view at mitral valve level.

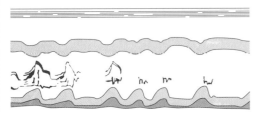

Mitral insufficiency due to chordal rupture involving posterior mitral leaflet. Discordant high-frequency oscillations.

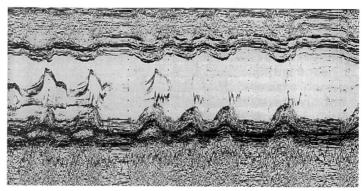

M-mode recording; left parasternal long-axis view; level of left ventricle and mitral valve apparatus.

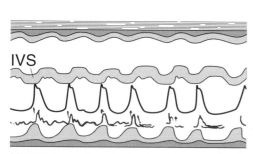

Mitral regurgitation due to chordal rupture involving the posterior mitral leaflet; flail sections can be seen between leaflet and posterior left ventricular wall.

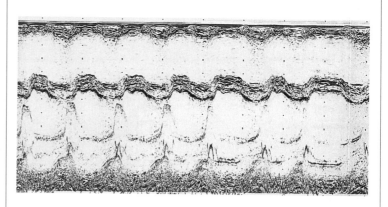

M-mode; left parasternal long-axis view; level of mitral valve apparatus.

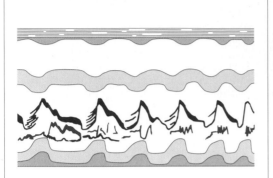

Mitral regurgitation due to chordal rupture in posterior leaflet. Chaotic motion of posterior leaflet causes chaotic echoes.

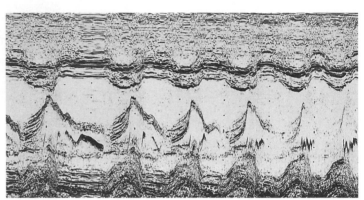

M-mode; left parasternal long-axis view; level of mitral valve apparatus and mitral valve.

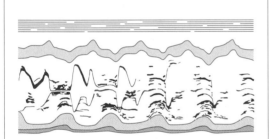

Mitral regurgitation due to chordal rupture in posterior leaflet. Multiple echos make it difficult to distinguish between anterior and posterior mitral leaflet echoes.

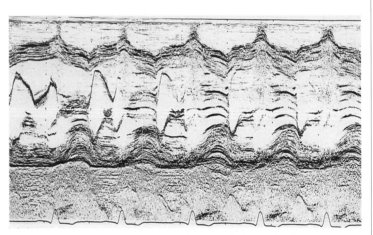

M-mode; left parasternal long-axis view; level of mitral valve apparatus and mitral valve.

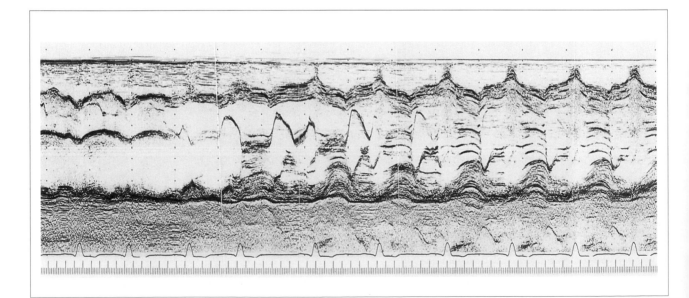

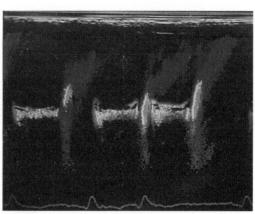

M-mode; left parasternal long-axis view; color flow imaging. Systolic image. Mild mitral insufficiency in patient with only a few ruptured chordae in the posterior mitral leaflet. Small yellow, turquoise and (aliasing) red mosaic area, flow directed away from the C and D line.

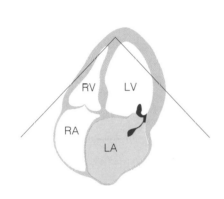

Moderately severe mitral insufficiency. Chaotic diastolic motion of posterior mitral leaflet due to considerable chordal rupture. Systolic leaflet echos detected in the left ventricle and left atrium.

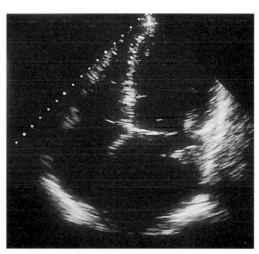

Apical four-chamber 2-D echocardiogram; systole.

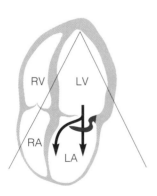

Same patient. Regurgitation due to maladaptation of tips of leaflet (initially small regurgitant orifice). Turbulent acceleration flow and aliasing.

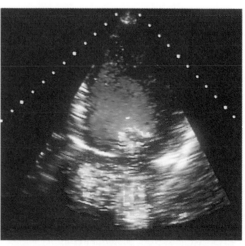

Color flow map of apical four-chamber 2-D echocardiogram; systole.

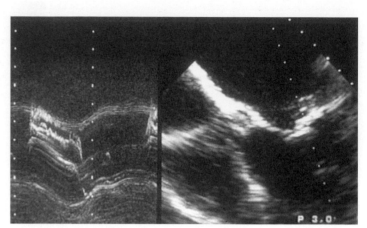

Mitral insufficiency due to chordal rupture in posterior leaflet. High-frequency oscillations from flail leaflet segments that flutter in the blood stream.

Transesophageal 2-D and M-mode echocardiograms; short-axis view at mitral valve level. Systole.

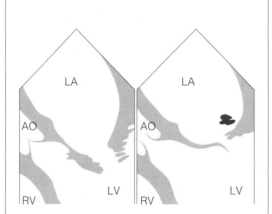

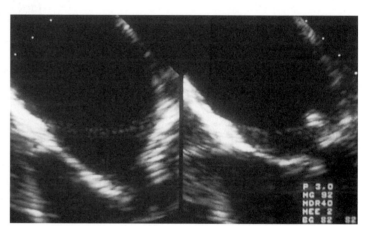

Same patient. Echos from posterior mitral segment in left atrium during systole. Chordal rupture in posterior mitral leaflet.

Transesophageal short-axis 2-D echocardiograms: Diastole and systole.

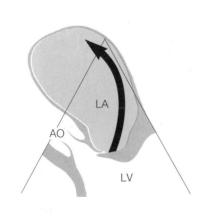

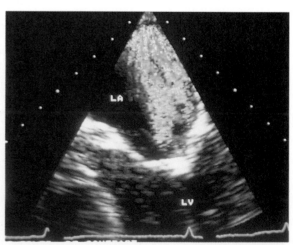

Moderately severe mitral insufficiency. Systolic reflux in left atrium extends from posterior mitral leaflet.

Color flow map of transesophageal short-axis view at mitral valve level. Systole.

The hemodynamics of perforated mitral leaflets is similar to that observed in chordal and papillary muscle ruptures. Thus, gross systolic fluttering of the flail leaflet frequently is also observed in patients with perforated mitral leaflets [40]. The direction in which the tip or the margins of the leaflet are pointing has been proposed as an index for distinguishing between these conditions and mitral valve prolapse syndrome. The tip of the leaflet points to the left atrium in perforated mitral leaflets, whereas the margin points to the left ventricle in mitral valve prolapse syndrome [65]. Furthermore, since leaflet perforation normally occurs only in conjunction with infective endocarditis, additional findings such as vegetations can be expected in that case.

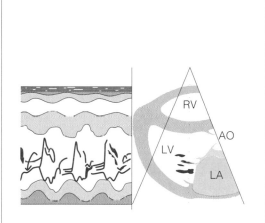

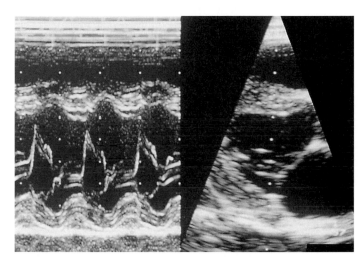

Mild mitral insufficiency in infective endocarditis and AIDS. Perforation of the anterior mitral leaflet. Note systolic fluttering of flail leaflet.

M-mode and 2-D; left parasternal long-axis view. Systole.

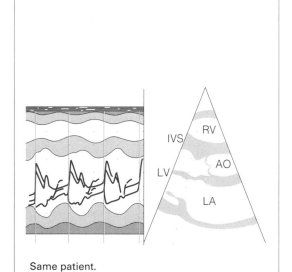

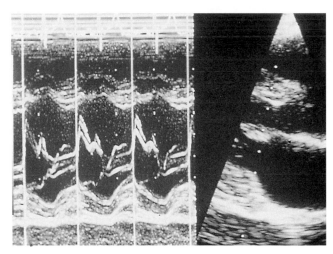

Same patient.

M-mode and 2-D; left parasternal long-axis view. ECG triggering. Diastole (2-D image).

Etiology of chronic mitral insufficiency

▸ Congenital
(atrioventricular defects, corrected transposition of great arteries with insufficiency of left-sided morphological tricuspid valve)
▸ Mitral valve prolapse syndrome
▸ Mitral annular calcification
▸ Rheumatic mitral insufficiency
▸ Ischemic mitral insufficiency
▸ "Functional" or dynamic mitral insufficiency
(regurgitation not primarily valve-related or exercise- induced)

10.3.1.2 Chronic Mitral Insufficiency
10.3.1.2.1 Mitral Valve Prolapse Syndrome

There are no standard criteria for diagnosis of mitral valve prolapse by cine-cardioangiography or echocardiography [21, 28, 67, 79, 86]. The following echocardiographic criteria for the diagnosis of mitral valve prolapse are used:

- *Systolic posterior motion of one or both mitral leaflets* below the C-D line (visualized in M-mode images from the left parasternal long axis view).
- *Systolic prolapse of one or both mitral leaflets* and/or their coaptation point toward the left atrial wall across the line drawn between their points of insertion (visualized in left parasternal long-axis 2-D echocardiograms).
- Similar *prolapse* seen from the apical four-chamber view.

Thus, different and nonuniform criteria are utilized. Furthermore, the nonplanar, saddle-shaped configuration of the mitral annulus can give rise to false-positive findings [30, 56]. Transesophageal biplane probes appears to be the most accurate method for diagnosis of mitral valve prolapse. If multiplane transesophageal echocardiography is not available, or if the use of semi-invasive techniques seems unjustified because the relation between the strain on the patient and the expected consequences of a positive result seems inadequate, at least the following recommendations should apply. Systolic prolapse must be visualized in at least *two* imaging planes. Detection in the apical four-chamber view is sensitive but relatively unspecific; it alone cannot be the sole basis for the diagnosis. *Two-dimensional imaging from the left parasternal long-axis view* is the most specific modality, but it is relatively insensitive. In equivocal cases, visualization of accelerated orthograde transmitral flow and a regurgitant jet that extends from the prolapsed leaflet and flows in the opposite direction within the left atrial cavity can support the diagnosis [102].

Echocardiographic detection of mitral valve prolapse does not mean that myxomatous degeneration of the mitral valve must exist. Mitral valve prolapse is also caused by an imbalance between left ventricular volume and the mitral annulus, as is seen in hypertrophic cardiomyopathy and atrial septal defect or in papillary muscle dysfunction attributable to ischemic and myocardial heart disease [12].

Considering all the effects of myxomatous degeneration, its association with mitral insufficiency, chordal rupture, infective endocarditis, and ischemic cerebral infarction has been shown to be more than coincidental. Isolated mitral valve disease with only mild to moderate regurgitation, however, seldom causes any symptoms other than iatrogenic anxiety syndrome [55].

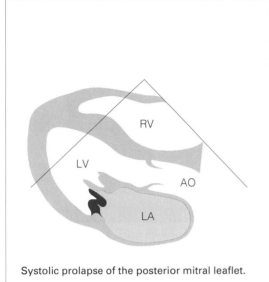

Systolic prolapse of the posterior mitral leaflet.

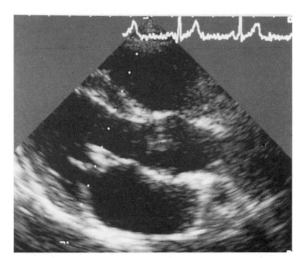

Left parasternal long-axis 2-D echocardiogram.

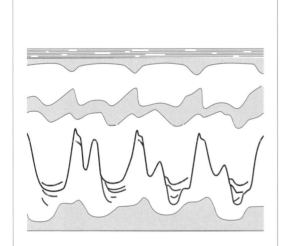

Holosystolic prolapse of posterior mitral leaflet.

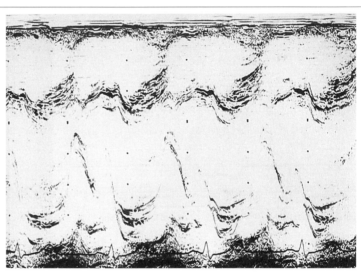

M-mode; left parasternal long-axis view at mitral valve level.

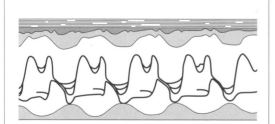

Telesystolic prolapse of posterior mitral leaflet in Marfan's syndrome.

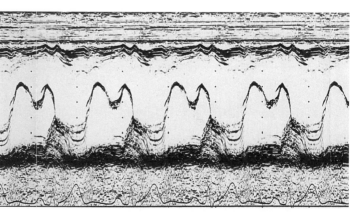

M-mode; left parasternal long-axis view at mitral valve level.

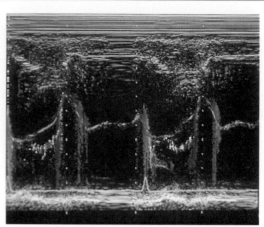

M-mode; left parasternal long-axis view at mitral valve level; color flow imaging. Systolic prolapse of posterior mitral leaflet. Turbulent yellow-encoded flow along the borders of the posteriorly displaced leaflet.

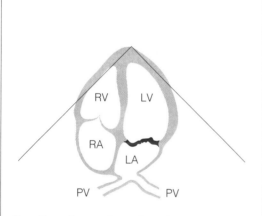

Systolic prolapse of anterior mitral leaflet with less prominent protrusion of posterior mitral leaflet.

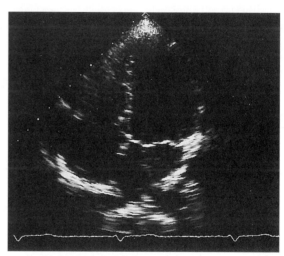

Apical four-chamber 2-D echocardiogram.

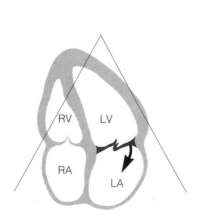

Mild mitral insufficiency with apicolateral to basoseptal direction of reflux in patient with systolic prolapse of posterior mitral leaflet.

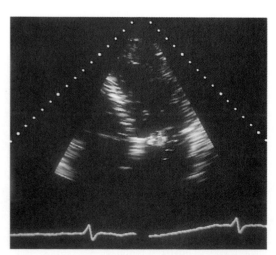

Color flow map of apical four-chamber 2-D echocardiogram.

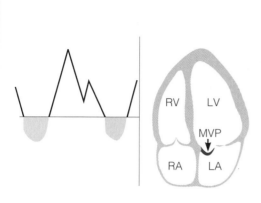

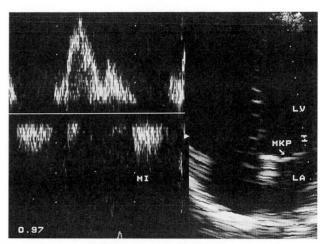

Mild mitral insufficiency in patient with systolic prolapse of anterior mitral leaflet. Poor spectral image without precise envelope curve. Image of dubious value.

PW Doppler recording and apical four-chamber 2-D echocardiogram.

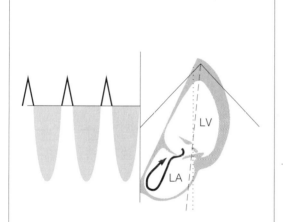

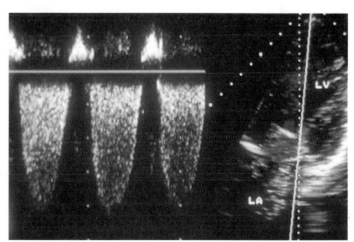

Chordal rupture in posterior leaflet in patient with mitral valve prolapse syndrome.

Color-encoded CW Doppler and apical four-chamber 2-D recordings.

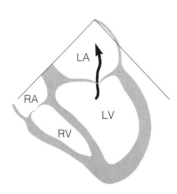

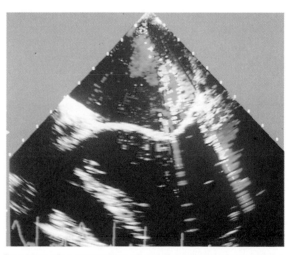

Mitral valve prolapse syndrome. ECG triggering; timed with R wave. Indistinct systolic prolapse of anterior mitral leaflet. Turbulent reflux in left atrium.

Color flow map of transesophageal short-axis 2-D echocardiogram.

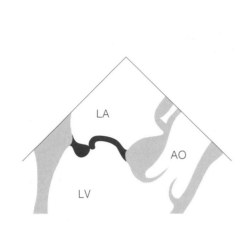

Same patient. ECG triggering 100 ms after R wave. Arch-shaped prolapse of anterior mitral leaflet into left atrial cavity.

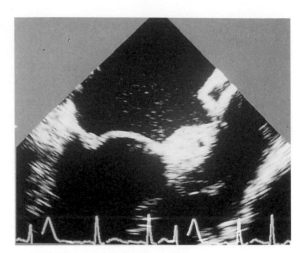

Transesophageal long-axis 2-D echocardiogram.

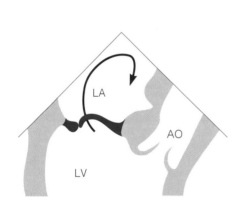

Same patient. ECG triggering 100 ms after R wave. Although systolic prolapse was demonstrated, the Doppler cursor is not properly parallel with the regurgitant jet is in the longitudinal scanning plane, as compared with transverse plane. The jet is therefore not visible.

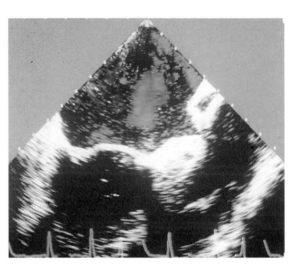

Color flow map of transesophageal long-axis 2-D scan.

10.3.1.2   Chronic Mitral Insufficiency
10.3.1.2.2   Mitral Annular Calcification

- *Highly echo reflective band* of annular calcification behind the posterior mitral leaflet, in some cases surrounding the entire base of the heart and extending into left atrium and to the mitral and aortic valves.
- *May be mistaken for mitral stenotic echoes.*

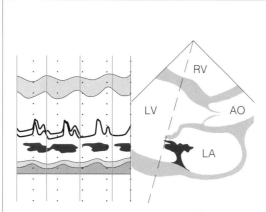

Mitral annular calcification. Highly echo reflective band behind posterior mitral leaflet is visualized in M-mode echocardiography. In 2-D echocardiograms, calcium echos are projected onto the posterior mitral leaflet. May be mistaken for mitral stenosis echoes.

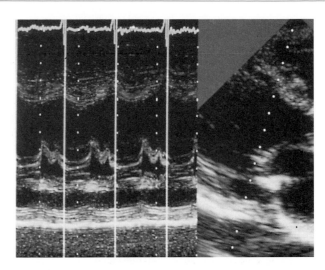

M-mode and 2-D; left parasternal long-axis view.

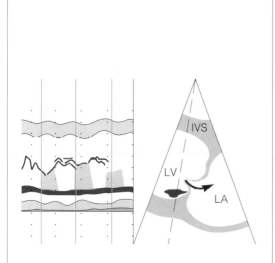

Mitral insufficiency in mitral annular calcification.

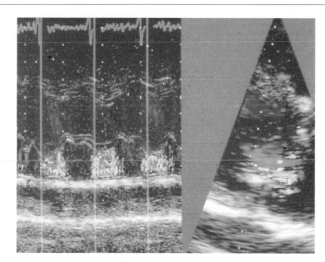

M-mode and 2-D; left parasternal long-axis view at mitral valve level; color flow imaging.

10.3.1.2   Chronic Mitral Insufficiency
10.3.1.2.3   Rheumatic Mitral Insufficiency

Rheumatic mitral valve disease with a predominant regurgitation component results from the highly inflammatory activity of recurring disease [62]. Anatomic abnormalities that cause rheumatic mitral insufficiency include:

- *Mitral valve prolapse with elongated chordae tendineae* and/or *dilated mitral annulus* in patients with pure mitral insufficiency.
- *Leaflet thickening and reduced closing velocity* [51] in late EF course expressing consecutive reparative processes which lead to hardening and scarred retraction.
- In some cases, *combined mitral lesions* with hemodynamically significant stenosis and/or multivalvular lesions.

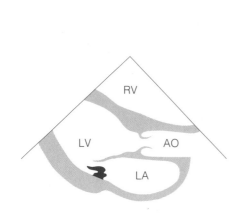

Combined mitral lesions, the predominant component being stenosis. Thickened anterior mitral leaflet. Early systole.

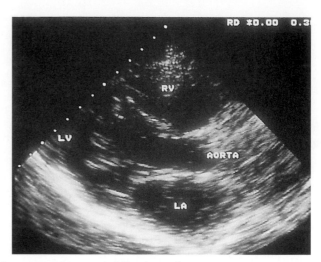

Left parasternal long-axis 2-D echocardiogram.

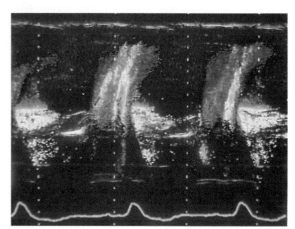

M-mode; left parasternal long-axis view at mitral valve level; color flow imaging. Combined mitral lesions with predominant regurgitation. Turbulent regurgitant flow detected during early systole.

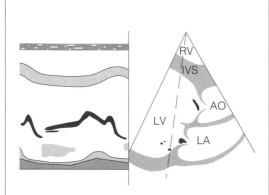

Moderate rheumatic mitral and aortic regurgitation. Latter seen especially well in color M-mode images. Aortic regurgitant jet located near septum.

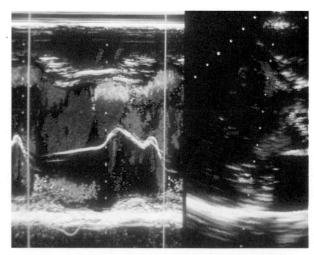

Color M-mode and 2-D images; left parasternal long-axis view.

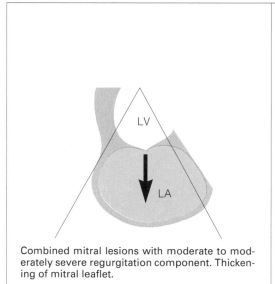

Combined mitral lesions with moderate to moderately severe regurgitation component. Thickening of mitral leaflet.

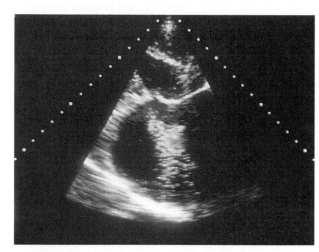

Apical four-chamber 2-D echocardiogram; color flow imaging.

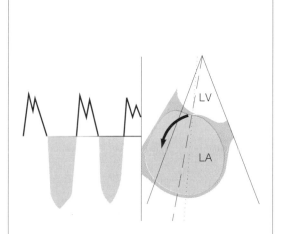

Same patient. Although there is highly turbulent orthograde flow attributable to increased stroke volume, stenotic component is not significant.

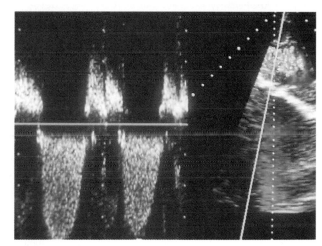

CW Doppler and color 2-D images; apical four-chamber view.

10.3.1.2 Chronic Mitral Insufficiency
10.3.1.2.4 Ischemic Mitral Insufficiency

Ischemic mitral insufficiency arises more frequently from inferior myocardial infarction than from anterior myocardial infarction [96]. In anterior myocardial infarction, a relative increase in the prevalence of mitral insufficiency is seen after two years, probably in response to dilation and remodelling of the left ventricle [4]. Some authors therefore postulate that global left ventricular function is a significant index for the development of incomplete mitral valve closure. This was supported by experiments in which individual variations in papillary muscle function and global ventricular function were studied [44]. The traditional concept of papillary muscle dysfunction is based on the hypothesis that regional disturbances in ventricular and papillary muscle function are responsible for ischemic mitral insufficiency [37]. This view is supported by textural analytical studies made after intracoronary administration of echo contrast medium [57] and after induction of ischemic mitral insufficiency via balloon inflation during percutaneous transluminal coronary angioplasty [22].

Both hypotheses assume that incomplete mitral valve closure is the final pathogenetic stage. However, controversy remains as to whether mitral insufficiency manifests in ischemia only in the presence of dilation of the left ventricular and reduction in its global function. Both hypotheses may describe acute [85] and chronic ischemia-induced mitral insufficiency, respectively, because total loss of papillary muscle function is followed by a change in left ventricular size and architecture and, thus, by a reduction in left ventricular function [26, 49].

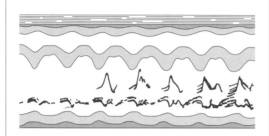

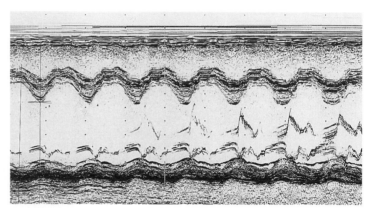

Severe mitral insufficiency in patient with chordal rupture in anterior leaflet five days after right coronary artery occlusion. Papillary muscle infarction. Pressure in left atrium = 40/30/90/5 mmHg, mean = 40 mmHg. Systolic separation of leaflets. High motion amplitude of interventricular septum as evidence of left ventricular volume overload.

M-mode; left parasternal long-axis view from level of mitral valve and mitral valve apparatus.

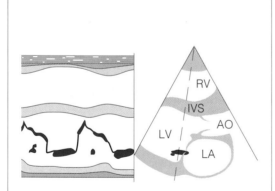

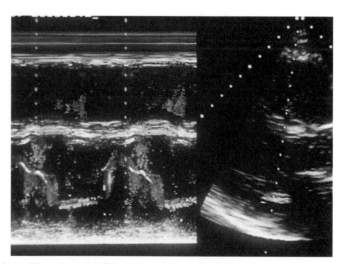

Mild ischemic mitral insufficiency without previous myocardial infarction. Reduced amplitude of contraction in interventricular septum and posterior wall.

Color M-mode and 2-D images; left parasternal long-axis view.

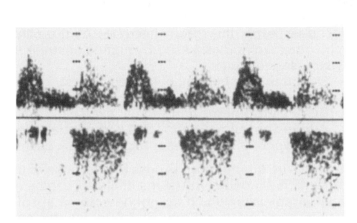

Same patient. CW Doppler frequency spectrum from apical position. Inhomogeneous signal intensity, unsatisfactory envelope curve. Angle between regurgitant jet and Doppler cursor is larger than 60°.

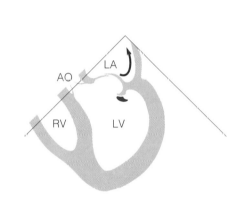

Same patient. Portions of the posterior mitral valve apparatus move towards anterior mitral leaflet during systole. Infarction of posterolateral papillary muscle (following posterior commissuroplasty).

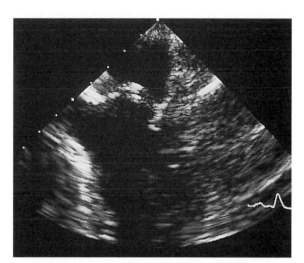

Transesophageal short-axis view at mitral valve level. Systole.

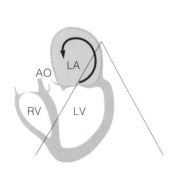

Same patient. Regurgitant flow due to maladaptation of both leaflet tips.

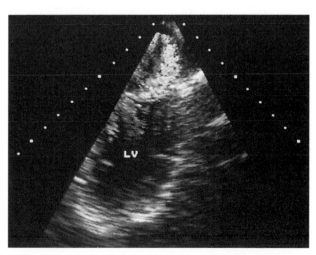

Color flow map of transesophageal short-axis echocardiogram.

Some ischemic mitral insufficiencies cause hemodynamically severe consequences even at rest, due to extensive anatomic abnormalities. However, many other types are characterized by recurrencies and transient periods of ischemia that more often arise from exercise-induced ischemia than from necrosis. As the name implies, exercise-induced regurgitation can be detected and assessed by means of stress echocardiography. The appropriate laboratory stressors include:

- Qualitative tests (*e.g.*, cold-pressor test, knee-bend exercise);
- Handgrip exercise
- Bicycle ergometry or treadmill exercise;
- Adenosine, angiotensin I and II, dipyridamole, dobutamine, dopamine, ergotamine; and
- Transvenous or transesophageal RV/LA pacing.

When no true quantitation is possible because of unfavorable scanning conditions, the severity of exercise-induced mitral insufficiency can be assessed on the basis of the initial hemodynamic parameters, which do not have to be absolute. Survival time decreases with increasing severity of exercise-induced mitral insufficiency. The five-year survival for risk patients (average age $\geq$ 65, coronary 3-vessel disease, Left ventricular ejection fraction $\leq$ 0.40) who received drug treatment was 49%, as compared with 77% in those who received coronary and mitral valve surgery [68]. In patients with and without revascularization, a trend was observed in favor of those operated on, whereas patients who undergo additional mitral valve surgery survive significantly longer. The prognosis of patients with mitral valve repair compared to those with a prosthetic mitral valve is even better [68].

When the echocardiographic examination is performed with the patient seated on an exercise bicycle, scans should be obtained using the subcostal two and four-chamber views. When the patient is lying down, scans should preferably be obtained from the parasternal short-axis view and apical two and four-chamber views immediately after the interruption of exercise. For off-line analysis we recommend the use of continuous video recordings that can be digitized for computer analysis. Most examiners recommend that continuous 12-lead ECG should be performed and standard reanimation equipment should be on hand any time when stress echocardiography is being performed.

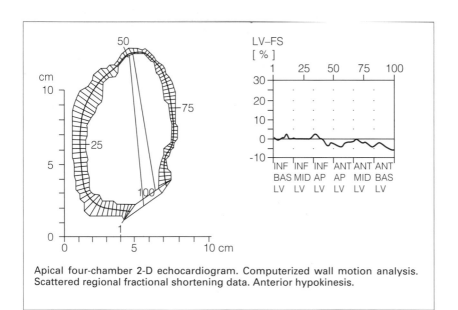

Apical four-chamber 2-D echocardiogram. Computerized wall motion analysis. Scattered regional fractional shortening data. Anterior hypokinesis.

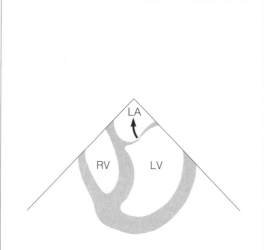

Mild turbulence near the margins of the posterior mitral leaflet. Minimal regurgitant flow at rest.

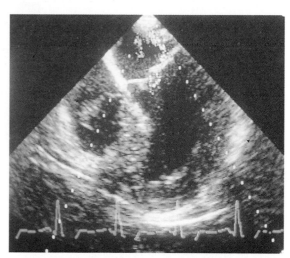

Color flow map of transesophageal short-axis 2-D scan. Baseline scan.

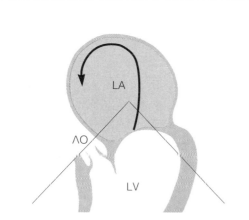

Same patient after stress is induced with a cumulative dose of 0.84 mg dipyridamole/kg. Broad-based highly turbulent regurgitant jet penetrating to the top of the atrium. Ischemic mitral insufficiency.

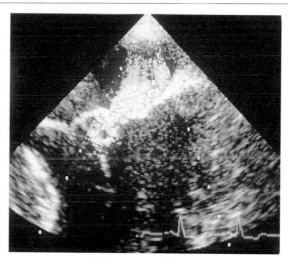

Color flow map of transesophageal short-axis 2-D echocardiogram (identical ECG triggering). Exercise frame.

10.3.1.2 Chronic Mitral Insufficiency
10.3.1.2.5 "Relative" and Dynamic Mitral Insufficiency

Remodelling of the left ventricle occurs in response to dilation [74]. In some cases, and the left ventricle becomes globular in shape [50]. Lateral displacement of papillary muscles and mitral annular dilation occur [48]. When these phenomena exceed a certain limit, "functional" mitral insufficiency, a condition in which the leaflets lose their ability to co-apt during systole, will occur. Mitral insufficiency is basically a function of the ruling load conditions. When mitral insufficiency is dynamic, its detection and severity can also be used as indices to guide follow-up and to assess the efficacy of therapy in patients with critical cardiac insufficiency [24, 45].

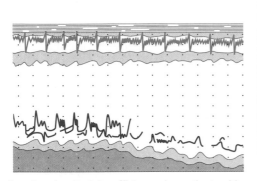

Functional mitral insufficiency in patient with dilated cardiomyopathy. Dilated left ventricle. Steep drop in EF slope. Decreased rapid filling phase.

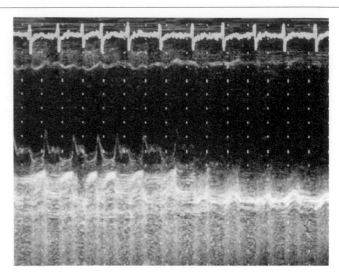

M-mode; left parasternal long-axis view.

Same patient (female). Here regurgitant flow is directed away from transducer and is therefore visualized well, even from the parasternal position.

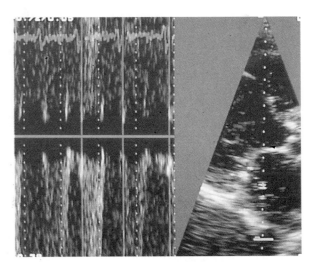

Color PW Doppler and left parasternal long-axis 2-D echocardiograms.

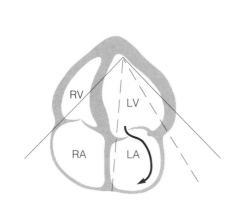

Regurgitant jet extending to free wall of left atrium. All four heart cavities are dilated.

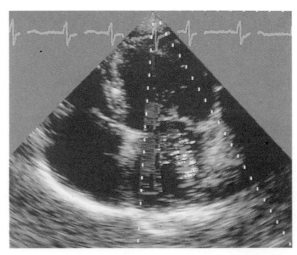

Apical four-chamber 2-D echocardiogram; color flow imaging.

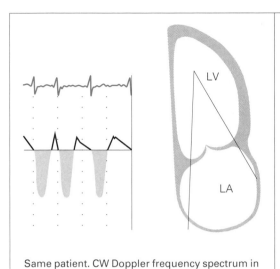

Same patient. CW Doppler frequency spectrum in patient with mild functional mitral insufficiency. Dilated cardiomyopathy.

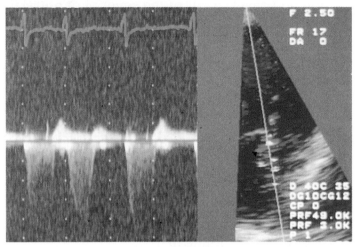

Color CW Doppler and apical four-chamber 2-D echocardiograms.

10.3.1   Mitral Insufficiency
10.3.1.3   Semiquantitation and Quantitation

In cardiac ultrasound diagnosis, the "royal path" to quantitation of the severity of mitral insufficiency is computation of the regurgitant fraction, obtained as a product of total and effective stroke volumes [38]. However, this method is complex and time-consuming. Calculations are based on the determined stroke volume and cross-sectional area of flow. If conditions for imaging are suboptimal and other problematic examination conditions exist, the quality of results will be diminished. In practice severity is often graded by qualitative visual assessment of the images and by comprehensive analysis of audio and spectral signals and/or color flow images in which the presence of regurgitation has been detected.

However, error will result when the amount of regurgitation is graded into more than two classes of severity (*e.g.* less severe - more severe). The classical hemodynamic grading scheme for mitral insufficiency divides regurgitations into four classes of severity according to regurgitant fraction range and a 1+ to 4+ cine-cardioangiographic contrast medium effect scale [29, 64].

Severity of Mitral Insufficiency. Grading Scheme

	Contrast medium effects	Regurgitant fraction
Mild	1+	$RF \leq 0.20$
Moderate	2+	$0.20 < RF \leq 0.40$
Moderately severe	3+	$0.40 < RF \leq 0.60$
Severe	4+	$0.60 < RF$

The following parameters have been proposed as Doppler echocardiographic indices for detection and assessment of the severity of mitral insufficiency:

Doppler echocardiographic indices for detection and assessment of mitral insufficiency
▸ Jet length and/or width (by conventional Doppler or PW-color Doppler) ▸ Regurgitant jet area (by color Doppler) ▸ Comparison of regurgitant jet slices from orthogonal planes ▸ Regurgitant jet length/width/area relative to left atrial length/width/area
▸ Maximum instantaneous diastolic flow velocity ▸ Regurgitant jet velocity at different sites ▸ Time-velocity integrals for flow across mitral valve or across mitral and aortic valves
▸ Doppler signal intensity (signal amplitude, audio signal, densitometry)
▸ Regurgitant fraction
▸ Special indices (*e.g.* reflux signal in right upper pulmonary vein)

The most common method of estimating the severity of mitral insufficiency is by relating severity to the visualized color jet length, width, and/or area. It remains unclear whether relating regurgitant jet length/width/area to left atrial length/width/area actually improves the validity of this technique.

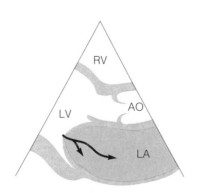

Divided regurgitant jet. Angle between jet sections and Doppler beam varies during systole. Planimetered regurgitant jet area = 686 mm², length = 192 mm. Semiquantitation results are dubious, because regurgitant flow geometry is unsuitable for assessment.

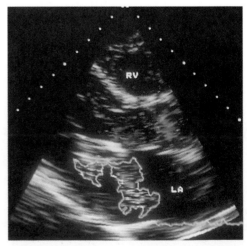

Color M-mode; left parasternal long-axis view at mitral valve level.

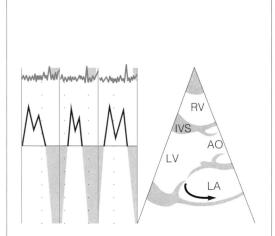

Here the Doppler cursor is satisfactorily parallel to the direction of regurgitant flow.

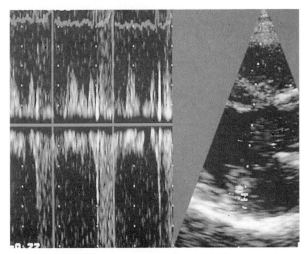

Color PW Doppler and left parasternal long-axis 2-D echocardiograms.

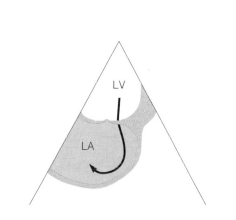

Planimetered regurgitant jet area and left ventricular area are 11.6 cm² and 30.9 cm², respectively. Regurgitant fraction = 0.38.

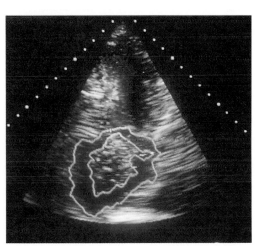

Apical four-chamber 2-D echocardiogram; color flow imaging.

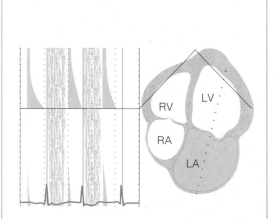

Sample volume immediately proximal to mitral valve. Strong reflux echo.

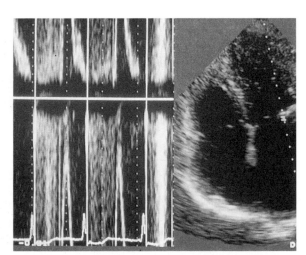

PW Doppler. Apical four-chamber view (mapping position 1).

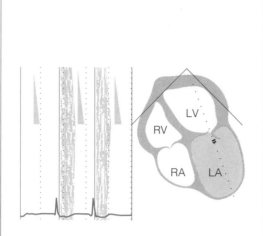

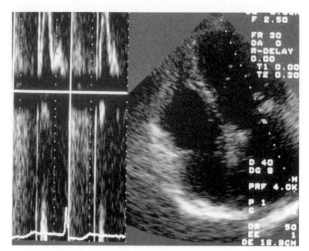

Sample volume 0.5 cm proximal to mitral valve. Low signal density.

PW Doppler. Apical four-chamber view (mapping position 2).

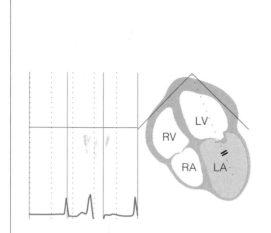

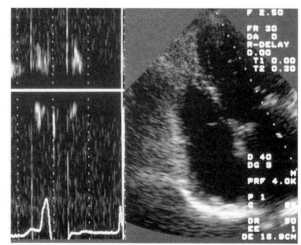

Sample volume 2 cm proximal to mitral valve. Poor reflux echoes.

PW Doppler. Apical four-chamber view (mapping position 3).

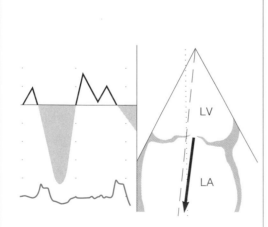

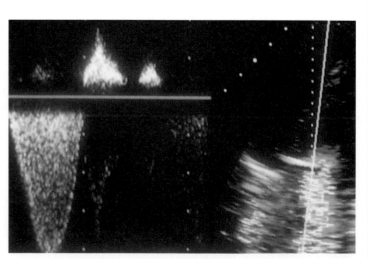

Parabolic Doppler frequency spectrum in patient with moderately severe mitral insufficiency.

Color CW Doppler and apical four-chamber 2-D echocardiograms.

In color flow images, the regurgitant jet is characterized by its turbulent core and laminar outer flow. Depending on whether the entire regurgitant jet or only its central area was planimetered, different correlations to the true regurgitant volume are obtained. The best results are obtained by planimetering the "total" flow in transthoracic scans and by planimetering only the central jet in transesophageal scans [10].

Regurgitation creates increased forward flow during mitral valve opening. In assessment of mitral insufficiency, the maximum instantaneous diastolic flow velocity is therefore utilized under the assumption that it is proportional with flow.

The smallest cross-sections of the central regurgitant jet as assessed in color flow imaging from the short axis view can be used to quantify mitral insufficiency [23], as is the regurgitant jet width in aortic regurgitation. This method provides helpful data for distinguishing between mild and severe lesions. Since very small flow volumes are involved, variations in the transducer angle can cause a large range of error. Thus, reproducibility is not always good.

Another interesting assessment technique is the *proximal isovelocity surface area* (PISA) method. Acceleration flow is visualized proximal to the regurgitant lesion using color flow mapping. Acceleration flow is identified as a homogeneous blue region of increasing brightness on the left ventricular side of the mitral valve; there is also a central mosaic area immediately proximal to the regurgitant orifice. Flow accelerates progressively as it converges toward the regurgitant orifice, at which point it reaches its maximum velocity. Various authors report that PISA is more specific than conventional assessments that relate jet area to left atrial size [2, 11, 69, 72, 94, 99, 100]. PISA functions on the assumption that ventricular flow in front of the regurgitant orifice corresponds with the atrial flow behind it. Errors due to small flow volumes and variations in the transducer angle are also encountered here.

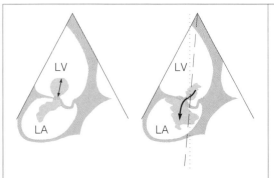

Homogeneous blue region of increasing brightness on the left ventricular side of the mitral valve and central red-yellow area proximal to the regurgitant orifice. Measured velocity reduced to 38 cm/s due to zero-baseline shift. Pulse repetition frequency = 25 kHz. Radius of proximal flow convergence = 18 mm. Peak instantaneous reversed flow velocity = 3.19 m/s; peak instantaneous reversed flow = 983 ml/s.

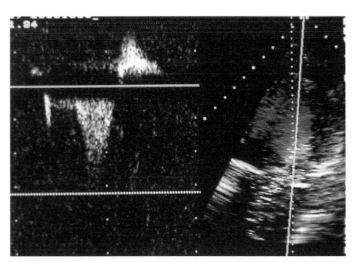

Color PW Doppler and apical four-chamber 2-D echocardiograms.

$Q_1 = 2\pi\, r^2\, V_r$ = Flow rate for any given isovelocity hemisphere

Q_1	Flow proximal to valve
$2\pi\, r^2$	Hemispheric surface area
v_r	Flow velocity at radiance distance r

A method for assessment of central regurgitant jets measures velocities proximal to the mitral orifice and velocities located more atrially, then determines the distance between the two sites [71]. A conversion equation is then used to transform the velocities into flow data. This method therefore provides a transition to quantitative measurement.

Since Doppler signal intensity increases as the number of echo-reflective, regurgitant corpuscular blood particles increases, the above statement also applies for assessment methods that make use of Doppler signal intensity, signal amplitude, audio reproduction, or densitometric techniques. The latter was demonstrated in a canine model comparing echo contrast medium densities in the left atrium and left ventricle [41]. Another study evaluated the relationship between systolic and diastolic Doppler signal amplitudes and length of time for outflow and inflow across the mitral valve [35].

Turbulence, an expression of flow variance, is assigned the color green in color flow imaging. Some investigators have attempted relate the severity of mitral insufficiency to the intensity of green pixels in the regurgitant jet or compared the pixel density of the outflow signal to that of the inflow signal using data obtained from digital images [61, 91].

In addition to these semiquantitative techniques, quantitative assessment of the severity of mitral insufficiency can be made using the total and effective stroke volumes. Methods which determine total and effective stroke volumes across the mitral and aortic valves (or pulmonary valve) correlate well with invasive measurements [104]. The effective stroke volume is derived as a product of cross-sectional area of the ascending aorta at the level of the aortic valve cusps (left parasternal long-axis 2-D echocardiograms), ejection time, and inflow velocity immediately proximal to the aortic valve (apical four-chamber view). The stroke volume can alternatively be measured using the cross-sectional area of the pulmonary trunk [73].

Effective Stroke Volume According to [73]

$$SV_{eff} = SV_{PA} = 0.5 \times A_{PA} \times V_{max,PA} \times ET$$

SV_{eff}	Effective stroke volume
SV_{PA}	Stroke volume across the pulmonary valve
A_{PA}	Systolic cross-sectional area of the pulmonary artery (between insertions of pulmonary valve cusps)
$V_{max,PA}$	Peak instantaneous flow velocity across the pulmonary valve
ET	Ejection time, measured outside the Doppler-spectrum (left parasternal short-axis view)

Total stroke volume through the mitral valve can be measured in 2-D, M-mode, and Doppler echocardiography as follows:

Total Stroke Volume According to [104]

$$SV_{total} = SV_M = TVI \times MVA_{corr}$$

$$MVA_{corr} = MVA_{max} \times \text{opening ratio}$$
$$\text{opening ratio} = \text{opening(mean)}/\text{opening(max)}$$
$$\text{opening(mean)} = \text{area(open)}/t_{D-C}$$
$$MVA_{corr} = MVA_{max} \times [\text{area(open)}/t_{D-C}]/\text{opening(max)}$$

SV_{total}	Total stroke volume
SV_M	Stroke volume through mitral valve
TVI	Time-velocity integral
MVA_{corr}	Corrected mitral valve area
MVA_{max}	Maximum corrected mitral valve area as measured from left parasternal short-axis view
area(open)	Area between mitral leaflets as measured in M-mode from left parasternal long-axis view
T_{D-C}	Time from mitral valve opening (D) to closing (C)
opening(max)	Maximum early diastolic mitral leaflet separation in left parasternal long-axis view (M-mode)

The regurgitant fraction can then be calculated out of effective and total stroke volumes. However, this method cannot be used when an additional stenotic component involving the mitral or aortic valve is present. Furthermore, reproducibility is somewhat limited by use of the imprecise parameter „area(open)".

An alternative method calculates the total stroke volume as a product of the diastolic mitral annular diameter measured in the apical four-chamber view, peak instantaneous velocity at the annular level, and filling time. In patients with sinus rhythm the peak instantaneous velocity and filling time for both parts of the Doppler spectrum, passive filling and atrial systole, are measured and added.

Total Stroke Volume According to [73]

$$SV_{total} = SV_M = 0.5 \times MVA \times v_{max, MV} \times FT$$

SV_{total}	Total stroke volume
SV_M	Stroke volume across mitral valve
MVA	Mitral valve area
$v_{max, MV}$	Peak instantaneous flow velocity at mitral annulus level
FT	Filling time

Similar techniques [92] utilize alternative calculations to obtain the mitral valve area. For example, the total stroke volume can be derived as the product of TVI of orthograde transmitral flow and MVA, as is shown in the following equation.

Total Stroke Volume According to [92]

$$SV_{total} = SV_M = TVI \times MVA$$

$$MVA = \pi/4 \times A \times B$$

SV_{total}	Total stroke volume
SV_M	Stroke volume across mitral valve
TVI	Time-velocity integral
MVA	Mitral valve area
A	Color jet width from apical two-chamber view
B	Color jet width from apical four-chamber view

The regurgitant fraction is derived as the quotient of the difference between total and effective stroke volume divided by total stroke volume. Methods for the assessment of severity using the continuity equation and pressure half-time in conjunction with cross-sectional area measurements still have to be developed.

In order to minimize error in cross-sectional area measurement, some authors propose quantification of mitral insufficiency using the TVI for mitral and aortic flow [58] or amplitude-weighted mean diastolic flow velocity [42]. The main theoretical limitations of the latter method are simultaneous constriction of the mitral and aortic valves leading to non-laminar flow, which can cause falsely high amplitudes across the stenotic valve. When the derived stroked volumes are not absolute but relative, it is not possible to quantitate the true stroke volume. Thus, concomitant aortic regurgitation will preclude reliable use of this method. On the other hand, it could still be used to quantitate isolated aortic regurgitation.

It is possible to differentiate between mild and hemodynamically significant mitral insufficiency using transesophageal Doppler echocardiography to detect turbulent reversed systolic flow in the upper pulmonary veins. When the regurgitant jet is eccentric, error may arise if only the left upper pulmonary vein is sampled [46].

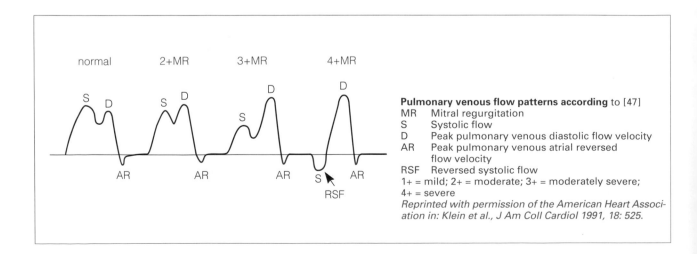

Pulmonary venous flow patterns according to [47]
MR   Mitral regurgitation
S   Systolic flow
D   Peak pulmonary venous diastolic flow velocity
AR   Peak pulmonary venous atrial reversed
      flow velocity
RSF   Reversed systolic flow
1+ = mild; 2+ = moderate; 3+ = moderately severe;
4+ = severe
Reprinted with permission of the American Heart Association in: Klein et al., J Am Coll Cardiol 1991, 18: 525.

Doppler echocardiography is a highly sensitive technique for detecting mitral regurgitation. Besides auscultation, the only comparable complementary techniques are invasive techniques using manometry and cine-cardangiography.

An unsolved dilemma with Doppler echocardiography, especially color flow mapping, is the visualization of mostly trivial regurgitation that does not correspond with auscultatory and angiographic findings. Relying heavily on the reliability of Doppler echocardiography, this could be interpreted as "physiologic" regurgitation [1]. On the other hand, one could also assume this reflects hemodynamically insignificant regurgitation due to yet unexplained standardization problems in color flow imaging. However, the accuracy of these assumptions remains unclear.

This becomes especially problematic in transesophageal echocardiography. In TEE visualization dilemmas such as regurgitant jets extending to the top of the atrium must be dealt with in addition to trivial regurgitations due, for example, to leaflet closure motion that leads to displacement and acceleration of blood immediately proximal to the tips of the leaflets.

The sheer number of proposed methods for assessing the severity of mitral insufficiency using cardiac ultrasound techniques makes it clear that this subject has come to an impasse.

The more commonly used formal methods - and also the most vehemently criticised - are those which attempt to relate the severity of mitral insufficiency to the regurgitant jet length, width, and/or area [9, 32]. Severity of regurgitation is thereby defined according to the how far the regurgitant jet extends towards the top of the atrium, which can be visualized in black-and-white PW Doppler or color Doppler "maps". The jet length at the origin of regurgitation or the regurgitant jet area can also be determined via color Doppler. These parameters can be set in relation to left atrial size to obtain a formal "regurgitant fraction", *i.e.*, the ratio between regurgitant flow and the regurgitant cavity.

These methods maintain that the severity of mitral insufficiency increases in proportion with the visualized maximal jet size. However, visualization of the jet is affected by acoustic impedance, topography, instrumentation factors, and the selected imaging position [84]. When Doppler monoplane techniques are used, only two-dimensional real-time images of regurgitation can be obtained, *i.e.*, there is a corresponding loss of the three-dimensionality. Regurgitant jets that flow at an excessive angle to the Doppler beam will therefore be underestimated or overlooked.

It follows that, when these Doppler techniques are used to assess the severity of mitral insufficiency, the most compromised results are obtained with nonuniform and divided regurgitant jets. These frequently occur in conjunction with mitral valve prolapse syndrome, flail leaflets due to lesions in the valve support apparatus, and with prosthetic valves. Attempts to circumvent these problems by using multiple orthogonal projections [32] usually fail, because no one has yet come up with an algorithm that can reasonably establish a relation between the various formal "regurgitant fractions" that are obtained from different transducer positions. Although it is imperative to sample the regurgitant jet from every possible imaging position, we still do not know whether the visualized maximal regurgitant jet length gives the best possible approximation of the regurgitant volume. When relating regurgitant jet area to atrial size, we also do not know whether this reflects the relationship between true regurgitant volume and true atrial volume.

The second significant error is associated with attempts to semiquantitate mitral insufficiency according the length of jet penetration into atrium. Jet penetration into the atrium is affected not so much by the *volume* of the jet as by its *velocity*. This, in turn, is influenced by the mitral valve regurgitation area and the compliance from the left ventricle and pulmonary venous bed.

When there is a great systolic pressure difference, small regurgitations form focused high-velocity jets. These can penetrate to the top of the atrium without necessarily having a large volume. Large regurgitations, on the other hand, form slower and more dispersed jets and display a truncated cone-shaped geometry when there is a low systolic pressure difference. They are shorter in length, although they have a large volume.

The third source of error is of great practical importance but is unfortunately difficult to quantify. This error arises when dynamic compliance from the left atrium and pulmonary venous bed are disregarded in computations [60].

A further problem associated with large atrial cavities and long regurgitant jets is the fact that Doppler signal intensity decreases as the distance from the transducer increases.

In view of these problems, it is easy to understand why some Doppler-derived estimations correlate well with the true regurgitation fraction while others do not.

All other methods either depend on excellent acoustic impedance since they are based on cross-sectional area calculation, or they have never become established despite their good correlation with invasive data.

A Canadian study [13] probably describes the quantitation dilemma best and the practical truth in most echocardiography laboratories most accurately. They found informal global visual assessment of the severity of mitral stenosis based on personal experience of the cardiologist to be superior to any individual formal method of jet measurement. The correlation between TEE and angiography was comparable to the correlation between two independent readings of angiography.

The most honest solution, then, is probably to use a restricted grading scale where lesions are graded only as "mild" or "severe". When further differentiation cannot be substantiated by the assessment method, the auscultatory findings and indication for surgery are only seemingly objectivized. The regurgitant volume itself cannot be measured, at least not accurately. Therefore, the severity of regurgitation can only be estimated [8].

In individual cases where the pathophysiology of regurgitation is known and imaging quality is good, an experienced echocardiographer can make good, valid grading assessments according to the four-grade Sellers grading system used in cine-cardangiography - that is, assuming that results of the different methods overlap. It is essential to interrogate from all possible scan planes, apply different methods of assessment, to critically evaluate the findings with the help of the auscultatory findings and the anatomic causes and hemodynamic effects detected by conventional echocardiography.

10.3.1   Mitral Insufficiency
10.3.1.5   Ventricular Function

Since the left ventricle functions as a double outlet chamber in mitral insufficiency, its afterload is therefore decreased. The use of afterload-dependent parameters of ventricular function will therefore result in overestimated values [43, 97, 98]. The end of the ejection phase, defined as minimal ventricular dimension or minimal ventricular volume, will then differ from end-systole.

This is because time until end-systole is reduced, whereas the time until end ejection remains the same due to reduced impedance. Pressure-volume relationships, calculated at the time of minimum dimension or volume, can therefore give rise to error in the assessment of ventricular performance [3, 6, 82].

The end-systolic pressure-volume relationship is based on the concept of time-dependent ventricular elastance and is relatively independent of ventricular load conditions [75, 76, 77]. Some authors have therefore suggested that this relationship or its stress-stain-transformation be used to differentiate between preserved and impaired ventricular function [14]. In addition to echocardiography-derived data, this method requires invasive ventricular pressure measurements and a pharmacologic variation in contractility. Controversy still exists as to whether it is necessary to standardize ventricular contractility in terms of size and mass [3, 34]. The current gold standard for experimental and clinical studies is probably determination of a standardized end-systolic pressure-volume relationship to describe ventricular function and to answer the question of whether contractile dysfunction produced by mitral regurgitation is reversible or not [36].

Various indices of ventricular function have been established by comparing pre- and post-operative ventricular function in patients undergoing mitral valve replacement [70, 105]. These indices can enable the clinician to predict favorable or unfavorable outcome, and are therefore useful at the time of surgery. The following indices were proposed.

Echocardiographic predictors of unfavorable postoperative functional performance after mitral valve replacement due to chronic mitral insufficiency, according to [70] and [105]
(1)   LVESD-I   > 26   mm/m^2 (2)   LVESWS-I   > 195   mmHg (3)   LVFS   < 0.31 Predictive: (1) with (3), (1) and (3) [(1) and (2)]
(1)   LVEST/LVESD   < 0.20 (2)   LA-I   > 70   mm Predictive: (1), (2)

LVESD-I   Left ventricular end-systolic dimension index
 	
LVESWS-I   Left ventricular end-systolic wall stress index
 	
               LVESWS-I = BP$_{RRsys}$ x (LVESR/LVEST)
 	
                     BP$_{RRsys}$ Systolic cuff pressure (Riva-Rocci)
                     LV-ESR   Left ventricular end-systolic radius
                     LV-EST   Left ventricular end-systolic wall thickness
 	
                     LVFS   Left ventricular fractional shortening

LVESD   Left ventricular end-systolic dimension
 	
LA-I   Left atrial index
 	
               LA-I = LADmax(transverse) x LADmax(longitudinal)
 	
                   LADmax(transverse)   maximal transverse left atrial dimension
 	
                   LADmax(longitudinal)   maximal longitudinal left atrial dimension
                                            (all measurements from apical four-chamber view)

The significance of left atrial size follows from the fact that, with the severity and duration, it reflects the "history" of the regurgitant lesion.

Invasively determined predictors of postoperative ventricular size and function, some of which can be obtained by echocardiographic techniques, include the ejection fraction, end-systolic volume index, and pulmonary artery pressure (including pulmonary arteriolar resistance).

Invasively determined predictors of unfavorable postoperative functional performance after mitral valve replacement due to chronic mitral insufficiency according to [17]

(1)	LVEF	< 0. 50 m
(2)	LVESV-I	> 50 ml/m^2
(3)	PAPmean	> 20 mmHg

LVEF	Left ventricular ejection fraction
LVESV-I	Left ventricular end-systolic volume index
PAPmean	Mean pulmonary artery pressure

One problem that remains in these attempts to define limit values is the effects of different mitral valve prostheses on outcome.

A significant factor in ventricular function is performance of the mitral subvalvular apparatus. Even when implanting a prosthetic valve, many surgeons now attempt to preserve portions of the posterior mitral leaflet and its supporting structures. The importance of this cannot be assessed in preoperative evaluations [7, 19, 27, 87, 103]. However, in postoperative follow-ups after conventional mitral valve replacement, fractional shortening of the left ventricle at the level of the subvalvular apparatus was reduced as compared with other sites [78].

Reduced left ventricular diastolic function is partially responsible for the clinical manifestation of cardiac insufficiency in patients with chronic mitral insufficiency and reduced systolic function [93]. Chronic adaptation to volume overload leads to reduced ventricular compliance or increased muscle stiffness. Reduced ventricular compliance occurs only when systolic function is preserved, and increased muscular stiffness occurs only when systolic function has already been compromised [15].

The decision to use either echocardiographic techniques or cardiac catheterization in following the patient and, when applicable, timing and planning surgical intervention depends on the following factors:

- Acuteness
- Etiology
- Severity
- Ventricular function
- Age of the patient

The decision is also centered around exclusion or proof of concomitant coronary heart disease.

- **Acuteness, etiology**
  The etiology of acute mitral insufficiency must be clarified beforehand [88]. In mitral insufficiency due to coronary artery disease, the need for revascularization must be assessed by means of coronary arteriography.
- **Severity of mitral insufficiency**
  If mitral insufficiency is more than moderate and if surgery is being considered, cardiac catheterization should be performed in patients in whom concomitant coronary artery disease has not been excluded or in whom the etiology of mitral insufficiency is still unknown.
- **Ventricular function**
  Reduced or borderline ventricular function requires further preoperative diagnostic testing (such as stress hemodynamics), because echocardiographic techniques frequently overestimate ventricular function in patients with mitral insufficiency.
- **Age of the patient**
  Coronary arteriography should be performed in patients in whom, due to their age, the possibility of clinically silent coronary artery disease exists.

When using ultrasound techniques to follow up patients with mitral insufficiency, the following rule applies: the larger the regurgitant fraction and the lower the left ventricular function, the shorter the interval between follow-up examinations. Patients with chronic mitral insufficiency secondary to mitral valve prolapse syndrome require serial long-term follow-ups [95].

In patients with paroxysmal or chronic atrial fibrillation, the atrial cavities must be interrogated for the presence of thrombi. The incidence of proximal pulmonary artery embolism in patients with hemodynamically significant mitral valve disease and pulmonary hypertension is 61% [83]. When potential thromboembolic foci are detected (preferably via TEE), anticoagulant therapy should be considered. If atrial thrombus has been diagnosed prior to surgery, the thrombus should be located and removed intraoperatively.

The timing of a surgical intervention should be planned with the help of exercise tests that include pressure-flow measurements (pulmonary artery and capillary pressure, cardiac index). These measurements should be compared with preoperative measurements from patients who required mitral valve replacement or reconstruction [52, 53]. Since the majority of patients retain pathologic stress hemodynamics after mitral valve replacement due to mitral insufficiency, the time of surgical intervention is, from a pathophysiologic point of view, predominantly too late.

When surgical intervention is indicated, mitral valve replacement or reconstruction are the two treatment options to be considered. Extensive destruction, stiffening or calcification of the mitral valve itself or ruptures in the commissural chordae or subvalvular apparatus of the anterior leaflet preclude the possibility of preserving the native valve. The location of these lesions is therefore an essential factor in the planning of surgery [80].

Intraoperative quality check of valve repair can be performed using either an epicardial [18, 90] or transesophageal approach [20, 54, 81], with or without the assistance of echo contrast medium. This is now state-of-the-art practice, even though the severity of residual regurgitation can be affected by temporary hemodynamic factors such as temporarily impaired ventricular function and reduced filling and by complications due to arrhythmias [63]. In addition to residual regurgitation, persistent leaflet fluttering and systolic anterior motion of the mitral valve with dynamic obstruction of the left ventricular outflow tract also require attention.

In the same vein, taking the patient off the heart-lung machine to evaluate the patency of the blood-filled, beating heart may also prove to be problematic. Before the valve becomes suitably competent, it may be necessary to go back on by-pass: Searching for a perfectly competent valve comes into conflict with the standards of modern myocardial protection.

10.3.1   Mitral Insufficiency
10.3.1.7   Sources of Error

Echocardiography detection of mitral insufficiency and assessment of its severity has inherent sources of error.

1. Regurgitant jets through the mitral valve are more frequently nonparallel to the transducer beam than in any other valves. The entire repertoire of technically possible transducer positions with or without semi-invasive access must therefore be used for proper assessment.
2. Grading of mitral insufficiency can be compromised by overestimation of hemodynamically insignificant regurgitations and underestimation of hemodynamically significant regurgitation. The theoretically correct methods of assessment are mostly very time-consuming and require good acoustic conditions. Thus, they have not found wide acceptance in clinical practice. The more practical methods, on the other hand, result in poorer or at least no better results that those of auscultation.

It is imperative that decisions concerning the timing and planning of surgery be based on classical findings such as left atrial size, left ventricular function, x-ray detection of pulmonary congestion, increased V wave in the PC or LA curve, and cine-cardangiographic classification data.

Morphometry and ventricular function

RVEDD   _____ mm
LADmax   _____ mm
LVEDD   _____ mm
LVESD   _____ mm

Ventricular function. Signs of concomitant ischemic heart disease?
Fractional shortening   _____
Wall motion analysis

Morphology and dynamics of tricuspid valve and its support apparatus

- ▸ Valvular tissue defects?
- ▸ Grade and extent of calcification of valve or subvalvular apparatus
- ▸ High DE amplitude, steep drop in EF slope, reduced rapid filling phase?
- ▸ Systolic separation of leaflets, possibly with color pattern indicative of turbulence between leaflets?
- ▸ Is a regurgitant orifice identifiable in systole?

Indirect indicators of abnormal hemodynamic situation

- ▸ Paradoxical motion of interventricular septum?
- ▸ Leftward protrusion of interatrial septum?

Ventricular function and pressure-flow relationships (Doppler echocardiography)

- ▸ Velocity measurements (m/s)
  - peak instantaneous velocity
  - mean transtricuspid velocity
- ▸ Regurgitant flow
  - qualitative visual assessment
  - semiquantitative or quantitative assessment if necessary
    Calculation
  - of regurgitant fraction derived from total and effective stroke volumes
  - of regurgitant volume derived from proximal isovelocity surface area
- ▸ Intracardiac pressure (mmHg)
  - $PA_{diastolic}$ with concomitant pulmonary regurgitation

Transesophageal echocardiography

- ▸ Detection of thrombus in the left atrium
- ▸ Valve morphology and dynamics
- ▸ Detection and classification of lesions in mitral valve support apparatus

Stress echocardiography in ischemic mitral insufficiency, when indicated

---

SYMPTOMATOLOGY / AUSCULTATION

ECHOCARDIOGRAPHY

Conventional echocardiography:

Morphometry (RA, RVEDD, LADmax, LVEDD, LVESD)
Ventricular function (LVFS, wall motion analysis)
Visualization of anatomic causes and hemodynamic effects
Valve morphology and dynamics

Doppler and transesophageal echocardiography:

Qualitative visual assessment; semiquantitative and/or quantitative assessment
Visualization of anatomic causes

Stress echocardiography:

When ischemic mitral insufficiency is suspected

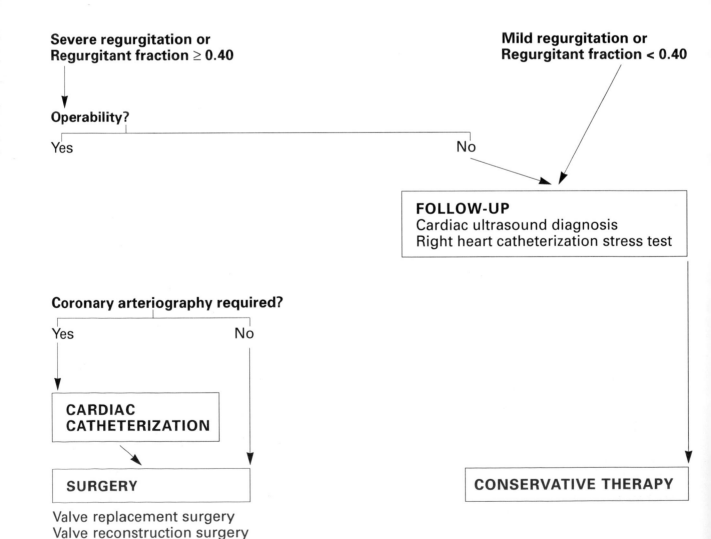

**Severe regurgitation or
Regurgitant fraction ≥ 0.40**

Operability?

Yes   No

**Mild regurgitation or
Regurgitant fraction < 0.40**

FOLLOW-UP
Cardiac ultrasound diagnosis
Right heart catheterization stress test

Coronary arteriography required?

Yes   No

**CARDIAC
CATHETERIZATION**

SURGERY

Valve replacement surgery
Valve reconstruction surgery

CONSERVATIVE THERAPY

1. Akamatsu S, Kagawa K, Terazawa E, Takeda T, Arakawa M, Dohi S. Physiological mitral regurgitation: A study with transesophageal Doppler echocardiography. Circulation 1990: 82 (suppl III): 0178.
2. Bargiggia GS, Tronconi L, Sahn DJ, Recusani F, Raisaro A, De Servi S, Valdes-Cruz LM, Montemartini C. A new method for quantitation of mitral regurgitation based an color flow Doppler imaging of flow convergence proximal to regurgitant orifice. Circulation 1991; 84: 1481-1489.
3. Berko B, Gaasch WH, Tanigawa N, Smith D, Craige E. Disparity between ejection and end-systolic indexes of left ventricular contractility in mitral regurgitation. Circulation 1987; 75: 1310-1319.
4. Biasucci LM, Lombardo A, Pennestri' F, Rinelli G, Coppola E, Loperfido F. Is long-term evolution of post myocardial infarction mitral regurgitation related to infarct location? Circulation 1990; 82 (suppl III): 1869.
5. Bibra H v, Becher H, Firschke C, Schlief R, Emslander HP, Baedeker W. SHU 508 for contrast color Doppler of left heart chambers. Improved evaluation of mitral regurgitation. Circulation 1991; 84 (suppl II): 1431.
6. Brickner ME, Starling MR. Dissociation of end systole from end ejection in patients with long-term mitral regurgitation. Circulation 1990; 81: 1277-1286.
7. Carabello BA. Preservation of left ventricular function in patients with mitral regurgitation: A realistic goal for the nineties. J Am Coll Cardiol 1990; 15: 565-565.
8. Carabello BA. What exactly is 2+ to 3+ mitral regurgitation? J Am Coll Cardiol 1992; 19: 339-340.
9. Castello R, Lenzen PM, Aguirre FV, Labovitz AJ. Quantitation of mitral regurgitation by transesophageal echocardiography with Doppler color flow mapping: correlation with cardiac catheterization. J Am Coll Cardiol 1992; 19: 1516-1521.
10. Castello R, Lenzen PM, Aguirre FV, Labovitz AJ. Quantitative comparison of transthoracic and transesophageal echocardiography in the evaluation of mitral regurgitation. Circulation 1990; 82 (suppl III): 2184.
11. Chen C, Koschyk D, Mehl C, Klarh^fer M, Kupper W, Bleifeld W. Comparison of quantifying mitral regurgitation using color Doppler proximal isovelocity surface area and angiography. Circulation 1991; 84 (suppl II): 2531.
12. Chesler E, Gornick CC. Maladies attributed to myxomatous mitral valve. Circulation 1991; 82: 328-332.
13. Cohen GI, Chan KL. Comparison of transesophageal echocardiography and angiography in the assessment of mitral regurgitation. Circulation 1990; 82 (suppl III): 2185.
14. Corin WJ, Monrad ES, Murukami T, Nonogi H, Hess OM, Krayenbuehl HP. The relationship of afterload to ejection performance in chronic mitral regurgitation. Circulation 1978; 76: 59-67.
15. Corin WJ, Murakami T, Monrad S, Hess OM, Krayenb,hl HP. Left ventricular passive diastolic properties in chronic mitral regurgitation. Circulation 1991; 83: 797-807.
16. Cormier B, Starkman C, Michel PL, Vahanian A, Acar J. Transesophageal echocardiography for the detection of rupture of chordae. Circulation 1990; 82 (suppl III): 1666.
17. Crawford MH, Souchek J, Oprian CA, Miller DC, Rahimtoola S, Giacomini JC, Sethi G, Hammermeister KE. Determinants of survival and left ventricular performance after mitral valve replacement. Circulation 1990; 81: 1173-1181.
18. Czer LSC, Maurer G, Bolger AF, Robertis M de, Resser KJ, Kass RM, Lee ME, Blanche C, Chaux A, Gray RJ, Matloff JM. Intraoperative evaluation of mitral regurgitation by Doppler color flow mapping. Circulation 1987; 76 (suppl III): III-108-III-116.
19. David TE, Ho WC. The effect of preservation of chordae tendineae on mitral valve replacement for post-infarction mitral regurgitation. Circulation 1986; 74 (suppl I): I-116.
20. de Bruijn NP, Clements FM, Kisslo JA. Intraoperative transesophageal color flow mapping: Initial experience. Anesth Analg 1987; 66: 386-390.
21. Engel PJ, Hickman JR Jr, Alpert BL, Adams DF. Quantitative angiographic diagnosis of mitral valve prolapse. Circulation 1978; 58 (suppl II): 122.
22. Fehrenbacher G, Feiring A, Bajwa T, Schmidt DH. Mitral regurgitation induced by ischemia. Circulation 1989; 80 (suppl II): 1349.
23. Fehske W, Heider C, Elfner R, Hammentgen R, Nitsch J, L,deritz B. Evaluation of different Doppler-echocardiographic methods for quantitation of mitral valve incompetence. Circulation 1989; 80, (suppl II): 2297.
24. Feldman Md, Beller GA. Is secondary mitral regurgitation in congestive heart failure a marker of clinical importance? J Am Coll Cardiol 1990; 15: 181-183.
25. Fraser AG, St,mper OFW, Herwerden LA van, Ho SY, Anderson RH, Roelandt JRTC. Anatomy of imaging planes used to study the mitral valve: Advantages of biplane transesophageal echocardiography. Circulation 1990; 82 (suppl III): 2653.
26. Gams E, Hagl S, Heimisch W, Meisner H, Mendler N, Schad H, Sebening F. Influence of papillary muscle function on the mitral valve and left ventricular mechanics. In: Vetter HO, Hetzer R, Schmutzler H, eds. Ischemic mitral incompetence. Darmstadt: Steinkopff; New York: Springer, 1991: 35-54.
27. Gams E, Heimisch W, Hagl S, Mendler N, Schad H, Sebening F. Significance of the subvalvular apparatus following mitral valve replacement. Circulation 1987; 76 (suppl IV): 2140.
28. Gillam LD, Radford MJ, Schulman P, Slowik DS, Munson JT. Mitral valve prolapse: A disease in need of universal diagnostic criteria. Circulation 1987; 76 (suppl IV): 2106.
29. Grossman W, Baim DS, ed. Cardiac catheterization, angiography, and intervention. 4nd ed. Philadelphia: Lea & Ferbiger, 1991: p.566.

30. Handschumacher MD, Hagege AA, Harrigan P, Sanfilippo AJ, Weyman AE, Levine RA. Direct demonstration of mitral leaflet annular relationships by three-dimensional echocardiography: Implications for the diagnosis of mitral valve prolapse. Circulation 1988; 77 (suppl A), 126A.

31. Harlamert E, Smith M, Booth D, Grayburn P, Kwan OL, DeMaria AN. Relationship of the murmur in mitral regurgitation to jet size, shape, and direction by Doppler flow imaging. Circulation 1987: 76 (suppl IV): 1261.

32. Helmcke F, Nanda NC, Hsiung MC, Soto B, Adey CK, Goyal RG, Gatewood, RP Jr. Color Doppler assessment of mitral regurgitation with orthogonal planes. Circulation 1987; 75: 175-183.

33. Himelman RB, Kusumoto F, Oken K, Lee E, Cahalan MK, Shah PM, Schiller NB. The flail mitral valve: Echocardiographic findings by precordial and transesophageal imaging and Doppler color flow mapping. J Am Coll Cardiol 1991; 17: 272-279.

34. Hsia HH, Starlin MR. Is standardization of left ventricular chamber elastance necessary? Circulation 1990; 81: 1826-1836.

35. Huhta JC, Ludomirsky A, Lee R. Is the average Doppler signal amplitude useful in grading mitral regurgitation? Circulation 1988; 78 (suppl II): 2432.

36. Ishihara K, Nakano N, Zile M, Spinale F, Kanazawa S, Smith A, Swindle M, Carabello B. Early mitral valve replacement reverses the contractile dysfunction produced by experimental mitral regurgitation. Circulation 1990; 82 (suppl III): 2253.

37. Izumi S, Miyatake K, Beppu S, Park Y-D, Nagata S, Kinoshita N, Sakakibara H, Nimura Y. Mechanism of mitral regurgitation in patients with myocardial infarction: A study using real-time two-dimensional Doppler flow imaging and echocardiography. Circulation 1987; 76: 777-785.

38. Jaffe WM, Roche AHG, Coverdale HA, McAlister HF, Ormiston JA, Greene ER. Clinical evaluation versus Doppler echocardiography in the quantitative assessment of valvular heart disease, Circulation 1988; 78: 267-275, tbl. 3 p. 271.

39. Jain S, Moos S, Awad M, Fan PH, Helmcke F. Assessment of mitral regurgitation severity using pulmonary venous flow by transesophageal color Doppler. Circulation 1989; 80 (suppl II): 2272.

40. Jamal N, Winters W; Nelson J, Echocardiographic features of flail mitral valve leaflets: ruptured chordae tendineae versus ruptured papillary muscle. Circulation 1978; 58 (suppl II): 157.

41. Jayaweera AR, Dent J, Watson DD, Glasheen WP, Kaul S. Contrast echocardiography can be used to quantitate the severity of mitral regurgitation. Circulation 1990; 82 (suppl III): 0376.

42. Jenni R, Ritter M, Eberli F, Grimm J, Krayenbuehl HP. Quantification of mitral regurgitation with amplitude-weighted mean velocity from continuous wave Doppler spectra. Circulation 1989; 79: 1294-1299.

43. Jeresaty RM. Left ventricular function in acute non-ischaemic mitral regurgitation. Europ Heart J 1991; 12 (suppl B): 19-21.

44. Kaul S, Spotnitz WD, Glasheen WP, Touchstone DA. Mechanism of ischemic mitral regurgitation. Circulation 1991; 84: 2167-2180.

45. Keren G, Katz S, Strom J, Sonnenblick EH, LeJemtel TH. Dynamic mitral regurgitation: An important determinant of the hemodynamic response to load alterations and inotropic therapy in severe heart failure. Circulation 1989; 80: 306-313.

46. Klein AL, Cohen GI, Davison MB, Marwick TM, Husbands K, Pearce GL. Importance of sampling both pulmonary veins in the transesophageal assessment of severity of mitral regurgitation. J Am Coll Cardiol 1991; 17 (suppl A): 199A.

47. Klein AL, Obarski TP, Stewart WJ, Casale PN, Pearce GL, Husbands K, Cosgrove DM, Salcedo EE. Transesophageal Doppler echocardiography of pulmonary venous flow: A new marker of mitral regurgitation severity. J Am Coll Cardiol 1991; 18: 518-526.

48. Kono T, Sabbah HN, Rosman H, Alam M, Jafri S, Stein PD, Goldstein S. The onset of functional mitral regurgitation during the course of evolving heart failure is associated with ventricular shape changes. Circulation 1991; 84 (suppl II): 1305.

49. Kono T, Sabbah HN, Rosman H, Mohsin A, Jafri S, Stein PD, Goldstein S. Mechanism of functional mitral regurgitation during acute myocardial ischemia. J Am Coll Cardiol 1992; 19: 1101-1105.

50. Kono T, Sabbah HN, Stein PD, Brymer JF, Khaja F. Role of left ventricular shape in the etiology of mitral regurgitation in patients with heart failure. J Am Coll Cardiol 1991; 17, (suppl A): 356A.

51. Konstantinov BA, Zaretskij VV, Bobkov VV, Sandrikov VA, Lukushkina EF. Ekhograficheskaia diagnostika revmaticheskoi nedostatochnosti mitral'nogo klapana (Echocardiographic diagnosis of rheumatic mitral insufficiency). Kardiologija 1977; 17: 28-33.

52. Kraus F, Dacian S, Rudolph W. Belastungsuntersuchungen bei valvul‰orer Herzerkrankung und Herzklappenersatz. Herz 1982; 7: 144-155.

53. Kraus F, Rudolph W. Symptoms, exercise capacity and exercise hemodynamics: Interrelationships and their role in quantification of the valvular lesions. Herz 1984; 9: 187-199.

54. Kyo S, Takamoto S, Matsumura M, Asano H, Yokote Y, Motoyama T, Omoto R. Immeadiate and early postoperative evaluations of results of cardiac surgery by transesophageal two-dimensional Doppler echocardiography. Circulation 1987; 76 (suppl V): V-113-V-121.

55. Leatham A, Brigden W. Mild mitral regurgitation and the mitral valve prolapse fiasco. Am Heart J 1980; 99: 659-664.

56. Levine RA, Triulzi MO, Harrigan P, Weyman AE. The relationship of mitral annular shape to the diagnosis of mitral valve prolapse. Circulation 1987; 75: 756-767.

57. Lim Y-J, Masuyama T, Kohama A, Hashimura K, Naito J, Nanto S. Role of papillary muscle perfusion abnormalities for mitral regurgitation in patients with myocardial infarction. Circulation 1990; 82 (suppl III): 2959.
58. Lsbre JP, Tribouilloy C. Echo-Doppler quantitative assessment of non-ischemic mitral regurgitation. Europ Heart J 1991; 12 (suppl B): 10-14.
59. Luxereau P, Dorent R, de Gevigney G, Bruneval P, Chomette G, Delahaye G. Aetiology of surgically treated mitral regurgitation. Europ Heart J 1991; 12 (suppl B): 2-4.
60. Maciel BC, Moises VA, Shandas R, Simpson IA, Beltran M, Valdes-Cruz L, Sahn DJ. Effects of pressure and volume of the receiving chamber on the spatial distribution of regurgitant jets as imaged by color Doppler flow mapping. Circulation 1991; 83: 605-613.
61. Maciel BC, Valdes-Cruz L, Murillo A, Moises V, Sahn DJ. Quantitative analysis of variance indices in mitral regurgitation: An in vitro color Doppler flow mapping study. Circulation 1988; 78 (suppl II): 0152.
62. Marcus RH, Sareli P, Pocock WA, Barlow JB. Mechanisms of rheumatic mitral valve disease. Influence of disease acitivity on valve lesion. Circulation 1988; 78 (suppl II): 1877.
63. Mihaileanu S, El Asmar B, Acar C, Lamberti A, Diebold B, Perier P, Dreyfus G, Bensasson D, Dang Y, Ilie-su D, Carpentier A. Intra-operative transesophageal echocardiography after mitral repair - specific conditions and pitfalls. Europ Heart J 1991; 12 (suppl B): 26-29.
64. Miller G. Invasive investigation of the heart. A guide to cardiac catheterization and related procedures. Oxford: Blackwell, 1989: p. 277.
65. Mintz GS, Kotler MN, Segal BL, Parry WR. Two-dimensional echocardiographic recognition of ruptured chordae tendineae. Circulation 1978; 57: 244-250.
66. Pearson AC, Vrain J St, Mrosek D, Labovitz AJ. Color Doppler echocardiographic evaluation of patients with a flail mitral leaflet. J Am Coll Cardiol 1990; 16: 232-239.
67. Ranganathan N, Silver MD, Robinson TI, Kostuk WJ, Felderhof CH, Patt NL, Wilson JK, Wigle ED. Angiographic-morphologic correlation in patients with severe mitral regurgitation due to prolapse of the posterior mitral valve leaflet. Circulation 1973; 48: 514-518.
68. Rankin JS, Hickey MSJ, Smith LR, DeBruijn NP, Sheikh KH, Sabiston DC Jr. Current concepts in the pathogenesis and treatment of ischemic mitral regurgitation. In: Vetter HO, Hetzer R, Schmutzler H, eds. Ischemic mitral incompetence. Darmstadt: Steinkopff; New York: Springer, 1991: 157-178.
69. Recusani F, Bargiggia GS, Yoganathan AP, Raisaro A, Valdes-Cruz LM, Sung HW, Bertucci C, Gallati M, Moises VA, Simpson IA, Tronconi L, Sahn DJ. A new method for quantification of regurgitant flow rate using color Doppler flow imaging of the flow convergence region proximal to a discrete orifice. Circulation 1991; 83: 594-604.
70. Reed D, Abbott RD, Smucker ML, Kaul S. Prediction of outcome after mitral valve replacement in patients with symptomatic chronic mitral regurgitation. Circulation 1991; 84: 23-34.
71. Rodriguez L, Vlahakes GJ, Cape EG, Yoganathan AP, Guerrero JL, Levine RA. In vivo validation of a new method for non-invasive quantification of mitral regurgitation. Circulation 1989; 80 (suppl II): 2289.
72. Rodriguez L, Vlahakes GJ, Yoganathan AP, Guerrero JL, Levine RA. Quantification of regurgitant flow rate using the proximal flow convergence method: In vivo validation. Circulation 1989; 80 (suppl II): 2275.
73. Rokey R, Sterling LL, Zoghbi WA, Sartori MP, Limacher MC, Kuo LC, Quinones MA. Determination of regurgitant fraction in isolated mitral or aortic regurgitation by pulsed Doppler two-dimensional echocardiography. J Am Coll Cardiol 1986; 7: 1273-1278.
74. Sabbah HN, Kono T, Rosman H, Jafri S, Stein PD, Goldstein S. Changes of left ventricular shape: A factor in the etiology of mitral regurgitation in heart failure. Circulation 1990; 82 (suppl III): 0445.
75. Sagawa K, Suga H, Shoukas A, Bakalar K. End-systolic pressure-volume ratio: A new index of ventricular contractility. Am J Cardiol 1977; 40: 748-753.
76. Sagawa K. The end-systolic pressure-volume relation of ventricle: Definition, modifications, and clinical use. Circulation 1981; 63: 1223-1227.
77. Sagawa K. The ventricular pressure-volume diagram revisited. Circ Res 1978; 43: 677-687.
78. Sakai K, Sakaki S, Hirata N, Nakano S. Assessment of postoperative left ventricular function after mitral valve repair. Circulation 1991; 84 (suppl II): 2298.
79. Sanfilippo AJ, Weyman AE, Levine RA. The problem of echocardiographic detection of mitral valve prolapse and determination of its true prevalence. Herz 1988; 13: 284-292.
80. Schmailzl KJG, Fleck E, Hetzer R. Timing mitral valve repair for regurgitant lesions: Transthoracal and - esophageal echo-Doppler findings with color flow mapping and hemodynamic evaluation. Heart Vessels 1987; 3 (suppl 3): 22.
81. Sheikh KH, Bengtson JR, Rankin JS, de Bruijn NP, Kisslo J. Intraoperative transesophageal Doppler color flow imaging to guide patient selection and operative treatment of ischemic mitral regurgitation. Circulation 1991; 84: 594-604.
82. Shimizu G, Hirota Y, Kita Y, Takeuchi A, Kawamura K. Evaluatoin of pre- and post-operative systolic function in chronic mitral regurgitation. Circulation 1990; 82 (suppl III): 2982.
83. Skoulagiris J, Essop R, Middlemost S, Nicola G di, Sarelli P. The incidence of proximal pulmonary thrombotic disease in patients with significant rheumatic mitral valve disease and pulmonary hypertension. Circulation 1989; 80 (suppl II): 0035.

84. Smith MD, Harrison MR, Pinton R, Kandil H, Kwan OL, DeMaria AN. Regurgitant jet size by transesophageal compared with transthoracic Doppler color flow imaging. Circulation 1991; 83: 79-86.

85. Smyllie JH, Sutherland GR, Geuskens R, Dawkins K, Conway N, Roelandt JRTC. Doppler color flow mapping in the diagnosis of ventricular septal rupture and acute mitral regurgitation after myocardial infarction. J Am Coll Cardiol 1990; 15: 1449-1455.

86. Spindola-Franco H, Bjork L, Adams DF, Abrams HL. Classification of the radiological morphology of the mitral valve: Differentiation between the true and pseudoprolapse. Brit Heart J 1980; 44: 30-36.

87. Spratt JA, Olsen CO, Tyson GS, Glower DD, Davis JW, Rankin JS. Experimental mitral regurgitation: Physiological effects of correction on left ventricular dynamics. J Thorac Cardiovasc Surg 1983; 86: 479 489.

88. Stewart WJ, Agler DA, Homa DA, Salcedo EE, Klein AL, Currie PJ, Lytle BW, Cosgrove DM. Predicting the mechanism of mitral regurgitation prior to repair: A system using leaflet motion and color Doppler jet direction. Circulation 1990; 82 (suppl III): 2188.

89. Stewart WJ, Chavez AM, Currie PJ, Gill CC, Salcedo EE, Agler DA, Schiavone WA, Lytle BW, Cosgrove DM. Echo determination of mitral pathology and feasibility of repair for mitral regurgitation. Circulation 1987; 76 (suppl IV): 1785.

90. Stewart WJ, Currie PJ, Salcedo EE, Lytle BW, Gill CC, Schiavone WA, Agler DA, Cosgrove DM. Intraoperative Doppler color flow mapping for decision-making in valve repair for mitral regurgitation. Circulation 1990; 81: 556-566.

91. Tak T, Goel S, Kulick D, Thaker K, Rahimtoola SH, Chandraratna PAN. Estimation of severity of mitral regurgitation by determining intensitiy of regurgitant signal. J Am Coll Cardiol 1991; 17 (suppl A): 148A.

92. Tanabe K, Yamagishi M, Nakatani S, Takamiya M, Miyatake K. A new method for quantitative assessment of regurgitant volume of isolated mitral insufficiency by color Doppler echocardiography. Circulation 1990; 82 (suppl III): 2191.

93. Tsutsui H, Urabe Y, Mann D, Kent R, Cooper G, Carabello B, Zile M. Effects of chronic mitral regurgitation on diastolic function in isolated cardiocytes. Circulation 1991; 84 (suppl II): 1775.

94. Utsunomiya T, Nguyen D, Doshi R, Patel D, Gardin JM. Regurgitant volume estimation in mitral regurgitation by color Doppler using the „Proximal Isovelocity Surface Area" method. Circulation 1989; 80 (suppl II): 2291.

95. Wilcken DEL, Hickey AJ. Lifetime risk for patients with mitral valve prolapse of developing severe valve regurgitation requiring surgery. Circulation 1988; 78: 10-14.

96. Williams MB, McMannia K, Gabel M, Hoit BD. Ischemic zone site, not size is the major determinant of acute ischemic mitral regurgitation. J Am Coll Cardiol 1991; 17 (suppl A): 356A.

97. Wisenbaugh T. Does normal pump function belie muscle dysfunction in patients with chronic severe mitral regurgitation? Circulation 1987; 76 (suppl IV): 0646.

98. Wisenbaugh T. Does normal pump function belie muscle dysfunction in patients with chronic severe mitral regurgitation? Circulation 1988; 77: 515-525.

99. Yamaura Y, Yoshikawa J, Yoshida K, Akasaka T, Hozumi T. Color flow Doppler quantitation of mitral regurgitation using an acceleration flow proximal to the orifice of a regurgitation jet. Circulation 1989; 80 (suppl II): 2290.

100. Yoshida K, Yoshikawa J, Hozumi T, Akasaka T, Yamaura Y, Tsukishima N. Value of acceleration flow signals in the quantitative assessment of prosthetic regurgitation in the mitral position. Circulation 1990; 82 (suppl III): 0065.

101. Yoshida K, Yoshikawa J, Yamaura Y, Hozumi T, Akasaka T, Fukaya T. Assessment of mitral regurgitation by biplane transesophageal color Doppler flow mapping. Circulation 1990; 82: 1121-1126.

102. Yoshida K, Yoshikawa J, Yamaura Y, Hozumi T, Shakudo M, Akasaka T, Kato H. Value of acceleration flows and regurgitant jet direction by color Doppler flow mapping in the evaluation of mitral valve prolapse. Circulation 1990; 81: 879-885.

103. Yun KL, Rayhill SC, Niczyporuk MA, Fann JI, Zipkin RE, Derby GC, Handen CE, Daughters GT, Ingels Jr NB, Bolger AF, Miller DC. Mitral valve replacement in dilated canine hearts with chronic mitral regurgitation. Circulation 1991; 84 (suppl III): III-112-III-124.

104. Zhang Y, Ihlen H, Myhre E, Levorstad K, Nitter-Hauge S. Measurement of mitral regurgitation by Doppler echocardiography. Brit Heart J 1985; 54: 384-391.

105. Zile MR, Gaasch WH, Carroll JD, Levine HJ. Chronic mitral regurgitation: Predictive value of preoperative echocardiographic indexes of left ventricular function and wall stress. J Am Coll Cardiol 1984; 3: 235-242.

Rheumatic fever is still the main cause of mitral stenosis. Isolated mitral stenosis typically results from the postinflammatory adhesive, fibrotic and degenerative changes that occur during the healing process. These changes lead to commissural fusion, scarring and consecutive contracture of leaflet tissue [32]. Chordae tendineae shortening may cause the two leaflets to form a funnel-shaped infundibulum, which typically has a wide inlet near the left atrium and a narrow outlet inside the left ventricle.

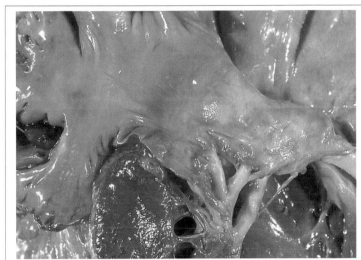

Morphological specimen: rheumatic mitral stenosis. Thickening, stiffening and fusion of chordae tendineae; atrial appendage thrombus.

Echocardiography is sometimes helpful in differentiating rheumatic mitral stenosis from non-rheumatic left atrial outflow tract obstruction.

Dysplasia or "parachute anomaly" in which both leaflets are connected via the chordae tendineae to a single large papillary muscle is rare in adults. The diagnosis is secured from the left parasternal short axis position.

Other non-rheumatic left atrial outflow tract obstructions include such intracardiac masses as thrombi, atrial tumors, and vegetations from infective endocarditis. Cardiac ultrasound is particularly helpful in detecting these masses.

Non-rheumatic obstruction of left atrial outflow
▸ Mitral valve dysplasia ▸ Mitral valve parachute anomaly ▸ Intracardiac masses

---

Cardiac Ultrasound Diagnosis

The preferred scan planes are the left parasternal long and short-axis views, the apical two and four-chamber views, and the subcostal four-chamber view.

Conventional Echocardiography

Visualization of anatomic causes:

2-D and M mode echocardiography:

- *Thickening and calcification of the mitral leaflets.* Compared to a normal valve in orthogonal view at maximum opening. Multiple, parallel echoes (M-mode).

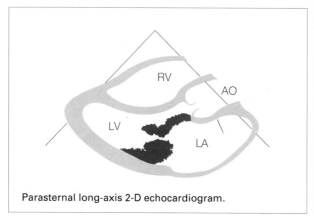

Parasternal long-axis 2-D echocardiogram.

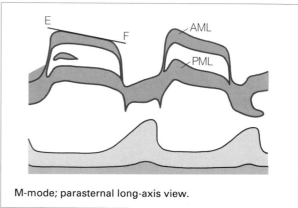

M-mode; parasternal long-axis view.

Nonspecific features and possible hemodynamic effects of mitral stenosis:

2-D echocardiography:

- *Leaflet mobility, the presence and extent of calcification, involvement of subvalvular apparatus;*
- *Diastolic doming of the mitral leaflets into the left ventricle.* The increased mitral valve gradient causes the body of the mitral leaflets to bulge, because fused cusp edges prevent complete opening;
- *Enlargement of the left atrium.*

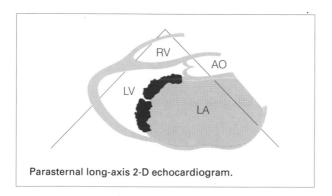

Parasternal long-axis 2-D echocardiogram.

- *Indication of pulmonary hypertension,* which causes rightward bulging of interatrial septum (best visualized in four-chamber view), and dilatation of the right ventricular outflow tract.

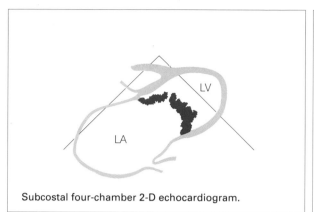

Subcostal four-chamber 2-D echocardiogram.

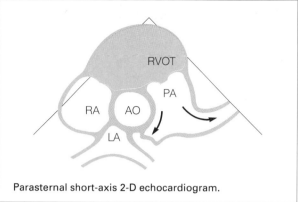

Parasternal short-axis 2-D echocardiogram.

M-mode echocardiography:

- *M-shaped motion pattern expressing anterior motion of the posterior mitral leaflet* due to commissural fusion. The posterior leaflet is pulled forward by the larger and more mobile anterior leaflet [12, 46].

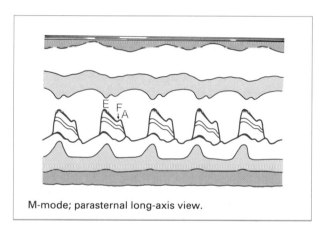

M-mode; parasternal long-axis view.

- A *flat EF slope* (< 36 mm/s) reflects a reduction in mitral valve closing velocity due to extended left ventricular filling time [13]. A sustained transmitral pressure gradient prolongs valve opening (albeit only slightly) [14].
  More severe stenosis is indicated only when the values drop below 10 mm/s. When there is less pronounced flattening, the EF slope correlates poorly with the degree of severity, but it does, to some extent, correlate with mitral annular movement. Since ventricular filling time and therefore EF slope are dependent on heart rate [15], single beats with extremely long diastoles occurring in conjunction with atrial fibrillation often give rise to error.

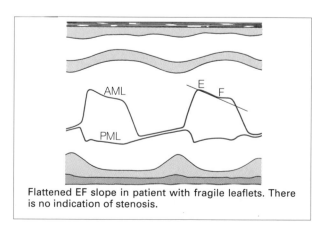

Flattened EF slope in patient with fragile leaflets. There is no indication of stenosis.

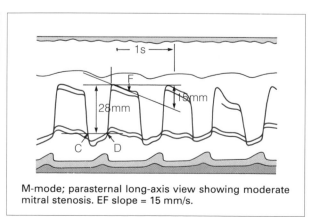

M-mode; parasternal long-axis view showing moderate mitral stenosis. EF slope = 15 mm/s.

- Interventricular septum has a *very deep early diastolic dip*. This is an expression of contraction-like, acute-angled movement to posterior that results from accelerated right ventricular filling during the rapid filling phase [52].

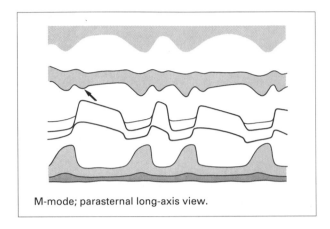

M-mode; parasternal long-axis view.

- *Flattened "A" wave with preserved sinus rhythm and reduced D-E amplitude.*

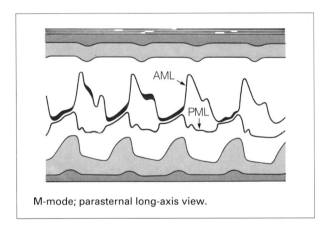

M-mode; parasternal long-axis view.

Quantification (conventional echocardiography):

Two-dimensional echocardiography:

- *Planimetry of the mitral valve area from the left parasternal short-axis view* [33].

Other conventional echocardiographic methods have lost their former significance since the advent of Doppler echocardiography.

Conventional Doppler Echocardiography

Pulsed-wave Doppler (PW Doppler):

- *Detection, velocity measurement, and "mapping" of diastolic stenotic flow jets at mitral valve level.*

Continuous-wave Doppler (CW Doppler):

- *Detection and velocity measurement of diastolic stenotic flow jets at mitral valve level.*

Mitral stenosis can be visualized in continuous or pulsed-wave Doppler recordings obtained from the apical transducer position. The CW Doppler beam is focused on the left ventricle at the base of transmitral inflow, whereas the sample volume of the PW Doppler is positioned proximal to the mitral valve orifice. As regards detection and quantification of mitral stenosis, Doppler echocardiography seems to be slightly advantageous to auscultation by an experienced examiner. Echocardiography can, however, provide useful information for determining whether to preserve the native valve or to implant a prosthetic valve [27].

Doppler Color Flow Imaging (2-D and M-mode)

- *Graphic representation of turbulent transmitral stenotic flow jets.*

Transesophageal Echocardiography (Single and Multiplane)

Transesophageal echocardiography has only slight advantages with respect to detection and assessment of mitral stenosis [35]. Transesophageal echocardiography can, however, better detect the anatomic causes of stenosis and provides better information for evaluating the feasibility of special treatment procedures. Furthermore, the mitral valve area can be planimetered using multiplane views.

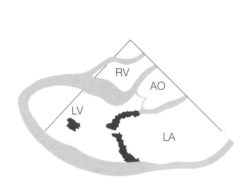

Doming of the anterior mitral leaflet and enlargement of the left atrium.

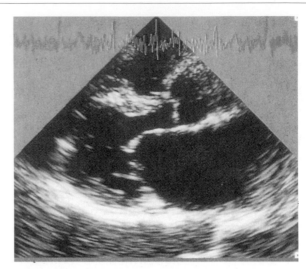

Left parasternal long-axis 2-D echocardiogram.

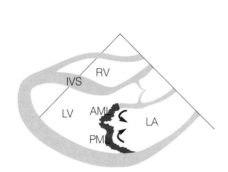

Early diastole. Transmitral outflow is encoded in red and blue due to obstruction in the vicinity of the anterior mitral leaflet. Jet inversion at the apex of the doming leaflet.

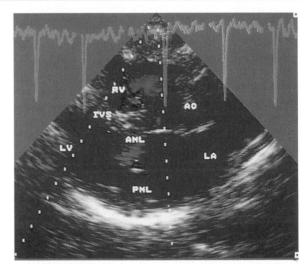

Color flow map of left parasternal long-axis view; early diastole.

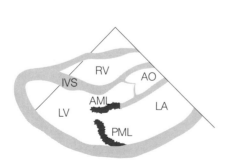

Turbulent flow near the anterior mitral leaflet as a result of increased flow obstruction. Stenosis expressed mainly as restricted movement of the anterior mitral leaflet.

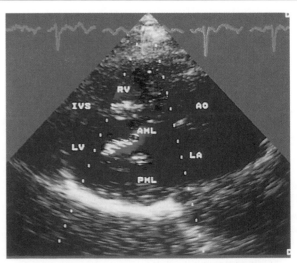

Color flow map of left parasternal long-axis view; late diastole.

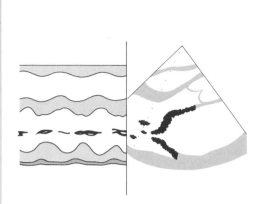

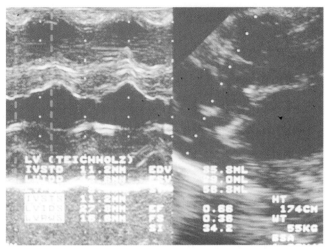

This images shows a left ventricle with normal dimension and normal systolic function, echo-dense mitral leaflets, and calcification of the mitral valve apparatus. The left atrium is slightly enlarged.

2-D and M-mode; left parasternal long-axis view at level of mitral valve apparatus. Morphometry.

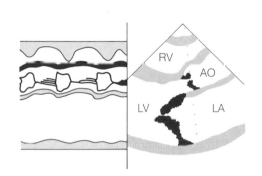

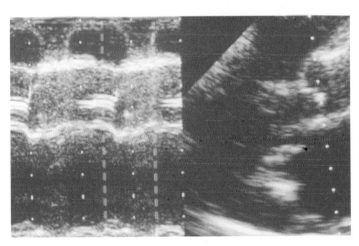

Left atrial enlargement, echo-dense anterior leaflet, calcified posterior leaflet and calcium deposits on the aortic wall. Calcification of the aortic valve is seen during diastole; opening amplitude is preserved.

2-D and M-mode; left parasternal long-axis view at level of the aortic valve.

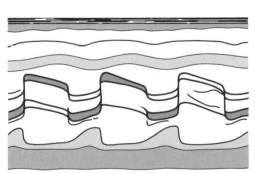

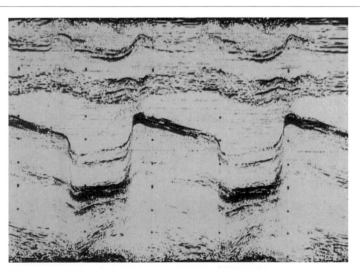

Thickening and calcification of mitral leaflet. The M-shaped movement of the posterior leaflet is concordant with that of the anterior leaflet. The EF slope is flattened with reduced diastolic separation of mitral leaflets and atrial fibrillation with extinction of the A wave.

M-mode; left parasternal long axis at mitral valve level.

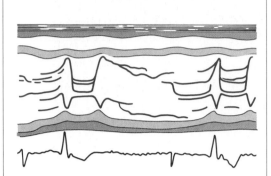

Thickened and partially calcified mitral leaflets. There is also sustained, anterior discordant W-shaped movement of posterior leaflet, atrial fibrillation with premature ventricular beats and variable duration of diastole. The EF slope is flattened during diastoles of normal duration. Reduced left ventricular size.

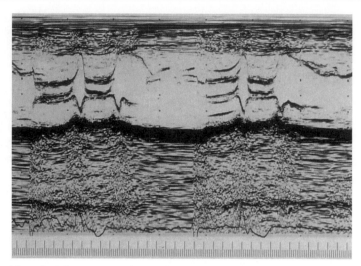

M-mode; left parasternal long axis at mitral valve level.

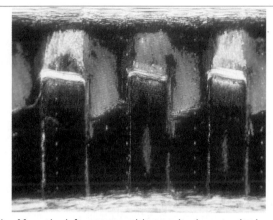

Color M-mode; left parasternal long-axis view at mitral valve. Note calcium-dense anterior mitral leaflet with flat EF slope; the A wave is absent during atrial fibrillation. Above rims of closed leaflets, blue colored outflow from LV extends to aorta in systole. Highly turbulent, accelerated transmitral flow near anterior mitral leaflet in diastole.

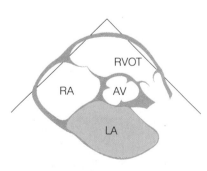

Left atrium enlarged due to mitral stenosis. The right atrium is also enlarged due to coexistent tricuspid regurgitation.

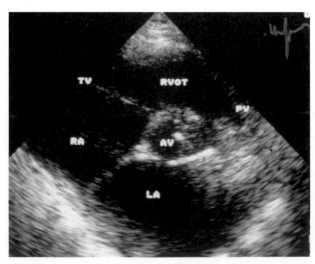

2-D left parasternal long-axis view at aortic valve level.

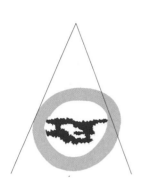

Findings: small left ventricle and calcified mitral valve that opens incompletely.

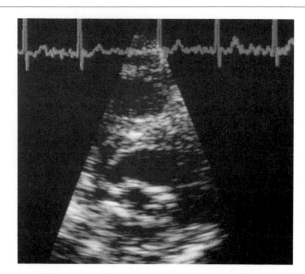

2-D left parasternal short-axis view at mitral valve level.

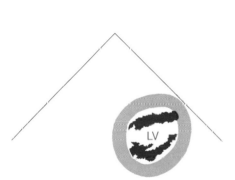

Early diastole. Slightly accelerated, yellow-red encoded transmitral flow. Red encoded inflow from right atrium is seen in the region of the right ventricle.

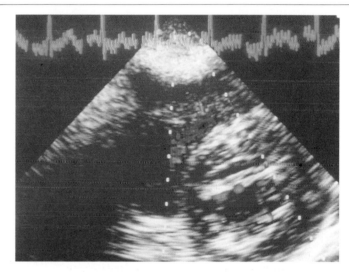

Color flow map, left parasternal short-axis view at mitral valve level.

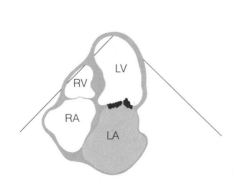

Findings: Normal-sized ventricles. Both atria are dilated, especially the left. The tip of posterior mitral leaflet is slightly thickened. Mild mitral stenosis.

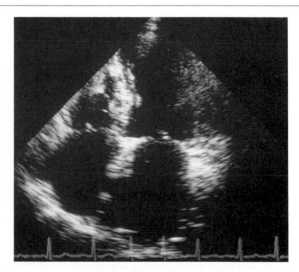

Apical four-chamber 2-D echocardiogram.

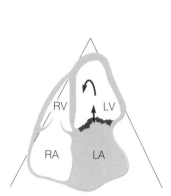

Mild mitral stenosis. Early diastole. Only minor increase in mitral valve echoes. Yellow-red encoded, accelerated and focused transmitral jet extends from left atrium to left ventricle.

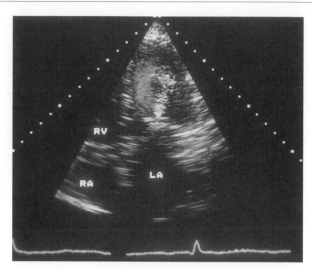

Apical four-chamber 2-D echocardiogram; color flow imaging.

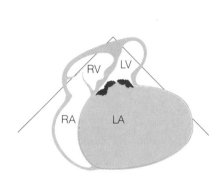

More severe mitral stenosis. Thickened posterior mitral leaflet, calcified anterior leaflet. Small ventricle. Severe enlargement of left atrium.

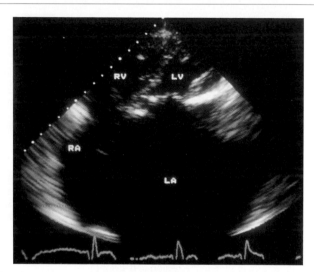

Apical four-chamber 2-D echocardiogram.

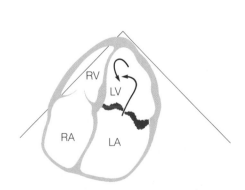

More severe mitral stenosis. Jetlike, focused, high-velocity turbulent transmitral stenotic flow jet that bounces against the lateral ventricle wall and proceeds from there to the apex. Color change from red to blue due to aliasing, with turbulent jet borders.

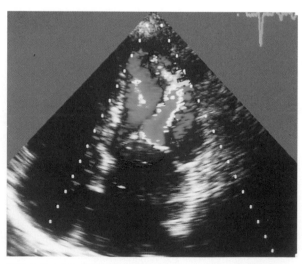

Apical four-chamber 2-D echocardiogram; color flow imaging.

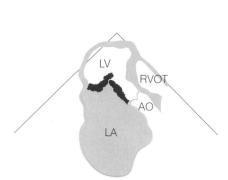

Severe mitral stenosis. Echocardiogram at onset of diastole shows mitral valve thickening, pronounced left atrial enlargement, and marked reduction in left ventricular size.

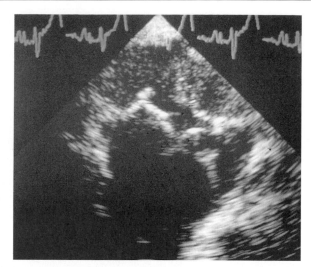

Apical two-chamber 2-D echocardiogram.

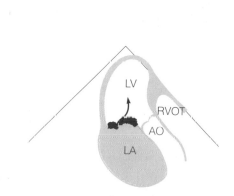

Echocardiogram showing highly turbulent stenotic mitral jet with prompt color change from red to blue resulting in turquoise-yellow mosaic pattern.

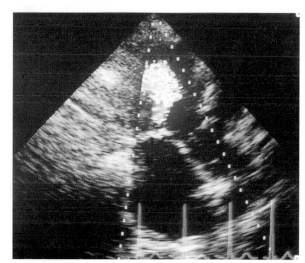

Apical two-chamber 2-D echocardiogram; color flow imaging.

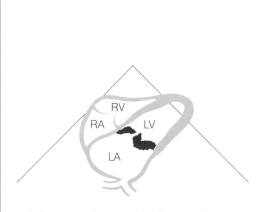

Calcified posterior mitral leaflet and dilated the left atrium.

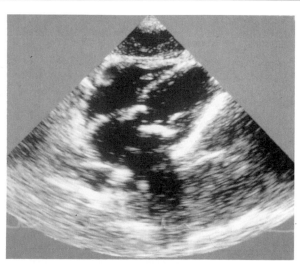

Subcostal four-chamber 2-D echocardiogram.

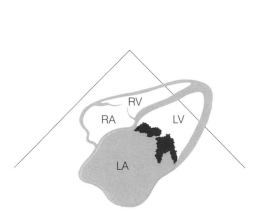

Severe mitral stenosis. Echocardiogram shows mitral valve calcification, considerable dilation of the left atrium, and a minimal mitral valve area. The jet changes color from red to light yellow with lancet-shaped flow geometry.

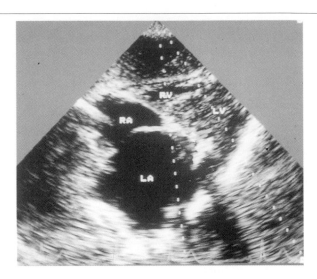

Color flow map of subcostal four-chamber 2-D echocardiogram.

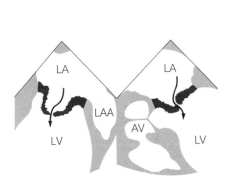

Moderately severe mitral stenosis. Aliasing with color change from blue to red in core of stenotic flow jet and peripheral turbulence can be seen. Variable jet cross sections are due to projection differences. (Tricuspid aortic valve from transverse plane).

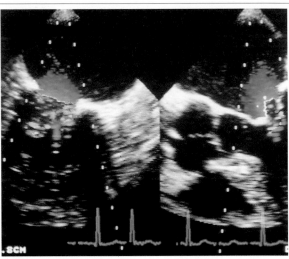

Biplane TEE with color flow mapping: long (left) and short-axis (right) views at mitral valve level, 0.36 s after R wave.

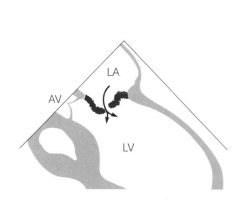

Moderate mitral stenosis. Thickening of mitral valve, doming of posterior leaflet, and aliasing. Jet has turbulent center and laminar outer flow. Slight, spontaneous contrast is seen in the left atrium.

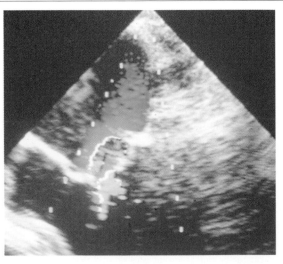

Transesophageal short-axis 2-D echocardiogram in diastole.

The normal mitral valve area is 4 to 6 cm². Obstruction is hemodynamically significant only when the orifice area is smaller than 2.5 cm². The pressure gradient must then increase significantly if proper filling of the left ventricle is to be maintained. According to the Gorlin hydraulic formula, a four-fold increase in the mean transmitral pressure gradient is required to double the cardiac output, assuming that the heart rate and diastolic filling period are constant. Tachycardia, which limits the time available for filling per beat, also causes the pressure gradient to increase. The heart's attempt to adjust its stroke volume or heart rate to additional perfusion requirements raises the pressure gradient as well as left atrial and pulmonary capillary pressure. A mitral valve area of 1.0 cm² is conventionally assessed as hemodynamically critical, because even a slight pressure increase can cause acute pulmonary venous hypertension.

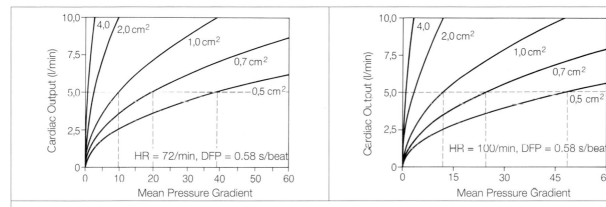

Relationship between cardiac output and the mean diastolic transmitral pressure gradient in mitral stenosis, measured via the Gorlin formula. The curves represent orifice areas of 4.0, 2.0, 1.0, 0.7 and 0.5 cm², respectively. The left and right panels show different flow-gradient relationships at different heart rates and diastolic filling periods. A cardiac output of 5 l/min can be maintained with an only slight increase in the pressure gradient when the MVA is still 2.0 cm². The pressure gradient rises proportionally with progressive restriction. An MVA of 1.0 cm² requires a pressure gradient of 8 to 10 mmHg at rest to sustain a cardiac output of 5 l/min with a normal heart rate of 72/min and a diastolic filling period of 0.58 s/beat. Even at this cardiac output level, tachycardia might cause the pressure gradient to rise steeply (right) due to the reduced diastolic filling time. *Reprinted with permission from: Grossman W, Baim DS: Cardiac catheterization, angiography and intervention. Philadelphia: Lea & Febiger, 4th ed., 1991.*

The perfusion requirement is dependent on the total vascular cross sectional area. Therefore, the mitral valve area index, *i.e.* the orifice area related to body surface area, is normally used for measurement. Traditionally, mitral stenoses are divides into four grades of severity; surgery is considered necessary when the orifice area is 1.5 to 1.0 cm² or smaller.

Mitral Stenosis. Grading Scheme

	Mitral valve orifice area [cm²]	Mitral valve orifice area index (cm²/m²)
Mild	2.50 - 1.50	2.30 - 1.50
Moderate	2.50 - 1.50	1.50 - 1.00
Moderately severe	1.50 - 1.00	1.00 - 0.50
Severe	< 1.00	< 0.50
Source: [28].		
Mild	2.50 - 2.00	1.45 - 1.15
Moderate	2.00 - 1.00	1.15 - 0.55
Severe	1.00 - 0.75	0.55 - 0.40
Critical	0.75 - 0.50	0.40 - 0.25
Source: [38].		

Pulmonary vessel complications in mitral stenosis usually occur when the mitral valve area is less than 1.0 cm². This corresponds to a mean left atrial pressure of 25 mmHg at rest.

Some cardiologists therefore wish to revise the prevailing grading systems and reset the intervention limit to include mitral valve areas of 1.50 cm². Under the prevailing methods for timing surgical interventional (and clinical severity), surgical intervention may come too late. In other words, the average postoperative patient will keep pathologic stress hemodynamics. The hemodynamic outcome is more favorable in postoperative patients who receive a commissurotomy or valvuloplasty [29] that in those who receive a mitral valve prosthesis. However, it remains unclear whether the former group is a suitable reference group for determining which hemodynamic stress characteristics might be good indicators for timing surgery. Such indicators would make it possible to identify patients in need of surgical intervention in the course of preoperative check-ups.

For ultrasound based quantitation of mitral stenosis the following methods are available:

Echocardiographic techniques for quantitation of mitral stenosis
1. Planimetry of the mitral valve area (MVA) from the left parasternal short-axis view.
2. Computation of MVA based on stenotic flow jet diameters using transesophageal short and long-axis views.
Doppler techniques for quantitation of mitral stenosis
3. Pressure half-time method
4. Continuity equation
5. Modified Gorlin formula
6. Special techniques

Morphological and hydraulic data describing mitral stenosis may vary: they may not necessarily be in agreement. The use of approximation relationships for adapting data may result in inadequate results. An unusual drop in pressure that leads to discrepancies between orifice area measurements obtained via planimetry, or via the pressure half-time method, the continuity equation and the Gorlin formula can hold a significant message. Finding out the reason for this discrepancy can be more helpful than simply disregarding it. The discrepancy may point to other causes of energy loss (*e.g.* reduced leaflet flexibility at the onset of transvalvular flow) or to irregularities in the valvular or perivalvular surface that can cause friction losses which may lead to turbulence and swirling. The hydraulically derived orifice area represents the total impedance of blood flow, whereas the planimetered orifice area describes pathomorphological narrowing at the mitral valve orifice [19].

Planimetry of the mitral valve area from the left parasternal short axis position proceeds along the inner edges of the valve leaflets, regardless of the thickness or mobility of the leaflets [23]. Correlation of planimetered data with invasive data obtained via the Gorlin formula in patients with pure mitral stenosis revealed only a moderate amount of agreement and a relatively high degree of scatter [56]. Since the visible orifice size is affected by the gain setting, poor lateral resolution (which can result in circumferential echo drop out, resulting in a certain degree of unreliability in planimetry), and dependence on the transmitral stroke volume, certain limitations do exist. Imaging of the mitral valve is unsuitable for planimetry in up to 10% of patients, because the orifice is eccentric and therefore cannot be visualized completely in a single plane [49].

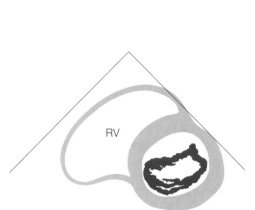

Hemodynamically insignificant mitral stenosis. Note mitral valve calcification. Planimetry of left ventricle and mitral valve was performed during diastole.

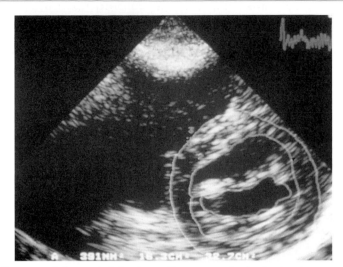

Parasternal short-axis 2-D echocardiogram at mitral valve level.

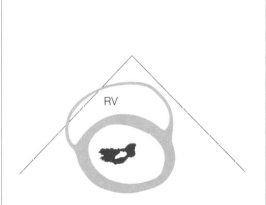

Severe mitral stenosis. Planimetry revealed MVA of 0.41 cm^2.

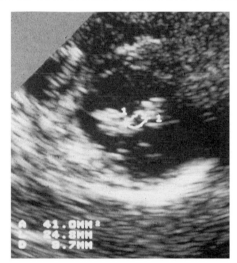

Parasternal short-axis 2-D echocardiogram at mitral valve level.

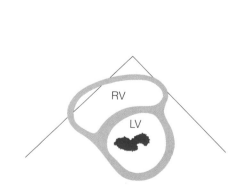

Mitral stenosis. Because of overmodulation, the mitral valve area cannot be measured.

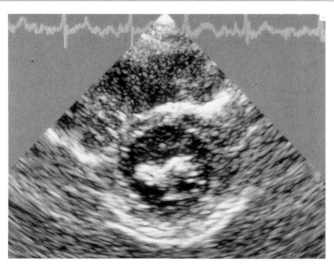

Parasternal short-axis 2-D echocardiogram at mitral valve level.

Alternatively, the MVA can be derived from stenotic flow jet diameters obtained in biplane transesophageal images [8].

While conventional echocardiographic techniques describe the morphologic features of mitral stenosis, Doppler pressure-flow relationships describe its functional status.

To obtain Doppler recordings, the transducer is positioned apically or slightly medial to the apex beat for visualization of the mitral valve. In the 2-D echocardiogram, the Doppler sample volume is positioned at the stenotic flow jet through the mitral orifice. Color flow can make it easier to locate the jet. By making slight adjustments in the angle and position of the transducer, maximum frequency shifts can be found using the audio signal; peak velocity can also be determined.

The pressure-velocity relationship across the mitral valve at any point in time (t) is defined by the *modified Bernoulli equation* as follows:

$$P_1 - P_2 = 4\ V_2^2, \hspace{4cm} \{A\}$$

in mitral stenosis, the relationship characterizing the diastolic pressure difference between left atrial (P_1) and left ventricular pressure (P_2) and the flow rate (V_2) within the stenotic flow jet at any time (t), except at the time of valve opening or closure, can be described as follows:

$$(P_1 - P_2)(t) = 4\ [V_2(t)]^2. \hspace{4cm} \{B\}$$

The *pressure half-time* (PHT) is defined as the time interval over which the pressure gradient $(P_1 - P_2)$ drops to one-half its early diastolic peak value (t=0):

$$(P_1 - P_2)(t = PHT] = 1/2 \times (P_1 - P_2)(t=0). \hspace{2.5cm} \{C\}$$

By setting {B} into {C}, it follows that:

$$4\ (V_2[t=PHT])^2 = 1/2 \times 4 \times (V_2[t=0])^2, \hspace{2.5cm} \{D\}$$

and solving to $V_2(t=PHT)$ yields:

$$V_2(t=PHT) = 1/\sqrt{2} \times V_2(t=0) \hspace{3.5cm} \{E\}$$

The pressure half-time, which is less than 60 ms in normals, ranges from 100 to 400 ms or more in patients with mild to severe mitral stenosis. The pressure half-time correlates with the mitral valve area. A proportional relationship was found to exist between pressure half-time and mitral valve areas measured at the time of surgery or autopsy [30, 31]. The pressure half-time also remains relatively unaffected by the transvalvular stroke volume. This makes it acceptable to infer the mitral valve area from the pressure half-time [22]. When the pressure half-time is greater than 220 ms, the MVA is usually less than 1.00 cm^2.

Similar mathematical correlations were derived from comparisons of invasively measured mitral valve areas and Doppler pressure half-time values.

MVA (cm^2) = 220/PHT (ms)
MVA   Mitral valve area PHT   Pressure half time

Differences in empirical constants (195-239) found by comparing invasive study data are probably attributable to technique differences and linear versus non-linear approximations. Due to the hyperbolic relationship between pressure half-time and the mitral valve area, the proportional relationship for short pressure half-times increases sharply.

This may lead to error, even when high-speed paper transport is used during signal recording.

The main advantage of the pressure half-time method is that it remains relatively unaffected by the flow rate. It is a valuable tool for the assessment of combined mitral valvular disease. In these patients, a steep drop in pressure may be attributable to 1) obstruction when the stenosis is the dominant lesion or to 2) a large transvalvular stroke volume when regurgitation is dominant. Given a prestenotic flow velocity of > 1 m/s, the latter can be described according to the Bernoulli equation as follows:

$$\Delta P = 4 \times (V_2^2 - V_1^2)$$

The same applies for patients with low output syndrome or small transvalvular stroke volumes. Then, if attention is focused solely on the low pressure gradient, the severity of obstruction may be underestimated.

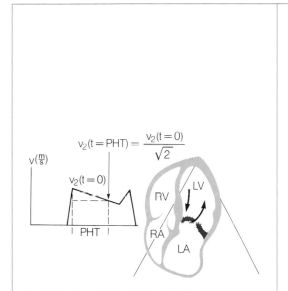

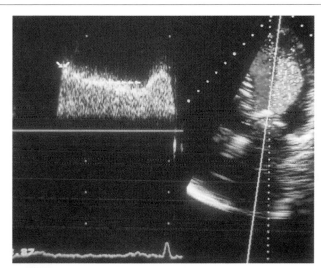

Color CW Doppler and 2-D echocardiograms; apical four-chamber view.

Calculation of pressure half-time (PHT). The PHT corresponds to the time interval over which the early diastolic peak velocity V_2 (t=0) drops to the reduced transmitral flow velocity of $V_2(t=0) / \sqrt{2}$.

The pressure half-time is calculated as the mean of the peak instantaneous velocities from five diastoles. Beat-to-beat changes in the pressure half-time are relatively low when taken as the mean value of five diastoles (7% on average). The figure is 8% in atrial fibrillation and slightly less (5%) with sinus rhythm [9].

The geometry of the spectral curves for Doppler frequency is reminiscent of the significance of EF slope in M-mode echocardiography. However, similar spectral curve slopes lead to completely different pressure half-times when peak instantaneous early diastolic flow velocities differ substantially. The higher the velocity, the steeper the slope, despite a significantly extended pressure half-time. The lower the velocity, the flatter may be the slope in the presence of a normal pressure half-time.

Although Doppler-derived pressure half-time values are routinely used to quantitate mitral stenosis, only few studies have been performed to validate the technique on the basis of direct pressure measurements. A recent study [10] comparing the mitral valve area measured from simultaneous LA-LV pressure measurements using the Gorlin formula and the pressure half-time method found that Doppler measurements correlated well, although the statistical curve was curvilinear. These results were contradicted by another study, which found a poor correlation between both invasive and Doppler pressure half-time measurements and results obtained using the Gorlin formula [50]. This may also be due to differences in methodology and patient characteristics as well as to differences in the approximation relationships used to derive the figures [51].

Limitations are known for both methods, due to particular hemodynamic constellations.

In volume overloaded conditions, the Gorlin formula tends to underestimate the mitral valve area, whereas the pressure half-time method tends to overestimate [16, 17, 39, 41, 55, 58].

When mitral stenosis is accompanied by more severe aortic regurgitation, the degree of error in the pressure half-time method apparently correlates with the severity of aortic regurgitation. The effects of aortic regurgitation on the pressure half-time may in addition to intermingling the mitral stenotic and aortic regurgitation jets be attributable to a steep increase in left ventricular diastolic pressure which, in turn, leads to a sharp drop in the transmitral pressure gradient. Similar overestimation of the mitral valve area may be expected when the pressure half-time method is used in patients with severely restricted left ventricular compliance due, for example, to ischemic or myocardial heart disease.

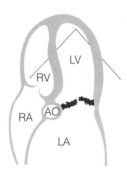

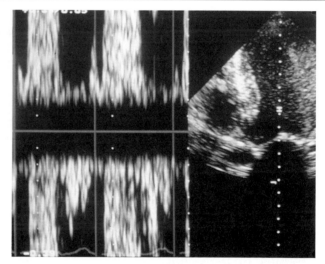

Mild to moderate mitral stenosis. Note diastolic doming of the mitral valve and aliasing in Doppler frequency spectrum with over-extended measurement range (accelerated transmitral inflow).

PW Doppler; apical 4-chamber 2-D echocardiogram; ECG triggering.

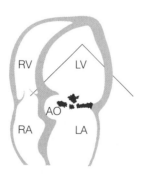

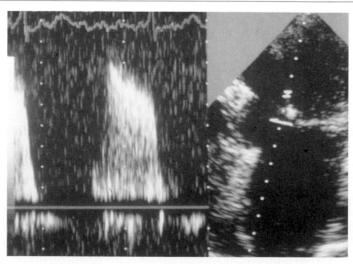

Moderate mitral stenosis. Calcification is seen on the tip of the anterior mitral leaflet. Sample volume was placed immediately proximal to leaflet tips. Enlargement of the left atrium was also found.

PW Doppler and apical four-chamber 2-D echocardiogram.

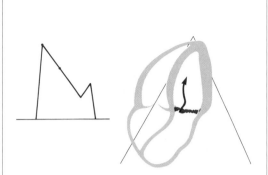

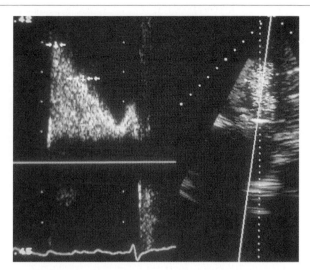

Mitral stenosis. Pressure half-time = 165 ms. Note twin peaked CW Doppler frequency spectrum in sinus rhythm. Early diastolic peak instantaneous velocity of 1.90 m/s. After 165 ms it drops to $1.90/\sqrt{2} = 1.35$ m/s.

Color PW Doppler and apical four-chamber 2-D echocardiograms.

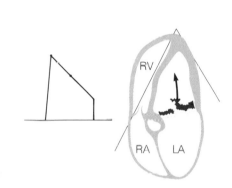

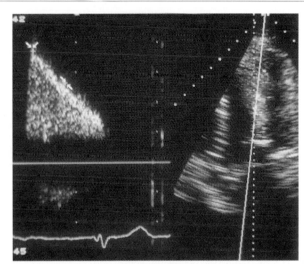

Mitral stenosis. Pressure half-time = 195 ms. Single peaked CW Doppler frequency spectrum in atrial fibrillation. Early diastolic peak instantaneous velocity = 1.83 m/s. After 195 ms it drops to $1.83/\sqrt{2} \approx 1.30$ m/s.

Color CW Doppler and apical four-chamber 2-D echocardiograms.

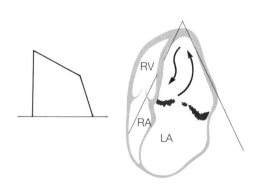

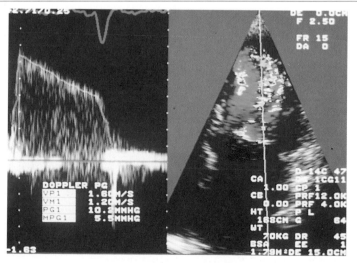

Planimetered CW Doppler frequency spectrum. Peak instantaneous flow velocity = 1.60 m/s. Mean flow velocity = 1.20 m/s. Peak instantaneous pressure gradient = 10.2 mmHg. Mean pressure gradient = 5.5 mmHg. Atrial fibrillation.

Color CW Doppler and apical four-chamber 2-D echocardiograms.

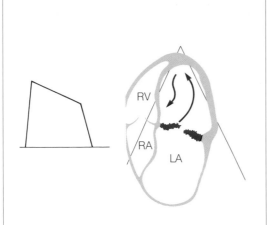

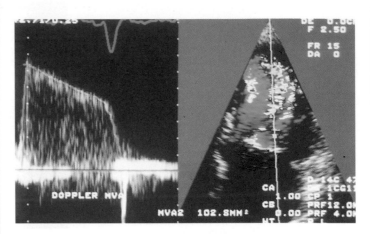

Same patient. Pressure half-time = 214 ms. MVA = 1.03 cm². MVA-I = 0.58 cm²; body surface area = 1.78 m².

Color CW Doppler and apical four-chamber 2-D echocardiograms.

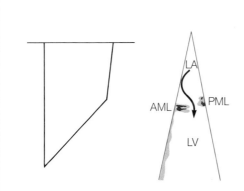

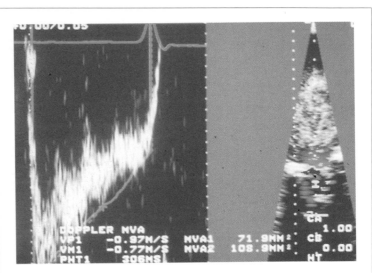

Mitral valve calcification with spontaneous contrast in left atrium. Sample volume placed directly distal to the mitral valve in left ventricle. PW Doppler frequency spectrum oriented downstream. Large range of scatter in MVA data (range = 0.72 to 1.09 cm²). Atrial fibrillation.

Color PW Doppler and transesophageal long-axis view.

The disadvantages of computing the mitral valve area using the Gorlin formula and the pressure half-time method become especially critical in conjunction with transluminal valvuloplasty or stress tests [5]. Use of the *continuity equation* (described below), which entails determination of the cross-sectional area (CSA) of the pulmonary valve region, the flow velocities there and in the mitral stenotic flow jet, was therefore recommended.

$$(A_1) \cdot (V_1) = (A_2) \cdot (V_2)$$

$$(A_{PA}) \cdot (V_{max, PA}) = (MVA) \cdot (V_{max, MS})$$

$$MVA\ [cm^2] \quad = (A_{PA}[cm^2] \cdot V_{max, PA}\ [m/s])/V_{max, MS}\ [m/s]$$

$A_1 = A_{PA}$	Systolic CSA of pulmonary trunk (diameter between the insertions of the pulmonary valve cusps)
$V_1 = V_{max, PA}$	Peak instantaneous flow velocity through the pulmonary valve
$A_2 = MVA$	Mitral valve area
$V_2 = V_{max, MS}$	Peak instantaneous flow velocity of mitral stenotic flow jet

The continuity equation is more time-consuming and its use in calculation of the cross sectional area (CSA) is sometimes questionable. However, the main disadvantage of the continuity equation is that it underestimates MVA in patients with coexistent mitral regurgitation [17, 39, 40].

The equation can be simplified to the ratio of time-velocity integrals of mitral flow and pulmonary flow (or aortic flow in absence of aortic disease) [40]. However, a considerable range of error will arise in certain cases.

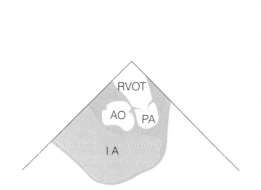

Calculation of MVA using the continuity equation: CSA in the region of the pulmonary valve is determined; systolic pulmonary trunk diameter at the level of the pulmonary valve cusps = 1.95 mm. Dilated left atrium.

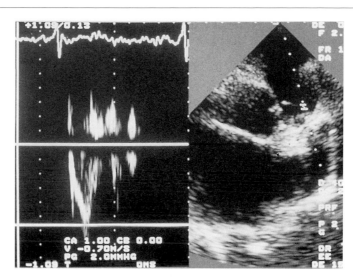

Parasternal short-axis 2-D echocardiogram.

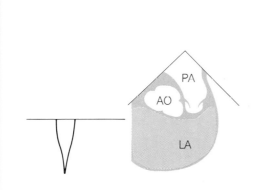

Calculation of MVA using the continuity equation: peak instantaneous flow velocity across the pulmonary valve = 0.70 m/s. Dilated left atrium.

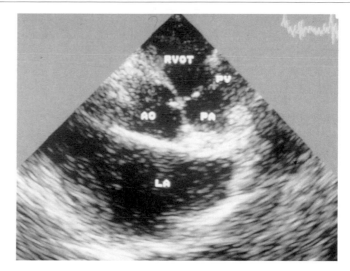

Left parasternal short-axis 2-D echocardiogram.

Example:

$$
\begin{aligned}
\text{MVA} &= (A_{PA})(V_{max,\,PA})/(V_{max,\,MS}) \\
&= \{[(1.95\ \text{cm}/2)^2 \times (3.14)] \times (0.70\ \text{m/s})\} / (1.71\ \text{m/s}) \\
&= [(0.95\ \text{cm}^2) \times (0.70\ \text{m/s})] / (1.71\ \text{m/s}) \\
&= (0.67\ \text{cm}^2\ \text{m/s}) / (1.71\ \text{m/s}) \\
&= 0.39\ \text{cm}^2
\end{aligned}
$$

(Planimetered minimal mitral valve area = 0.41 cm². Mitral orifice area determined by pressure half-time method = 0.86 cm² (mean value of 5 measurements): severe (= "critical") mitral stenosis, moderate aortic regurgitation.)

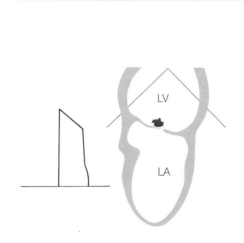

Calculation of mitral valve area using the continuity equation. Peak instantaneous flow velocity, as measured through the mitral valve = 1.71 m/s.

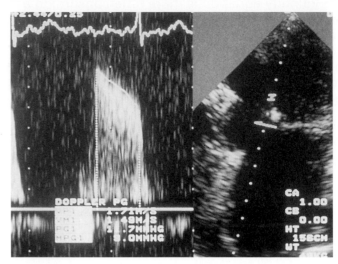

PW Doppler and apical four-chamber 2-D echocardiograms.

Simplified Gorlin Formula [2, 21, 42]:

$MVA \ (cm^2) = CO \ (l/min) \ \sqrt{\Delta P_m} \ (mmHg)$

MVA	Mitral valve area
CO	Cardiac output
ΔP_m	Transmitral pressure gradient

The simplified Gorlin formula permits non-invasive assessment of mitral stenosis while disregarding diastolic filling time, frequency and constants. As compared with the original formula [41], discrepancies in mitral valve area measurement (due mainly to heart rate variability) do arise in approximately 50% of all patients examined. However, since the measurements and calculations required for applying the simplified Gorlin formula are often routinely incorporated into other measurement programs, additional comparison data is usually on hand in equivocal cases.

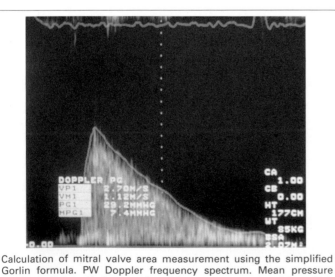

Calculation of mitral valve area measurement using the simplified Gorlin formula. PW Doppler frequency spectrum. Mean pressure gradient = 7.4 mmHg (mean value of five measurements = 6.8 mmHg).

Example:

$MVA = CO/\sqrt{\Delta P_m}$

$MVA = (3.50 \text{ l/min})/(\sqrt{6.80 \text{ mm Hg}}) = (3.50 \text{ l/min})/(2.61 \text{ mmHg})$

$MVA = 1.35 \text{ cm}^2$

Minimum mitral valve area detected by planimetry = 1.68 cm². Mitral orifice area via pressure half-time method = 1.33 cm² (mean of five measurements): moderately severe (moderate) mitral stenosis.

One color Doppler quantification technique assesses the assumed elliptical origin of the mitral stenotic flow jet from two perpendicular planes [26]. Another first measures proximal acceleration flow until the onset of color aliasing to obtain a product based on the Nyquist limit and peak instantaneous transmitral flow velocity [44]. These methods correlate acceptably with invasive date. Additional techniques for Doppler quantification of mitral stenosis have also been described. Some use a combination of Doppler and invasive techniques [24]. Others are unsuitable for assessing severe mitral stenosis, because the given parameters are restricted by aliasing in pulsed-wave Doppler recordings [11, 25, 53].

10.3.2   Mitral Stenosis
10.3.2.2   Sources of Error

In conventional echocardiographic techniques for assessment of mitral stenosis, errors can arise due to:
- Diminished EF slope caused by mitral annular motion or simulated by an extremely long diastole in patients with atrial fibrillation;
- Reduced diastolic mitral leaflet separation due to low stroke volume and low cardiac output;
- Motion variance in interventricular septum due to necrosis causing a dyskinetic motion pattern or due to conduction disturbances mimicking a very deep early diastolic dip.

When planimetering the mitral valve area from the left parasternal short-axis view, errors can be systematically avoided by first determining the maximum vertical diastolic separation of the leaflet tips from the left parasternal long-axis view, then rotating the transducer 90° to the short-axis position. From there, the transducer should be angled and panned along the long axis of the left ventricle toward the papillary muscles, then angled to the point where the mitral leaflet tips first reappear. Proper gain adjustment is essential for obtaining clear images; too much gain will result in underestimation of the mitral orifice area. Furthermore, the valve must be imaged at the level of the tips of the mitral valve leaflets; imaging at the base of the mitral valve funnel will result in overestimation of the orifice area.

Minimize error in Doppler quantification of mitral stenosis in patients with:
- *atrial fibrillation* by obtaining measurements from as many beats as possible, then calculating the mean value from them.
- *coexistent regurgitation* by using prestenotic flow velocity of >1 m/s to calculate the pressure gradient across the mitral valve using the Bernoulli equation.
- *increased cardiac output* by using, in addition to the pressure half-time method, the continuity equation, the simplified Gorlin formula, and planimetry of the mitral valve area from the left parasternal short-axis view for comparison and control.

In addition to hypertension, left atrial hemodynamic consequences of mitral stenosis also include an increase in end-systolic volume and a reduced ejection fraction with normal or increased stroke volume [4]. Although the reduced left ventricular filling phase in atrial fibrillation may be caused by loss of the atrial contribution, it is more likely to be caused by the increased ventricular heart rate [37].

Hemodynamic findings in the left ventricle include reduced cardiac output with increased total peripheral resistance and a reduced ejection fraction. Approximately one-third of all patients with mitral stenosis have reduced ventricular function in the ejection phase due to increased afterload in conjunction with reduced preload. In other words, the Frank-Starling relation is altered [54]. The systolic myocardial properties of the left ventricle, assessed as endsystolic pressure-volume relationship, are normal. In other words, the change in left ventricular performance results from preload and afterload changes and from the reduced ventricular size, whereas the muscle function remains basically unchanged [7, 20]. In fact, left ventricular systolic function does not appear to have a significant influence on the natural course of mitral stenosis or on the outcome of surgery.

The subvalvular apparatus essential for ventricular function plays a less important role in prosthetic mitral valve replacement due to mitral stenosis than in preexisting mitral regurgitation [45].

The diastolic pressure-volume relationship in patients with mitral stenosis is displaced to the left due to reduced end-diastolic volume.

10.3.2   **Mitral Stenosis**
10.3.2.4   **Follow-up and Treatment Considerations**

When left untreated, rheumatic mitral stenosis usually progresses gradually, but rapid progression is sometimes seen. Rapid progression is more likely to occur in patients with high transmitral pressure gradients, those with severely thickened, calcified and mobility-restricted leaflets, and in those with severe scarring and contracture of the subvalvular apparatus. These patients therefore require more frequent follow-up examinations [18].

Follow-up of patients with mitral stenosis has to look for:
1. Worsening of obstruction, determined by comparing MVA measurements;
2. Severe pulmonary hypertension, determined by measuring pressure in the lesser circulation at rest and under stress and by measuring pulmonary arteriole resistance;
3. Risk factors such as thrombo-embolic complications (*e.g.* left atrial thrombus, paroxysmal or chronic atrial fibrillation) and accompanying diseases that may influence survival.

The use of ultrasound in follow-up examinations has to answer the questions of the physician who must act upon the provided findings.

As regards points (1) and (3), the cardiac ultrasound examination can provide information essential for treatment [48].

To point 1: The progression of mitral stenosis can be determined by comparing data with previous MVA/MVA-I measurements. Surgery is indicated in severe or moderately severe mitral stenosis.

To point 2: Factors that increase perioperative mortality and worsen the postoperative prognosis include patient age, severity of the condition assessed according to the New York Heart Association's classification scheme, increased pulmonary arteriole resistance, and a reduced cardiac index due to reduced ventricular function primarily attributable to secondary cardiac diseases.

To point 3: The incidence of proximal pulmonary artery embolism in patients with hemodynamically significant mitral disease and pulmonary hypertension is 61% [47]. Two factors that affect the prognosis are cerebral and recurring peripheral embolism. The sensitivity and specificity of transthoracic echocardiography for detecting left atrial thrombi is 56% and 94%, respectively. That of transesophageal echocardiography is 89% and 98%, respectively. Thrombus was found in the left atrial appendage in 10% and 90% of these cases, respectively. Thrombi weighing less than 15 g were found in 33% and 78%, respectively.

The debate over the best timing of surgery in mitral stenosis has been refuelled by the advent of valvuloplasty. The procedure is now performed earlier and more freely, because it does not cause complications in later surgery. New criteria to define patient suitability were therefore required.

Leaflet thickening, calcification, motility and/or flexibility, as well as subvalvular apparatus involvement have been systematically studied and compared. The resulting echocardiographic indices were evaluated for their suitability for use in predicting the patient's suitability for valvuloplasty [1, 3, 34]. Of these variables, *leaflet thickness* and *involvement of the subvalvular apparatus* proved to be the best morphological predictors of the most extensive enlargement of the orifice area.

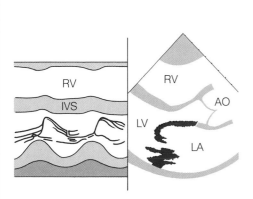

Mild leaflet calcification with moderate involvement of the subvalvular apparatus. Annular calcification in the vicinity of the posterior leaflet, the motility of which is not significantly impaired. Absence of mitral regurgitation. Conditions are favorable for percutaneous transluminal valvuloplasty.

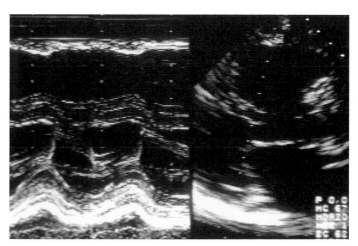

2-D and M-mode; left parasternal long-axis view at mitral valve level.

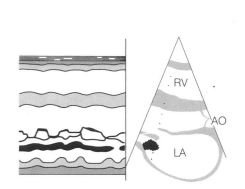

Moderate calcification, particularly in posterior mitral leaflet. There is significant involvement of the subvalvular apparatus with massive annular calcification, severe impairment of motility in both leaflets, and moderate mitral regurgitation. These conditions are unfavorable for percutaneous transluminal valvuloplasty.

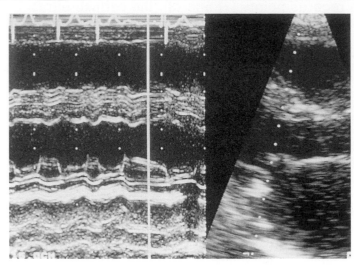

2-D and M-modes; left parasternal long-axis view at mitral valve level.

Though the effective balloon dilation area and probably the underlying heart rhythm, too, are of relatively greater importance in predicting the maximum increase in the orifice area than those scores.

10.3.2   Mitral Stenosis
10.3.2.5   Critical Evaluation of Results and Comparison With Those
of Complementary Diagnostic Techniques

Cardiac ultrasound can provide decisive findings for grading mitral stenosis and for planning the best possible treatment. The most significant parameters are the mitral valve area index, the mean transmitral pressure gradient, a descriptive analysis of valve morphology and dynamics, and morphometric data. In some cases, planimetry of the mitral valve area from the left parasternal short-axis view and computations derived from the continuity equation and the Gorlin formula provide significant comparison data.

In right heart catheterization, pressure-flow measurements in the lesser circulation obtained during stress testing can provide important information for surgical planning and timing.

Left heart catheterization is performed only when it is necessary to exclude or confirm suspected concomitant ischemic heart disease that may require additional revascularization at the time of surgery. The patient's medical history and symptoms do not play a decisive role in determining the necessity of surgical intervention [28].

Morphometry and ventricular function

RVEDD   _____ mm
LADmax   _____ mm
LVEDD   _____ mm
LVESD   _____ mm

Fractional shortening   _____

Signs of concomitant ischemic heart disease?
- wall motion analysis

Signs of pulmonary hypertension?
- Right lateral bulging of interatrial septum observed in subcostal four-chamber view
- RVOT-EDD   _____ mm

Valve morphology and dynamics

▸ Thickening and/or calcification of mitral leaflets,
  Grade and extent of calcification?
▸ Concordant M-shaped movement of posterior and anterior mitral leaflets?
▸ EF slope < 36 mm/s? or < 10 mm/s?
▸ Reduced motility or doming of mitral leaflets?
▸ Involvement of subvalvular apparatus?

Ventricular function and pressure-flow relationship (Doppler echocardiography)

▸ Velocity measurements (m/s)
  - peak instantaneous transmitral velocity
  - mean transmitral velocity
▸ Pressure gradients (mmHg)
  - peak instantaneous transmitral pressure gradient
  - mean transmitral pressure gradients
▸ Mitral valve orifice area (cm^2), orifice area index (cm^2/m^2)
  - derived from pressure half-time method
  - derived from continuity equation
  - planimetered from left parasternal short-axis view
    in patients with coexistent aortic regurgitation
  - derived from simplified Gorlin formula as a control when results seem dubious
▸ Regurgitant jet
  - qualitative visual assessment
▸ Intracardiac pressure (mmHg)
  - $PA_{systolic}$ with coexisting tricuspid regurgitation

Transesophageal echocardiography

▸ Left atrial thrombus?
▸ Valve morphology and dynamics

SYMPTOMATOLOGY / AUSCULTATION

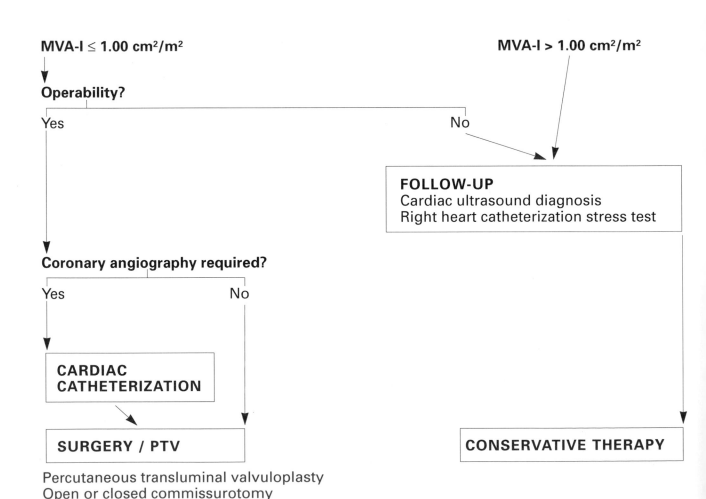

ECHOCARDIOGRAPHY

Conventional echocardiography:

Morphometry (RVEDD, RVOT-EDD, LADmax, LVEDD, LVESD),
Ventricular function (LVFS, wall motion analysis);
Visualization of underlying anatomic causes and hemodynamic effects

Doppler and transesophageal echocardiography (TEE):

Mitral valve area (MVA), Mitral orifice area index (MVA-I) according to
pressure half-time method
± Planimetry from left parasternal short-axis view
± Use of continuity equation in patients with coexistent aortic regurgitation

Paroxysmal or chronic atrial fibrillation?
TEE for exclusion/detection of left atrial thrombus

MVA-I ≤ 1.00 cm²/m²

Operability?

Yes ──────────── No

MVA-I > 1.00 cm²/m²

FOLLOW-UP
Cardiac ultrasound diagnosis
Right heart catheterization stress test

Coronary angiography required?

Yes ──── No

CARDIAC CATHETERIZATION

SURGERY / PTV

Percutaneous transluminal valvuloplasty
Open or closed commissurotomy
Valve replacement surgery

CONSERVATIVE THERAPY

1. Abascal VM, Wilkins GT, O'Shea JP, Choong CY, Palacios IF, Thomas JD, Rosas E, Newell JB, Block PC, Weyman AE. Prediction of successful outcome in 130 patients undergoing percutaneous balloon mitral valvotomy. Circulation 1990; 82: 448-456.
2. Angel J, Soler-Soler J, Anivarro I, Domingo E. Hemodynamic evaluation of stenotic cardiac valves: II.Modification of the simplified formula for mitral and aortic valve area calculation. Cathet Cardiovasc Diagn 1985; 11: 127-138.
3. Babic UU, Pejcic P, Djurisic Z, Vucinic M, Grujicic SN. Percutaneous transarterial balloon mitral valvuloplasty: 30 months experience. Herz 1988; 13: 91-99.
4. Boudoulas H, Barrington W, Wooley CF. Left atrial dynamics in mitral stenosis. Circulation 1988; 78 (suppl II): 1878.
5. Braverman AC, Lee TH, Lee RT. Mitral valve area determination during minor changes in hemodynamic state: Superiority of the continuity equation. J Am Coll Cardiol 1991; 17 (suppl A): 155A.
6. Brogan WC, Lange RA, Hillis LD. Limitations of the simplified formula for calculating valve area in patients with mitral stenosis. J Am Coll Cardiol 1991; 17 (suppl A): 254A.
7. Chang MS, Kass DA, Ting CT, Liu CP, Lawrence W, Maughan WL. Left ventricular function in mitral stenosis: A shrunken chamber. Circulation 1990; 82 (suppl III): 0959.
8. Chen C, Schneider B, Sievers B, Koschyk D, Meinertz T, Hamm C, Kupper W. Estimation of mitral valve area using biplane transesophageal color Doppler echocardiography. Circulation 1991; 84 (suppl II): 0515.
9. Dennig K, Rudolph W. Doppler-echokardiographische Bestimmung des Schweregrades der Mitralstenose. Herz 1984; 9: 222-230.
10. Denys BG, Reddy PS, Herrera L. Is the pressure half-time a valid technique to measure mitral valve area? Circulation 1990; 82 (suppl III): 0967.
11. Diebold B, Theroux P, Bourassa MG, Thuillez C, Peronneau P, Guermonprez JL, Xhaard M, Waters DD. Non-invasive pulsed Doppler study of mitral stenosis and mitral regurgitation: preliminary study. Brit Heart J 1979; 42: 168-175.
12. Duchak JM, Chang S, Feigenbaum H. The posterior mitral valve echo and the echocardiographic diagnosis of mitral stenosis. Am J Cardiol 1972; 29: 628-623.
13. Edler I, Gustafson A. Ultrasonic cardiogram in mitral stenosis. Acta Med Scand 1957; 159: 85-90.
14. Edler I. Ultrasound-cardiogram in mitral valvular disease. Acta Chir Scand 1956; 11: 230-231.
15. Edler I. Ultrasoundcardiography in mitral valve stenosis. Am J Cardiol 1967; 19: 18-31.
16. Flachskampf FA, Weyman AE, Gillam L, Chun-Ming L, Abascal VM, Thomas JD. Aortic regurgitation shortens Doppler pressure half-time in mitral stenosis: Clinical evidence, in vitro simulation and theoretic analysis. J Am Coll Cardiol 1990; 16: 396-404.
17. Gillam LD, Choong CY, Wilkins GT, Marshall JE. The effect of aortic insufficiency on Doppler pressure half-time calculations of mitral valve area in mitral stenosis. Circulation 1986; 74 (suppl II): II-217.
18. Gordon SPF, Douglas PS, Manning WJ. Echo-Doppler determinants of progressive stenosis in patients with rheumatic mitral valve disease. J Am Coll Cardiol 1991; 17 (suppl A): 298A.
19. Gorlin R, Gorlin WB. Further reconciliation between pathoanatomy and pathophysiology of stenotic cardiac valves. J Am Coll Cardiol 1990; 15: 1181-1182.
20. Goto S, Handa S, Akaishi M, Abe S, Ogawa S. Left ventricular ejection performance in patients with mitral stenosis. Circulation 1991; 84 (suppl II): 0160.
21. Hakki AH, Iskandrian AS, Bemis CE, Kimbiris D, Mintz GS, Segal BK, Brice C. A simplified valve formula for the calculation of stenotic cardiac valve areas. Circulation 1981; 63: 1050-1055.
22. Hatle L, Angelsen B. Doppler-ultrasound in cardiology. Physical principles and clinical applications. Lea & Febiger, Philadelphia 1982.
23. Henry WL, Griffith JM, Michaelis LL, McIntosh CL, Morrow AG, Epstein SE. Measurement of mitral orifice area in patients with mitral valve disease by real-time, two-dimensional echocardiography. Circulation 1975; 51: 827-831.
24. Holen J, Aaslid R, Landmark K, Simonson S, Ostrem T. Determination of effective orifice area in mitral stenosis from noninvasive ultrasound Doppler data and mitral flow rate. Acta Med Scand 1977; 201: 83-88.
25. Kalmanson D, Veyrat C, Bouchareine F, Degroote A. Noninvasive recording of mitral valve flow velocity patterns using pulsed Doppler echocardiography. Application to diagnosis and evaluation of mitral valve disease. Brit Heart J 1977; 39: 517-528.
26. Kawahara T, Tamai J, Mitani M, Seo H, Yamagishi M, Miyatake K. A new method for determination of mitral valve area in mitral stenosis by color Doppler flow imaging technique. Circulation 1989; 80 (suppl II): 2659.
27. Kotlewski A, McKay CR, Harrison EC, Kawanishi DT, Reid CL, Chandraratna PAN, Bhandari A, Elkayam U, Niland J, Rahimtoola SH. Incremental value of clinical examination, echocardiography, and cardiac catheterization in the evaluation of mitral valve disease. Circulation 1987; 76 (suppl IV): 0350.
28. Kraus F, Rudolph W. Symptoms, exercise capacity and exercise hemodynamics: Interrelationships and their role in quantification of the valvular lesions. Herz 1984; 9: 187-199.

29. Lee GW, Hsu TL, Chang MS, Chen CY, Wang SP, Chang BN, Pandian N. Exercise Doppler echocardiography aids in the assessment of the functional severity of mitral stenosis and the efficacy of balloon mitral valvuloplasty. J Am Coll Cardiol 1991; 17 (suppl A): 68A.
30. Libanoff AJ, Rodbard S. Atrioventricular pressure half-time. Measure of mitral valve orifice area. Circulation 1968; 38: 144.
31. Libanoff AJ, Rodbard S. Evaluation of the severity of mitral stenosis and regurgitation. Circulation 1966; 33: 218-226.
32. Marcus RH, Sareli P, Pocock WA, Barlow JB. Mechanisms of rheumatic mitral valve disease. Influence of disease acitivity on valve lesion. Circulation 1988; 78 (suppl II): 1877.
33. Martin RP, Rakowski H, Kleimann JH, Beaver W, London E, Popp RL. Reliability and reproducibility of two-dimensional echocardiographic measurement of the stenotic mitral valve orifice area. Am J Cardiol 1979; 43: 560-568.
34. Marwick TH, Stewart WJ, Salcedo EE, Casale PN, Lytle BW, Loop FD, Cosgrove DM. Echo splitability score predicts the requirement for valve replacement vs repair for mitral stenosis. Circulation 1989; 80 (suppl II): 0665.
35. Matsumura M, Kyo S, Shah P, Yokote Y, Omoto R. A new look at mitral valve pathology with bi-plane color Doppler transesophageal probe. Circulation 1989; 80 (suppl II): 2298.
36. Matsumura M, Shah P, Kyo S, Omoto R. Advantages of transesophageal echo for correct diagnosis on small left atrial thrombi in mitral stenosis. Circulation 1989; 80 (suppl II): 2693.
37. Meisner JS, Keren G, Pajaro OE, Mani A, Strom JA, Frater RWM, Laniado S, Yellin EL. Atrila contribution to ventricular filling in mitral stenosis. Circulation 1991; 84: 1469-1480.
38. Miller G. Invasive investigation of the heart. A guide to cardiac catheterization and related procedures. Oxford: Blackwell, 1989: p. 271, tbl. 15.1b und p. 274.
39. Moro E, Nicolosi GI, Burelli C, Zanuttini D, Roelandt J. Aortic regurgitation in patients with mitral stenosis: influence on determination of pressure half-time for mitral valve area calculation. Circulation 1986; 74 (suppl II): II-231.
40. Nakatani S, Masuyama T, Kodama K, Kitabatake A, Fuji K, Kamada T. Value and limitations of Doppler echocardiography in the quantification of stenotic mitral valve area: comparison of the pressure half-time and the continuity equation methods. Circulation 1988; 77: 78-85.
41. Nakatani S, Masuyama T, Sato H, Ohara T, Uematsu M, Kodama K. Noninvasive estimation of stenotic mitral valve area: Comparison of pressure half-time and continuity equation methods. Circulation 1987; 76 (suppl IV): 1411.
42. Nigri A, Martuscelli E, Mangieri E, Voci P, Danesi A, Sardella R, Feroci L, Reale A. Nomogram for calculation of stenotic cardiac valve areas from cardiac output and mean transvalvular gradient. Cathet Cardiovasc Diagn 1984; 10: 613-618.
43. Robson DJ, Flaxman JC. Measurement of the end-diastolic pressure gradient and mitral valve area in mitral stenosis by Doppler ultrasound. Europ Heart J 1984; 5: 660-667.
44. Rodriguez L, Levine RA, Monteroso VH, Thomas JD, Abascal VM, Mueller L, Weyman AE. Validation of valve area calculation using the proximal isovelocity surface area in patients with mitral stenosis: A color Doppler study. Circulation 1989; 80 (suppl II): 2691.
45. Salter, DR, Murphy CE, Brunsting TA, Pellom GL, Goldstein JP, Wechsler AS. Mitral valve replacement in the failing ventricle. Circulation 1989; 80 (suppl II): 1686.
46. Shiu M, Jenkins BS, Webb-Peploe MM. Echocardiographic analysis of posterior mitral leaflet movement in mitral stenosis. Brit Heart J 1978; 40: 372-376.
47. Skoulagiris J, Essop R, Middlemost S, Nicola G di, Sarelli P. The incidence of proximal pulmonary thrombotic disease in patients with significant rheumatic mitral valve disease and pulmonary hypertension. Circulation 1989; 80 (suppl II): 0035.
48. Slater J, Gindea AJ, Freedberg RS, Chinitz LA, Tunick PA, Rosenzweig BP, Winer HE, Goldfarb A, Perez JL, Glassman E, Kronzon I. Comparison of cardiac catheterization and Doppler echocardiography in the decision to operate in aortic and mitral valve disease. J Am Coll Cardiol 1991; 17: 1026-1036.
49. Smith HD, Handshoe R, Handshoe S, Dwan OL, DeMaria AN. Comparative accuracy of two-dimensional echocardiography and Doppler pressure half-time methods in assessing the severity of mitral stenosis in patients with and without prior commissurotomy. Circulation 1986; 73: 100-107.
50. Smith MD, Gurley JC, Spain MG, Wisenbaugh T. Accuracy of pressure half-time in quantifying mitral stenosis in a clinically relevant range: Comparison with micromanometer catheter recordings. Circulation 1987; 76 (suppl IV): 1410.
51. Tabbalat RA, Haft JI. Doppler pressure half-time is more accurate than the Gorlin equation in patients with mitral stenosis and severe pulmonary hypertension. Circulation 1990; 82 (suppl III): 0966.
52. Thompson CR, Kingma I, MacDonald RPR, Belenkie I, Tyberg JV, Smith ER. Transseptal pressure gradient and diastolic ventricular septal motion in patients with mitral stenosis. Circulation 1987; 76: 974-980.
53. Thuillez C, Theroux P, Bourassa MG, Blanchard D, Peronneau P, Guermonprez JL, Diebold B, Waters DD, Maurice P. Pulsed Doppler echocardiographic study of mitral stenosis. Circulation 1980; 61: 381-387.
54. Toutoutzas P. Left ventricular function in mitral valve disease. Herz 1984; 9: 297-305.
55. Walling A, Foster A, Richards KL, Crawford MH, Cannon SR, Archibeque DC. Effect of altering left ventricular volume on mitral valve orifice area during exercise. J Am Coll Cardiol 1991; 17 (suppl A): 69A.

56. Weyman AE, Wann LS, Rogers EW, Godley RW, Dillon JC, Feigenbaum H, Green D. Five-year experience in correlating cross-sectional echocardiographic assessment of the mitral valve area with hemodynamic valve area determinations. Am J Cardiol 1979; 43: 386.
57. Winer H, Slater J, Chinitz L, Glassman E, Spencer F, Earls J, Post J. Predictors of surgical outcome in isolated mitral stenosis. Circulation 1988; 78 (suppl II): 1518.
58. Wisenbaugh T, Berk M, Essop R, Middlemost S, Sareli P. Effect of mitral regurgitation and volume loading on pressure half-time before and after balloon valvotomy in patients with mitral stenosis. Circulation 1990; 82 (suppl III): 1986.

10.4	**Aortic Valve Disease**
10.4.1	**Aortic Insufficiency**
	(Irmtraut Kruck)

Aortic insufficiency is caused by diseases involving the aortic valve or aortic root. Various etiologies are listed below.

Chronic aortic insufficiency

- ► Rheumatic aortic valve lesions
- ► Degenerative-myxomatous aortic valve lesions
- ► Infective Endocarditis
- ► Inflammatory diseases of the aorta and the aortic valve
  (aortitis syndromes, e.g. bacterial aortitis and mycotic aneurysm, other "nonspecific" aortitis syndromes, luetic aortitis, systemic Lupus erythermatosus, rheumatoid arthritis, ankylosing spondylitis, Reiter's syndrome, Jaccoud's arthropathy, Whipple's disease, Crohn's disease and diseases of the aorta such as Takayasu's giant cell arteriitis syndromes of the aortic arch)
- ► Congenital aortic disease
- ► Bicuspid aortic valve
- ► Aortic valve prolapse
- ► Ventricular septal defect
- ► Aneurysm of a sinus of Valsalva
- ► Overstretching of the annular ring in connective tissue disorders (aortic ectasia, senile media degeneration, kryptogenic cystic media degeneration in Marfan's syndrome, Ehlers-Danlos syndrome)
- ► Atherosclerosis and arterial hypertension
- ► Aortic dissection

Acute aortic insufficiency

- ► Infective endocarditis
- ► Acute aortic dissection
- ► Ruptured aneurysm of a sinus of Valsalva
- ► Traumatic aortic insufficiency
- ► Acute prosthetic valve incompetence after valve and/or ascending aorta replacement

As in mitral regurgitation, one also differentiates between acute and chronic aortic insufficiency. The chronic form is seen mainly in degenerative or rheumatic etiologies, luetic or degenerative aortic aneurysms, and in bicuspid valves. Acute aortic insufficiency most commonly arises during or after infective endocarditis or due to acute dissecting aortic aneurysms. Echocardiographic evaluation of the aortic valve is performed from the parasternal long and short-axis views, apical "five-chamber view", and apical long-axis view. Aortic cusps and morphological features of the aorta can be evaluated from subcostal and suprasternal views.

Conventional Echocardiography

Two-dimensional echocardiography:

- Assessment of morphological features and motion of the aortic cusps. *Diastolic separation* or an *eccentric diastolic closure echo* are nonspecific signs of aortic regurgitation.

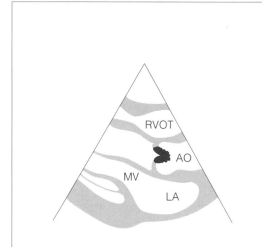

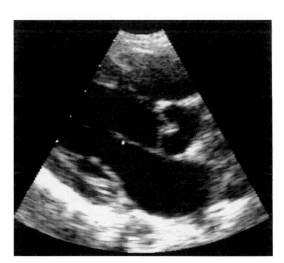

Aortic regurgitation. Thickened aortic valves with double contour lines. Dilated aortic root. Normal-sized left ventricle.

Parasternal long-axis 2-D echocardiogram.

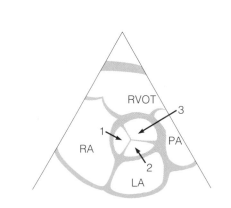

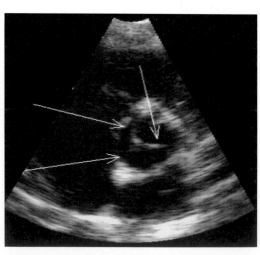

Aortic cusps are delicate and eccentrically located in the diastolic closure position. The right (arrow 1) and noncoronary (arrow 2) aortic cusps are relatively small, whereas the left coronary cusp (arrow 3) is clearly higher.

2-D parasternal short-axis view at aortic valve level.

- *Diastolic fluttering* of the mitral valve is not clearly identifiable in 2-D echocardiograms because of poor resolution quality. Regurgitation frequently causes abnormal mitral valve motion that is echocardiographically similar to mitral valve prolapse (reversed doming). Prolapse of the aortic cusps can be detected in the parasternal long-axis view as well as in the apical two and five-chamber views [11, 31, 62].

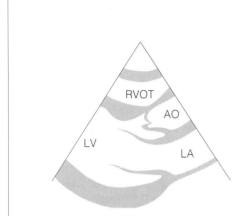

The aortic cusps (AKP) that are closed during diastole (right and noncoronary cusps) prolapse into the left ventricular outflow tract (arrow). The cusps are not calcified.

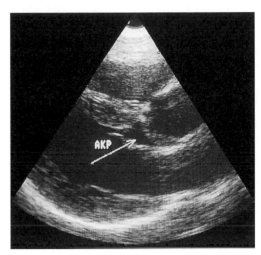

Parasternal long-axis 2-D echocardiogram.

- 2-D echocardiography can also be used to determine *width of the aortic root* and to detect *aneurysmal dilatation of the sinuses of Valsalva.*

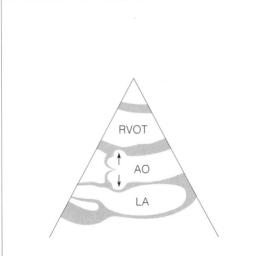

Slight bulging of anterior and posterior sinuses of Valsalva. Normal sized heart cavities.

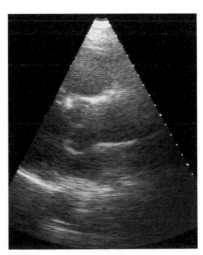

Parasternal long-axis 2-D echocardiogram in systole.

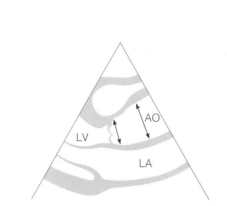

The base of the proximal aortic root is of normal size (arrow a), but the root broadens distally (arrow b). No double contours are seen in the aortic wall region; aneurysmal dilatation of the ascending aorta.

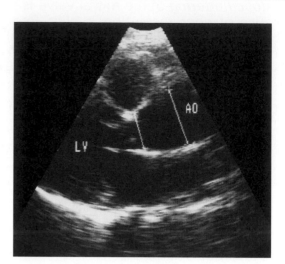

Parasternal long-axis 2-D echocardiogram.

Two-dimensional echocardiography can also detect *proximal aneurysm* or *dissection*.

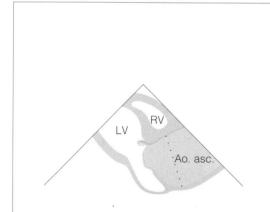

Massive dilatation of the ascending aorta (diameter = 70 mm), which displaces the left atrium (LA). Due to this dilation, the left ventricle (LV) is also high arched = aneurysm of the ascending aorta with no evidence of dissection in this

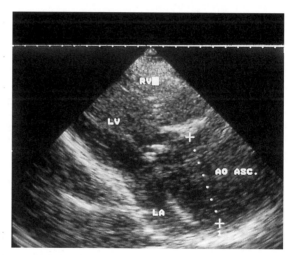

2-D parasternal long-axis view at aortic valve level.

Left ventricular size and contractility can be assessed in apical 2-D echocardiograms.

M-mode echocardiography:

- Although *diastolic separation of the aortic cusps* is suggestive of aortic regurgitation, the finding is frequently observed in normals and may simply result from view-related distortion.

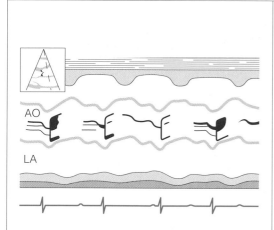

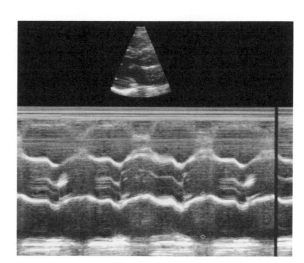

Aortic cusps are slightly thickened; opening is diminished but sufficient. Parallel echoes are detected in diastole. The left atrium is not enlarged.

M-mode; parasternal long-axis view at aortic valve level.

A characteristic feature of aortic insufficiency is high-frequency *diastolic fluttering of the anterior mitral leaflet*. Depending on the jet direction, similar fluttering may also be seen in the posterior mitral leaflet, ventricular septum or posterior wall [9, 26, 40].

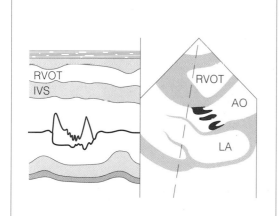

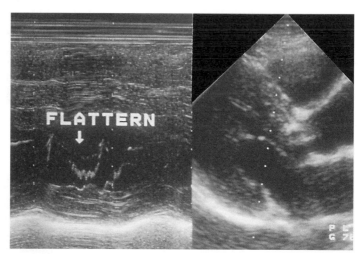

Thickened aortic cusps. In diastole the anterior mitral leaflet displays the zigzag motion pattern typical of aortic insufficiency. No fluttering of the posterior mitral leaflet is detected.

M-mode and 2-D; parasternal long-axis view at mitral valve level.

Diastolic fluttering of the anterior mitral leaflet is a highly specific feature that is observed in 90% of all cases of confirmed aortic insufficiency, whereas endocardial fluttering from the septum and anterior wall are observed in only 50% of cases. Neither the intensity nor duration of fluttering correlates with the severity of regurgitation. When the regurgitant jet is directed towards the septum, mitral valve fluttering may be completely absent. No fluttering occurs in patients with severe mitral stenosis or mitral valve replacement, either [30]. Severe aortic insufficiency can lead to diminished early diastolic opening of the mitral valve [20]; a reduced or absent DE amplitude can then be detected in M-mode scans.

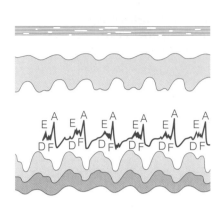

Anterior mitral valve opening in early diastole is clearly smaller than at end-diastole. The left ventricle is dilated. The mitral valve itself is thin. Mitral valve fluttering is detected in early diastole. No fluttering detected in interventricular

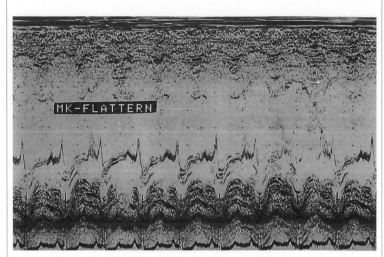

M-mode; parasternal long-axis view at mitral valve level.

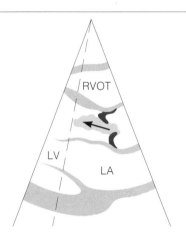

The aortic cusps are thickened. In diastole there is turbulent backward flow in the left ventricular outflow tract, a sign of aortic insufficiency.

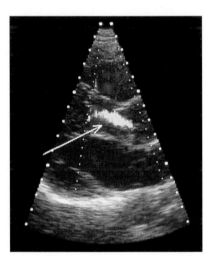

Color flow map of parasternal long-axis 2-D echocardiogram.

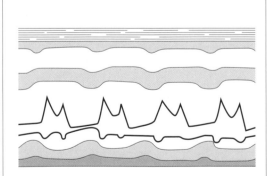

Same patient. The mitral valve motion pattern is completely normal in the presence of aortic insufficiency (AI).

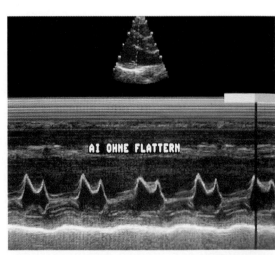

2-D and M-mode; parasternal long-axis view at mitral valve level.

In severe aortic insufficiency, the left ventricular end-diastolic pressure exceeds left atrial pressure. This leads to *premature mitral valve closure* and *premature aortic cusp opening*, particularly in acute cases [36]. However, these signs are no longer recognizable in patients with tachycardia. As the severity of aortic insufficiency progressively increases, *progressive dilatation of the left ventricle* ultimately occurs. M-mode echocardiography is particularly useful in detecting this.

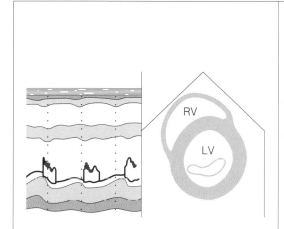

The left ventricle is hypertrophic and dilated. The contractile function of the ventricle is already diminished. The anterior mitral leaflet shows no signs of fluttering.

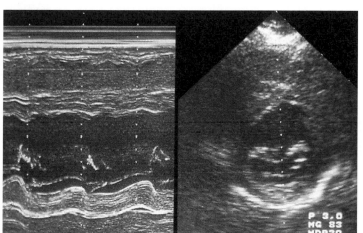

M-mode and 2-D; parasternal short-axis view at mitral valve level.

These findings, together with pathological or increased mitral-septal separation, are suggestive of progressive left ventricular failure [52].

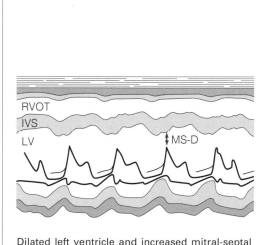

Dilated left ventricle and increased mitral-septal separation distance (MS-D).

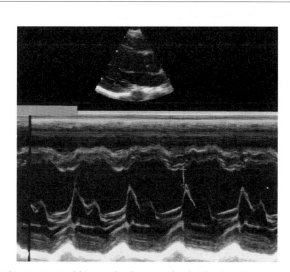

M-mode; parasternal long-axis view at mitral valve level.

Left *ventricular hypercontractility* initially occurs as a manifestation of volume overload [33, 34], whereas the shortening fraction usually remains within the normal range.

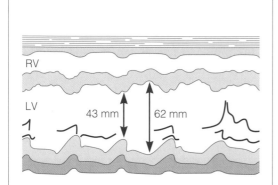

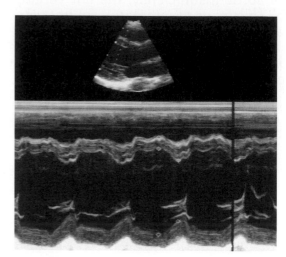

The left ventricle is dilated (diameter = 62 mm at end-diastole and 43 mm at end-systole). The interventricular septum and posterior wall of the left ventricle display marked systolic excursion as a sign of left ventricular volume overload. There is no hypertrophy.

M-mode; parasternal long-axis view at level of the ventricle.

As dilatation progresses, the left ventricle becomes more globular in shape. Both over- and underestimation of volume calculations may then occur [2, 5]. If dilatation continues, enlargement of the left atrium will occur. The muscle mass of the left ventricle increases in the presence of hemodynamically significant aortic regurgitation, and eccentric hypertrophy may develop [28].

Conventional Doppler Echocardiography

Pulsed-wave Doppler (PW Doppler):

- *Detection, velocity measurement, "mapping", and follow up of regurgitant jets in the left ventricular outflow tract.*

PW Doppler mapping and assessment of the extent, *i.e.* length, of the regurgitant signal in the left ventricle is performed from the parasternal long-axis view and the apical long-axis and five-chamber views; the sample volume is thereby placed in the left ventricular outflow tract. A determination of the extent of aortic regurgitation can also be made using the systolic-diastolic flow velocity relationship obtained from the suprasternal view through the ascending or descending aorta. The sample volume can alternatively be positioned in the abdominal aorta.

Continuous-wave Doppler (CW Doppler):

- *Detection, velocity measurement, semiquantitation, and follow up of aortic insufficiency.*

In CW Doppler regurgitant echoes are normally detected and quantified from the apical window and more infrequently from the right parasternal or suprasternal windows.

Doppler Color Flow Imaging (M-mode and 2-D)

- *Graphic representation of regurgitations and irregular turbulent flow.*

    The color Doppler hallmark of aortic regurgitation is a *turbulent diastolic regurgitant jet* in the left ventricular outflow tract. Color flow imaging can define the jet direction and the jet length and width, as measured from the base of the jet.

Transesophageal Echocardiography (Single and Multiplane):

- *Image quality better than that of transthoracic echocardiograms.*

    Sub- and supravalvular structures and changes can be imaged in much better detail with transesophageal echocardiography (TEE). TEE must often be used to obtained an unequivocal diagnosis of aortic valve prolapse. Because the left ventricular outflow tract lies at an unfavorable angle for assessment via TEE, transesophageal color and conventional Doppler techniques seldom provide any additional diagnostic information, except when the regurgitant jet is eccentric.

| 10.4.1 | Aortic Insufficiency |
| 10.4.1.1 | Quantitation and Semiquantitation |

PW Doppler is a useful method of identifying and semiquantitating aortic insufficiency. With the PW Doppler sample volume positioned in the left ventricular outflow tract, the presence of turbulent diastolic flow signals confirms the presence of aortic insufficiency.

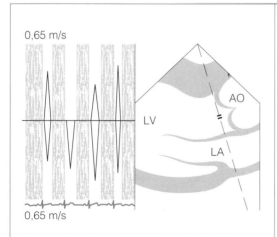

The sample volume (SV) is located in the left ventricular outflow tract. A diastolic flow signal is obtained on both sides of the zero baseline as an expression of aortic insufficiency (AI).

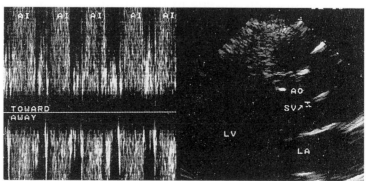

PW Doppler and parasternal long-axis 2-D echocardiograms.

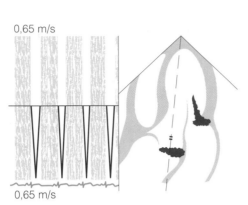

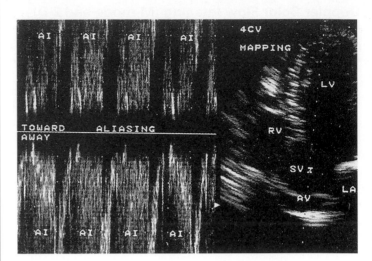

The sample volume (SV) is located immediately proximal to the aortic valve (AV). The aortic cusps and the posterior mitral annulus are thickened. Diastolic echoes registered on both sides of the zero baseline represent diastolic aortic insufficiency (AI).

PW Doppler and apical five-chamber 2-D echocardiograms.

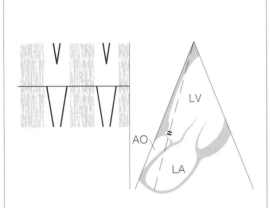

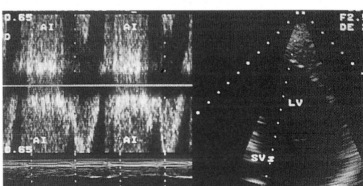

The sample volume in the left ventricle is now located further proximal, but still near the septum. Strong diastolic aortic insufficiency signals are detected on both sides of the zero baseline.

PW Doppler and apical five-chamber 2-D echocardiograms.

Aortic regurgitant signals in the left outflow tract are "mapped" from the parasternal long-axis, apical "RAO-equivalent", and apical "five-chamber view".

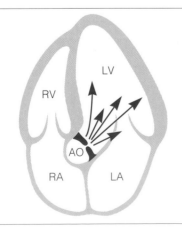

The direction of aortic regurgitant jets may vary greatly depending on the changes that have taken place in the aortic valve. The jet may flow along the interventricular septum, but may also flow laterally towards the anterior mitral leaflet or towards the lateral wall. The absence of mitral valve fluttering is to be expected when the regurgitant jet flows towards the septum.

The severity of aortic insufficiency can be estimated using the extent of detected diastolic turbulent flow [1, 18, 60]. Although it is much more sensitive and has better temporal resolution than Doppler color flow imaging, PW Doppler is more tedious and time-consuming; its use requires a high degree of skill and experience [21, 37]. Significant variation in the location of the sample volume may occur due to respiratory movement and heart rotation. Error may therefore arise when assessing eccentric regurgitant jets, especially when they flow towards the mitral valve or lateral wall.

The more surprising, PW Doppler estimates often correlate excellent with the angiographically assessed severity of aortic insufficiency [10, 48]. The good correlation of regurgitant fraction and regurgitant volume measurements is similarly surprising, especially since volume computations based on two-dimensional echocardiograms are fraught with potential error. The regurgitant fraction (RF) can be derived as the difference between the stroke volume across the aortic (ASV) and pulmonary valves (PSV) [15, 16].

$$RF = (ASV - PSV) / ASV$$

Nonetheless, this method has not gained wide acceptance, because the stroke volume across the pulmonary valve is often difficult to quantitate. PW Doppler recordings obtained from the suprasternal notch probably provide the most reliable measurements. As the severity of aortic insufficiency increases, the Doppler signal becomes stronger and can be detected further into the aorta. Pulsed-wave Doppler records systolic-diastolic signals in the ascending or descending aortae [27, 57, 59]. These signals can be planimetered and set in relation to one another.

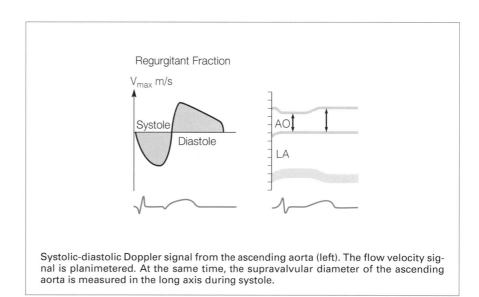

Systolic-diastolic Doppler signal from the ascending aorta (left). The flow velocity signal is planimetered. At the same time, the supravalvular diameter of the ascending aorta is measured in the long axis during systole.

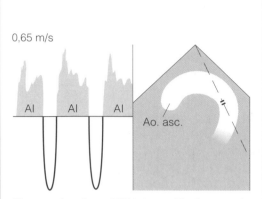

0,65 m/s

AI   AI   AI

Ao. asc.

The sample volume (SV) is located in the ascending aorta (Ao. asc.). The Doppler signal is recorded on the left. In diastole a turbulent aortic insufficiency (AI) signal is detected above the zero baseline. The Doppler forward flow signal lies below the baseline.

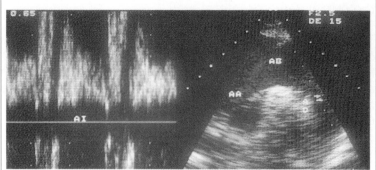

PW Doppler and suprasternal 2-D echocardiograms of the aorta.

However, this method is also subject to underestimation and other sources of error. Furthermore, it should be used only in patients with pure aortic insufficiency [16]. Diastolic retrograde flow may also be detected in patients with a ruptured sinus of Valsalva, patent ductus arteriosus, or coronary fistula. For optimal results, no significant systolic-diastolic changes in aortic diameter should occur, and flow velocities across the cross-sectional area should also remain constant. Since neither of these two conditions can be fulfilled, the appropriate precautions must be taken [35]. The fact that slight diastolic reflux in the proximal descending aorta can occur even in normals is a significant limitation. This technique of semiquantitation should not be used when the forward flow velocity is low. A similar limitation applies to PW Doppler recordings from the abdominal aorta. In that case, the assumption is made that systolic-diastolic signals in the abdominal aorta are detectable only when aortic insufficiency is severe.

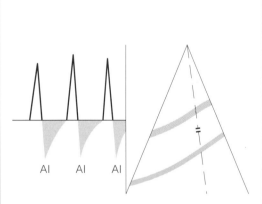

AI   AI   AI

The sample volume is located in the abdominal aorta. PW Doppler detects not only systolic forward flow, but also diastolic backward flow, which extends as far as the abdominal aorta. This is a sign of severe aortic insufficiency (AI).

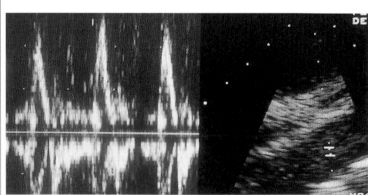

PW Doppler recording of the abdominal aorta.

In aortic insufficiency the peak diastolic retrograde flow velocity is dependent on the difference between left ventricular pressure and aortic pressure. The best signals are obtained from the apical window, but recording is sometimes performed from the suprasternal or right parasternal positions. Slight trivial reflux, also called "physiologic" regurgitation, is also found in normals and in individuals with a morphologically normal aortic valve with a low peak flow velocity [35]. Generally, flow velocities in aortic insufficiency usually range from 3 to 6 m/s, and can therefore be measured only with CW Doppler.

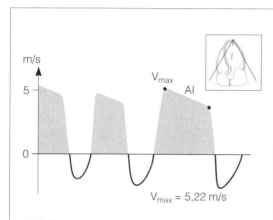

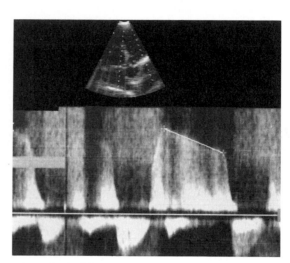

CW Doppler detects both the systolic signal below the zero baseline and the diastolic regurgitant signal of aortic insufficiency (AI), which produces a trapezoid configuration above the baseline. The strong signal is indicative of hemodynamically significant regurgitation.

CW-Doppler and apical five-chamber 2-D echocardiograms.

The turbulent signal observed in aortic insufficiency has a broad spectrum. Depending on the severity of regurgitation, the intensity of the signal ranges from weak to strong.

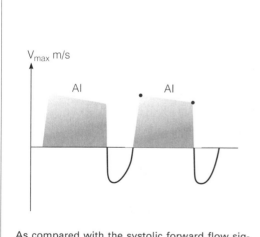

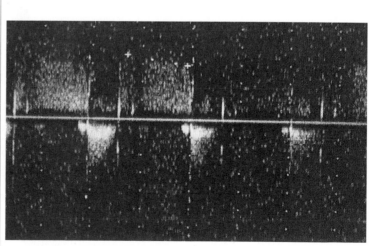

As compared with the systolic forward flow signal, the CW Doppler signal intensity in retrograde flow is relatively weak, which indicates only mild aortic insufficiency (AI).

CW Doppler recording.

Doppler-derived diastolic blood velocities provide useful information on the diastolic pressure in the left ventricle. The difference between left ventricular pressure and aortic pressure at end-diastole can be calculated directly from the aortic regurgitant signal velocity at end-diastole. When end-diastolic pressures are equal, no regurgitant flow is detected at end-diastole. Plotting the flow velocity signal allows differentiation between acute severe, subacute, or chronic aortic insufficiency. Acute aortic insufficiency is characterized by a sharp drop in the Doppler signal velocity.

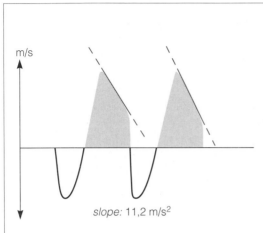

slope: 11,2 m/s²

A very strong CW Doppler flow velocity signal was recorded in diastole. The sharp drop in signal velocity indicates acute aortic insufficiency in a patient with aortic valvular endocarditis.

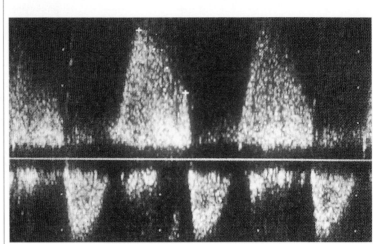

CW Doppler recording.

Chronic aortic insufficiency is characterized by a more gradual decline in the Doppler signal velocity curve.

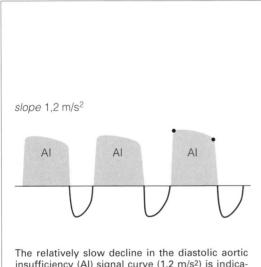

slope 1,2 m/s²

AI   AI   AI

The relatively slow decline in the diastolic aortic insufficiency (AI) signal curve (1.2 m/s²) is indicative of chronic aortic insufficiency (clinical stage I).

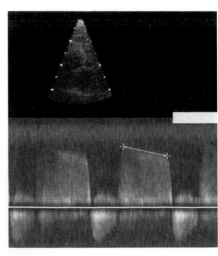

CW Doppler recording.

As in mitral stenosis, the pressure half-time (in ms) for aortic insufficiency can be derived from the flow velocity signal [38, 39]. The pressure half-time (PHT) is time interval over which the velocity falls from its maximum value (V_{max}) to its maximum value divided by the square root of 2 ($V_{max}/\sqrt{2}$).

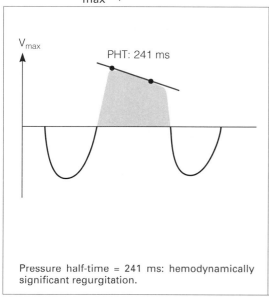

Pressure half-time = 241 ms: hemodynamically significant regurgitation.

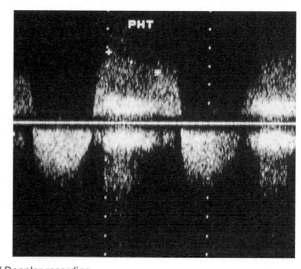

CW Doppler recording.

The lower the pressure half-time, the more severe the aortic insufficiency. A similar parameter is the flow velocity slope (m/s²), *i.e.*, its decline. The slope can be determined directly by generating a tangent across points of the flow velocity profile. A rapid decline in velocity results in a high slope, and a slower decline gives a lower slope.

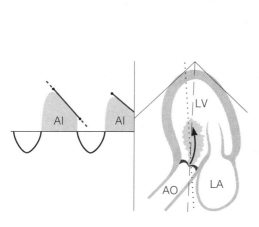

Acute aortic insufficiency (AI). The slope of 11.2 m/s² is highly pathological. Turbulent flow in the left ventricular outflow tract was detected in the Doppler color flow map on the right.

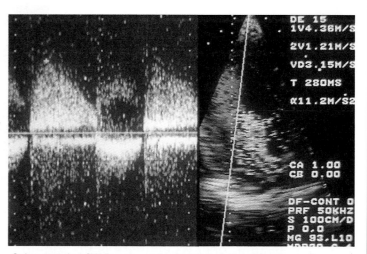

Color-encoded CW Doppler and apical 5-chamber 2-D echocardiograms.

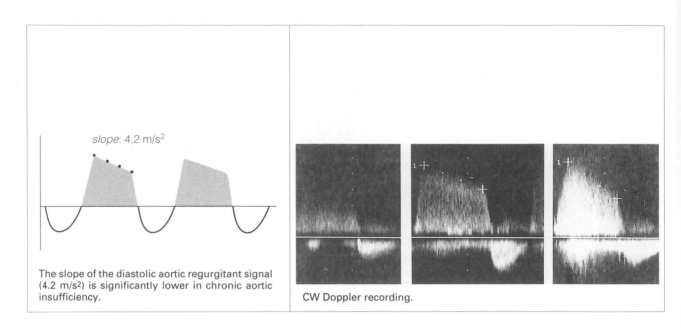

slope: 4,2 m/s²

The slope of the diastolic aortic regurgitant signal (4.2 m/s²) is significantly lower in chronic aortic insufficiency.

CW Doppler recording.

Factors such as stroke volume, peripheral resistance, and left ventricular compliance also affect the flow velocity profile.

These two methods should be used only if there is a good Doppler signal and a well-defined envelope curve.

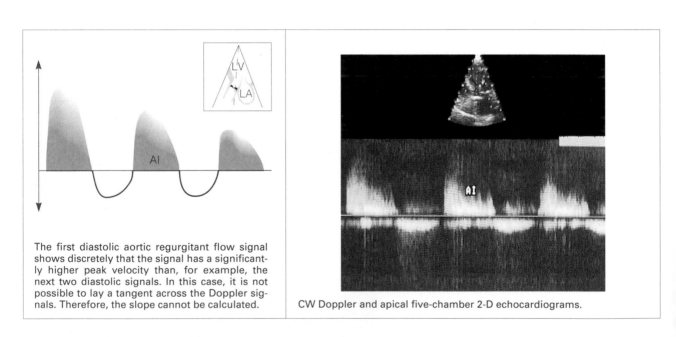

AI

The first diastolic aortic regurgitant flow signal shows discretely that the signal has a significantly higher peak velocity than, for example, the next two diastolic signals. In this case, it is not possible to lay a tangent across the Doppler signals. Therefore, the slope cannot be calculated.

CW Doppler and apical five-chamber 2-D echocardiograms.

The reliability of semiquantitative assessments using the pressure half-time and slope methods is assured only when there is no additional disease affecting left ventricular function. Since scatter is relatively large as compared with angiographic findings, precautions should be taken when making quantitative assessments using these methods [29, 32, 63].

The CW-Doppler signal intensity can also be used to semiquantitate the severity of aortic insufficiency [63], especially when it is compared with the systolic forward flow signal.

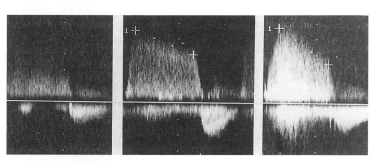

I = weak diastolic signal (left panel); II = moderately strong regurgitant signal (middle panel); III = very strong diastolic regurgitant signal corresponding to acute aortic insufficiency (right panel).

As was previously described for the pulsed Doppler technique, CW Doppler can be used to calculate the regurgitant fraction by relating the diastolic and systolic flow signals in the aorta as measured from the suprasternal position. In most patients, flow signals can be obtained only by using a pencil transducer, which requires a high degree of skill and experience [7].

In Doppler color flow imaging, aortic insufficiency is seen as a mosaic-like diastolic flow signal pattern in the left ventricular outflow tract. The turbulent color flow signals may vary greatly from one imaging plane to another, depending on the direction of the regurgitant jet. The main advantage of color Doppler flow imaging is that it provides at a glance information on the linear extent and width of regurgitant flow. Images of the left ventricular outflow tract can be obtained from the parasternal long and short-axis views as well as from the apical "RAO-equivalent" view and apical "five-chamber" view.

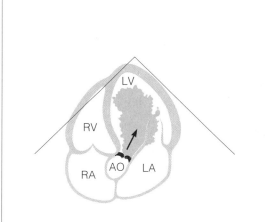

A massive, broad-based regurgitant jet is detected in the left ventricle in diastole. Turbulence extends up to the apex.

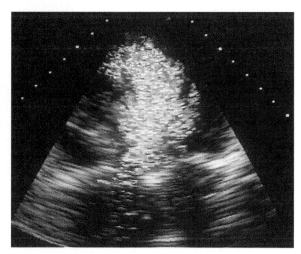

Color flow map of apical five-chamber 2-D echocardiogram.

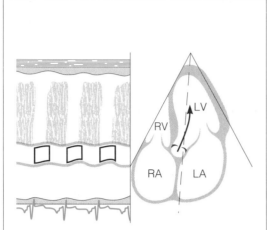

Extensive diastolic turbulent retrograde flow (right). Turbulence extends up to the apex. The diastolic Doppler signals are typical of aortic insufficiency.

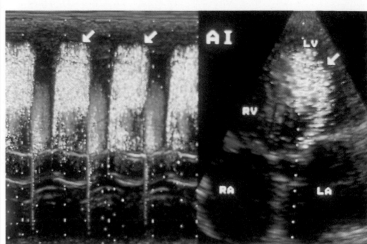

Color M-mode and 2-D echocardiograms; apical 5-chamber view.

Detection of the regurgitant jet depends on the patient-related and equipment-related imaging conditions [43]. The sensitivity and specificity of Doppler color flow imaging techniques for detection of aortic regurgitation is comparable to that of PW Doppler [38, 42].

It is sometimes difficult to distinguish an aortic regurgitant jet from turbulent flow due to mitral stenosis or mitral valve prostheses [17]. Color M-mode echocardiography, which provides better temporal resolution, can be particularly helpful in this case.

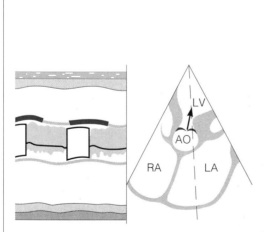

Lateral turbulence in the aorta (right). The M-mode cursor is positioned through this region. The aortic regurgitant jet is broad and highly turbulent.

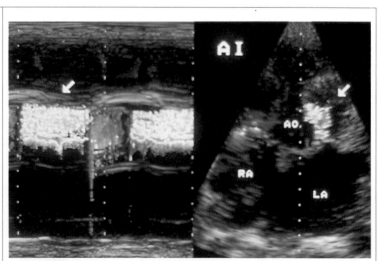

Color M-mode and 2-D echocardiograms, parasternal short-axis view at aortic valve level.

Diastolic color Doppler flow signals must be distinguished from wall motion artifacts and valve artifacts. The color-encoded regurgitant flow is quantitated by measuring the maximal linear extent, *i.e.* planimetry, of the regurgitant jet [4, 8, 14, 91, 46, 47, 61].

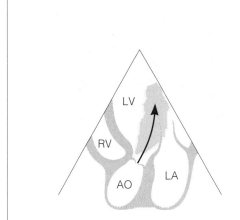

The area of turbulence due to aortic regurgitation in the left ventricle is circumscribed and measured. This area can now be set in relation to the area of the left ventricle.

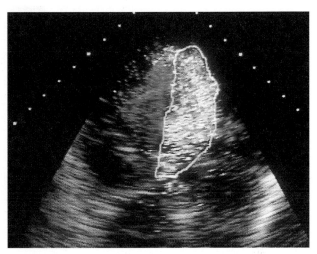

Color flow map of apical five-chamber 2-D echocardiogram.

The planimetered regurgitant area can also be set in relation to the area of the left ventricle. Alternatively, the base jet width can be measured and related to the maximal height of the left ventricular outflow tract [51, 53]. Clinical studies of this technique have reported greatly variable correlations to angiographic findings. Quantitation of eccentric jets is not possible.

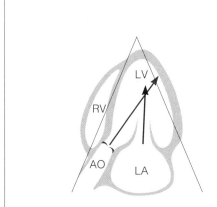

Very eccentric aortic regurgitant jet that extends to the lateral wall of the left ventricle. In the middle of the left ventricle, turbulence transsects the laminar diastolic inflow from the mitral valve.

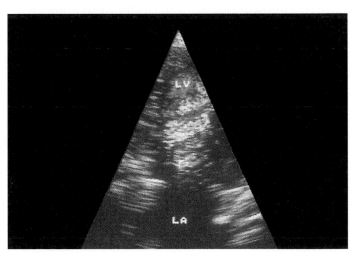

Color flow map of apical five-chamber 2-D echocardiogram.

Use of the color jet width measured along the long or short axis directly below aortic valve level, or measured in the *vena contracta* region has also been proposed for semiquantitation.

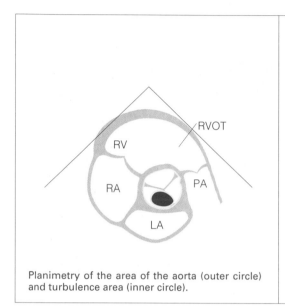

Planimetry of the area of the aorta (outer circle) and turbulence area (inner circle).

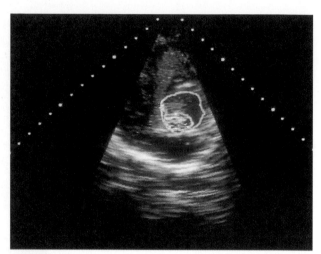

Parasternal short-axis 2-D view at aortic valve level; color flow mapping.

An *in vitro* study of color jets concludes that quantification results are improved by multiplying the jet area with the time interval until which the maximal variance is reached [41]. The limitations and sources of error in color Doppler semiquantitation techniques are similar to those discussed for the pulsed-wave Doppler technique.

Problems in quantitation arise primarily from the fact that the regurgitant volumes measured in angiography are compared with Doppler flow velocity relationships. The regurgitant volume is dependent on the size of the defect and the pressure gradient at the aortic valve. The color jet area and the flow velocity distribution can, in turn, vary greatly [55]. It remains to be proven whether the PISA method (proximal isovelocity surface area) which measures the color jet area proximal to the regurgitant valve combined with the aortic flow velocity integral permits reliable quantitation of aortic insufficiency, especially in routine diagnostic examinations [45, 56].

When using Doppler color flow imaging in clinical practice, one should keep in mind that the technique allows only semiquantitation, not quantitation, of regurgitation [13]

Because aortic regurgitant jets usually lie at an unfavorable angle to the Doppler beam in transesophageal echocardiography, this imaging modality is used only to provide additional information in cases where the regurgitant jet runs a very eccentric course and in patients with aortic insufficiency secondary to aneurysm of the sinuses of Valsalva or dissecting aneurysm.

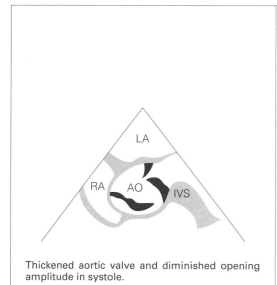

Thickened aortic valve and diminished opening amplitude in systole.

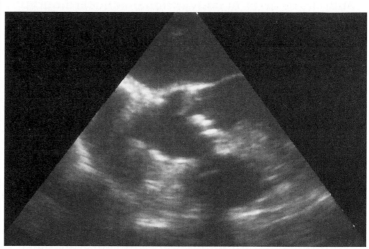

Transesophageal long-axis 2-D echocardiogram.

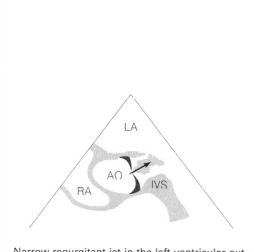

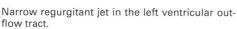

Narrow regurgitant jet in the left ventricular out-flow tract.

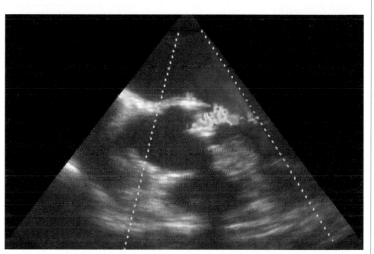

Color flow map of transesophageal short-axis 2-D echocardiogram.

As compared with conventional echocardiographic techniques, Doppler echocardiography is a much more sensitive and reliable method for qualitative diagnosis and quantitative assessment of aortic insufficiency.

Aortic insufficiency (modified from [21])		
	Specificity	Sensitivity
Auscultation	92 %	73 %
2-D echocardiography	91 %	43 %
Mitral valve fluttering	81 %	46 %
Doppler echocardiography	96 %	96 %

Sources of error in conventional echocardiography

- Absence of mitral valve fluttering in the presence of eccentric aortic regurgitant jets (*e.g.* directed towards the interventricular septum)
- Echo-dense aortic valve despite parallel diastolic echoes
- Echo-dense aortic valve despite eccentrically located diastolic echo
- Absence of left ventricular dilatation in highly acute aortic insufficiency

---

Sources of error in Doppler echocardiography

- Eccentric aortic regurgitation jets are difficult to detect, which leads to underestimation of severity
- Respiration and rotation-dependent variability in measurement volume location complicates quantification and reproducibility
- Echocardiographer must be highly skilled and experienced
- Aortic regurgitant signal may be masked by wall or valve artifacts

CW Doppler

- Eccentric jets do not allow optimal positioning of the CW Doppler beam
- The regurgitant signal used for slope or pressure half-time computation cannot be demarcated precisely.
- The severity of regurgitation is overestimated when there is associated mitral stenosis

Doppler Color Flow Imaging

- Poor imaging conditions to poor-quality color-encoding
- Quantitation by color flow imaging can lead to over- or underestimation of severity
- Eccentric aortic regurgitant jets lead to reduced quality of color encoding
- The color jet may be masked by concomitant mitral stenosis or by flow signals from a prosthetic mitral valve
- The systolic jet due to obstruction, *e.g.* in hypertrophic-obstructive cardio-myopathy, may be mistaken for the diastolic retrograde flow of aortic regurgitation

---

10.4.1   **Aortic Insufficiency**
10.4.1.3   **Ventricular Function**

Valvular incompetence gives rise to diastolic retrograde flow from the aorta into the left ventricle. The regurgitant volume is dependent on the size of the valve leak, the difference between left ventricular pressure and aortic pressure, and the heart rate. In mild incompetence the end-diastolic volume is not increased and, in turn, the left ventricle does not become enlarged. Hyperkinesis of left ventricular wall segments occurs as an expression of severe volume overload, and fractional shortening is at the upper limits of normal. As volume overload increases the end-diastolic and end-systolic diameters increase, but fractional shortening usually remains in the normal range. Severe regurgitation lead to an increase in the total stroke volume. This results in an increase in left ventricular muscle mass and a decrease in contractile function. This is more severe in patients with aortic insufficiency with associated aortic stenosis or hypertension [44, 49].

As the natural course continues, elevated end-diastolic left ventricular filling pressure leads to atrial enlargement and ultimately to right ventricular dilatation. In acute aortic insufficiency, however, wall thickness and left ventricular diameters are normal. Left ventricular hypertrophy is more pronounced in patients with concomitant aortic stenosis or arterial hypertension.

| 10.4.1 | Aortic Insufficiency |
| 10.4.1.4 | Follow-up and Treatment Considerations |

Subjective complaints manifest much earlier in pure or predominant aortic insufficiency than in aortic stenosis. The mean 10-year survival rate for patients with mild aortic insufficiency ranges from 85 to 90 %. Most patients are asymptomatic, but some report dyspnea at higher levels of exertion [22]. Patients with moderate aortic insufficiency usually experience symptoms of dyspnea on exertion; angina pectoris symptoms are more infrequent. Blood pressure is usually elevated, the carotid pulse is increased, and the apex beat is raised. In severe aortic insufficiency, dyspnea and angina pectoris symptoms manifest even at low levels of exertion. 39% of the patients with severe aortic insufficiency that required surgical treatment survived 5 years after surgery. One-third of the patients survived 10 years after surgery. After left ventricular decompensation occurred, the 2-year survival rate dropped to 10%. The expected survival in patients with angina pectoris symptoms is ca. 4 years [25]. When right ventricular overload occurs, not even surgery is able to provide satisfactory recompensation in most cases. Since the overall long-term prognosis for patients with aortic insufficiency is relatively good, it is difficult to determine the optimum time for surgical intervention [50, 54]. Echocardiography can provide useful information for making this decision, especially when left ventricular dilatation progresses rapidly. Patients with mild aortic insufficiency should be checked once a year to once every two years. Patients with moderate to moderately severe aortic insufficiency should be checked bianually, and asymptomatic patients with severe insufficiency should be checked quarterly. The use of the index "preoperative left ventricular systolic diameter $\geq$ 55 mm" could not be substantiated [12, 23, 24]. The essential echocardiographic follow-up parameters include: left ventricular end-systolic and end-diastolic diameter, left atrial size, fractional shortening, ejection fraction, fluttering of septum and anterior wall, width and linear extent of color jet as measured in multiple imaging planes, alternative PW Doppler "mapping", CW Doppler signal intensity, slope or pressure half-time derived from the CW Doppler signal.

| 10.4.1 | Aortic Insufficiency |
| 10.4.1.5 | Critical Evaluation of Results and Comparison with Those of Complementary Techniques |

Aortic insufficiency is usually graded either semiquantitatively according to Sellers system or quantitatively according to the regurgitant fraction. Increased left ventricular end-diastolic pressure is, of course, also measured in acute and severe acute aortic insufficiency. Symptomatic patients under age 40 with clear Doppler echocardiographic signs of regurgitation do not require left heart catheterization. In patients with angina pectoris, coronary angiography must be performed in order to exclude the possibility of associated coronary artery disease.

Radionuclide angiography enables evaluation of left ventricular pump function in resting and exercise conditions [3, 6]. A decrease in the ejection fraction under exertion is a sign of imminent decompensation; many patients still have no symptoms at this time.

Right heart catheterization stress testing is of little value in assessing the severity of aortic insufficiency. Magnetic resonance imaging (MRI) can also provide real-time images of aortic regurgitation. When used for quantitation of aortic insufficiency, however, MRI is subject to problems similar to those of Doppler echocardiography. Therefore, MRI is inferior to the more convenient echocardiographic diagnostic techniques in routine diagnostic examinations. The promising preliminary results of stress echocardiography must be further investigated before an assessment can be made.

Morphometry and ventricular function

LADmax	_____	mm
LVEDD	_____	mm
LVESD	_____	mm
Fractional shortening	_____	
Ejection fraction	_____	
Mitral-septal distance	_____	mm
AREDD	_____	mm

Hyperkinesis of septum or anterior wall?
Signs of concomitant ischemic heart disease?
Wall motion analysis

Valve morphology and dynamics
▸ Thickening or calcification of aortic valve?
  - Parallel diastolic echoes?
  - Eccentric diastolic valve closure echo?
  - Aortic valve prolapse?
  - Diastolic oscillation of mitral valve, septum and/or anterior wall?
  - Premature aortic valve closure, premature mitral valve opening?
▸ Assessment of aortic root, ascending and descending aorta:
  - aortic ectasia, aneurysm and/or dissection?
  - aneurysm of sinuses of Valsalva?
▸ Hemodynamic consequences
  - (dilatation of the left ventricle)

Ventricular function and pressure-flow relationships (Doppler echocardiography)
▸ Qualitative visual assessment
▸ Detection, velocity measurement, "mapping", and follow-up
▸ Graphic (color-encoded) visualization
▸ Peak instantaneous orthograde transaortic flow velocity (m/s)
▸ Slope of the Doppler aortic regurgitant curve (m/s^2)
▸ Pressure half-time (ms)
▸ Regurgitant orifice area (cm^2)
▸ Width at base of regurgitant jet, linear extent and area in different imaging planes (cm, cm^2)

Transesophageal echocardiography
▸ Assessment of valve morphology and dynamics, morphology of aortic root and ascending aorta up to supradiaphragmatic segments, morphology of descending aorta

---

HISTORY / SYMPTOMATOLOGY / AUSCULTATION

Exertional dyspnea, palpitations, angina pectoris?

ECHOCARDIOGRAPHY

Conventional echocardiography:

Morphometry (LADmax, LVEDD, LVESD, AREDD, asc. aorta)
Ventricular function (LVFS, wall motion analysis including)
Visualization of anatomic causes and resulting complications:
Valve morphology and dynamics, primary aortic disease?

Doppler and transesophageal echocardiography:

Slope
Pressure half-time
CW Doppler signal intensity, PW Doppler mapping
Color jet width, length, and area as measured in multiple scan planes

Transesophageal echocardiography:
Exclusion or proof of primary aortic disease

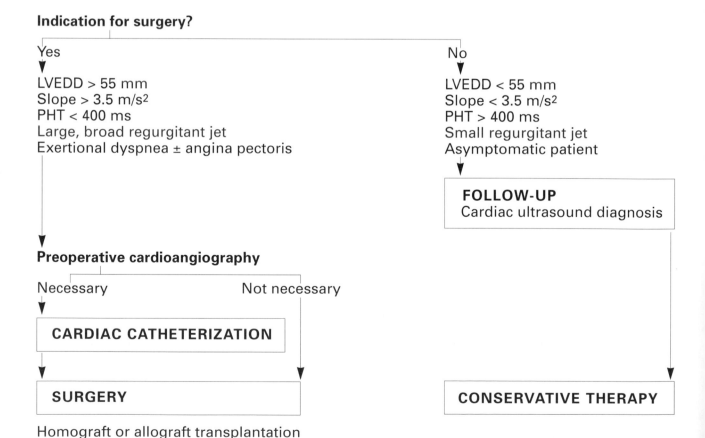

Indication for surgery?

Yes

LVEDD > 55 mm
Slope > 3.5 m/s^2
PHT < 400 ms
Large, broad regurgitant jet
Exertional dyspnea ± angina pectoris

No

LVEDD < 55 mm
Slope < 3.5 m/s^2
PHT > 400 ms
Small regurgitant jet
Asymptomatic patient

FOLLOW-UP
Cardiac ultrasound diagnosis

Preoperative cardioangiography

Necessary   Not necessary

CARDIAC CATHETERIZATION

SURGERY

CONSERVATIVE THERAPY

Homograft or allograft transplantation
Valve replacement surgery

1. Abbasi AS. The role of Doppler echocardiography in valvular insufficiency. In: Berger M (ed). Doppler echocardiography in heart disease. Dekker 1986; 133-177.
2. Abdulla AM, Frank, MJ, Canedo MI, Stefadouros, MA. Limitations of echocardiography in the assessment of the left ventricular size and function in aortic regurgitation. Circulation 1980; 61: 148-155.
3. Baxter RH, Becker LC, Alderson PQ, Rogo P, Wagner HN, Weisfeldt ML. Quantification of aortic valvular regurgitation in dogs by nuclear imaging. Circulation 1980; 61: 404-410.
4. Becher H, Grube E, Lüderitz B. Beurteilung der Aorteninsuffizienz mittels Farbdopplerechokardiographie. Z Kardiol 1987; 76: 8-14.
5. Biamino G, Wessel J, Schlag W, Schröder R. Echocardiographic pattern of motion of the aortic root as a correlate of changes in volume of the left atrium. Am J Cardiol 1980; 36: 191-200.
6. Borer JS, Bacharach SL, Green MV, Kent KM, Henry WL, Rosing DR, Seides SF, Johnston GS, Epstein ES. Exercise-induced left ventricular dysfunction in symptomatic and asymptomatic patients with aortic regurgitation: assessment with radionuclide cineangiography. Am J Cardiol 1987; 42: 193-199.
7. Bouchard A, Blumlein S, Schiller NB, Schlitt S, Byrd BF, Pots T, Chatterjee K. Measurements of left ventrilcular stroke volume using continous wave Doppler echocardiography of the ascending aorta and m-mode echocardiography of the aortic valve. J Am Coll Cardiol 1987; 9: 75-83.
8. Byard CE, Perry GJ, Roitman DI, Nanda NC. Quantitative assessment of aortic regurgitation by color Doppler. Circulation 1985; 72 (suppl III): III-146.
9. Chia BL. Mitral valve fluttering in aortic insufficiency. J Clin Ultrasound 1981; 9: 198-200.
10. Ciubanu M, Abbasi M, Allen A, Hermer M, Spellberg R. Pulse doppler echocardiography in the diagnosis and estimation of the aortic insuffieciency. Am J Cardiol 1984; 54: 857-868.
11. Craig BG, Smallhorn JF, Burrows P, Trusler GA, Rowe RD: Cross-sectional echocardiography in the evaluation of aortic valve prolapse associated with ventricular septal defect. Am Heart J 1986; 112: 800-804.
12. Daniel WG, Hood WP, Siart A, Hausmann D, Nellessen U, Oelert H, Lichtlen P. Chronic aortic regurgitation: reassessment of the prognostic value of preoperative left ventricular end-systolic dimension and fractional shortening. Circulation 1985; 71: 669-680.
13. DeMaria AY, Smith M. Quantification of Doppler color flow recordings: an oxymoron? J Am Coll Cardiol 1992; 439-440.
14. Dennig K, Hennecke S, Dacian S, Rudolph W. Zur Schweregradbestimmung von Aortenklappenregurgitationen mit Hilfe der Farb-Doppler-Echokardiographie. Herz 1987; 12: 204-211.
15. Diebold B, Perroneau P, Blanchard D, Colonna G, Guermonprez JL, Froman J, Seier P, Maurice P. Non-invasive quantification of aortic regurgitation by Doppler echocardiography. Br Heart J 1983; 49: 167-173.
16. Diebold B, Touati R, Delouche A. Guglielmi JP, Forman J, Guermonprez JL, Perroncau P. Doppler imaging of regurgitant jet in aortic insufficiency: expermimental validation and preliminary clinical evaluation. Eur Heart J 1987; 8 (suppl C): 45-52.
17. Dittmann,H, Karsch KR, Seipel L. Die Doppler-echokardiografische Diagnose und Schweregradeinteilung der Aorteninsuffizienz bei Patienten mit Aortenstenosen und Mitralfehlern. Z Kardiol 1986; 75: 522-527.
18. Esper RJ. Detection of mild aortic regurgitation by range-gated pulsed Doppler echocardiography. Am J Cardiol 1982; 50: 1037-1043.
19. Galassi AR, Nihoyannopoulos P, Pupita G, Odwadara H, Crea F, McKenna WJ. Assessment of colour flow imaging in the grading of valvular regurgitation. Eur Heart J 1990; 11: 1101-1108.
20. Glasser SP. Late mitral valve opening in aortic regurgitation. Chest 1981; 70: 70-74.
21. Grayburn PA, Smith MD, Handshoe R, Friedman BJ, DeMaria AN. Detection of aortic insufficiency by standard echocardiography, pulsed Doppler echocardiography, and auscultation. Ann Intern Med 1986; 104: 599-605.
22. Haerten K, Dohn V, Dohn G. Natürlicher Verlauf opertionswürdiger Aortenklappenvitien bei konservativer Therapie. Z Kardiol 1980; 69; 757-782.
23. Henry WL, Bobow RO, Rosing DR, Epstein SE. Observation of the optimum time for operative intervention for aortic regurgitation (II). Circulation 1980; 484-492.
24. Henry WL, Bonow RO, Borer JS, Ware JH, Kent KM, Redwood DR, McIntosh C, Morrow AG, Epstein SE. Observations on the optimum time for operation intervention for aortic regurgitation (I). Circulation 1980; 61: 471-483.
25. Horstkotte D, Loogen F. Erworbene Herzklappenfehler. Urban & Schwarzenberg, München 1987; 111-112.
26. Johnson AD, Gosink BB, Forsythe J, Grandjean N. Oscillation of left ventricular structures in aortic regurgitation. J Clin Ultrasound 1977; 5: 21-24.
27. Kitabatake A, Ito H, Inoue M, Tanouchi J, Ishihara K, Morita T, Fujii K, Yoshida Y, Masuyma T, Yoshima H. A new approach to noninvasive evaluation of the aortic regurgitant fraction by two-dimensional Doppler echocardiography as compared with cineangiography. Circulation 1985; 72: 523-529.
28. Kotler MN, Mintz GS, Parry WR, Segal BL. M-mode and two-dimensional echocardiography in mitral and aortic regurgitation: Pre- and postoperative evaluation of volume overload of the left ventricle. Am J Cardiol 1980; 46: 1144-1148.
29. Labovitz AJ, Ferrara MJ. Kern RJ, Bryg DG, Mrosek GA. Quantitative evaluation of aortic insufficiency by countinous wave Doppler echocardiography. JAMA 1986; 8: 1341-1347.

30. Louie EK, Mason TJ, Shah TR, Bieniarz T, Moore AM. Determinants of anterior mitral leaflet fluttering in pure aortic regurgitation from pulsed Doppler study of the early diastolic interaction between the regurgitant jet and mitral inflow. Am J Cardiol 1988; 61: 1085-1091.
31. Mardelli TJ, Morganroth J, Naito M, Chen C. Cross-sectional echocardiographc detection of aortic valve prolapse. Am Heart J 1980; 10: 295-301.
32. Masuyama TK, Kodama AK Kitabatake A, Nanto S, Sato H, Uematsu M, Inoue M, Kamada T. Noninvasive evaluation of aortic regurgitation by continous-wave Doppler echocardiography. Circulation 1986; 73: 460-466.
33. McDonald IG, Jelinek VM. Serial m-mode echocardiography in severe chronic aortic regurgitation. Circulation 1980; 62: 1291-1296.
34. McDonald IG. Echocardiographic assessment of left ventricular function in aortic valve disease. Circulation 1976; 53: 860-864.
35. Meltzer S, Finkelstein A. Regurgitation of all four cardiac valves detected by Doppler echocardiogrpahy. Am J Cardiol 1986; 58: 169-174.
36. Meyer D, Sareli P, Pocock A, Dean H, Epstein M, Barlow J. Echocardiografic and hemodynamic correlates of diastolic closure of mitral valve and diastolic opening of aortic valve in severe aortic regurgitation. Am J Cardiol 1985; 56: 811-814.
37. Meyers DG, Olson TS, Hansen DA. Auscultation, m-mode echocardiography and pulsed Doppler echocardiography compared with angiography for diagnosis of chronic aortic regurgitation. Am J Cardiol 1985; 56: 811-814.
38. Miyatake K, Okamoto M, Kinoshita N, Izumi S, Owa M, Takao S, Sakakibara H, Yasuhara N. Clinical applications of a new type of real-time two-dimensional Doppler flow imaging system. Am J Cardiol 1984; 54: 857-868.
39. Moro E, Nicolosi L, Zanuttini D, Cerveato E. Influence of aortic regurgitation on the assessment of the pressure halftime and derived mitral valve area in patients with mitral stenosis. Eur Heart J 1988; 9: 1010-1017.
40. Nakao S, Tanaka H, Tahara M, Yoshimura H, Sakurai S, Tei Ch, Kashima T. A regurgitant jet and echocardiographic abnormalities in aortic regurgitation. Circulation 1983; 67: 860-865.
41. Ohman EM, Helmy SH, Shaughenessy ED, Adams DB, Kisslo J. In vitro analysis of jets by Doppler colour flow imaging: the importance of time to maximum jet area. Eur heart J 1990; 11: 361-367.
42. Omoto R, Yokote Y, Tkamoto S, Tamura F, Asano H, Manekawa K, Kasai C, Tsukamoto M, Koyana A. The development of real-time two-dimensional Doppler echocardiography and its clinical significance in acquired valvular disease with special reference to the evaluation of valvular regurgitation. Jap Heart J 1984; 25: 325-340.
43. Omoto R. Color atlas of real-time two-dimensional Doppler echocardiography. Shindan-To-Chiryosha, Tokyo 1984.
44. Osbakken M, Bove A, Spann JF. Left ventricular function in chronic aortic regurgitation with reference to end-systolic pressure, volume and stress relations. Am J Cardiol 1981; 47: 193-199.
45. Perry GJ, Helmcke F, Kan MN, Tracy W, Kirklin JK, Moss N, Nanda NC. Determination of regurgitant volume by combined color and continous wave Doppler in a dog model of aortic insufficiency. Circulation 1987; 76 (suppl IV): IV-139.
46. Perry GJ, Helmcke F, Nanda NC, Byard C, Soto B. Evaluation of aortic insufficiency by Doppler color flow mapping. J Am Coll Cardiol 1987; 9: 952-959.
47. Perry GJ, Nanda NC. Diagnosis and quantification of valvular regurgitation by color Doppler flow mapping. Echocardiography: A review of cardiovascular ultrasound 1986; 3: 493-503.
48. Quinones MA, Young JB, Waggoner D, Ostojic MC, Ribeiro GT, Miller RR. Aessment of pulsed Doppler echocardiography in detection and quantification of aortic and mitral regurgitation. Br Heart J 1980; 44: 612-620.
49. Rakley CE, Dalldorf FG, Hood, WP jr, Wilcox BR. Sarcomere lenght and left ventricular function in chronic heart disease. Am J Med Sci 1970; 65: 501-509.
50. Rapaport E. Natural history of aortic and mitral valve disease. Am J Cardiol 1975; 35: 221-228.
51. Reynolds T, Abate J, Tenney A, Warner MG. The JH/LVOH method in the quantification of aortic regurgitation: how the cardiac sonographer may avoid an important potential pitfall. J Am Soc Echo 1991; 4: 105-108.
52. Rosoff MH, Cohen MV. Significance of E point-septal separation by m-mode echocardiography in patients with aortic regurgitation. Am J Cardiol 1985; 56: 809-811.
53. Seder JD, Burke JF, Pauletto FJ. Prevalence of aortic regurgitation by color flow Doppler in relation to aortic root size. J Am Soc Echo 1990; 3: 316-319.
54. Segal J, Harvey WP, Hufnagel CL. A clinical study of one hundred cases of severe aortic insufficiency. Am J Med 1956; 21: 200-207.
55. Simpson IA, Sahn DJ. Quantification of valvular regurgitation by Doppler echocardiography. Circulation 1991; 84 (suppl I): I-188-I-192.
56. Stewart EE, Schiavone WA, From JA, Castel T, Salcedo EE. In vitro studies of Doppler color flow mapping: dependence of spatial distribution on instrument settings. Circulation 1985; 72 (suppl III): III-98.
57. Stewart WA, Jiang L, Mich R, Pandian N, Guerrero JL, Weyman AE. Variable effects of changes in flow rate through the aortic, pulmonary, and mitral valves on valve area and flow velocity: impact on quantitative Doppler flow calculations. J Am Coll Cardiol 1985; 6: 653-662.

58. Teague SM, Heinsimer JA, Anderson JL, Sublett K, Olson EG, Voyles WF, Thandani U. Quantification of aortic regurgitation utilizing continous wave Doppler ultrasound. JAMA 1986; 8: 592-599.
59. Touche T, Prasquier R, Nitenberg A, Zuttere DD, Rgourgon. Asessment and follow-up of patients with aortic regurgitation by an updated Doppler echocardiographic measurement of the aortic regurgitant fraction in the aortic arch. Circulation 1985; 72: 819-824.
60. Veyrat C, Lessana AC, Abitbol G, Ameur A, Benaim R, Kalmanson D. New indices for assessing aortic regurgitation with two-dimensional Doppler echocardiographic measurement of the regurgitant aortic valvular area. Circulation 1983; 68: 998-1005.
61. Vigua C, Russo A, Salvatori MP, Laurenzi F, Perna G, Villella A, Langialonga T, Fanelli R, Loperfido F. Color and pulsed wave Doppler study of aortic regurgitation in systemic hypertension. Am J Cardiol 1988. 61: 928-929.
62. Whipple RL, Morris DC, Felner JM, Merill AJ, Miller JI. Echocardiographic manifestation of a flail aortic valve leaflet. J Clin Ultrasound 1977; 5: 417-422.
63. Wilkenshoff U. Inauguraldissertation der Freien Universität Berlin. 1992; 60.

10.4	**Aortic Valve Disease**
10.4.2	**Aortic Stenosis**
	(Kurt J.G. Schmailzl)

Rheumatic fever and infective endocarditis are no longer the predominant causes of aortic stenosis. The most common types of hemodynamically significant aortic stenosis today are calcifying degeneration of one or more cusps in the senium [19], and a congenital bicuspid aortic valve in patients under the age of 30, respectively [24]. Due to the architecture of the bicuspid aortic valve, highly turbulent flow arises. This traumatizes the valve cusps and subsequently leads to reactive fibrosis and calcification.

Etiopathogenetic types of left ventricular outflow tract obstruction

▸ Valvular aortic stenosis
     Congenital aortic stenosis
         – unicuspid, bicuspid, tricuspid, or multicuspid malformation
         – dome-shaped membrane
     Acquired aortic stenosis
         – rheumatic aortic stenosis
         – degenerative calcifying aortic stenosis
         – atherosclerotic diseases of the aortic valve and the aorta

▸ Supravalvular aortic stenosis
▸ Subvalvular aortic stenosis
▸ Hypertrophic obstructive cardiomyopathy

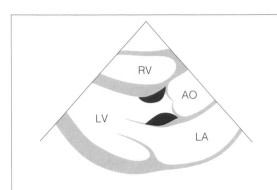

Subvalvular aortic stenosis. Parasternal long-axis 2-D echocardiogram.

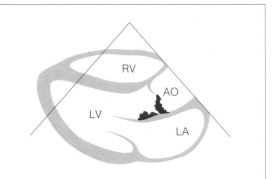

Calcification of aortic valve, aortic annulus, and mitral valve. Parasternal long-axis 2-D echocardio-

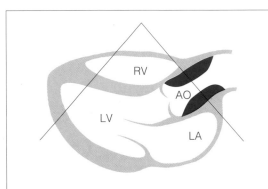

Tunnel-shaped subaortic stenosis. Parasternal long-axis 2-D echocardiogram.

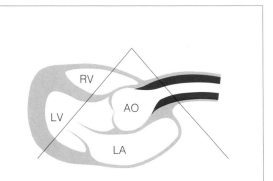

Supravalvular aortic stenosis. M-mode, parasternal long-axis view.

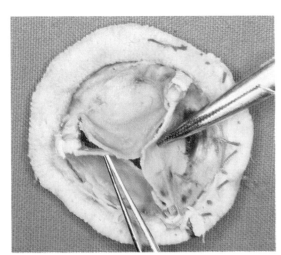

Morphological specimen: aortic stenosis.

10.4   **Aortic Valve Disease**
10.4.2   **Aortic Stenosis**
       563

Cardiac Ultrasound Diagnosis

Imaging of the aortic valve and flow velocity measurement in the region of the aortic valve and left ventricular outflow tract should preferably be performed from the left parasternal long and short-axis views, apical two and four-chamber views, right parasternal and suprasternal views, and transesophageal long-axis views.

Conventional Echocardiography

Visualization of anatomic causes:

Two-dimensional and M-mode echocardiography:

- *Thickened and/or calcified aortic cusps* (as compared with a normal valve or to echoes of a normal aortic wall from an orthograde plane), frequently with multiple parallel echoes (M-mode).

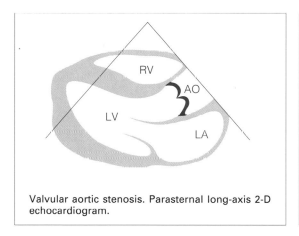

Valvular aortic stenosis. Parasternal long-axis 2-D echocardiogram.

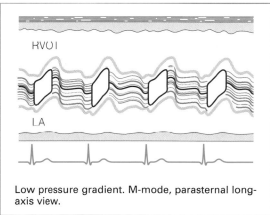

Low pressure gradient. M-mode, parasternal long-axis view.

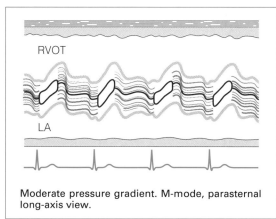

Moderate pressure gradient. M-mode, parasternal long-axis view.

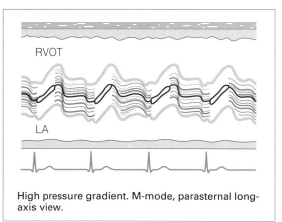

High pressure gradient. M-mode, parasternal long-axis view.

Nonspecific features and possible hemodynamic consequences of aortic stenosis:

Two-dimensional echocardiography:

- *Motility of valve cusps, severity and extent of calcification;*
- *Diminished systolic aortic cusp separation (<< 15 mm);*
- *Systolic protrusion (doming) of aortic cusps into the aorta.* The bodies of the cusps spread to a dome-like configuration in the blood stream, because their free edges no longer allow complete opening (noncalcifying congenital or rheumatic aortic stenosis with commissural fusion);
- *Concentric left ventricular hypertrophy.*

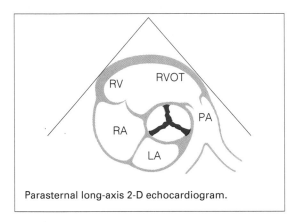

Parasternal long-axis 2-D echocardiogram.

- *Dilatation of the left ventricle* in reduced systolic LV performance in some cases.

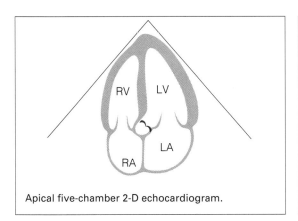

Apical five-chamber 2-D echocardiogram.

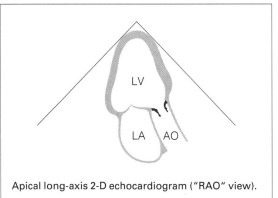

Apical long-axis 2-D echocardiogram ("RAO" view).

Conventional Doppler Echocardiography

Pulsed-Wave Doppler Echocardiography (PW Doppler):

- *Detection, velocity measurement and "mapping" of systolic stenotic flow jets at aortic valve level.*

Continuous-Wave Doppler Echocardiography (CW Doppler):

- *Detection and velocity measurement of systolic stenotic flow jets at aortic valve level.*

Aortic stenosis can be detected in CW and PW Doppler recordings obtained from the apical, suprasternal, and right parasternal transducer positions. In detection and assessment of the severity of aortic stenosis, Doppler echocardiography is significantly superior to auscultation, because the loudness of systolic murmurs does not always allow reliable grading.

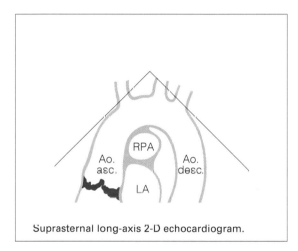

Suprasternal long-axis 2-D echocardiogram.

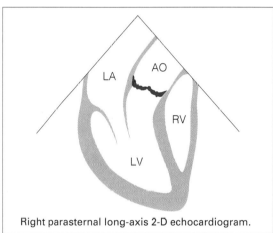

Right parasternal long-axis 2-D echocardiogram.

Doppler Color Flow Imaging (2-D and M-mode)

- *Graphic (color-encoded) representation of transaortic turbulent stenotic jet.*

Unsatisfactory spectral (or color) Doppler signals can be enhanced by using transpulmonary echocontrastography agents [16].

Transesophageal Echocardiography (Single and Multiplane)

Transesophageal echocardiography can improve detection and assessment of the severity of aortic stenosis. With transesophageal echocardiography it is also possible to assess sub- and supravalvular regions and to planimeter the aortic valve orifice area.

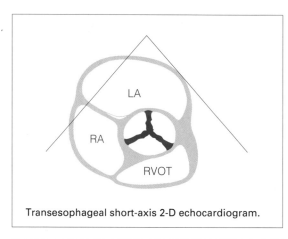

Transesophageal short-axis 2-D echocardiogram.

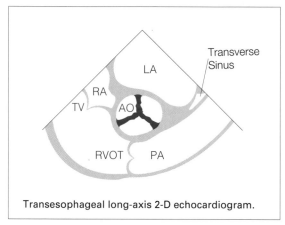

Transesophageal long-axis 2-D echocardiogram.

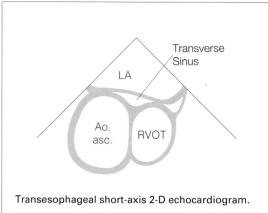

Transesophageal short-axis 2-D echocardiogram.

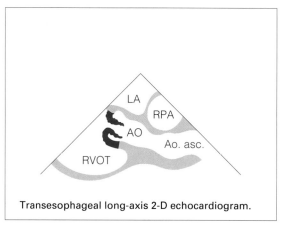

Transesophageal long-axis 2-D echocardiogram.

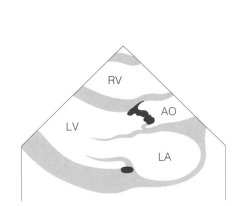

Aortic stenosis. Calcium-dense aortic cusps. Doming of aortic valve cusps. Mitral annular calcification.

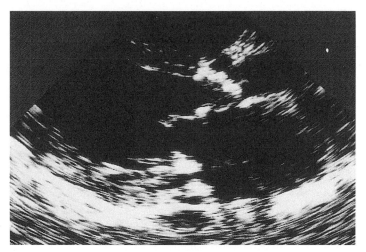

2-D left parasternal long-axis view at aortic valve level.

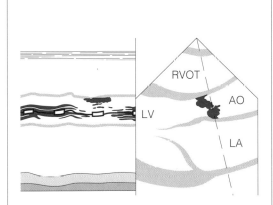

Aortic stenosis. Aortic cusps abnormally thickened and calcified as compared with anterior aortic wall. Multiple parallel echo bands. No separation is detected.

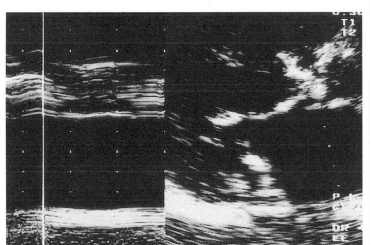

M-mode and 2-D; left parasternal long-axis view at aortic valve level.

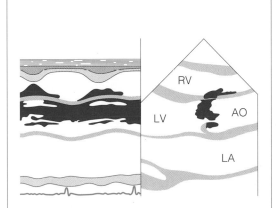

Moderately severe aortic stenosis. Aortic cusps abnormally thickened and calcified as compared with posterior aortic wall. Multiple parallel echo bands. No separation is detected.

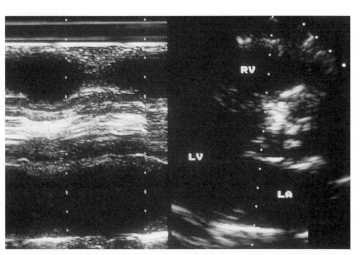

M-mode and 2-D; left parasternal long-axis view at aortic valve level.

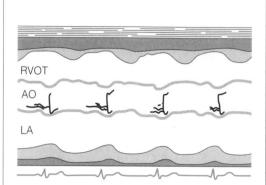

Bicuspid aortic valve with thickened cusps and hemodynamically significant stenotic component. Diastolic aortic valve echo displaced to posterior.

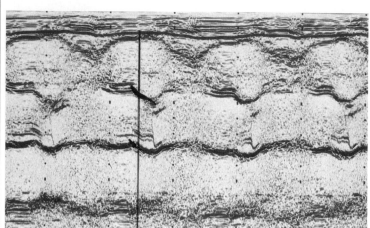

M-mode; left parasternal long-axis view at aortic valve level.

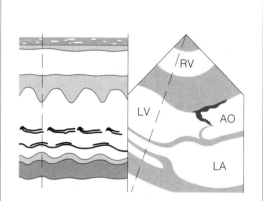

Concentrically hypertrophied and dilated left ventricle in combined aortic lesions. Multiple parallel echo bands in view at aortic valve level; no massive traces of calcium.

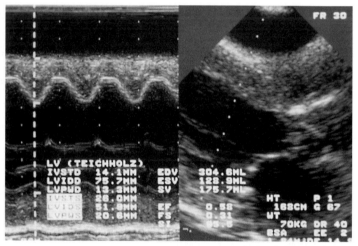

M-mode and 2-D; left parasternal long-axis view. Morphometry.

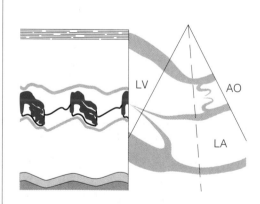

Combined aortic lesions in infected bicuspid aortic valve. Increased echoes from 0right coronary aortic cusp. Doming. Turbulent transvalvular flow.

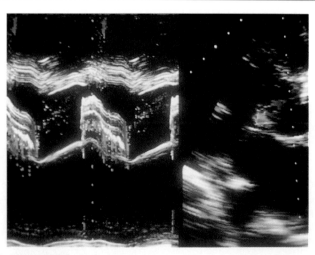

Color M-mode and 2-D; left parasternal long-axis view at aortic valve level.

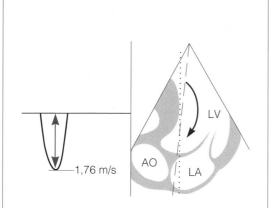

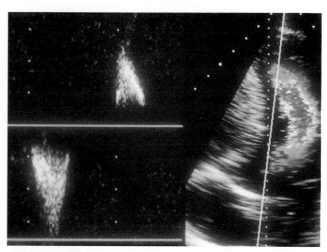

Acceleration flow from left ventricle to aorta without hemodynamically significant aortic stenosis. Peak instantaneous flow velocity is still within reference range. Aliasing with color change from blue to red. High output state.

Color flow mapping of CW Doppler and apical five-chamber 2-D echocardiograms. Mitral and aortic Doppler frequency spectra.

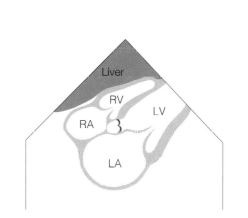

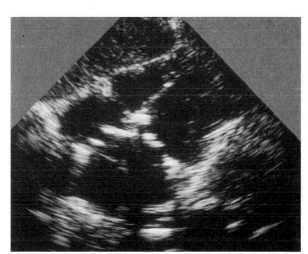

Moderate aortic stenosis. Calcium-dense echoes in view through aortic valve.

Subcostal five-chamber 2-D echocardiogram.

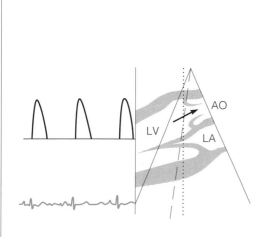

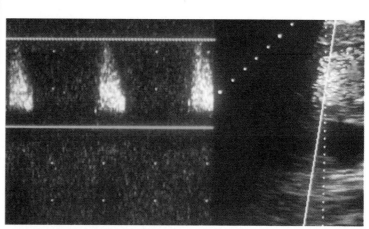

Moderate aortic stenosis.

CW Doppler. Right parasternal long-axis view.

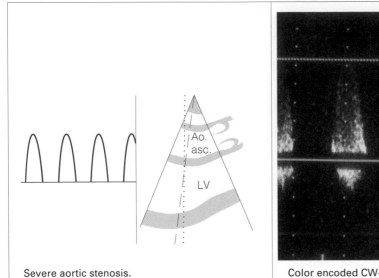

Severe aortic stenosis.

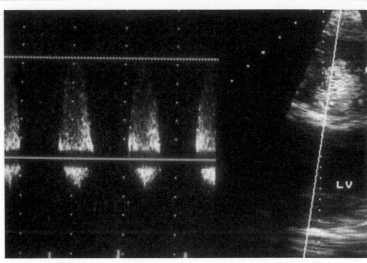

Color encoded CW-Doppler. Right parasternal long axis view.

10.4.2 Aortic Stenosis
10.4.2.1 Quantitation

The normal aortic valve area is 2 to 3 cm². Characteristic problems are encountered in the quantitation of aortic stenosis. They are determined by the natural course of the disease, by the fact that it may not cause symptoms for decades, and by the fact that the average survival time after the occurrence of angina pectoris or exertional syncopes is two years. These problems determine the indications for surgical intervention.

Aortic Stenosis. Grading Schemes		
	Aortic Valve Area (cm²)	**Aortic Valve Area Index (cm²/m²)**
Mild	> 1.50	**1.20 - 0.90**
Moderate	1.50 - 1.00	**0.90 - 0.60**
Moderately severe	1.00 - 0.50	**0.60 - 0.30**
Severe	< 0.50	**< 0.30**
According to [11].		
Mild	> 1.00	**> 0.60**
Moderate	1.00 - 0.75	**0.60 - 0.40**
Moderately severe	0.75 - 0.50	**0.40 - 0.30**
Critical	< 0.55	**< 0.30**
According to [6] and [12].		

The following techniques can be used for ultrasound based quantitative assessment of aortic stenosis.

Echocardiographic Quantitation of Aortic Stenosis
1. Planimetry of the aortic valve area from transesophageal short and long-axis views.
Doppler Echocardiographic Quantitation of Aortic Stenosis
2. Continuity equation.
3. Simplified Gorlin formula.

When resolution across the entire circumference is good, transesophageal planimetry of the aortic valve area from short and long-axis views provides reproducible results. Aortic valve area assessment is more satisfactory than mitral valve area planimetry assessment, probably because of the geometry of the aortic valve is less complicated. However, when the aortic valve is severely calcified, its architecture becomes more irregular, and planimetry gives unreliable results.

Doppler echocardiography is the standard noninvasive technique for quantitation of aortic stenosis. The peak gradient calculated from the Doppler-assessed peak blood flow velocity represents the peak instantaneous gradient and not a peak-to-peak gradient measured at cardiac catheterization, nor the mean gradient obtained from Doppler or invasive measurements, nor the Doppler-derived ("effective") gradient.

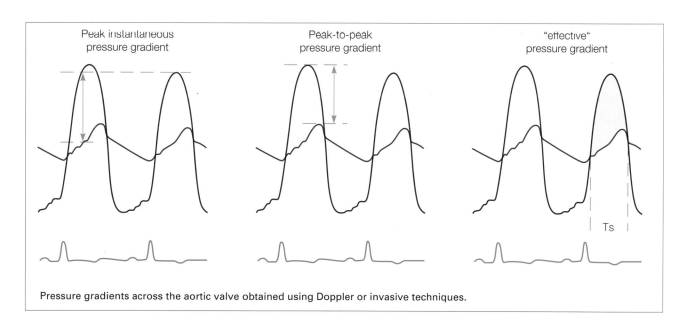

Pressure gradients across the aortic valve obtained using Doppler or invasive techniques.

The peak instantaneous pressure gradient represents the maximum difference between left ventricular pressure and aortic pressure at any time during the ejection period. The time at which it occurs varies from patient to patient.

$$\Delta p_{peak} = \Delta p_{max,inst} = \Delta p_{max}(t=i)$$

The peak-to-peak gradient represents the differences between the peak left ventricular and peak aortic pressures during the ejection period:

$$\Delta p_{pp} = (p_{max,LV} - p_{max,AS})(t=ET)$$

The "effective" gradient, which represents the difference between the left ventricular pressure and aortic pressure integrated separately throughout the ejection period, is a fictitious constant pressure value for the ejection period.

$$\Delta p_{eff} = \int(p_{LV})/ET - \int(p_{AS})/ET$$

The mean gradient represents the difference between left ventricular and aortic pressure, measured at equally spaced times (interval as small as possible) throughout the ejection period. The individual values are averaged to obtain the mean systolic gradient:

$$\Delta p_{mean} = \int(p_{LV} - p_{AS})/ET$$

The differences and incompatibilities between gradients obtained by Doppler and invasive measurements occur, on the one hand, because the Doppler-derived peak instantaneous gradient exceeds the peak-to-peak gradient measured at cardiac catheterization by an unknown figure. On the other hand, the often falsely termed "mean" gradient obtained by Doppler does not correspond to the true mean gradient. Furthermore, since the geometry of the stenotic aortic orifice is often bizarre and irregular, the assumed geometric conditions often are not met. Also, eccentric stenotic jets may flow at an excessive angle to the Doppler beam. When there are multiple stenotic jets, the jet assessed by Doppler does not necessarily correspond to the "representative" main jet. When a stenotic jet is dispersed into multiple single jets after passing through the irregularly shaped calcific tunnel, the velocity of each jet is determined by the diameter of its respective passageway. Theoretically, 90% of the cardiac output might flow through a residual orifice of 0.75 cm^2, yet the jet is eccentric and difficult to detect. In that case, the Doppler beam might more easily detect the other 10% output jet that flows at a more favorable angle to the beam and consider it to be "representative". Depending on whether it passes through a smaller or larger orifice, the true degree of stenosis would then be either over- or underestimated.

It is therefore essential that velocity measurements be performed from all possible scan planes. It remains unclear whether 3-dimensional reconstruction can obviate this source of error.

The clinical severity of aortic stenosis is defined by the aortic valve area and the transvalvular pressure gradient, which is dependent on transvalvular flow. The common practice of simply using the transvalvular pressure gradient without the aortic valve area to define severity ignores this fact. A pressure gradient of 25 mmHg with a cardiac output of 2 l/min can reflect severe aortic stenosis requiring surgical intervention, whereas a pressure gradient of 50 mmHg with a cardiac output of 15 l/min reflects only mild aortic stenosis. Cardiac output is determined not only by ventricular function, but also by the existing load conditions, heart rate, and the treatment received. Particularly when a decision must be made as to whether to surgically intervene or merely to follow the patient, the assessment of the severity of aortic stenosis should not be based on the transvalvular pressure gradient alone.

The aortic valve area can be calculated using the continuity equation.

First, the diameter of the left ventricular outflow tract is measured immediately proximal to the aortic valve [14]. Next, flow velocities are measured proximal to the stenosis and within the stenotic flow jet.

$$A_1 V_1 = A_2 V_2$$

$$A_{LVOT} \times V_{max, LVOT} = AVA \times V_{max, AS}$$

$$AVA = (A_{LVOT} \times V_{max, LVOT}) / V_{max,AS}$$

$A_1 = A_{LVOT}$	Systolic diameter area of the left ventricular outflow tract (cm2) (Measured between insertions of aortic cusps)
$V_1 = V_{LVOT}$	Flow velocity in left ventricular outflow tract (m/s)
$A_2 = AVA$	Aortic valve area (cm2)
$V_2 = V_{AS}$	Flow velocity of aortic stenotic flow jet (m/s)

A fictitious parameter is obtained when the peak instantaneous flow velocity is incorporated in this relation, as is the case when using flow velocity curves integrated from the ejection period [3, 21, 26, 28]. The former is not the "peak" aortic valve area, since the two velocity peaks do not occur at the same time. The latter can be more accurately described as the "effective" instead of the mean aortic valve area, since this relation describes an area that remains constant throughout the ejection period. In order to obtain the mean aortic valve area, the envelope curves must be digitized and the quotients V1/V2 must be averaged from measurements made at the smallest possible time intervals [2]:

$$AVA_{mean} = A_{L-OT} \int(V_1/V_2)/ET = A_{LVOT} \int(V_1/V_2)/ET$$

The difference between the aortic valve area derived from peak instantaneous velocities or from integrated flow velocities from the ejection period and the mean aortic valve area becomes smaller and smaller as the aortic valve area measured throughout the ejection period becomes more constant. Since determination of the mean aortic valve area is more tedious, the two alternative methods are more commonly used, except in cases where the degree of calcification is very slight.

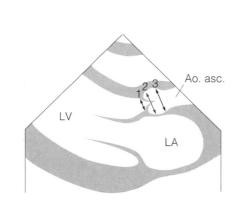

Computation of aortic valve area using the continuity equation: First the diameter of the left ventricular outflow tract is determined. The systolic diameter, measured at the aortic cusp insertions, is 20.6 mm.

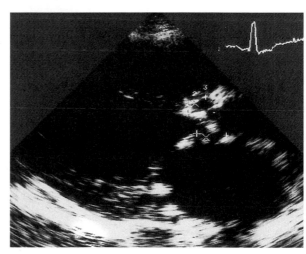

Parasternal long-axis 2-D echocardiogram.

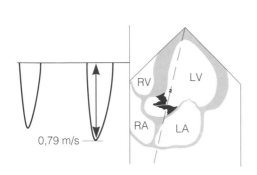

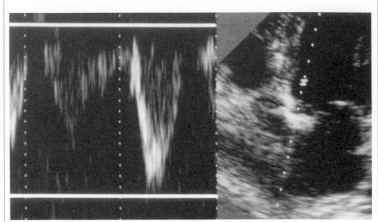

Determination of aortic valve area using the continuity equation: Peak instantaneous flow velocity in the left ventricular outflow tract = 0.79 m/s.

Apical five-chamber 2-D echocardiogram. The PW Doppler sample volume is located 1 cm proximal to the aortic valve.

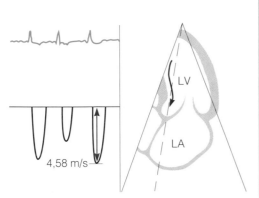

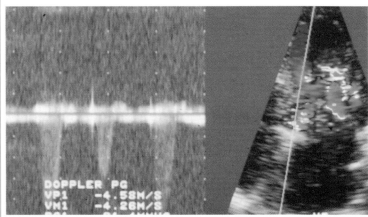

Determination of aortic valve area using the continuity equation: Peak instantaneous flow velocity across the aortic valve = 4.58 m/s.

CW Doppler and apical five-chamber 2-D echocardiograms.

Example:

$$AVA = (A_{LVOT} \, V_{max,LVOT})/V_{max,AS}$$

$$AVA = \{[(2.06 \text{ cm}/2)^2 \times 3.14] \times 0.78 \text{ m/s}\} / 4.58 \text{ m/s}$$

$$AVA = (3.33 \text{ cm}^2 \times 0.78 \text{ m/s}) / 4.58 \text{ m/s}$$

$$AVA = 3.33 \text{ cm}^2 \text{ m/s} / 3.57 \text{ m/s}$$

$$AVA = 0.93 \text{ cm}^2$$

Determination of the aortic valve area according to the Gorlin formula - using either the modified Bernoulli equation [18] or flow across the pulmonary valve [10, 27] and simplifying assumptions -

$$AVA = CO/\sqrt{\Delta P_m}$$

AVA	aortic valve area (cm2)
CO	cardiac output (l/min)
ΔP_m	mean transaortic pressure gradient (mmHg)

or:

$$AVA = SV/(0.9 V_{AS} \times ET)$$

AVA	aortic valve area (cm2)
SV	stroke volume (l/min)
V_{AS}	velocity of aortic stenotic jet (m/s)
ET	ejection time (s)

also makes it possible to make a noninvasive assessment of the severity of aortic stenosis.

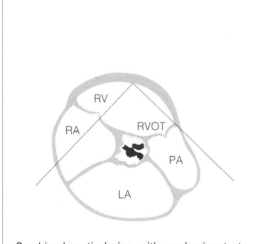

Combined aortic lesion with predominant stenotic component. Planimetry of the aortic valve area is attempted.

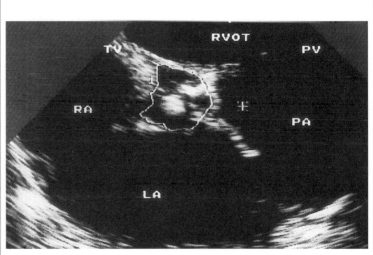

2-D left parasternal short-axis view at aortic valve level.

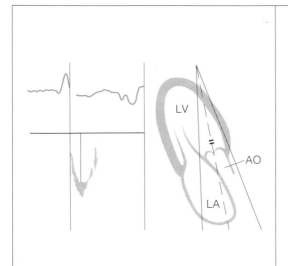

Diameter of the left ventricular outflow tract.

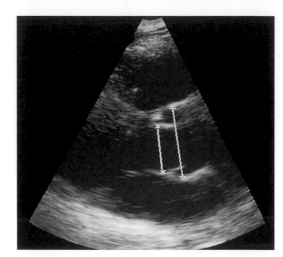

Parasternal long-axis 2-D echocardiogram.

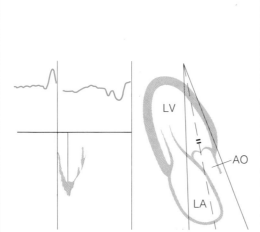

Sample volume is located 1 cm proximal to the aortic valve. Measured flow velocities = 0.35 and 0.25 m/s.

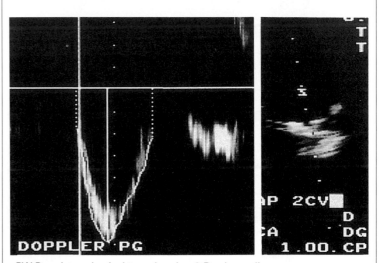

PW Doppler and apical two-chamber 2-D echocardiograms.

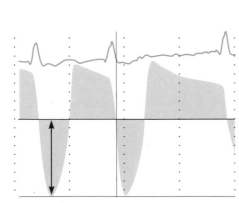

4,29 m/s ≙ 74 mmHg

Combined aortic lesion. Peak instantaneous flow velocity = 4.29 m/s; peak instantaneous pressure gradient = 74 mmHg.

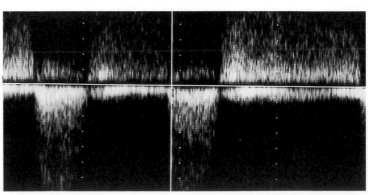

CW Doppler spectrum.

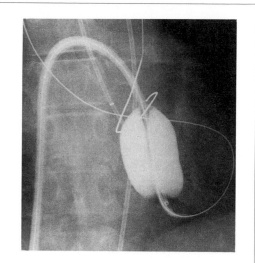

Percutaneous transluminal balloon vacuumplasty of the aortic valve.
Image shows inflated balloon in the aortic valve.

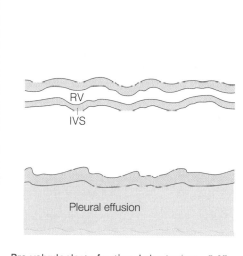

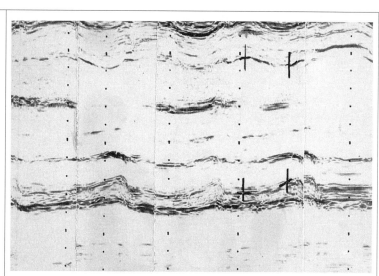

Pre-valvuloplasty fractional shortening = 0.18.

M-mode; left parasternal long-axis view from level of the ventricle.

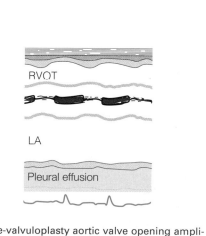

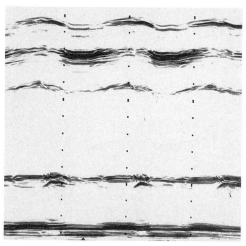

No pre-valvuloplasty aortic valve opening amplitude could be detected.

M-mode; left parasternal long-axis at from aortic valve level.

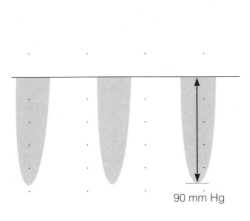

Pre-valvuloplasty peak instantaneous flow velocity = 4.74 m/s; peak instantaneous pressure gradient = 90 mmHg.

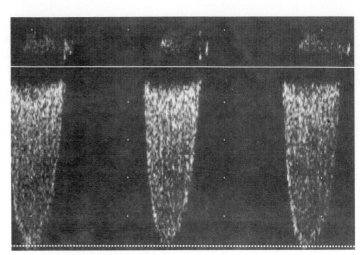

CW Doppler image at aortic valve level.

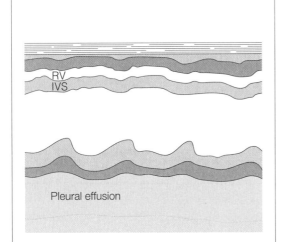

Post-valvuloplasty fractional shortening = 0.28.

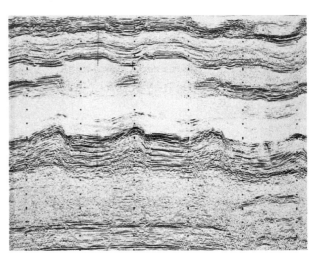

M-mode; left parasternal long-axis view from level of the ventricle.

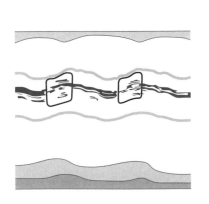

Post-valvuloplasty aortic valve opening amplitude > 15 mm.

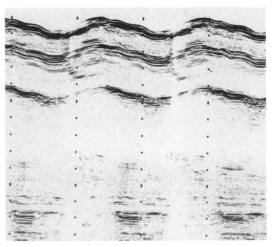

M-mode; left parasternal long-axis view at aortic valve level.

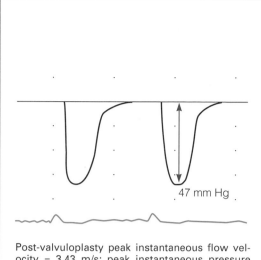

Post-valvuloplasty peak instantaneous flow velocity = 3.43 m/s; peak instantaneous pressure gradient = 47 mmHg.

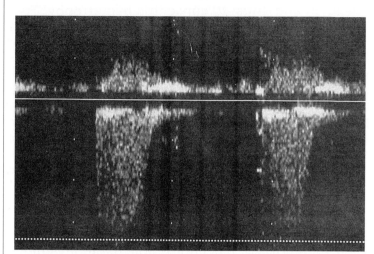

CW Doppler recording.

10.4.2   **Aortic Stenosis**
10.4.2.2   **Sources of Error**

Error may arise in the following areas when using conventional echocardiographic techniques for detection of aortic stenosis:
- Interpretation of noncalcifying aortic stenosis;
- Interpretation of reduced systolic separation of the aortic cusps, due to small stroke volume and small cardiac output.

Error can be minimized in Doppler quantitation of aortic stenosis:
- By using multiple imaging positions (*e.g.* apical five and two-chamber views, suprasternal and right parasternal views, additional transesophageal views if necessary).
- By taking the prestenotic flow velocity of > 1 m/s into account when computing the pressure gradient using the Bernoulli equation in cases with a concomitant regurgitant component.
- By making multiple measurements of the left ventricular outflow tract diameter and excluding outliers before calculating the mean.
- By measuring the prestenotic flow velocity at the same site where the left ventricular outflow tract diameter was measured.

The increase in systolic wall stress associated with aortic stenosis leads to parallel sarcomere replication and, thus, to concentric hypertrophy. The intracellular consequences include the formation of large cytoplasmatic regions lacking contractile material and interstitial proliferation of fibroblasts and collagen fibers. Since hypertrophy compensates for the increase in systolic wall stress, the ejection fraction will remain constant as long as the compensatory mechanism is still working [8]. In some patients, a progressive reduction in the ejection fraction signalises insufficient or inadequate hypertrophy (afterload mismatch) [25] and primary failure of the compensatory mechanism in the presence of normal contractile function. In other patients, however, a reduced ejection fraction results from reduced contractility and a secondary breakdown of the compensatory mechanism [4]. Both an increased afterload and altered contractility can reduce left ventricular performance (stroke index, cardiac index, stroke work, cardiac work) [9]. Therefore, it is essential to set the ventricular function parameters from the ejection period in relation to wall stress, particularly when making a prognosis concerning postoperative outcome.

Although compensatory hypertrophy is a key mechanism against the pressure stress caused by aortic stenosis, it has undesirable pathophysiologic consequences, namely an increase in diastolic stiffness. As a result, intracavitary pressure increases in order to maintain ventricular filling. The increase in overall chamber stiffness associated with aortic stenosis occurs simply due to an increase in myocardial mass in absence of increased myocardial stiffness. In other patients, both the overall chamber stiffness and the myocardial stiffness increase, causing a subsequent increase in ventricular filling pressure. Although overall chamber stiffness usually returns to normal after surgical intervention, myocardial stiffness seldom does. The extent of interstitial fibrosis is said to play a role in this phenomenon. In patients with extensive fibrosis, myocardial stiffness increases in the postoperative phase due to regressive hypertrophy and the lack of reduction in fibrosis [7, 15].

Left ventricular dilatation does not occur in aortic stenosis until ventricular contractility is significantly reduced. Dilatation then shifts the diastolic pressure-volume curve in another attempt to gain time for compensating for systolic pressure-volume conditions [22]. As left ventricular performance continues to decrease, compensatory hypertrophy and dilatation are no longer able to maintain a normal antegrade stroke volume. Dilatation and progressively reduced contractility lead to an increase in systolic wall stress (preload-afterload mismatch), which in turn leads to increased left ventricular end-diastolic pressure, diminished ejection fraction, and decreased cardiac output [23].

10.4.2   Aortic Stenosis
10.4.2.4   Treatment and Follow-up Considerations

In the natural course of aortic stenosis, the prognosis is significantly reduced after the onset of symptoms. The average survival time is two years after the manifestation of heart failure, three years after the manifestation of syncopes, and five years after the manifestation of angina pectoris [5]. Therefore, asymptomatic patients with mild aortic stenosis should have an annual echocardiographic follow-up examination, and those with moderate aortic stenosis should have echocardiographic follow-ups every six months. In patients with moderately severe to severe aortic stenosis, follow-up examinations should be performed by means of right and left heart catheterization [17].

Treatment is goverend by:
1. Pressure gradients, aortic valve area, and aortic valve area indices.
2. Left ventricular size and function.

There is still disagreement as to whether an increase in the "functional" aortic valve area, which can be assessed during stress testing, is a reliable predictor of the onset of symptoms [20].

New aspects have been added to the discussion concerning the optimal timing of surgical intervention for aortic stenosis since the advent of valvuloplasty and due to the results of studies on the natural course of the disease. As long as there is no definitive decision on the role of asymptomatic yet hemodynamically significant higher-grade lesions, stress hemodynamics should be evaluated thoroughly and the possibility of concomitant coronary disease should be excluded before a decision against surgical intervention is made. There is a reserved attitude about performing valvuloplasty. It is usually performed only in otherwise inoperable cases, and frequently is performed as an interim solution before surgery, because of the apparently rapid and regular occurrence of restenosis.

10.4.2   **Aortic Stenosis**
10.4.2.5   **Critical Evaluation and Comparison with the Results**
                   of Complementary Diagnostic Techniques

Echocardiographic techniques can provide technical and diagnostic information that is decisive for the assessment of aortic stenosis and for deciding how to treat it. The most important parameters provided by echocardiography include the aortic valve area index, the mean transaortic pressure gradient, and morphometric data.

Right heart catheterization, which can provide essential pressure-flow data from the lesser circulation under stress, is an important tool for timing surgical interventions.

Left heart catheterization is required only for the exclusion or confirmation of suspected concomitant ischemic heart disease, which may require same-time revascularization. The patient history and symptoms are important factors in planning the optimal time of surgical intervention.

Morphology and ventricular function

LADmax	_____	mm
LVEDD	_____	mm
LVESD	_____	mm

Fractional shortening   _____
LVEF   _____

Signs of concomitant ischemic heart disease?
Wall motion analysis

Valve morphology and dynamics

- ▸ Thickening and/or calcification of aortic cusps?
  - degree and extent of calcification
- ▸ Doming of aortic cusps?
- ▸ Poststenotic dilatation?

Valvular function and pressure-flow relationships (Doppler echocardiography)

- ▸ Velocity measurements (m/s)
  - peak instantaneous velocity
  - mean transaortic velocity
- ▸ Pressure gradients (mmHg)
  - peak instantaneous pressure gradient
  - mean transaortic pressure gradient
- ▸ AVA (aortic valve area, cm^2); AVA index (cm^2/m^2)
  - according to continuity equation
  - according to simplified Gorlin equation (as a control)
- ▸ Regurgitant jets
  - qualitative visual assessment
- ▸ Intracardiac pressure (mmHg)
  - LVEDP (Δ AV-RR$_{dia}$)

Transesophageal echocardiography

- ▸ Valve morphology and dynamics
- ▸ Planimetry of aortic valve area from short and long-axis views

SYMPTOMATOLOGY / AUSCULTATION

ECHOCARDIOGRAPHY

Conventional echocardiography:

Morphometry (LADmax, LVEDD, LVESD)
Ventricular function (LVFS, LVEF, wall motion analysis)
Visualization of structural causes and hemodynamic consequences

Doppler and transesophageal echocardiography:

Aortic valve area (AVA), valve area index (AVA-I)
calculated according to the continuity equation

Transesophageal echocardiography:
Planimetry of the aortic valve area

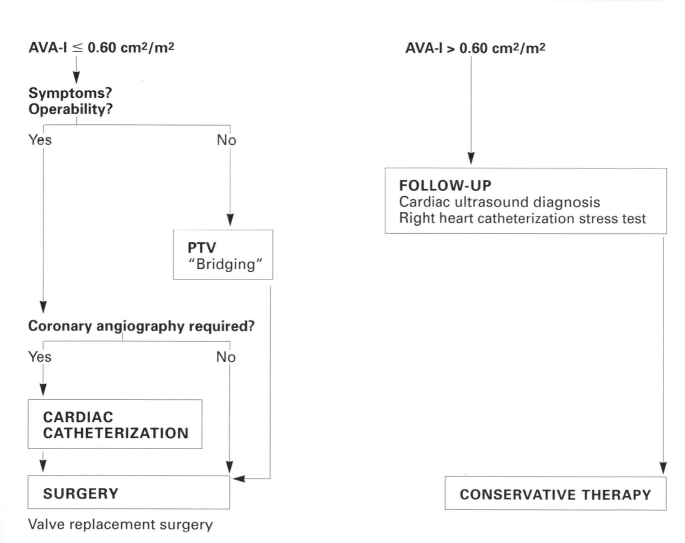

AVA-I $\leq$ 0.60 cm2/m2

Symptoms?
Operability?

Yes   No

PTV
"Bridging"

Coronary angiography required?

Yes   No

CARDIAC CATHETERIZATION

SURGERY

Valve replacement surgery

AVA-I > 0.60 cm2/m2

FOLLOW-UP
Cardiac ultrasound diagnosis
Right heart catheterization stress test

CONSERVATIVE THERAPY

1. Braunwald E. Pathophysiology of heart failure. In: Braunwald E (ed). Heart disease. 4th ed. Philadelphia: WB Saunders,1992: 393-418.
2. Dennig K, Kraus F, Rudolph W. Doppler-echokardiographische Bestimmung der Öffnungsfläche bei Aortenklappenstenose unter Anwendung der Kontinuitätsgleichung. Herz 1986; 11: 309-317.
3. Dennig K, Rudolph W. Doppler-echokardiographische Bestimmung der Öffnungsfläche bei Aortenklappenstenose nach der Kontinuitätsgleichung. Z Kardiol 1986; (suppl 1): 118.
4. Dodge HT, Baxley WA. Left ventricular volume and mass and their significance in heart disease. Am J Cardiol 1969; 23: 528.
5. Frank S, Johnson A, Ross J jr. Natural history of valvular aortic stenosis. Br Heart J 1973; 35: 41.
6. Grossman W, Baim DS (eds). Cardiac catheterization, angiography and intervention. 4th ed. vgl. (1) Philadelphia: Lea & Ferbiger, 1991: 569.
7. Hess OM, Ritter M, Schneider J et al. Diastolic stiffness and myocardial structure in aortic valve disease before and after replacement. Circulation 1984; 69: 855.
8. Hood WP jr, Rackley CE, Rolett EL. Wall stress in the normal and hypertrophied human left ventricle. Am J Cardiol 1968; 22: 550.
9. Huber D, Grimm J, Koch R, Krayenbuehl HP. Determinants of ejection performance in aortic stenosis. Circulation 1981; 64: 126.
10. Kosturakis D, Allen HD, Goldberg SJ, Sahn DJ, Valdes-Cruz LM. Noninvasive quantification of stenotic semilunar valve areas by Doppler echocardiography. J Am Coll Cardiol 1984; 3: 1256.
11. Kraus F, Rudolph W. Symptoms, exercise capacity, and exercise hemodynamics: Interrelationships and their role in the quanification of the valvular lesions. Herz 1984; 9: 187-199.
12. Miller G. Invasive intestigation of the heart. A guide to cardiac catheterization and related procedures. Blackwell, Oxford 1989; 282.
13. Moreno PR, Jang IK, Palacios IF. Does percutaneous balloon valvuloplasty have a role in patients with cardiogenic shock and critical aortic stenosis? J Am Coll Cardiol 1933; 21 (suppl A): 215A.
14. Moscucci M, Weinert L, Karp RB, Neumann A. Prediction of aortic annulus diameter by two-dimensional echocardiography. Circulation 1991; 84 (suppl III): III-76-III-80.
15. Murakami T, Hess OM, Gage JE et al. Diastolic filling dynamics in patients with aortic stenosis. Circulation 1986; 73: 1162.
16. Neudert J, Sutherland G, Bibra HV, Becher H. Usefulness of contrast enhanced Doppler echocardiography for the evaluation of aortic valve disease. J Am Coll Cardiol 1993; 21 (suppl A): 215A.
17. O'Fallon WM, Weidman WH (eds). Longterm follow-up of congenital aortic stenosis, pulmonary stenosis and ventricular septal defect. Circulation 1993; 87 (suppl I): I-1-I-126.
18. Ohlson J, Wranne B. Noninvasive assessment of valve area in patients with aortic stenosis. J Am Coll Cardiol 1986; 7: 501.
19. Olsson MC, Dalsgaard CJ, Haegerstrand AN, Nilsson JC, Rosenqvist M, Rydén LE. Accumulation of T-lymphocytes and expression of interleukin-2 receptors in non-rheumatic stenotic aortic valves. J Am Coll Cardiol 1993; 21 (suppl A): 215A.
20. Otto CM, Burwash IG, Pearlman AS, Gardner CJ, Healy NL, Schwaegler R. Exercise Doppler-hemodynamics may predict symptom onset in valvular aortic stenosis. J Am Coll Cardiol 1933; 21 (suppl A): 216A.
21. Otto CM, Pearlman AS, Comess KA, Reamer RP, Janko CL, Huntsman LL. Determination of the stenotic aortic valve area in adults using Doppler echocardiography. J Am Coll Cardiol 1986; 7: 509.
22. Rackley CE, Hood WP jr. Aortic valve disease. In: Levin HJ (ed). Clinical cardiovascular physiology. New York: Grune & Stratton, 1976: 493.
23. Rackley CE, Edwards JE, Wallace RB, Katz NM. Aortic valve disease. In: Hurst JW (ed). The heart. 7th ed. New York: McGraw Hill, 1990: 797.
24. Roberts WC. The congenitally bicuspid aortic valve stenosis. Am J Cardiol 1970; 26: 72.
25. Ross J jr. Afterload mismatch and preload reserve: a conceptual framework for the analysis of ventricular function. Progr Cardiovasc Dis 1976; 18: 255.
26. Skjaerpe T, Hegrenaes L, Hatle L. Noninvasive estimation of valve area in patients with aortic stenosis by Doppler ultrasound and two-dimensional echocardiography. Circulation 1985; 72: 810.
27. Warth DC, Stewart WJ, Block PC, Weyman AE. A new method to calculate aortic valve area without left heart catheterization. Circulation 1984; 70: 978.
28. Zoghbi WA, Farmer KL, Soto JG, Nelson JG, Quinones MA. Accurate noninvasive quantification of stenotic aortic valve area by Doppler echocardiography. Circulation 1986; 73: 452.

The main focus of functional assessment in the follow-up of prosthetic cardiac valves is to exclude or detect regurgitation or restenosis in order to differentiate between valvular malfunction and ventricular dysfunction whenever clinical deterioration occurs. In addition to auscultation, cinefluoroscopy and cardiac catheterization, cardiac ultrasound diagnosis is able to describe and, in part, quantitate prosthetic valve malfunction similar to its use in native valve assessment. This includes evolution of transprosthetic pressure gradient, measurement of the effective prosthetic valve orifice area, and detection and assessment of central and paraprosthetic regurgitations. Functional assessment of prosthetic valve function is complicated by the prosthesis-specific nature of prosthetic valve flow patterns and hemodynamics, which results in a multitude of different echo characteristics and flow profiles.

Cardiac Ultrasound Diagnosis

Echocardiographic studies should preferably be performed from the parasternal long and short-axis views and apical and subcostal two and four-chamber views. Aortic valve prostheses are best visualized from suprasternal and right supraclavicular positions. Transesophageal echocardiography should, in all cases, be used to clarify suspected prosthetic valve malfunction.

11.1 Mitral Valve Prostheses
11.1.1 Normally Functioning Prosthetic Valves

Conventional Echocardiography

Caged-Ball Valves:

(*e.g.* Starr-Edwards Model 6120, Smeloff-Cutter)

2-D and M-mode echocardiography:

- To visualize poppet motion, determine the ball opening and closing velocities, and to identify impaired cage opening due to thrombus (M-mode).

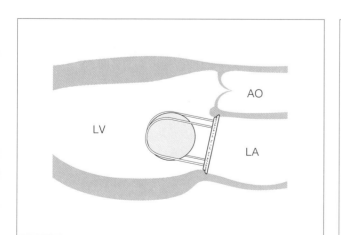

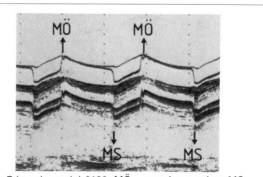

Starr-Edwards model 6120. MÖ = opening motion; MS = closure motion. *Reprinted with permission from: Biamino G, Lange L. Aktuelles Wissen. Echocardiographie, Hoechst AG, 1983.*

Disk Valves:
1. Central occluder disk valves (*e.g.* Kay-Shiley, Starr-Edwards Model 6500).
2. Tilting disk valves (*e.g.* Björk-Shiley, Lillehei-Kaster, Medtronic Hall (previously known as Hall-Kaster), Omnicarbon, Omniscience).
3. Bileaflet valves (*e.g.* Duromedics, Medtronic-Hall, St. Jude Medical).

2-D and M-mode echocardiography:
Central occluder disk valves:
Motion pattern similar to that of ball valves. Their lower excursion amplitude makes it difficult to distinguish between the disk and the cage.
Tilting disk valves:
The larger portion of the disk tilts into the ventricle, the smaller (which usually remains out of view) *tilts into the atrial cavity. Posterior motion of the disk occurs in diastole, and anterior motion occurs in systole. This results in a sharp point E.* In systole, multiple parallel echoes from the sewing ring make it difficult to determine the onset of disk excursion (maximum 60 to 70 % of the prosthetic valve diameter). Therefore, abnormally reduced motility can be difficult to identify. In atrial fibrillation, diastolic pressure fluctuations create "notches" in the disk echo traces and lead to variable closing velocities. This does not necessarily mean the prosthetic valve is malfunctioning.
Bileaflet prosthetic valves:
The anterior leaflet opens transducer-fugal towards posterior, and the posterior leaflet opens transducer-petal towards anterior. In diastole both leaflets appear as fine adjacent lines. Multiple echoes that extend to the posterior wall of the left ventricle may be recorded behind the posterior leaflet. Implantation-related differences in prosthetic valve alignment make it difficult to assess prosthetic leaflet motility. The diastolic leaflet motion can be assessed in the subcostal four-chamber view.

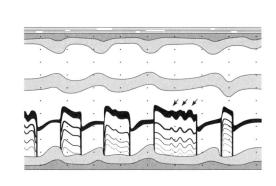

Björk-Shiley mitral valve prosthesis.

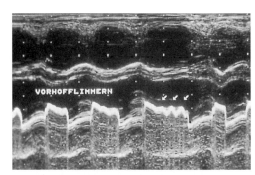

Opening velocity > 600 mm/s; closing velocity > 700 mm/s. Atrial fibrillation (= Vorhofflimmern). Diminished EF slope.

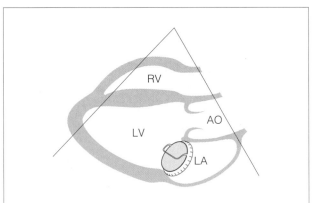

Björk-Shiley mitral valve prosthesis.

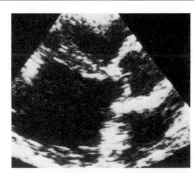

Scattered systolic echoes from sewing ring. *Reprinted with permission from: Biamino G, Lange L. Aktuelles Wissen. Echocardiographie, Hoechst AG, 1983.*

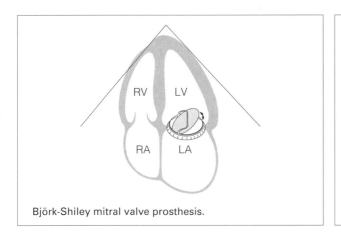

Björk-Shiley mitral valve prosthesis.

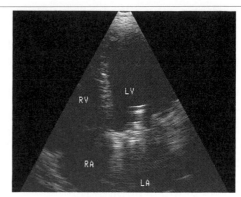

The disk is visible in diastole.

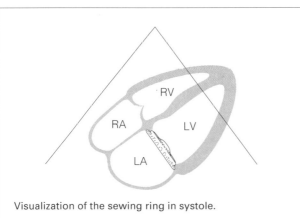

St. Jude Medical mitral valve prosthesis.

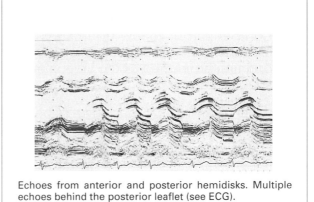

Echoes from anterior and posterior hemidisks. Multiple echoes behind the posterior leaflet (see ECG).

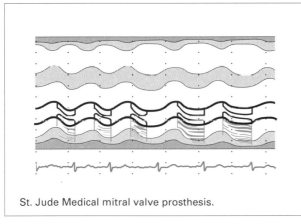

Visualization of the sewing ring in systole.

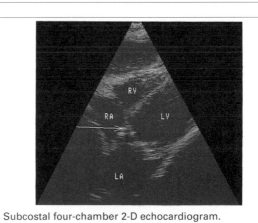

Subcostal four-chamber 2-D echocardiogram.

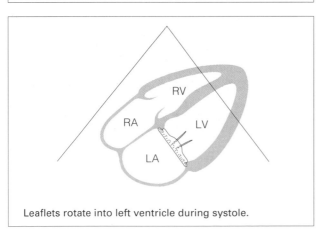

Leaflets rotate into left ventricle during systole.

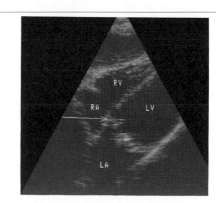

Subcostal four-chamber 2-D echocardiogram.

Bioprosthetic valves (hetero- and homografts)

In heterografts (animal tissue) and homografts (human tissue), biological transplant material is removed from the aortic or pulmonary region and can be transplanted to any other region.

Two-dimensional echocardiography:

- T*wo of the three stents can be identified,* but not when there is excessive rocking motion, *i.e.* partial dehiscence. The *stents should have smooth contours* without irregularities (as would be found with thrombus). The prosthetic valve should remain in its *axis of implantation.* Abnormal excursion may be due to paravalvular leakage or dehiscence.

M-mode echocardiography:

- In aortic valve prostheses implanted in the *reverse* (mitral) position, *two of the three valve cusps create the characteristic parallelogram-shaped M-mode motion pattern* (dense and wide echo band behind the anterior and posterior sections of the sewing ring).
- Comparison of follow-up images with the initial postoperative images is essential for identification of degeneration, thrombus, or endocarditic vegetations. Echodensity, opening amplitude or the steepness of the return movement of the sewing ring are non-specific criteria.

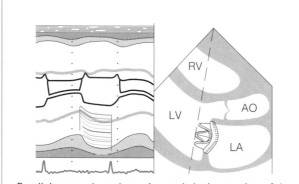

Parallelogram-shaped opening and closing motion of the prosthetic valve.

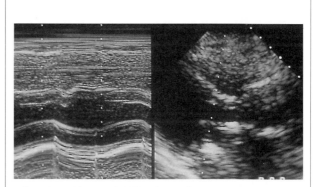

Parasternal long-axis 2-D echocardiogram.

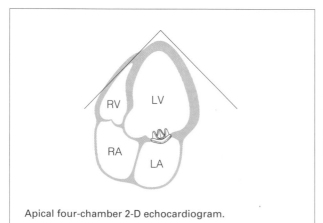

Apical four-chamber 2-D echocardiogram.

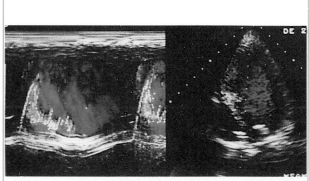

Stents are visualized, but cusps are not.

**Semiquantitation and Quantitation of Prosthetic Valve Function
(Conventional and Color Doppler Flow Imaging)**

- *Mean transprosthetic flow velocity, mean transprosthetic pressure gradient, and mitral prosthetic valve orifice area, "mapping" prosthesis-related central regurgitations or paraprosthetic leaks with pulsed-wave Doppler, with or without color Doppler flow imaging.*

Methods for semiquantitation or quantitation of prosthetic valve function must take into account that the prosthesis itself is associated with a certain degree of stenosis or regurgitation. This should not be misinterpreted as prosthetic valve malfunction.

Since the prosthesis fits inside the native annulus, the sewing ring and parts located inside the passageway reduce the effective orifice area. Prosthesis-related obstruction is therefore unavoidable.

The hemodynamic performance of the prosthetic valve is of greater significance in atrioventricular than in semilunar valve replacement, because even mild stenosis within the low pressure system can have significant consequences.

Doppler findings in various mitral prosthetic valves
(adapted from [24])

	Björk-Shiley (n = 24)	St. Jude-Medical (n = 30)	Duromedics (n = 20)	CE/H/MF (n = 20)
V_{max} (m/s)	1.68 ± 0.28	1.5 ± 0.25	1.54 ± 0.26	1.69 ± 0.29
V_{mean} (m/s)	1.04 ± 0.17	0.91 ± 0.20	0.96 ± 0.16	1.06 ± 0.21
Δp_{max} (mmHg)	11.9 ± 3.7	9.2 ± 3.0	9.7 ± 3.2	1.06 ± 0.21
Δp_{mean} (mmHg)	4.6 ± 1.5	3.5 ± 1.6	3.8 ± 1.2	4.7 ± 1.9
PHT (ms)	88 ± 31	71 ± 12	75 ± 21	95 ± 23
MPVA (cm2)	2.75 ± 0.82	3.21 ± 0.57	3.11 ± 0.66	2.44 ± 0.61

CE Carpentier-Edwards, H = Hancock, MF = Mitroflow
V_{max} Maximum (peak) instantaneous transprosthetic flow velocity
V_{mean} Mean transprosthetic flow velocity
Δp_{max} Maximum instantaneous transprosthetic pressure gradient
Δp_{mean} Mean transprosthetic pressure gradient
PHT   Pressure half time
MPVA   Mitral prosthetic valve area

It is essential to know the size of the prosthesis when performing Doppler studies of prosthetic valve function. As the size of the prosthesis decreases, the prosthesis-related transprosthetic flow velocities and pressure gradients increase. Mitral valve prostheses smaller than 28 mm are classified as relatively small [30].

In vivo hemodynamics of mitral prosthetic valves (adapted from [20]).

Type	d	Flow	Δp	A_t	A_{geo}	A_{eff}	
Star Edwards Model 6120	30	157 ± 50 251 ± 77	6.3 ± 2.0 11.9 ± 3.6	7.07	2.86	1.8 ± 0.4 2.0 ± 0.4	R 30 W
Björk-Shiley Standard	29	161 ± 40 316 ± 39	4.5 ± 1.6 9.4 ± 2.8	6.61	4.40	2.2 ± 0.5 2.8 ± 0.6	R 30 W
Medtronic-Hall	29	148 ± 41 329 ± 93	5.2 ± 3.3 16.5 ± 1.7	6.61	4.52	1.9 ± 0.5 2.3 ± 0.6	R 30 W
St. Jude-Medical	29	167 ± 42 291 ± 73	2.3 ± 0,6 6.4 ± 3.0	6.61	4.52	3.1 ± 0.8 3.4 ± 0.7	R 30 W
Ionescu-Shiley	29	149 ± 46 274 ± 31	5.3 ± 1.6 11.2 ± 2.3	6.61	5.07	1.9 ± 0.8 2.1 ± 0.9	R 30 W

d	Outer diameter of sewing ring (mm)
Δp	Transprosthetic pressure gradient (mmHg) (= Δp_{mean})
A_t	Total prosthetic valve area $(d/s)^2 \times \pi$
A_{geo}	Geometric prosthetic valve area (prosthetic valve area ignoring the body of the valve)
A_{eff}	Effective prosthetic valve area (SV / 51.6 x $\sqrt{\Delta p}$ (= MPVA)
R	Resting
30 W	30 watt exercise
SV	Transprosthetic stroke volume (ml)

These size 29 to 30 mm mitral valve prostheses have an effective prosthetic valve area of 1.81 to 3.1 cm² at rest and 2.0 to 3.4 cm² with mild exercise (30 W). Therefore, even when functioning properly, these relatively large prostheses will cause mild to moderate stenosis [25, 29].

The evaluation of prosthetic valve function is based on morphological data, mean transprosthetic flow velocity, mean transprosthetic pressure gradient, and the prosthetic valve area derived from the pressure half-time. Because the flow profile of practically all prosthetic valves is nonparabolic, peak instantaneous flow velocity and pressure gradients are often erroneous. Therefore, these parameters should not be used for functional assessment.

Doppler quantitation of inherent stenosis of mitral valve prostheses [8, 10]

- ► Pressure half-time method
- ► Simplified Gorlin formula
- ► Continuity equation

The mitral prosthetic valve area, like the native valve orifice area, is calculated using the pressure half-time method.

MPVA = 220/PHT

MPVA	mitral prosthetic valve area (cm²)
PHT	pressure half-time (ms)

Using the simplified Gorlin formula, which neglects the diastolic filling time, frequency, and constants [2, 17, 33], one can make a semiquantitative, relatively rough, assessment of prosthetic valve function [5].

$$MPVA = CO/\sqrt{\Delta P_m}$$

MPVA	Mean prosthetic valve area (cm^2)
CO	Cardiac output (l/min)
ΔP_m	Mean transprosthetic pressure gradient (mmHg)

When using the continuity equation, the prosthetic ring area listed by the manufacturer can be used as the paraprosthetic cross-sectional area A_1. This obviates the need for tedious and imprecise echocardiographic measurement. Since the preprosthetic flow velocity V_1 is difficult to quantitate in mitral prosthetic valves, this parameter is not used as often as in the assessment of aortic valve prostheses.

Criteria for distinguishing normal prosthesis-related regurgitation from pathological regurgitation are based on the spatial orientation of the regurgitant jets [14]. In tilting disk prostheses, prosthesis-related regurgitation is characterized by a large central jet and one or more smaller, often symmetrical jets in the periphery. In bileaflet prostheses, normal prosthesis-related regurgitation is characterized by multiple jets that arise from the hinges. The jets appear to converge when the beam is parallel to the jet direction, and diverge in orthogonal planes.

Transesophageal echocardiography (single and multiplane)

- *Transesophageal echocardiography can be used for graphic display and (semi) quantitation of prosthetic valve function or malfunction.*

Virtually all morphologically detectable prosthetic valve dysfunction can be suggested, but not proven, by transthoracic echocardiography. Functional assessment of mitral prosthetic valves is one of the primary indications for transesophageal echocardiography [32, 40]. Multiplane and high-frequency transducers can be expected to make transesophageal echocardiography even more effective.

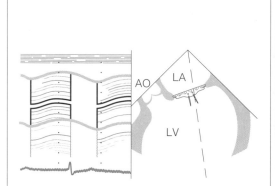

St. Jude Medical valve in the mitral valve position. The leaflets are visible in diastole. The valve is functioning properly. Reverberations posterior to the prosthesis are observed in diastole.

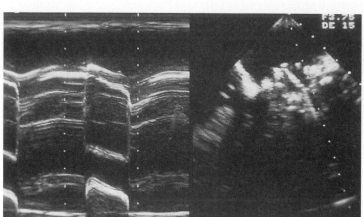

Transesophageal short-axis M-mode and 2-D echocardiograms.

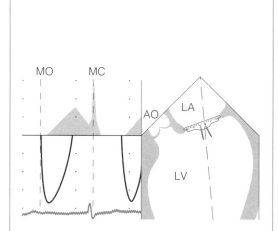

Same patient. Normal transprosthetic flow in diastole and "closure volume" in systole.

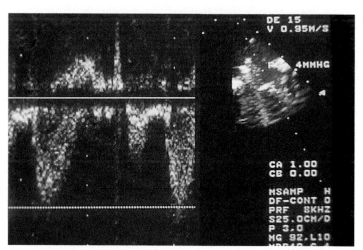

Transesophageal PW Doppler and 2-D recordings with color flow mapping.

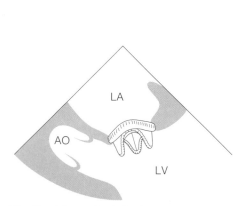

Mitroflow bioprosthesis in the mitral valve position. The stents are readily visible. The prosthesis is functioning properly.

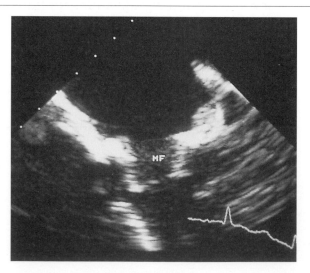

Transesophageal short-axis echocardiogram.

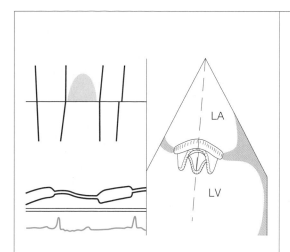

Same patient. Highly turbulent diastolic flow, aliasing in the prosthetic valve plane, and typical bioprosthetic valve "closure volume".

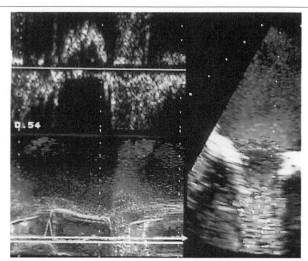

Transesophageal short-axis 2-D echocardiogram (right) and PW Doppler (upper left) and M-mode (bottom left) recordings, with color flow imaging.

11.1   Mitral Valve Prostheses
11.1.2   Prosthetic Valve Dysfunction

Dysfunction of mitral prosthetic valves can be caused by periprosthetic thrombus, prosthetic valve endocarditis, paraprosthetic leakage, mechanical malfunction and (partial) dehiscence of the prosthetic valve, or degeneration and degradation of the biological material.

False-positive findings due to reverberations and other artifacts must be differentiated from dysfunction due to hemodynamically significant obstruction. The evaluation of prosthetic valve dysfunction should not be based solely on conventional echocardiographic findings such as increased periprosthetic echoes, or delayed, intermittent, impaired, or incomplete opening of the valve. A non-prosthesis-related, high transprosthetic valve mean pressure gradient is of greater significance. Although it is of interest to determine whether the gradient is higher than average (> 5 mmHg for modern disk and bileaflet valves, > 25 mmHg for caged-ball prostheses), it is more important to know whether the gradient is higher than the initial baseline postoperative gradient. Taking into account the day-to-day variability, the threshold should be around +50%. Restenosis can be proven and quantitated using the prosthetic mitral valve orifice area.

Prosthetic valve endocarditis can be diagnosed in transthoracic scans only when the vegetations are massive. Therefore, when endocarditis is suspected, transesophageal echocardiographic studies are indicated.

Paraprosthetic leakage and regurgitation must be differentiated from normal prosthesis-related (usually) central regurgitation by identifying the characteristic prosthesis-related flow profile and by demonstrating the jet directions. The total prosthetic valve volume loss (the prosthesis specific regurgitant volume) can be calculated from the *closure volume* (volume regurgitant flow until the valve is fully closed) and the *leakage volume* (volume of regurgitant flow after the valve is fully closed). In normal prosthetic valves, the total volume loss is up to 10% of the forward stroke volume [18].

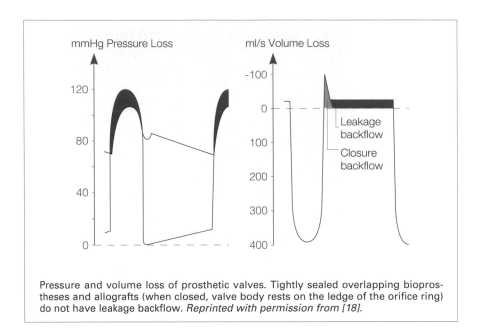

Pressure and volume loss of prosthetic valves. Tightly sealed overlapping bioprostheses and allografts (when closed, valve body rests on the ledge of the orifice ring) do not have leakage backflow. *Reprinted with permission from [18].*

One of the first indications of paraprosthetic leakage is "rounding off" of the E wave in early diastole in the M-mode echocardiogram. The systolic anterior motion of the valve is longer; it overlaps with the beginning of diastolic motion towards posterior. Therefore, the initial diastolic motion curve appears to be "rounded".

A second indication is a "very high" diastolic flow velocity with a normal pressure half-time and normal prosthetic mitral valve orifice area.

CW Doppler has the highest predictability for pathological regurgitation. Transesophageal echocardiography is essential to locate the origin of leakage.

Every mitral prosthetic valve exhibits model-specific regurgitant flow characteristics in transesophageal echocardiography. Disk prostheses exhibit pansystolic closure and leakage backflow and usually have more than two jets of eccentric origin [11]. Bileaflet prostheses have a central jet and two peripheral jets. Bioprosthetic valves usually have one central jet [31]. Color M-mode echocardiography permits differentiation of pathological, paraprosthetic leakage [23].

Degeneration and degradation of a bioprosthesis should be suspected 1. when there is evidence of restenosis or pathological regurgitation, or 2. when there is localized diastolic-systolic leaflet fluttering due to tearing and perforation, increased leaflet thickening and reduced motility or localized calcification (initially in the region of the commissures and the sewing ring).

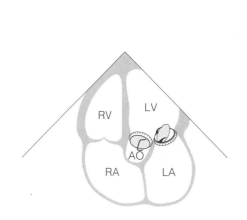

Mitral and aortic valve replacement with Lillehei-Kaster and Björk-Shiley prostheses, respectively. Mild combined tricuspid lesion. Mitral restenosis.

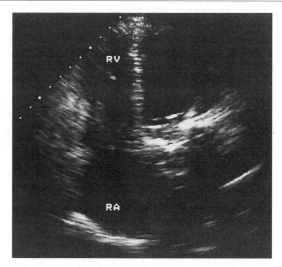

Apical four-chamber 2-D echocardiogram.

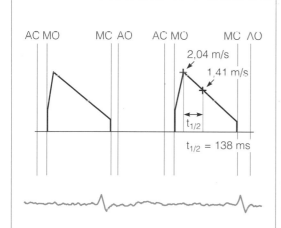

Same patient. The peak instantaneous transprosthetic valve pressure gradient is 17 mmHg. The pressure half-time is 138 ms, and the effective prosthetic mitral valve orifice area is 1.59 cm².

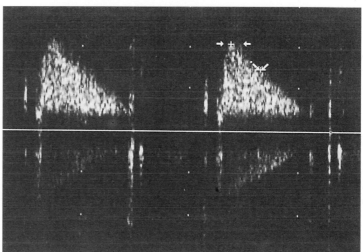

CW Doppler spectral display.

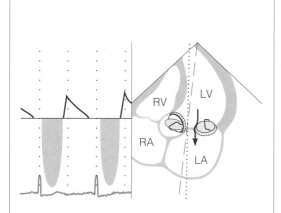

Paraprosthetic leakage from a Björk-Shiley mitral prosthetic valve after mitral and aortic valve replacement. Fast and turbulent regurgitant jet.

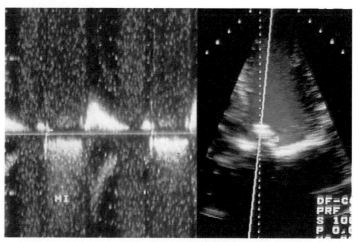

Apical four-chamber view. Color encoded CW-Doppler.

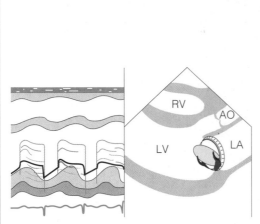

Partial thrombotic occlusion of Lillehei-Kaster mitral valve prosthesis. Finding confirmed intraoperatively.

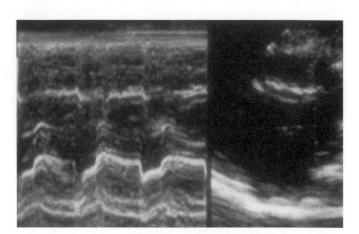

Parasternal long-axis M-mode and 2-D echocardiograms.

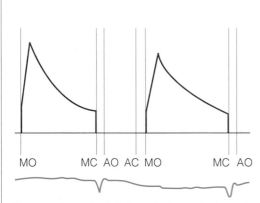

Same patient. Partial thrombotic occlusion of Lillehei-Kaster mitral valve prosthesis. High transprosthetic valve flow velocity and high transprosthetic valve pressure gradient, but normal pressure half-time. Findings confirmed intraoperatively.

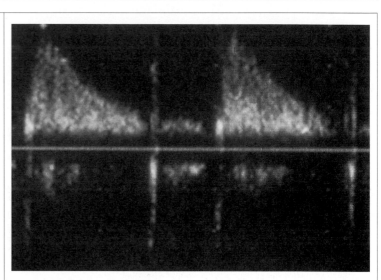

CW Doppler spectral display.

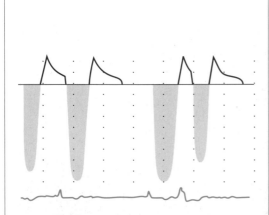

Paraprosthetic leak (Leck) in Duromedics mitral valve prosthesis. Rapid and turbulent regurgitant jet. MI = mitral insufficiency.

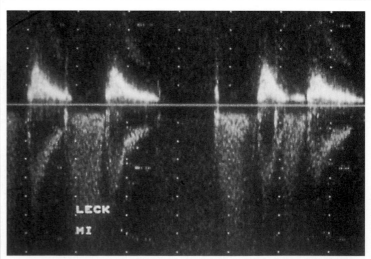

CW Doppler spectral display.

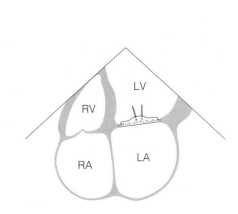

Paraprosthetic leakage in a Duromedics mitral valve prosthesis. Primarily normal prosthetic valve morphology and dynamics.

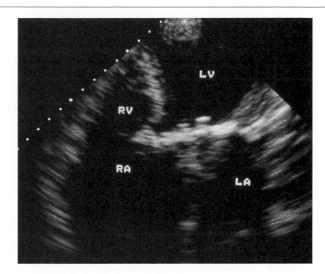

Apical four-chamber 2-D echocardiogram.

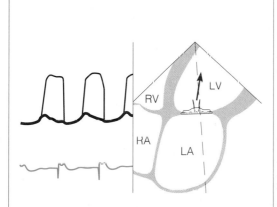

Continued. In the color flow map, no prosthetic incompetence can be detected from this angle.

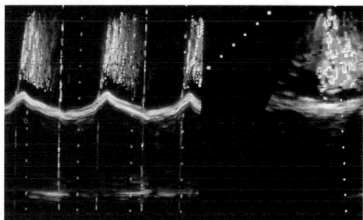

Color flow maps, M-mode and 2-D. Apical four-chamber view.

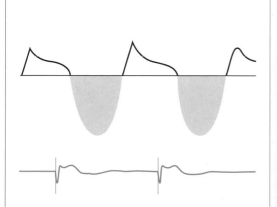

Continued. Prosthetic valve incompetence is demonstrated by CW Doppler.

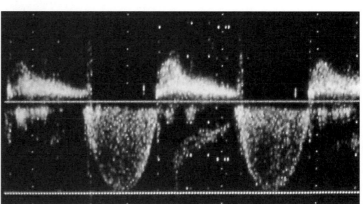

CW Doppler spectral display.

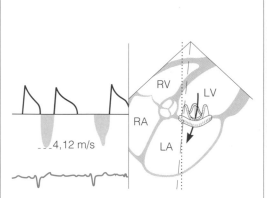

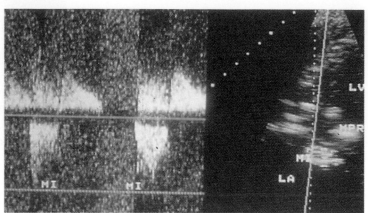

Mitral valve bioprosthesis. Central regurgitation. Poor envelope, but relatively fast regurgitant jet is detected.

Color flow maps of CW Doppler recording and apical four-chamber 2-D scan.

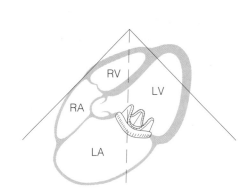

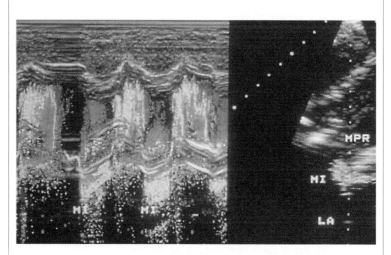

Paraprosthetic leakage in a mitral bioprosthesis. Rocking motion of the prosthesis is detected in color M-mode. Highly turbulent regurgitant jet. Regurgitation is paravalvular instead of central.

Apical four-chamber view. M-mode and 2-D with color flow mapping.

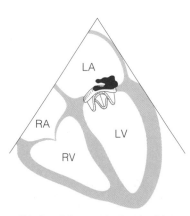

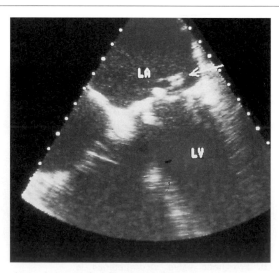

Endocarditis involving a mitral valve bioprosthesis. A vegetation is attached lateral to the prosthesis.

Transesophageal short-axis 2-D echocardiogram.

Conventional Echocardiography

Caged-Ball Prostheses:

(*e.g.* Starr-Edwards 1260, Smeloff-Cutter)

2-D and M-mode echocardiography:

- *Motion and amplitude of excursion of the ball from apical, suprasternal, and/or right supraclavicular transducer positions (2 D), opening and closing velocity of the ball and reduced opening motion due to thrombotic occlusion of the cage (M-mode).*

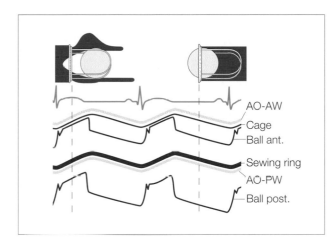
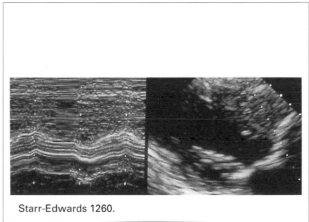

Starr-Edwards 1260.

Disk prostheses:

1. Central occluding disk prostheses
2. Tilting disk prostheses (*e.g.* Björk-Shiley, Björk-Shiley Monostrut, Hall-Kaster, Lillehei-Kaster, Omnicarbon, Omniscience).
3. Bileaflet prostheses (*e.g.* Duromedics, Medtronic-Hall, St. Jude Medical).

2-D and M-mode echocardiography:

To point 1: Motion pattern similar to that of ball prostheses, but with lower excursion amplitude. Therefore, it is difficult to differentiate between the struts and the disk.

To point 2: At the time of peak opening, the sewing ring moves abruptly towards posterior. In systole, multiple parallel echoes from the sewing ring make it difficult to determine the onset of disk excursion, which leads to uncertainties in determining if motility is pathologically impaired. When there is atrial fibrillation, diastolic pressure fluctuations create "notches" in the echo line of the disk, and lead to changes in the flow velocity.

To point 3: The anterior leaflet opens transducer-fugal towards posterior, and the posterior leaflet opens transducer-petal towards anterior. In diastole, the two leaflets appear as fine, adjacent lines. Because of implantation-related differences in valve alignment, it is difficult to determine whether leaflet motion is impaired. In 2-D echocardiography, diastolic leaflet motion can be assessed from the subcostal four-chamber view.

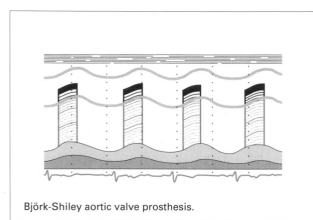

Björk-Shiley aortic valve prosthesis.

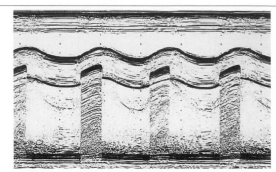

Opening and closing velocity around 700 mm/s. The greater half of the disk moves towards the transducer (anterior) in systole.

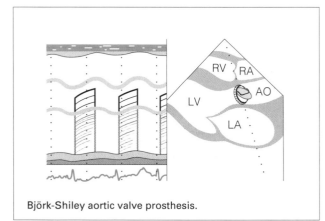

Björk-Shiley aortic valve prosthesis.

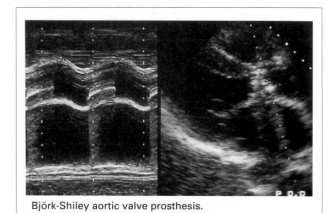

Björk-Shiley aortic valve prosthesis.

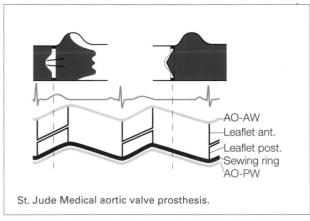

Björk-Shiley aortic valve prosthesis.

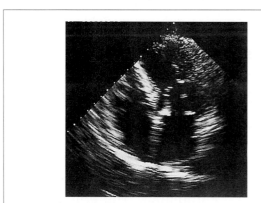

Björk-Shiley aortic valve prosthesis.

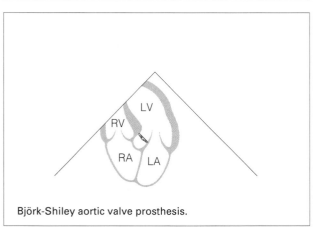

AO-AW
Leaflet ant.
Leaflet post.
Sewing ring
AO-PW

St. Jude Medical aortic valve prosthesis.

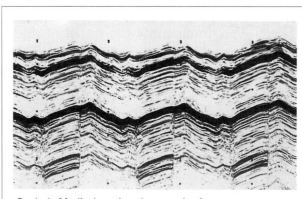

St. Jude Medical aortic valve prosthesis.

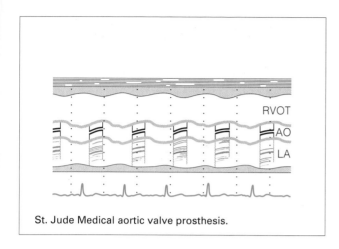

St. Jude Medical aortic valve prosthesis.

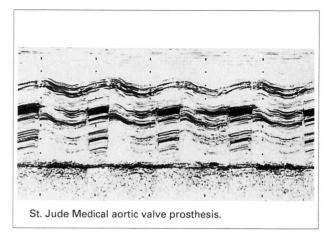

St. Jude Medical aortic valve prosthesis.

Prostheses made of biological material (hetero- and homografts)

Heterograft (animal) and homograft (human) transplants from aortic and (more infrequently) pulmonary positions can be used in any other position.

Two-dimensional echocardiography:

- *The prosthesis does not rock out of its axis of implantation* (as compared to prostheses with paraprosthetic leakage or a partial dehiscence). *Two of the three stents can be visualized.* The contours of the stents are smooth (as compared to prostheses with thrombus).

M-mode echocardiography:

- *Two of the three stents of the aortic valve prosthesis* (after the anterior and before the posterior part of the sewing ring - a dense and broad echo band) *appear* on M-mode recordings *as a typical parallelogram-shaped aortic valve motion pattern.*
- In order to diagnose degenerative, thrombotic, or endocarditic changes, it is essential to have baseline immediate postoperative echo images. Echo density, opening amplitude, and steepness of the return motion of the sewing ring are less important, as they are unspecific criteria.

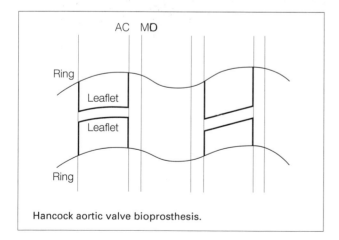

Hancock aortic valve bioprosthesis.

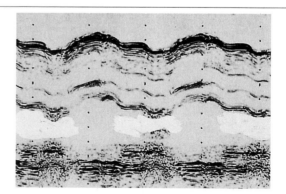

Parallelogram-shaped opening and closing motion of the prosthesis.

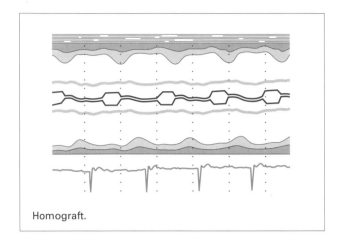

Homograft.

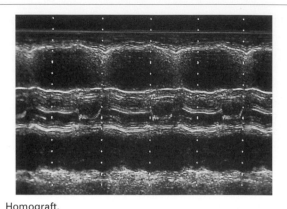

Homograft.

Semiquantitation and Quantitation of Prosthetic Valve Function (Doppler and Color Doppler Flow Imaging)

- *Transprosthetic valve pressure gradient, calculation of prosthetic aortic valve orifice area, mapping with black-and-white and color Doppler after prosthesis-related central regurgitation or paraprosthetic leakage.*

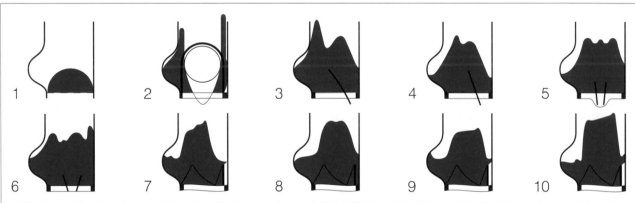

1. Native aortic valve; 2. Starr-Edwards ball valve prosthesis; 3. Björk-Shiley and 4. Medtronic-Hall disk prostheses; 5. St-Jude Medical and 6. Duromedics bileaflet prostheses; 7. Hancock and 8. Carpentier-Edwards bioprostheses; 9. Mitroflow and 10. Ionescu-Shiley bioprostheses; 2-6 are allografts; 7-8 are porcine heterografts, and 9-10 are bovine heterografts.
Reprinted with permission from: Horstkotte D, Loogen F: Erworbene Herzklappenfehler, Urban & Schwarzenberg, Munich-Vienna 1987, 247.

The flow characteristics of a prosthetic valve are dependent on the construction design and on the alignment of the prosthesis within the valve plane, which is determined at the time of implantation. The flow profile describes the individual transprosthetic flow contributions determined by the end-systolic position of the valve body and stents. Because these portions of flow differ in direction, velocity, and volumetric flow, the single Doppler-derived portion is not identical with the mean flow profile across the effective prosthetic valve orifice area, the greater the calculation error that can result. This is more critical in semilunar valve prostheses, which regulate high velocity flows over greatly variable pressure gradients, than in atrioventricular valve prostheses.

In vivo hemodynamics of aortic valve prostheses (adapted from [19])

Prosthesis	d	Flow	Δp	A_t	A_{geo}	A_{eff}	
Starr-Edwards 1260	24	301 ± 61 457 ± 53	25.1 ± 4.7 37.0 ± 8.4	4.52	1.79	1.4 ± 0.2 1.7 ± 0.2	R 30 W
Björk-Shiley Standard	23	284 ± 82 441 ± 111	18.9 ± 5.2 28.5 ± 6.5	4.15	2.55	1.5 ± 0.3 1.9 ± 0.3	R 30 W
St. Jude Medical	23	299 ± 52 433 ± 64	9.6 ± 3.1 15.7 ± 3.2	4.15	2.55	2.2 ± 0.3 2.5 ± 0.3	R 30 W
Ionescu-Shiley	23	204 ± 14 324 ± 13	10.8 ± 1.6 17.3 ± 1.6	4.15	2.96	1.6 ± 0.1 2.1 ± 0.1	R 30 W

d	Outer diameter of the sewing ring (mm)
Δp	Transprosthetic pressure gradient (mmHg; = mean Δp)
A_t	Total prosthetic valve orifice area (prosthetic ring area): $(d/2)^2 \times \pi$
A_{geo}	Geometric prosthetic valve area (prosthetic valve area disregarding the valve body)
A_{eff}	Effective prosthetic valve area (SV/51.6 x $\sqrt{\Delta p}$ (= APVA)
R	Resting
30 W	Exercise at 30 Watts
SV	Transprosthetic stroke volume

In these size 23 and 24 mm aortic valve prostheses, the effective prosthetic valve orifice area is 1.4 to 2.2 cm² at rest and 1.7 to 2.5 cm² with slight (30 Watts) exercise. Therefore, even when these prostheses are functioning normally, slight stenosis results [25, 28]. Aortic valve prostheses with a size of 25 mm or less are classified as relatively small [30].

Doppler echocardiographic quantitation of inherent stenosis associated with aortic valve prostheses

Mean transprosthetic pressure gradient [27, 34, 38]

Continuity equation [6, 9, 12, 15, 39]

▸ Standard continuity equation: APVA = SV/TVI_{CW}

▸ Simplified continuity equation: APVA = $(A_t \times VLVOT) / V_{APV}$

▸ Doppler index: APVA = $V_{max, LVOT} / V_{max, APV}$ [6, 41]

Simplified Gorlin equation [2, 17, 33]

Assessment based on the pressure drop across the prosthesis alone is subject to the same limitations as in native valves, because this parameter is dependent on the stroke volume across the valve and, thus, on the cardiac output and ventricular function [16, 37]. Thus, the mean transprosthetic pressure gradient is only an estimate of the hemodynamic effects of prosthetic valve stenosis. It should be taken as a compromise solution for cases where the effective orifice area of the prosthesis cannot be reliably determined.

The problem with the continuity equation in the functional assessment of a native aortic valve is its range of error in measurement of aortic valve ring diameter for determination of the pre-stenotic cross-sectional area flooded by blood. When applying the continuity equation in aortic valve prostheses, the "total" prosthetic ring area (i.e. the area including the sewing ring) as indicated by the manufacturer can be used as the preprosthetic cross-sectional area A_1. Difficult and imprecise echocardiographic assessments can thereby be avoided.

$$A_1\, v_1 = A_2\, v_2$$

$$A_t \times v_{LVOT} = APVA \times v_{APV}$$

$$APVA\ (cm^2) = (A_t\ [cm^2] \times v_{LVOT}\ [m/s])/v_{APV}\ (m/s)$$

$A_1 = A_t$	Total aortic prosthetic valve ring area
$v_1 = v_{LVOT}$	Preprosthetic flow velocity
$A_2 = A_{PVA}$	Aortic prosthetic valve area
$v_2 = v_{APV}$	Flow velocity of the transprosthetic jet

The preprosthetic flow velocity is measured with the PW Doppler sample volume in the left ventricular outflow tract, immediately proximal to the prosthesis, from an apical transducer position. The flow velocity of the transprosthetic jet is determined by CW Doppler from an apical, right parasternal, or suprasternal transducer position. The PW Doppler sample volume is positioned using the audio signal, and the CW Doppler cursor is position using the measured peak velocity signal.

The prosthetic valve orifice area A_2 is calculated at the time of peak flow as the product of the prosthetic valve ring area A_1 and the peak preprosthetic flow velocity v_1, divided by the maximum transprosthetic flow velocity v_2 at the time of the peak of the curve of prestenotic flow velocity v_2.

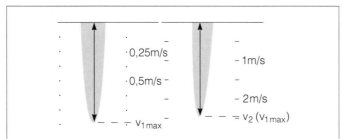

Pre- and transprosthetic flow velocities of an aortic valve prosthesis. Determination of peak of the curve of the preprosthetic flow velocity (v_1) and peak of the curve of transprosthetic flow velocity (v_2) at the time $t = v_{1max}[v_2(t=v_{1max})]$.

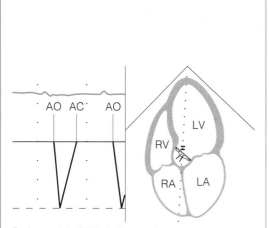

Patient with SJM 25A prosthesis in the aortic valve position presenting with considerable aortic insufficiency. V_{LVOT} = 0.86 m/s.

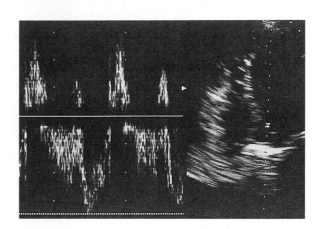

PW Doppler. Sample volume is positioned in the left ventricular outflow tract (LVOT). Apical four-chamber view.

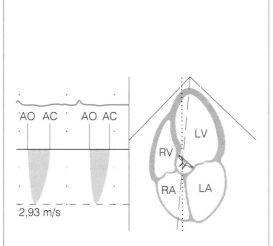

Same patient. V_{APV} = 2.93 m/s.

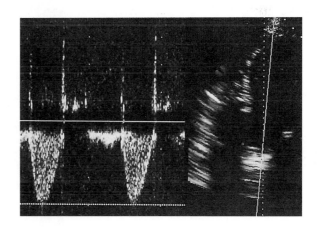

CW Doppler recording and apical four-chamber 2-D echocardiogram.

Example 1:

Patient with aortic valve replacement (SJM 25A-101) who presented with moderatly severe aortic insufficiency.

$$APVA = (A_t \times V_{LVOT}) / V_{APV}$$

$$APVA = (4.91 \text{ cm}^2 \times 0.86 \text{ m/s}) / 2.93 \text{ m/s}$$

$$APVA = 4.22 \text{ cm}^2 / 2.93$$

$$APVA = 1.44 \text{ cm}^2$$

A_t	Prosthetic valve ring area; SJM 25A-101 = 4.91 cm2)
V_{LVOT}	0.86 m/s
V_{APV}	2.93 m/s

Diagnosis: Normally functioning prosthetic valve without pathological stenosis.

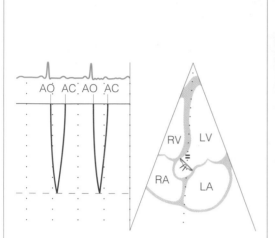

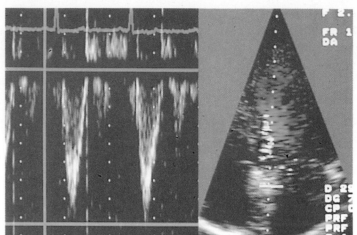

Patient with SJM 23A-101 aortic valve replacement presented with moderately severe aortic stenosis. V_{LVOT} = 1.04 m/s.

Color encoded of apical four-chamber view echocardiogram and PW Doppler recording with sample volume positioned in the left ventricular outflow tract.

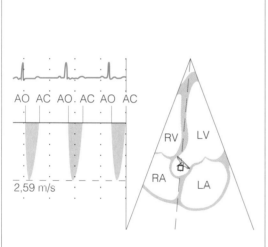

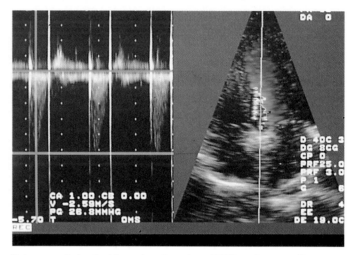

Same patient. V_{APV} = 2.59 m/s.

Color encoded apical four-chamber view. CW Doppler recording.

Example 2:

Patient with aortic valve replacement (SJM 23A-101) presenting with moderately severe aortic stenosis.

$$APVA = (A_t \times V_{LVOT}) / V_{APV}$$

$$APVA = (4.15 \text{ cm}^2 \times 1.04 \text{ m/s}) / 2.59 \text{ m/s}$$

$$APVA = 4.32 \text{ cm}^2 / 2.59$$

$$APVA = 1.67 \text{ cm}^2$$

A_t	Prosthetic ring area of SJM 23A-101 = 4.15 cm²
V_{LVOT}	1.04 m/s
V_{APV}	2.59 m/s

Diagnosis: mild aortic stenosis.

Grading the severity of stenosis in aortic valve prostheses, as in native valves, is warranted by the curvilinear relationship between the transprosthetic pressure gradient and the prosthetic valve area: A prosthetic valve effective orifice area that is sufficient for a small, physically inactive patient, usually is not sufficient for a large, physically active patient [36]. Even in relatively large prostheses, stroke volume increases of only $\leq 50\%$ can be expected at maximum physical exercise [13].

Measured prosthetic ring area in commonly implanted prostheses

Aortic valve prostheses: Starr-Edwards (SE) models 1200 and 1260, Björk-Shiley (BS) Standard, -60° CC and Monostrut, -70° CC, Medtronic-Hall (MH), model A 7700), St. Jude Medical (SJM) model A-101, Duromedics (DMS), Ionescu-Shiley (IS) Standard and Low Profile, Carpentier-Edwards (CE) model 2625, and Hancock II (HC) model T 505.

A_1 (A_t) (cm^2)

	SE1200	SE-1260	BS	MH	SJM	DMS	IS	CE	HC
A21			3.46	3.46	3.46				
A23	4.15		4.15	4.15	4.15	4.15	4.15	4.22	
A24		4.52							
A25			4.90	4.91	4.91	4.90	4.90	4.90	4.90
A26		5.31							
A27		5.73	5.73	5.72	5.73	5.73			
A29			6.60			6.60			

Scatter associated with calculated "effective" orifice areas [A_2 (A_{eff})] of normally functioning aortic prosthetic valves on to *in vitro* measurements is probably attributable to implantation-related differences in alignment of the artificial valve [1].

Transesophageal echocardiography (single and multiplane)

- *Provides a graphic display and (semi) quantitation of prosthetic valve function or dysfunction.*

Advantages of transesophageal echocardiography over transthoracic echocardiography in the assessment of prosthetic valve function are improved visualization of the prosthesis and of prosthesis movement, which makes it easier to identify prosthesis-related thrombus, vegetations [3], and regurgitation. The use of multiplane transducers has greatly improved the technique [7].

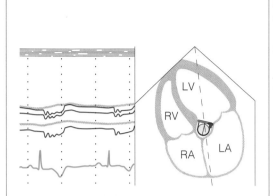

Starr-Edwards 1260 aortic valve prosthesis. Restenosis and unspecific ball vibrations (systole).

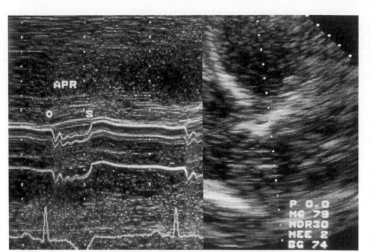

Apical four-chamber M-mode and 2-D echocardiograms.

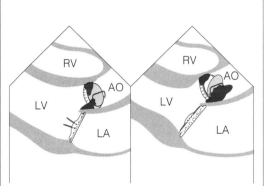

Björk-Shiley aortic valve prosthesis and St. Jude Medical mitral valve prosthesis. Partial prosthetic obstruction of the ring of the aortic valve prosthesis. However, scans are not conclusive.

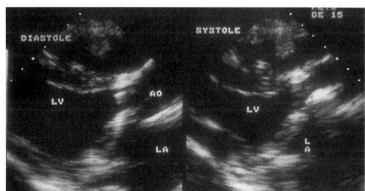

Parasternal long-axis 2-D echocardiograms.

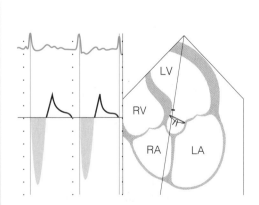

Duromedics bileaflet aortic valve replacement. The mean transprosthetic pressure gradient is 57 mmHg. Using a 2.0 MHz pencil transducer, the derived peak instantaneous pressure gradient was 135 mmHg.

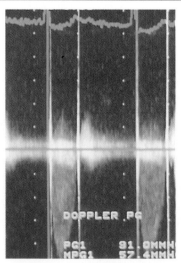

CW Doppler recording from apical four-chamber 2-D echocardiogram.

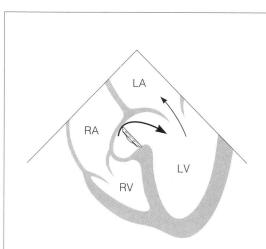

Paraprosthetic leakage in a Duromedics aortic valve prosthesis. There is a broad, pandiastolic regurgitant jet.

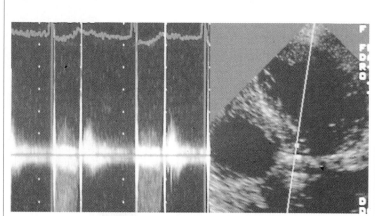

Apical four-chamber view. CW-Doppler.

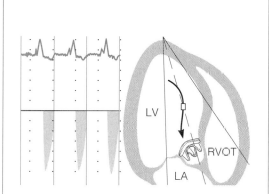

Patient with aortic valve replacement with Hancock bioprosthesis. Findings: bioprosthesis degeneration and restenosis. Peak instantaneous transprosthetic flow velocity ca. 4 m/s.

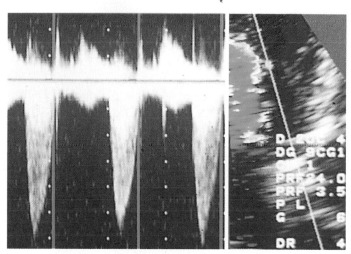

Apical long-axis view with color flow mapping and CW Doppler recording.

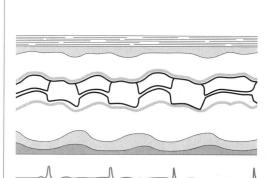

Aortic valve replacement with bioprosthesis. Findings: bioprosthesis degeneration, restenosis, and progressive prosthetic valve insufficiency. Despite the differences between the Doppler findings and the findings at cardiac catheterization, patient was reoperated on due to recurring pulmonary edema.

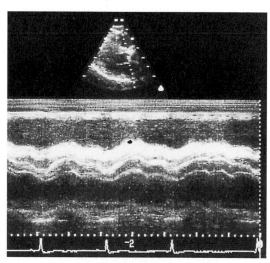

M-mode, parasternal long-axis recording.

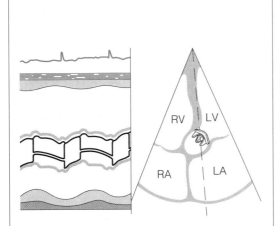

Same patient with aortic valve replacement with bioprosthesis. Findings: bioprosthesis degeneration, restenosis, and progressing prosthetic valve insufficiency.

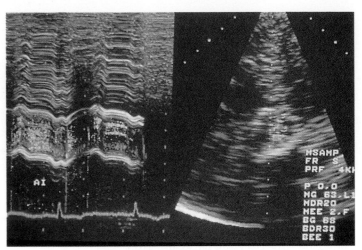

Apical four-chamber view M-mode and 2-D with color flow mapping.

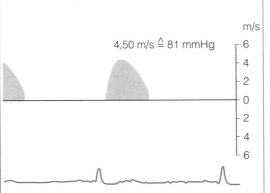

4,50 m/s ≙ 81 mmHg

Same patient, continued. Peak instantaneous pressure gradient = 81 mmHg, mean gradient = 44 mmHg. Mean pressure gradient at cardiac catheterization = 30 mmHg. Degeneration of the bioprosthesis was confirmed during surgery.

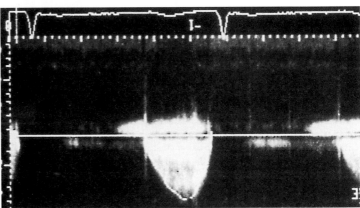

CW Doppler. Stenotic jet detected from the right supraclavicular position.

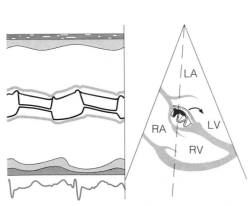

Patient with aortic valve replacement using Hancock bioprosthesis. Diagnosis: Early-onset prosthetic valve endocarditis with prosthetic insufficiency.

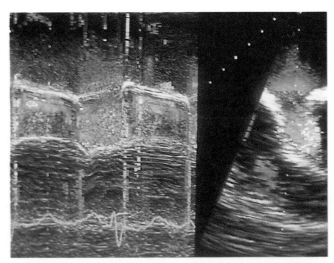

Transesophageal short-axis. Color M-mode and 2-D echocardiograms.

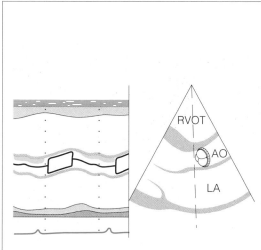
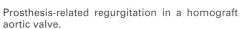

Prosthesis-related regurgitation in a homograft aortic valve.

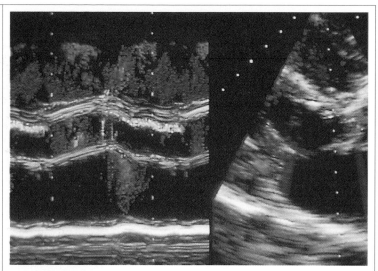

Parasternal long-axis color M-mode and 2-D echocardiograms.

11.   Assessment of Prosthetic Valve Function
11.3   Tricuspid Valve Management and Special Problems Associated with Reconstructive Valve Surgery - Valve-supporting Conduits

Usually, tricuspid valve replacement is indicated only in severe tricuspid stenosis and, in rare cases, tricuspid valve endocarditis. Since the intrinsic stenotic component of all prosthetic valves comes to fruition in this low pressure region, postoperative right heart failure is common. Valve repair makes it possible to preserve the native valve, diminish prosthesis-related problems, and spare ventricular function.

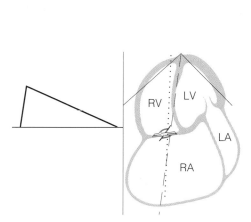

Patient with tricuspid valve replacement (Björk-Shiley tilting disk prosthesis). The effective orifice area of the prosthesis, calculated using the pressure half-time, is 1.12 cm².

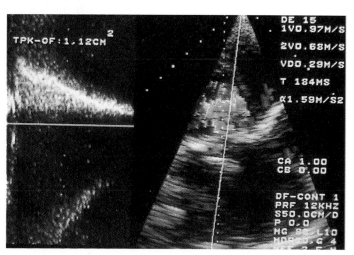

Color encoded apical four-chamber 2-D view. CW Doppler.

11.   **Assessment of Prosthetic Valve Function**   **612**
11.3   **Tricuspid Valve Management and Special Problems Associated**
         with Reconstructive Valve Surgery - Valve-supporting Conduits

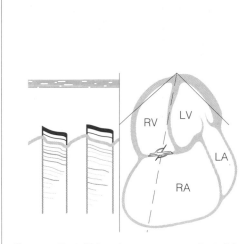

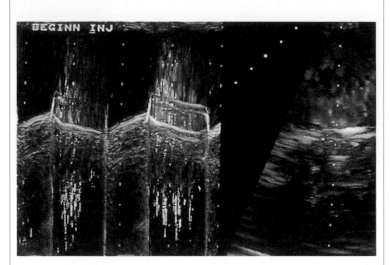

Same patient. Valve demonstrates typical tilting disk prosthesis motion pattern. Color flow mapping was enhanced by an injection of 10 ml echo contrast agent.

Apical four-chamber view (Color M-mode and 2-D).

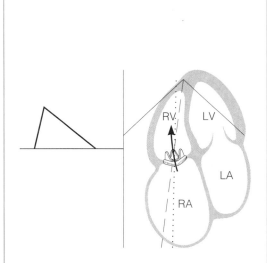

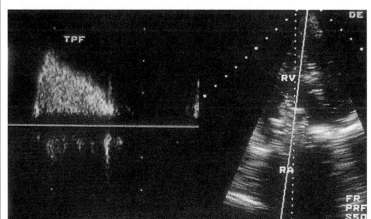

Tricuspid valve replacement (bioprosthesis). The stents are visible in diastole.

Color encoded apical four-chamber view. CW Doppler.

The success of valve reconstruction ist dependent on the intraoperative assessment of result. This is carried out in part by direct inspection of the valve after atrial filling and, to a greater extent, by cardiac ultrasound examination. Transesophageal echocardiography is the gold standard for such intraoperative assessment of result. The main disadvantage of transesophageal echocardiography is that the patient must be taken off the heart-lung machine before transesophageal echocardiography can be performed and, if the results of reconstruction are unsatisfactory, the procedure must be repeated again (see Chapter 5.4).

11. **Assessment of Prosthetic Valve Function**
11.3 **Tricuspid Valve Management and Special Problems Associated**
with Reconstructive Valve Surgery - Valve-supporting Conduits

613

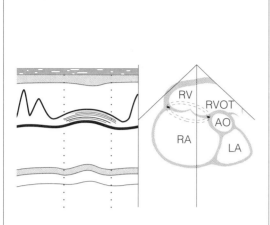

Prosthetic ring implantation for tricuspid valve repair. Residual regurgitation can be visualized only in color M-mode recordings and after administration of echo contrast agent.

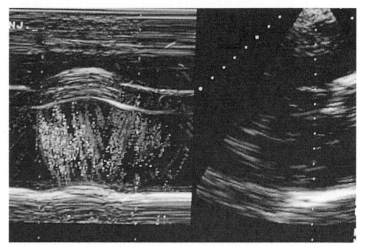

Color flow maps of parasternal short-axis M-mode and 2-D echocardiograms recorded at the level of the aorta and tricuspid valve.

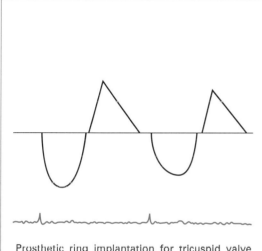

Prosthetic ring implantation for tricuspid valve repair. Residual regurgitation and moderate stenosis can be seen in the CW Doppler recording.

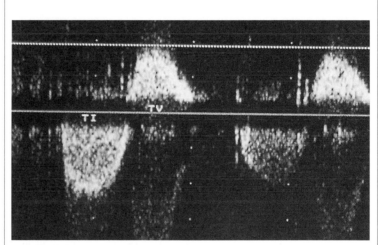

CW Doppler recording (non-imaging pencil transducer).

In addition to correction of congenital heart diseases (*e.g.* the Fontan procedure), conduits are usually implanted in aortic valve replacement with simultaneous replacement of the ascending aorta, in the context of type A aortic dissection and aortic valve endocarditis with annular and mural abscesses. Frequently, the native aorta is wrapped around the conduit, which can lead to false interpretation of the double wall contours, especially when the interstice is filled with residual blood postoperatively.

The assessment of valve reconstruction is no different from the assessment of mitral valve replacements or of solitary aortic valve replacements *(see Chapter 11.2 and Chapter 12)*.

All prostheses have a highly echo reflective sewing ring made of synthetic or metallic material. Because of its eccentric motion pattern, the angle of the sewing ring changes with respect to the ultrasound beam, giving rise to broad, dense echo bands that overshadow the opening and closing motion of the prosthetic valve mechanism. Usually, one attempts to direct the ultrasound beam through the opened valve, in order to reduce the number of spurious echoes. Such echoes make it harder to visualize and identify thrombi or vegetations, and makes it more difficult to assess their motion during the cardiac cycle. Some prostheses have additional echo reflective parts such as struts and a ball or disk, which can also impede assessment attempts.

Furthermore, the velocity of ultrasound differs in non-totally reflecting synthetic material and tissue. Therefore, one cannot expect that the echo topography will accurately reflect the true structures. Posterior parts of valves made of synthetic materials may be visualized posterior to the posterior sewing ring.

Due to the above-mentioned reasons, conventional echocardiography is able to provide only little reliable information on the functional state of prosthetic valves. Moreover, this data is often unspecific and can hardly be considered pathognomic.

Doppler echocardiography provides the instrumentation for (semi) quantitation of prosthetic valve dysfunction upon which follow-up studies can be based. If the model and size of the prosthesis are unknown, critical assessment of the measured transprosthetic flow velocities and the derived calculation parameters is neither possible nor acceptable.

The flow characteristics of any prosthetic valve is determined by its construction-related flow profile (which is reflected in the echo pattern) and the alignment of the prosthetic valve in the valve plane, which is determined at implantation. The flow characteristics describe the individual components of transprosthetic flow. Because these differ in the flow velocity and (volumetric) flow, the individual Doppler-determined components are not identical with the mean flow profile across the effective orifice area of the prosthetic valve, which is essential for quantitation. The validity of the measurements depends on the representativeness of the region included in the Doppler beam.

Peak instantaneous flow velocities and pressure gradients should be avoided or used with caution. These measurements are subject to great intra- and interindividual fluctuations. They may also be falsely high due to pathological regurgitation from the prosthesis.

| 11. | Assessment of Prosthetic Valve Function |
| 11.5 | Ventricular Function |

Ventricular function is an important factor in the assessment of prosthetic valve function for the following three reasons:

1. In ventricles with severely impaired function, the use of conventional echocardiographic criteria of prosthetic valve dysfunction (*e.g.* excursion amplitude, opening and closing velocity) and of Doppler-derived parameters (*e.g.* flow velocities and pressure gradients) is no longer acceptable. In low flow states, the transprosthetic stroke volume no longer suffices for complete opening. Despite the relatively low flow velocities and pressure gradients, hemodynamically significant obstruction may be present.

2. In high flow states, "relative" stenosis can develop without causing prosthetic valve dysfunction that would require reoperation.
3. Low intracardiac flow velocities are not detected well in color flow mapping. Therefore, some relevant pathological regurgitations may go undetected.

| 11. | Assessment of Prosthetic Valve Function |
| 11.6 | Follow-up and Treatment Considerations |

Patients with prosthetic valve replacements may have symptoms suggestive of prosthetic valve dysfunction. However, the same symptoms may also be due to fixed increased pulmonary arteriole resistance, left ventricular dysfunction, and prosthesis-related hemolytic anemia, or they may simply reflect the unavoidable inherent stenosis associated with artificial valves [30].

Complete non-invasive diagnostic testing is indicated in prosthetic valve recipients when a new heart murmur is heard or when a change in the original prosthesis-specific flow sounds and opening and closing clicks is observed. If the suspicion of prosthetic valve dysfunction persists, invasive testing is indicated [35].

Resting electrocardiogram	Conduction disturbances Left ventricular hypertrophy Myocardial infarction
Chest x-ray	Change in prosthesis position Enlarged heart silhouette Signs of pulmonary congestion
Cardiac ultrasound diagnosis	Prosthesis motility Thrombus Vegetations Transprosthetic pressure gradient Effective orifice area of the prosthesis Regurgitation Left ventricular function
Nuclear cardiology	Left ventricular function
Cardiac catheterization	Prosthetic valve dysfunction Coronary artery morphology Left ventricular function

The availability of immediate postoperative baseline findings is of great importance when assessing prosthetic valve dysfunction. Baseline measurements and, images can be compared with later measurements and images. Therefore, the patient and/or the doctor treating the patient should be given a record of baseline immediate postoperative measurements (transprosthetic flow velocity, transprosthetic pressure gradient, effective orifice area of the prosthesis, and data concerning prosthesis-related regurgitation), prosthetic valve identification data (type, model, and size of the prosthesis), and other important data (indication for surgery, date of surgery, hospital, etc.).

The key to planning therapy or for deciding on whether a change of prosthesis is necessary is to evaluate any signs of new or progressive heart failure and prosthetic valve endocarditis.

Prosthesis-related congestive heart failure that is progressive or resistant to conservative treatment, due to:
▸ Thrombotic occlusion of the prosthesis
▸ Calcific degeneration of a bioprosthesis
▸ Severe prosthetic valve insufficiency

Prosthetic valve endocarditis, especially when there is associated progressive congestive heart failure, septic embolism, and infection not curable with antibiotics, with
▸ Persistent bacteremia
▸ Continuous changes in heart sounds and murmurs
▸ New occurrence of conduction disturbances
▸ Progressive prosthetic valve insufficiency

The decision to reoperate is affected by the rapidly worsening prognosis in delayed second operations. In reoperation for prosthetic valve dysfunction, the mortality rate for aortic valve reoperation is 5.9%, and is 19.6% for mitral valve reoperation. The mortality rate for reoperation increases to 25% when there is active prosthetic valve endocarditis, and is more than 50% in early-onset prosthetic valve endocarditis [4, 21, 22].

---

11.   Assessment of Prosthetic Valve Function
11.7   Critical Assessment and Comparison of Results with Those
         of Complementary Diagnostic Techniques

Usually, prosthetic valve dysfunction can be diagnosed clinically and by means of cardiac ultrasound.
Fluroscopy, which can detect excessive diastolic-systolic motion of the sewing ring of the prosthetic valve (> 10°), is indicated when dehiscence is suspected [2].

Cardiac catheterization is indicated only when there is continued, but otherwise unconfirmable, suspicion of prosthetic valve dysfunction. Problems may arise when the catheter is passed through an allograft valve with asymmetrical parts [24], especially in patients with both mitral and aortic valve replacement. Use of the Gorlin formula is no longer acceptable when dysfunction of more than one prosthetic valve is suspected.

Therefore, one should first attempt to use all available techniques of cardiac ultrasound diagnosis to establish a definitive diagnosis.

Morphometry and Ventricular Function

RAV	_____	ml
RVEDD	_____	mm
LADmax	_____	mm
LVEDD	_____	mm
LVESD	_____	mm

LVFS   _____   (fractional shortening)

Evidence of concomitant ischemic heart disease??
- Wall motion analysis

RVEF   _____

Evidence of pulmonary hypertension?
- Rightward protrusion of the interatrial septum observed in the subcostal four-chamber view.
- RVOT-EDD   _____   mm

Valve Morphology and Dynamics

▸ Thickening (thrombus, calcification) or "degeneration" of the prosthesis?
▸ Motility of the prosthesis and its movable parts intact?

Valve Function and Pressure-Flow Relationships (Doppler Echocardiography)

▸ Velocity measurements (m/s)
- Mean transprosthetic velocities
▸ Pressure gradients (mmHg)
- Mean transprosthetic pressure gradients
▸ Prosthetic valve orifice area (cm^2), prosthetic valve orifice area indices (cm^2/m^2)
- using the pressure half-time method
- using the continuity equation
- using the simplified Gorlin formula for comparison, when other results seem implausible
▸ Regurgitation
- qualitative visual proof
▸ Exclusion of other valvular dysfunctions
▸ Intracardiac pressure values (mmHg)
- $PA_{systolic}$ in associated tricuspid insufficiency
- $PA_{diastolic}$ in associated pulmonary insufficiency

Transesophageal Echocardiography

▸ Valve morphology and dynamics
▸ Detection of vegetations
▸ To differentiate between central and paraprosthetic leakage

Causes of prosthetic valve malfunction
1. Thrombotic occlusion and fibrous tissue ingrowth
▶ Exclusion of false-positive echo findings due to reverberations and other artifacts
▶ Echo-dense mass in the vicinity of the prosthetic valve, with total absence of valve body motion (disk, ball, etc.)
▶ Intermittent, incomplete, or delayed opening of the valve
▶ Prostheses-unrelated high transprosthetic mean pressure gradient (higher (ca. + 50%) as the immediate postoperative pressure gradient), and more than mild to moderately reduced prosthetic mitral valve orifice area
2. Prosthetic valve endocarditis
3. Paraprosthetic leakage and regurgitation
▶ Exclusion of false-positive echocardiographic findings in patients with impaired ventricular function
▶ Evidence of volume overload in connected chambers on the outflow side
▶ Doppler echocardiographic proof of prosthetic (central) or paraprosthetic regurgitation - Doppler color flow imaging - CW Doppler - Mismatch of high diastolic flow velocity and normal pressure half-time (mitral position)
▶ Transesophageal (Doppler) echocardiography
▶ Early diastolic rounding of the E wave (M-mode) in paraprosthetic leakage of a mitral valve prosthesis: the systolic anterior motion of the valve is extended and overlaps with the onset of diastolic posterior motion (rounding of the initial diastolic motion)
▶ Diastolic fluttering of the mitral valve and premature mitral valve closure in severe prosthetic aortic valve insufficiency
4. Mechanical dysfunction and (partial) dehiscence of the prosthetic valve
5. Degeneration and degradation of bioprostheses
▶ Increased leaflet thickness and reduced motility
▶ Localized diastolic-systolic leaflet fluttering due to tearing or perforation
▶ Localized calcification (initially in the region of commissures and sewing ring)

SYMPTOMATOLOGY / AUSCULTATION

ECHOCARDIOGRAPHY

Conventional echocardiography:

Morphometry (RVEDD, RVOT-EDD, LADmax, LVEDD, LVESD)
Ventricular function (LVFS, wall motion analysis)
and
Visualization of structural causes and hemodynamic effects

Doppler and transesophageal echocardiography:

Prosthetic valve orifice area (PVA), PVA index (PVA-I)
using the pressure half-time method
± the continuity equation

Transesophageal echocardiography:
For visualization and assessment of valve morphology and dynamics
For detection of vegetations
To differentiate between central and paraprosthetic leakage

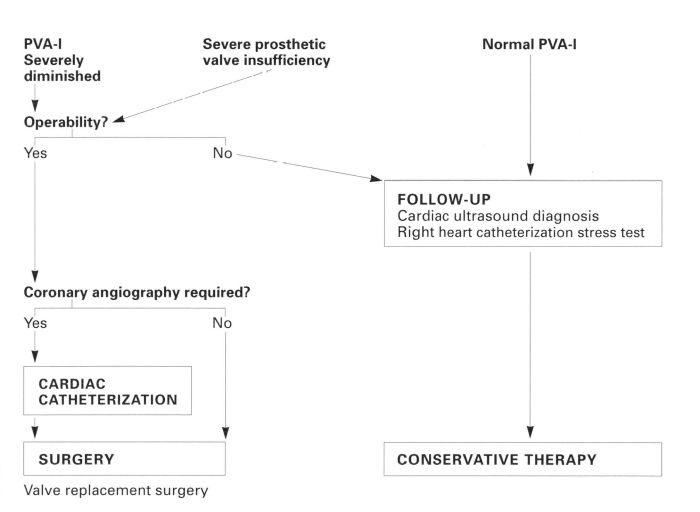

**PVA-I
Severely
diminished**

**Severe prosthetic
valve insufficiency**

Normal PVA-I

Operability?

Yes   No

Coronary angiography required?

Yes   No

FOLLOW-UP
Cardiac ultrasound diagnosis
Right heart catheterization stress test

**CARDIAC
CATHETERIZATION**

SURGERY
Valve replacement surgery

CONSERVATIVE THERAPY

1. Aaslid R, Levang O, Fröysaker T, Skagseth E, Hall KV. 'In situ' evaluation of the aortic pivoting disc valve prosthesis. Scand J Thorac Cardiovasc Surg 1975; 9: 81-84.

2. Angel J, Soler Soler J, Anivarro I, Domingo E. Hemodynamic evaluation of stenotic cardiac valves: II. Modification of the simplified valve formula for mitral and aortic valve area calculation. Cathet Cardiovasc Diagn 1985; 11: 127-138.

3. Bansal RC, Graham B, Jutzky K, Shakudo M, Shah PM. Left ventricular outflow tract to left atrial communication secondary to rupture of mitral-aortic intervalvular fibrosa in infective endocarditis: Diagnosis by transesophageal echocardiography and color flow imaging. J Am Coll Cardiol 1990; 15: 499-504.

4. Baumgartner WA, Miller DC, Reitz BA, Oyer PE, Jamieson SW, Stinson EB, Shumway NE. Surgical treatment of prosthetic valve endocarditis. Ann Thorac Surg 1983; 35: 87-104.

5. Brogan WC, Lange RA, Hillis LD. Limitations of the simplified formula for calculating valve area in patients with mitral stenosis. J Am Coll Cardiol 1991; 17 (suppl A): 254A.

6. Chafizadeh ER, Zoghbi WA. Doppler echocardiographic assessment of the St. Jude Medical prosthetic valve in the aortic position using the continuity equation. Circulation 1991; 83: 213-223.

7. Chan KL, Walley VM. Accuracy of transesophageal echocardiographic detection of cusp tears in degenerated bioprosthetic valves. J Am Coll Cardiol 1991; 17: 371.

8. Dennig K, Rudolph W. Dopplerechokardiographische Evaluierung von Mitralklappenprothesen. Z Kardiol 74 (suppl 3), 1985; 113.

9. Dennig K, Rudolph W. Nichtinvasive Bestimmung der Öffnungsfläche von Aortenklappenprothesen mit Hilfe der Doppler-Echokardiographie. Herz 1986; 11: 341-345.

10. Dianzumba SB, Cornman CR, Joyner CR. Estimation of mitral prosthetic valve area by Doppler echo cardiography. J Am Coll Cardiol 1985; 5: 526 A.

11. Dittrich HC. Clinical transesophageal echocardiography. St. Louis: Mosby-Year Book, 1992: 79.

12. Dumesnil JG, Honos GN, Lemieux M, Beauchemin Jocelyn. Validation and applications of indexed aortic prosthetic valve areas calculated by Doppler echocardiography. J Am Coll Cardiol 1990; 16: 637-643.

13. Dumesnil JG, Honos GN, Lemieux M, Beauchemin Jocelyn. Validation and applications of indexed aortic prosthetic valve areas calculated by Doppler echocardiography. J Am Coll Cardiol 1990; 16: 641, fig. 5.

14. Flachskampf FA, O'Shea JP, Griffin BP, Guerrero L, Weyman AE, Thomas JD. Patterns of normal transvalvular regurgitation in mechanical valve prostheses. J Am Coll Cardiol 1991; 18: 1493-1498.

15. Fuji K, Kitabake A, Asao M, Tanouchi J, Ishihara K, Morita T, Masuyama T, Ito H, Hori M, et al. Non-invasive evaluation of valvular stenosis by a quantitative Doppler technique. J Cardiovasc Ultrason 1984; 3: 201-208.

16. Gray RJ, Chaux A, Matloff JM, DeRobertis M, Raymond M, Stewart M, Yoganathan A. Bileaflet, tilting disc and porcine aortic valve substitutes: In vivo hydrodynamic characteristics. J Am Coll Cardiol 1984; 3: 321-327.

17. Hakki AH, Iskandrian AS, Bemis CE, Kimbiris D, Mintz GS, Segal BK, Brice C. A simplified valve formula for the calculation of stenotic cardiac valve areas. Circulation 1981; 63: 1050-1055.

18. Horstkotte D, Loogen F. Erworbene Herzklappenfehler. München: Urban & Schwarzenberg, 1987: 249.

19. Horstkotte D, Loogen F. Erworbene Herzklappenfehler. München: Urban & Schwarzenberg, 1987: 250.

20. Horstkotte D, Loogen F. Erworbene Herzklappenfehler. München: Urban & Schwarzenberg, 1987: 259.

21. Husebye DG, Pluth JR, Piehler JM, Schaff HV, Orszulak TA. Reoperation on prosthetic heart valves. An analysis of risk factors in 552 patients. J Thorac Carqdiovasc Surg 1983; 86: 543-552.

22. Ivert TS, Dismukes WE, Cobbs CG, Blackstone EH, Kirklin JW, Bergdahl LA. Prosthetic valve endocarditis. Circulation 1984; 69: 223-232.

23. Khandheria BK, Seward J, Oh J, Freeman WK, Nichols BA, Sinak LJ, Miller FA Jr, Tajik AJ. Value and limitations of transesophageal echocardiography in assessment of mitral valve prostheses. Circulation 1991; 83: 1956-1968.

24. Kober G, Hilgermann R. Catheter entrapment in a Bjork-Shiley prosthesis in aortic position. Cathet Cardiovsc Diagn 1987; 13: 262-265.

25. Kraus F, Rudolph W. Symptoms, exercise capacity and exercise hemodynamics: Interrelationships and their role in quantification of the valvular lesions. Herz 1984; 9: 187-199.

26. Kruck I, Biamino G. Quantitative Methoden der M-Mode-, 2D- und Doppler-Echokardiographie. Boehringer Mannheim GmbH, 1988: 114.

27. Lesbre JP, Chassat C, Lespérance J, Petitclerc R, Bonau R, Dyrda I, Pasternac A, Bourassa MG. Continuous wave Doppler evaluation of normally functioning new pericardial aortic prosthetic valves. J Am Coll Cardiol 1986; 7: 188 A.

28. Miller G. Invasive investigation of the heart. A guide to cardiac catheterization and related procedures. Oxford: Blackwell, 1989: 270, tbl 15.1a und 282.

29. Miller G. Invasive investigation of the heart. A guide to cardiac catheterization and related procedures. Oxford: Blackwell, 1989: 271, tbl 15.1b und 274.

30. Miller G. Invasive investigation of the heart. A guide to cardiac catheterization and related procedures. Oxford: Blackwell, 1989: 289.
31. Mohr-Kahaly S, Kupferwasser I, Erbel R, Oelert H, Meyer J. Regurgitant flow in apparently normal valve prostheses: Improved detection and semiquantitative analysis by transesophageal two-dimensional color-coded Doppler echocardiography. J Am Soc Echo 1990; 3: 187-195.
32. Nellesen U, Schnittger I, Appleton C, Masuyama T, Bolger A, Fischell TA, Tye T, Popp RL: Transesophageal two-dimensional echocardiography and color Doppler flow velocity mapping in the evaluation of cardiac valve prostheses. Circulation 1988; 78: 848-855.
33. Nigri A, Martuscelli E, Mangieri E, Voci P, Danesi A, Sardella R, Feroci L, Reale A. Nomogram for calculation of stenotic cardiac valve areas from cardiac output and mean transvalvular gradient. Cathet Cardiovasc Diagn 1984; 10: 613-618.
34. Panidis IP, Ross J, Mintz GS. Normal and abnormal prosthetic valve function as assessed by Doppler echocardiography. Circulation 1985; 72 (suppl II): II-101.
35. Rackley CE, Katz NM, Wallace RB. Artificial valve disease. In: Hurst JW, ed. The heart.New York: McGraw Hill, 1990: tbl. 45-1, 873.
36. Rahimtoola SH. The problem of valve prosthesis-patient mismatch. Circulation 1978; 58: 20-24.
37. Reisner SA, Meltzer RS. Normal values of prosthetic valve Doppler echocardiographic parameters: A review. J Am Soc Echo 1988; 1: 201-210.
38. Rothbart RM, Smucker ML, Gibson RS. Pulsed and continuous wave Doppler examination of prosthetic valves: correlation with clinical and cardiac catheterization data. Circulation 1985; 72 (suppl III): III-737.
39. Skjaerpe T, Hegrenaes L, Hatle L. Noninvasive estimation of valve area in patients with aortic stenosis by Doppler ultrasound and two-dimensional echocardiography. Circulation (1985); 72: 810-818.
40. Taams MA, Gussenhoven EJ, Cahalan MK, Roelandt JR, van Herwerden LA, The HK, Bom N, de Jong N. Transesophageal Doppler color flow imaging in the detection of native and Bjork-Shiley mitral valve regurgitation. J Am Coll Cardiol 1989; 13: 95 99.
41. Zoghbi WA, Farmer KL, Soto JG, Nelson JG, Quinones MA. Accurate noninvasive quantification of stenotic aortic valve area by Doppler echocardiography. Circulaton 1986; 73: 542-492.

Infective endocarditis can occur on all endocardial surfaces, but it most commonly affects the cardiac valves - in decreasing order of frequency: the aortic, mitral, tricuspid, and pulmonary valves. Other sites of predilection are the region between the valve rings (jet lesions), the interventricular septum and vascular walls. Amongst these, a ventricular septal defect, patent ductus arteriosus, and coarctation of the aorta, are associated with increased risk. Jet lesions [18] are sites with endothelial roughening and reactive fibrosis, where a turbulent regurgitant jet meets the endothelium. They are most commonly found between the aortic and mitral valve rings in aortic valve endocarditis. These are sites of predilection when there is secondary migration of infectious material from regurgitation through the primarily involved valve.

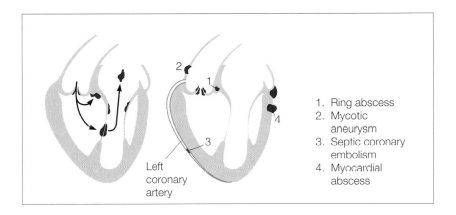

These are nosologically differentiated from non-infective endocardial diseases:

Infective and non-infective endocarditic diseases
▶ *Non-infective endocarditis* Non-infective thrombotic endocarditis Marantic endocarditis Libman-Sacks endocarditis in systemic lupus erythematosus

▶ *Infective endocarditis*
Native valve endocarditis
    – Right-side endocarditis
    – Left-side endocarditis
Prosthetic valve endocarditis

Platelet aggregation is found occasionally on normal valves. However, it is more commonly found on previously damaged valves in congenital or rheumatic heart diseases [2].

"Marantic" endocarditis can complicate consumptive diseases [9].

In 1924, long before systemic lupus erythematosus was recognized as a systemic disease, Libman and Sacks [28] described a „verrucous" endocarditis with sterile vegetations as a special form of non-infective endocarditis.

Such non-infective endocarditis can be secondarily colonized by circulating organisms and can lead to infective endocarditis.

The echomorphology of non-infective and infective endocarditis is largely identical:

"White" thrombi composed of coral-reef and sandbank-like platelet aggregates located one behind the other, and which are surrounded by fibrin nets in which erythrocytes, leukocytes, and bacteria are caught [7], *i.e.* "vegetations", on the cardiac valves are the most common manifestation. The left-sided valves are more frequently affected than the right valves, whereby vegetations predominantly arise downstream on the proximal side of the leaflets and cusps. This coincides with the observation that, if one pumps a bacterial aerosol through an ever narrowing tube into a low-pressure space, the bacteria will settle on the tube wall directly beyond the obstruction [40].

It is widely known that certain preexisting valve abnormalities are increasingly predisposed to colonization by virulent organisms - and a considerable amount of literature has been devoted to this risk stratification. However, previously healthy hearts are not immune, and normal hearts are more common than abnormal ones. The majority of urgent aortic valvular surgery is necessary in cases of Streptococcus viridans endocarditis with in younger men bicuspid valve, who previously knew as little as their physicians did about this abnormality [37, 40, 50].

Nosocomially acquired infective endocarditis is common (up to 28%), which is a less known fact [38], and has been observed in conjunction with iatrogenic endocardial injuries. Infective endocarditis has been reported to occur in 2 to 6 % of all long-term dialysis patients [16].

Cardiac Ultrasound Diagnosis

The echocardiographic diagnosis of infective endocarditis is based predominantly on the evidence of vegetations, *i.e.*, of foreign structures of varying echogenicity that adhere to cardiac structures and exhibit independent motion.

Two difficulties associated with the method are 1. the fact that the vegetations must be large enough to be visualized and 2. their interpretation as infective and virulent infective material. However, differentiation between acute and subacute forms now is largely of only historical interest, and does not play a role in echocardiographic diagnosis today.

Conventional Echocardiography

2-D and M-mode echocardiography:

- *Hazy, cloud-like structures* (vegetations) *that move independently* in the bloodstream *during diastole and/or systole and adhere to such endocardial surfaces as valves* (or heart and vessels walls). In contrast to fibrotic changes, vegetations *do not restrict valve motion* [8, 13, 20, 31]. Furthermore, their *echogenicity differs* from that of the valve and endocardial background. The topographical orientation and size of the vegetations can be demonstrated in various projections by 2-D echocardiography.
- Signs of *chordal rupture* and/or leaflet *perforation* (cannot be reliably differentiated from vegetations);
- *Prolapsing of vegetations* across the plane of the valve ring;
- *Dilatation* and *wall separation (spliss)* in the region of the aortic root, *i.e.* perivalvular echo-free spaces or an abnormal perivalvular echogenicity > 10 mm [26]. This is an indication of mycotic aneurysm or abscess.
- *Hemodynamic consequences* of valvular lesions (dilatation of volume-overloaded heart cavities, consequences attributable to irregular flows, etc.).

Conventional Doppler Echocardiography

Pulsed-wave Doppler (PW Doppler):
- *Detection, measurement of flow velocity, mapping and follow-up of regurgitations.*

Continuous-wave Doppler (CW-Doppler):
- *Detection, measurement of flow velocity, mapping and follow-up of regurgitations.*

Doppler Color Flow Imaging (M-mode and 2-D)

- *Graphic display of regurgitations and irregular, turbulent flows in the region of vegetations.*

Transesophageal echocardiography (single and multiplane)

- *Superior imaging quality compared to transthoracic echocardiography.*

Transesophageal echocardiography is indicated whenever there is suspicion of infective endocarditis [29,46]. Transesophegeal echocardiography can often visualize vegetations that were poorly visualized or not visualizable from the transthoracic route, and can detect complications in need of surgery (*e.g.* abscesses penetrating into neighboring cardiac ventricles).

12.1 Native Valve Endocarditis
12.1.1 Right-side Endocarditis

Right-sided endocarditis, which generally occurs in only 5 to 15 % of all cases [5], is seen predominantly in individuals with a history of intravenous drug abuse [25]. In these patients, involvement of the endocardial surface is distributed as follows: right heart valves - 50 to 66%, left heart valves - 30 to 40%, other endocardial surfaces - ca. 10%. Isolated pulmonary valve endocarditis is rare and occurs in only approximately 1% of all patients with infective endocarditis. In septic pulmonary embolism, the findings are eclipsed by the echocardiographical picture of acute cor pulmonale.

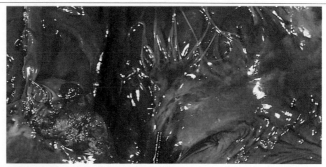

Morphological preparation demonstrating
endocarditis ulceropolyposa of the tricuspid valve.

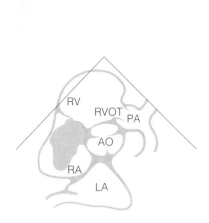

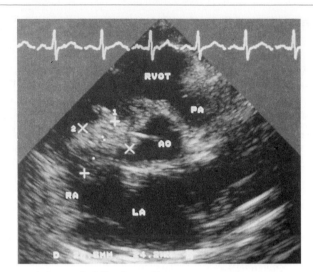

Vegetation measuring 28.6 x 24.2 mm on the posterior side of the septal tricuspid leaflet. ECG triggering 0.34 s after R wave. Early diastole.

Parasternal short-axis 2-D echocardiogram.

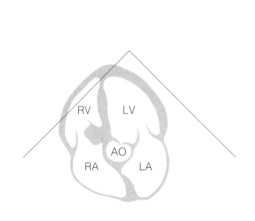

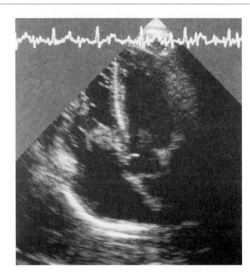

Poorly defined, cloud-like foreign structure on the septal tricuspid leaflet. Oblique cut of left ventricular outflow tract and left atrium. Diastole.

Apical four-chamber 2-D echocardiogram.

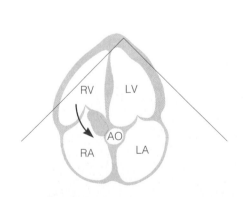

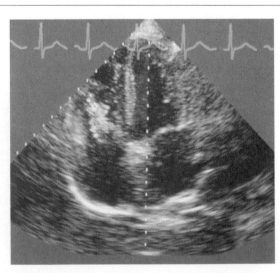

ECG triggering 0.34 s after R wave: Early diastole. Accelerated transtricuspid flow due to obstructive vegetation: Color change from red to red-yellow to blue.

Color flow map of apical four-chamber 2-D echocardiogram.

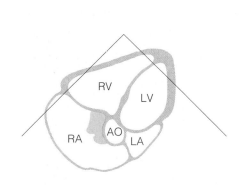

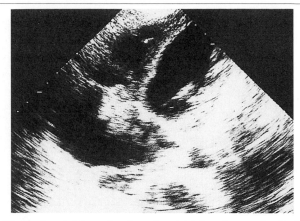

Large vegetation on the septal tricuspid leaflet. Fragile anterior tricuspid leaflet. Right atrium larger than the left atrium.

Modified subcostal four-chamber view (atrial septum and mitral valve level cut obliquely).

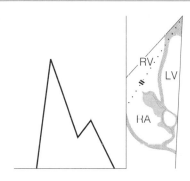

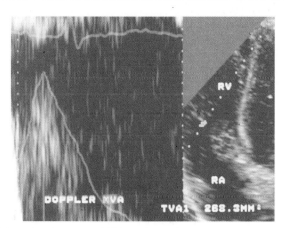

Tricuspid valve endocarditis with septal leaflet vegetation that flutters in the bloodstream during diastole. Pressure half-time of 82 ms corresponds to a tricuspid valve orifice area of 2.68 cm². Clinically insignificant flow obstruction.

Apical four-chamber view. PW Doppler, color encoded.

12.1 **Native Valve Endocarditis**
12.1.2 **Left-side Endocarditis**

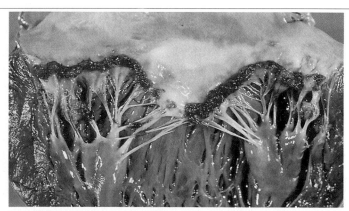

Morphological specimen: *endocarditis verrucosis* of the mitral valve.

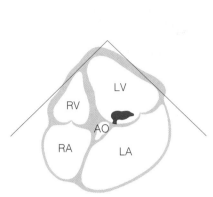

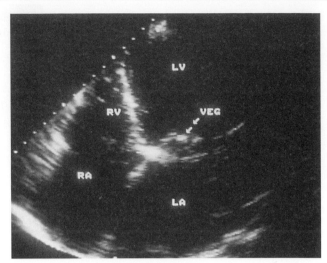

Vegetation on the anterior mitral leaflet moves freely in systole and diastole. It contains areas of increased echo-density and cannot be differentiated from old, partially calcified vegetation. Dilated left atrium.

Apical four-chamber 2-D echocardiogram.

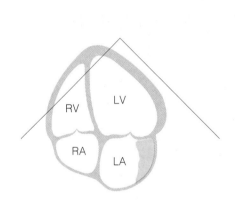

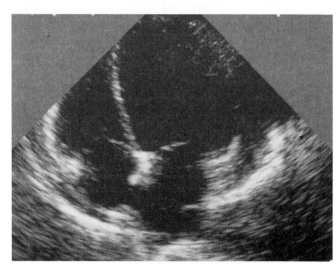

Poorly defined, cloud-like foreign structure in scan of the posterior side of the posterior mitral leaflet. Wall artifact must be differentially diagnosed. Clinical hyperacute mitral valve endocarditis.

Apical four-chamber 2-D echocardiogram.

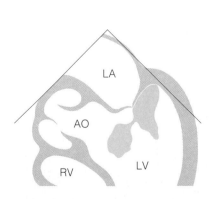

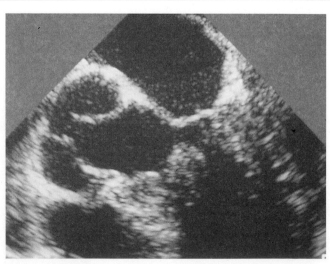

A large vegetation adheres to the posterior side of the posterior mitral leaflet. It is a poorly defined, cloud-like foreign structure that does not restrict leaflet motility. Thin aortic valve leaflets.

Transesophageal short-axis 2-D scan at end-diastole.

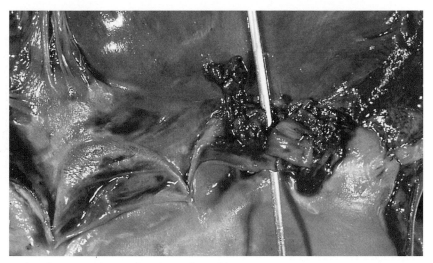

Morphological preparation demonstrating aortic valve endocarditis.

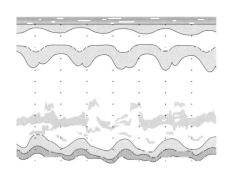

Differential diagnosis: vegetations and/or chordal rupture in mitral valve endocarditis versus diastolic oscillations in aortic insufficiency. Findings: Aortic valve endocarditis with moderate aortic insufficiency and jet lesion of the mitral valve. Oblique cut through the interventricular septum.

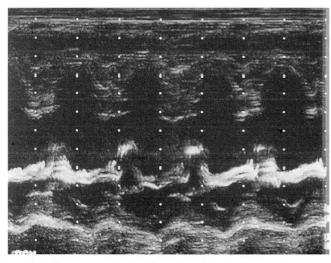

M-mode; left parasternal long-axis view at mitral valve level.

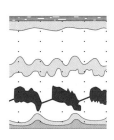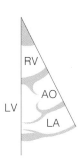

Same patient. Aortic regurgitant jet (2-D echo) that extends from the non-coronary cusp, and strikes the mitral valve in diastole. Flow pattern indicates turbulence between the mitral leaflets, that are set into oscillation and exhibit impaired opening. Dense mitral valve echos.

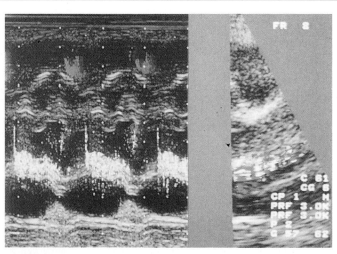

Color flow maps of parasternal long-axis M-mode and 2-D echocardiograms at mitral valve level at the junction of the aorta.

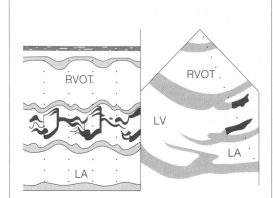

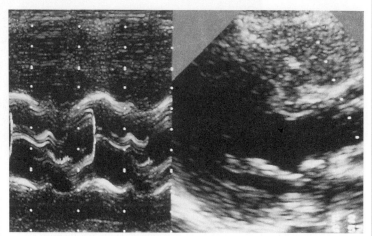

Aortic valve endocarditis. Intraoperative findings: vegetations on the right coronary and non-coronary valve cusps, perforation of the non-coronary valve cusp. No restriction of valvular motion. LAX = long-axis.

M-mode and 2-D scans, parasternal LAX view at aortic valve level.

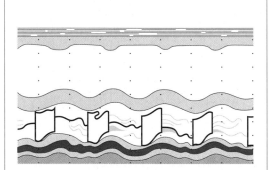

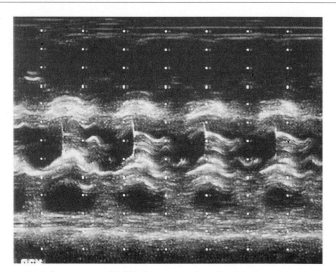

Aortic valve endocarditis. Poorly defined, partially cloud-like multiple echos in the region of the aortic wall and of aortic valve, which move normally. Wall separation in the region of the aortic root as evidence of suppuration.

M-mode, left parasternal LAX view at aortic valve level.

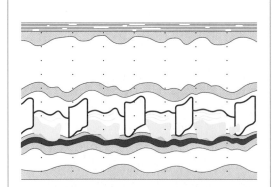

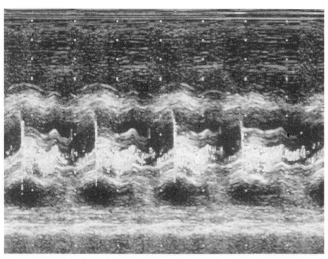

Same patient. Vegetations on the right coronary and non-coronary cusps. Perforation of the non-coronary cusp. Highly turbulent diastolic reflux is encoded yellow and turquoise; it extends from the perforated non-coronary cusp.

Color M-mode, left parasternal LAX view at aortic valve level.

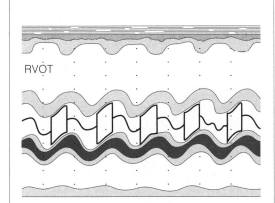

Aortic valve endocarditis. Thin aortic valve opening pattern with completely intact motility and unrestricted opening amplitude. Separation of the posterior aortic wall indicates aneurysmal widening and abscess of the aortic annulus.

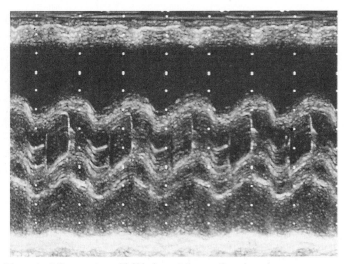

M-mode, left parasternal LAX view at the aortic valve plane.

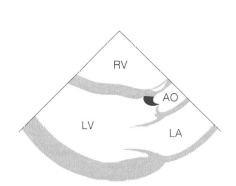

Aortic valve endocarditis. Aortic valve appears thickened: diagnosis of vegetations is not possible. Echo-free space with border lamella in the region of the anterior aortic wall as an indication of abscess (arrow).

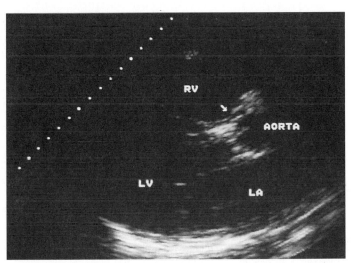

Left parasternal long-axis echocardiogram.

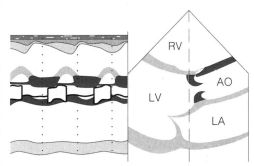

Same patient. Aortic wall exhibits calcium-dense echoes. Non-restricted valve opening amplitude. Cloud-like echoes in recording of valve. Separation of the anterior aortic wall with echo-free space. Findings indicate abscess of the aortic annulus. Abscess membrane sometimes delicately and sometimes sharply defined, and partially overshadowed by vegetations.

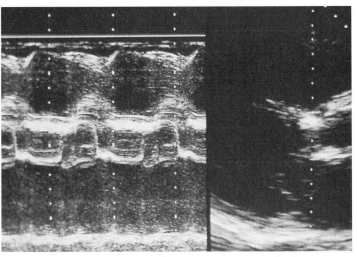

M-mode and 2-D, left parasternal LAX view at aortic valve level.

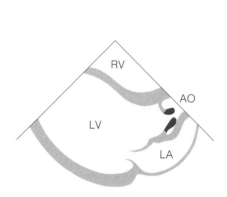

Early systole. Echo-dense anterior aortic wall. Cloud-like right coronary aortic cusp and echo-dense non-coronary aortic cusp. Dilated left ventricle with aortic insufficiency. Questionable aortic valve endocarditis.

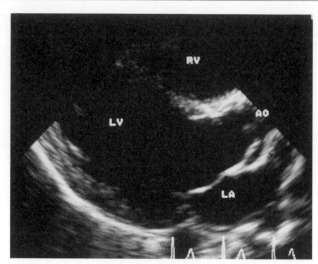

Left parasternal long-axis 2-D echocardiogram.

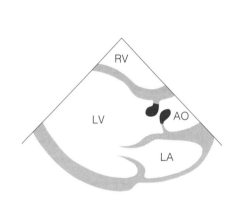

Same patient. Echo-dense structure in scan of the aortic valve. Suspicion of vegetation. Early diastole.

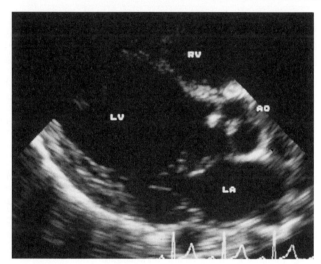

Left parasternal long-axis 2-D echocardiogram.

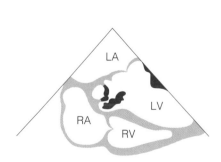

Same patient. Echo-dense structure in scan of the aortic valve. Suspicion of vegetation. Early diastole.

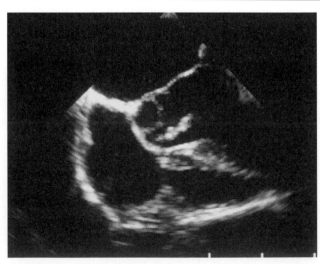

Transesophageal short-axis 2-D echocardiogram.

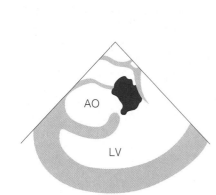

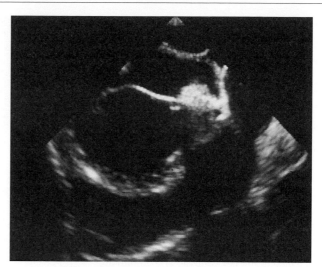

Same patient. Cloud-like structure on the aortic valve prolapses into the left ventricular outflow tract. Diastolic image. Findings indicate aortic valve endocarditis.

Transesophageal long-axis 2-D echocardiogram.

In aortic valve endocarditis, secondary metastatic infections can occur on jet lesions. They are brought into effect by the collision of the intermittent septic aortic regurgitant jet with intervalvular connective tissue between the aortic and mitral valves or the anterior mitral leaflet.

Infection of the subaortic region between the valve rings gives rise to subaortic abscess or pseudoaneurysm of the left ventricular outflow tract. The abscess or pseudoaneurysm can consequently rupture into the left atrium, whereby blood from the left ventricular outflow tract will eject into the left atrium in systole. Transthoracic Doppler color flow imaging reveals a signal that is similar to an eccentric mitral regurgitant jet originating from the left ventricular outflow tract. The transesophageal access usually permits exact diagnosis by visualizing the shunt from the left ventricular outflow tract to the left atrium. This can simulate mitral insufficiency clinically and on transthoracic scans.

Should the satellite infection affect the anterior mitral leaflet, an abscess can develop at this site and thereby result in perforation of the leaflet with consecutive mitral insufficiency or leaflet aneurysm.

These two complications are treated differently. Mitral valve replacement is indicated in severe mitral insufficiency, whereas a communication between the left ventricular outflow tract and the left atrium above the mitral valve plane cannot be corrected by a isolated mitral valve surgery [4].

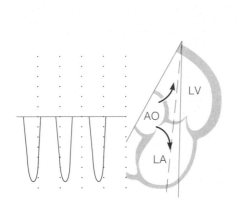

Aortic valve endocarditis with penetration of the posterior aortic wall across the base of the anterior mitral leaflet into the left atrium. Diastolic jets are detected in the left ventricle and left atrium, due to the aortic wall rupture.

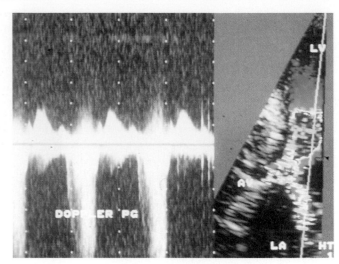

Apical four-chamber view. Color coded CW Doppler.

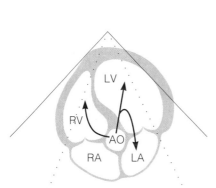

Aortic valve endocarditis with aortic insufficiency. Penetration of the aortic wall. At the beginning of diastole (0.31 s after R wave) highly turbulent jets are seen in the right ventricle and the left atrium.

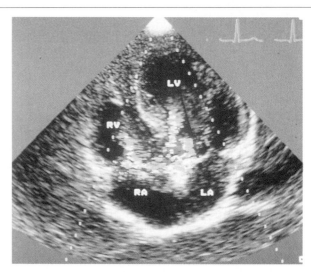

Apical four-chamber 2-D echocardiogram with color flow mapping.

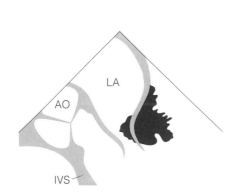

Mitral valve endocarditis. End-diastole. Independently moving vegetations that flutter in the bloodstream are attached to the posterior mitral leaflet. Opening restricted due to size of vegetation.

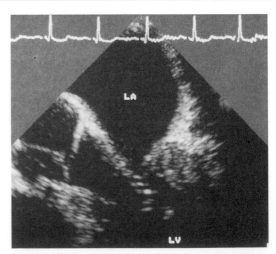

Transesophageal short-axis 2-D echocardiogram of the aortic valve, left atrium, mitral valve, and left ventricular outflow tract.

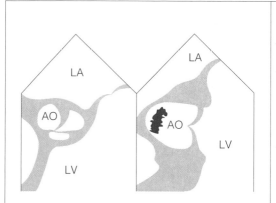

Differential diagnosis of thickened aortic valve (mid-systole: 0.21 s after R wave). Only in the long-axis view in mid-systole was thickening in the region of the noncoronary aortic cusp identified by its independent motion as a vegetation.

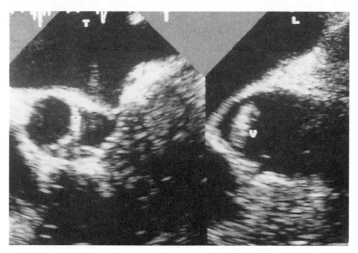

Transesophageal SAX (left) and LAX (right) views through the aortic valve.

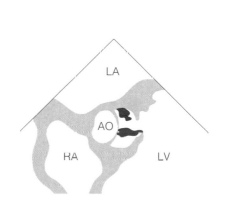

Same patient. End-systole (0.30 s after R wave): Vegetation that moves independently is located on the non-coronary aortic cusp. Left coronary aortic cusp is calcified.

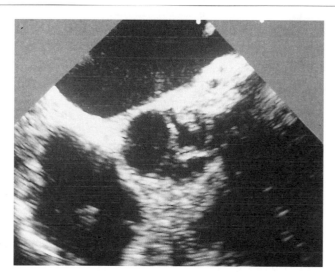

Transesophageal short-axis view through the aortic valve.

| 12. | Infective Endocarditis |
| 12.2 | Prosthetic Valve Endocarditis |

Prosthetic valve endocarditis

► Early-onset prosthetic valve endocarditis
► Late-onset prosthetic valve endocarditis

Early-onset prosthetic valve endocarditis is defined as an infection occurring within 3 months after cardiac valve replacement. The differentiation between early and late-onset prosthetic valve endocarditis is justified by the different bacteriological patterns and mortality rates associated with their respective bacterial spectra.

Early and late-onset prosthetic valve endocarditis can be expected to occur in 0.83% and 1.50%, respectively, of all patients who receive prosthetic valves [49]. The incidence is approximately the same in biological and non-biological prostheses. The mortality rate is 68 to 80% and 36 to 53%, respectively [15,21]. The leading causes of infection are Staphylococcus, Streptococci of the serogroup D (Enterococci), and gram-negative bacteria in early-onset prosthetic valve endocarditis, and Streptococci with α-hemolysis in the late-onset prosthetic valve endocarditis.

In early-onset prosthetic valve endocarditis, incomplete endothelialization leads to direct involvement of the artificial valves and sutures sites [17]. In late-onset prosthetic valve endocarditis, on the other hand, tissue infiltration caused by the bacteria usually occurs.

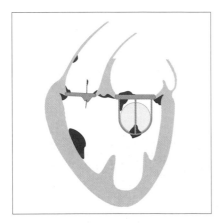

Suppurative aortic prosthetic valve endocarditis spreads to the bordering structures and usually sets in at the periaortic space and the atria, seldom in the anterior mitral leaflet or the interventricular septum [23]. The treatment of choice appears to be *allograft* or *homograft* replacement of the aortic root. This eliminates abscesses and the fragile, infected aortic annulus which is exposed to high systemic pressure [41].

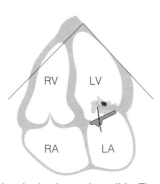

Prosthetic mitral valve endocarditis. The subvalvular apparatus of the posterior leaflet was left in place. At this site, cloud-like, floating foreign structures are visible above the dense, stationary echoes. Findings correspond to perivalvular abscess.

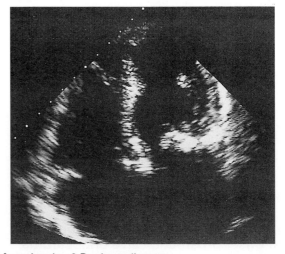

Apical four-chamber 2-D echocardiogram.

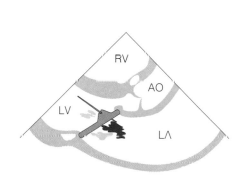

Same patient. Discontinuity of the posterior wall of the left ventricle: Abscess. Echo-dense structure at the level of the prosthetic mitral valve, which opens normally.

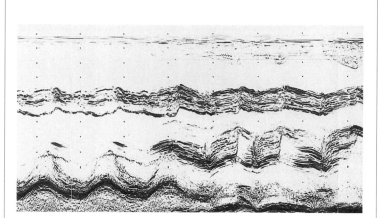

M-mode, left parasternal LAX view at mitral valve prosthesis level.

Same patient. Vegetation on the mitral valve prosthesis. Echofree spaces in the posterior wall of the left ventricle in the region of the basal posterior mitral leaflet, as well as in the anterior aortic wall correspond to abscesses. Secondary involvement of the aortic valve and of its ring.

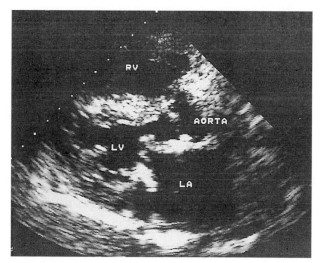

Left parasternal long-axis 2-D echocardiogram.

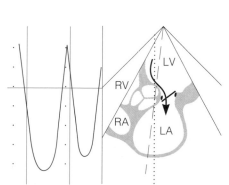

Early-onset prosthetic valve endocarditis involving the mitral valve. At the beginning of systole, a narrow, turbulent paravalvular regurgitant jet that proceeds, in the direction of the atrial septum.

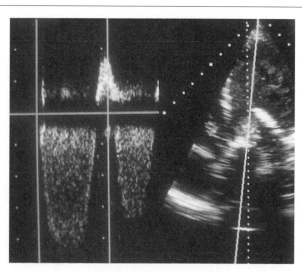

Apical four-chamber view. Color coded CW Doppler.

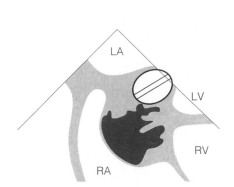

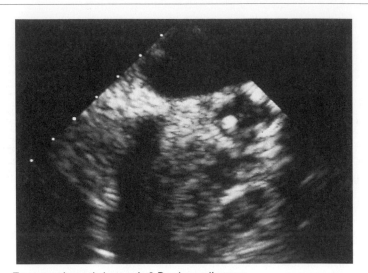

Aortic prosthetic valve endocarditis that occurred after replacement of the aortic valve and ascending aorta by a SJM-A29-conduit. Abscess between the aortic valve prosthesis and the origin of the main stem of the left coronary artery with minimal paravalvular leak. CT showed no evidence of abscess.

Transesophageal short-axis 2-D echocardiogram.

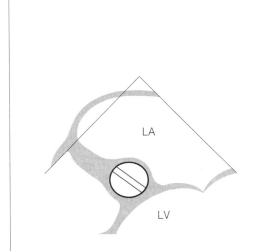

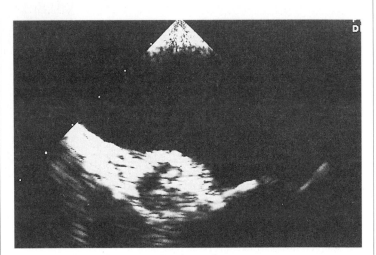

Same patient.

Transesophageal short-axis 2-D echocardiogram.

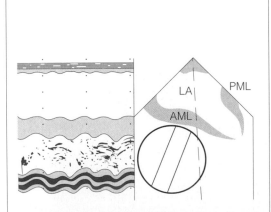

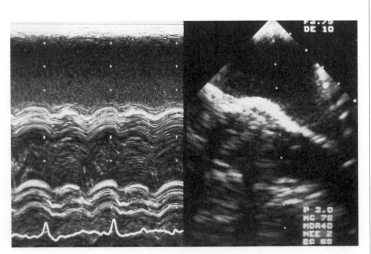

Same patient. Wall separation. Independently moving, filamentous foreign structures (vegetations) that flutter in the bloodstream during diastole.

Transesophageal short-axis M-mode and 2-D echocardiograms.

Aortic prosthetic valve endocarditis (prosthesis made of biological material): echo-dense structures in M-mode recording of the non-coronary aortic valve cusp and the anterior aortic wall. Cloud-like echoes in recording of the open aortic valve. Difficult to differentiate from noise. Unclear findings.

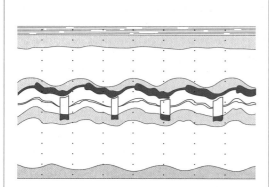

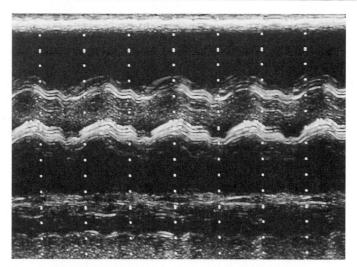

M-mode, left parasternal long-axis view at aortic valve level.

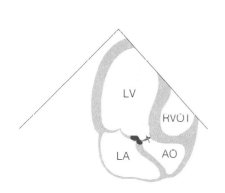

Same patient. Echo-dense structure in the region of the aorta and anterior mitral leaflet. Unclear findings.

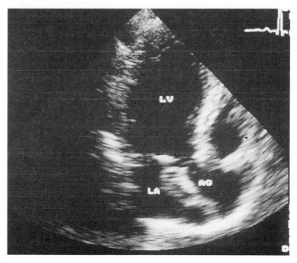

Apical long-axis 2-D echocardiogram.

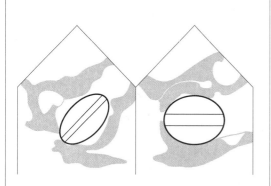

Same patient. Strong suspicion of vegetations and suppurations (echo-free spaces); prosthetic valve endocarditis.

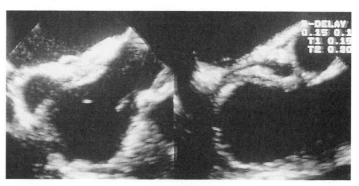

Transesophageal short and long-axis 2-D echocardiograms.

The reported sensitivity of echocardiography in detection of infective endocarditis ranges widely, from 50 to 100 % [1, 6, 10, 22, 30, 32, 36, 42]. This is due to several reasons. One is that the course of the disease may vary, and the vegetations are not always morphologically detectable. A second reason is that attempts to identify the vegetations come at different stages of the disease. In current echocardiographic systems, vegetations as small as 1 to 5 mm in size can be detected. Another reason for differences in sensitivity is that there is some variation in the patient population of different hospitals. Other reasons for poor sensitivity are the use of improper machine settings and improper acoustic windows. This is also the reason why the reported minimum size at which vegetations can be detected varies. Small vegetations can be identified retrospectively on echocardiograms when the echocardiographer has prior knowledge of their existence. However, it is difficult to unequivocally differentiate small vegetations from noise.

Pooled data sets show that conventional echocardiography detected vegetations larger than 5 mm in size almost 75% of all cases, and transesophageal access was able to detect them in as many as in 90% of all cases [19, 35]. The sensitivity for detection of perivalvular abscesses was similar [12, 39].

Conversely, the high specificity of echocardiography in endocarditis of native valves with non-primary morphological changes must be emphasized. In the clinical picture of infective endocarditis, the diagnosis can be made on the basis of echocardiographic evidence of vegetations, valvular destruction and perivalvular abscess. This is subject to the limitations in previously altered or artificial valves with metal components that can lead to total reflection and/or artifacts. Preexisting conditions such as thickening of sclerotic, myxomatous or rheumatically altered valves, oscillation and fluttering of valvular segments due to tears in the leaflet or cusp, rupture of the support apparatus, non-infective endocarditis, thrombus and neoplasms can easily lead to false-positive findings and can compromise the specificity of the echocardiographic diagnosis.

When considering the prevalence and specificity of echocardiographically demonstrated vegetations, the definition of the term is ultimately decisive. Many other abnormalities with a low specificity can be excluded when, by definition, the foreign structures suspected to be a vegetation a) must be attached to an endocardial surface, b) must exhibit independent motion, c) must not restrict the motility of the involved valve, d) must be visible in multiple imaging planes, and e) must exhibit echogenicity that differs distinctly from that of the valve or endocardial background.

Avoidable false-negative findings arise when the echocardiographer neglects to visualize all individual valve leaflets and cusps, neglects to utilize the transesophageal approach [27], neglects to perform follow-up exams despite continuing clinical suspicion (one negative echocardiographic study does not rule out infective endocarditis) [29]. Avoidable false-positive findings arise predominantly from ignorance of patient history, symptomatology and complementary diagnostic procedures. False-positive findings are bound to occur when the suspicious structure is evaluated only from one view, or if the above-mentioned criteria for ultrasound diagnosis of cardiac vegetations are neglected.

Despite the progress in antibiotic therapy, the mortality rate of infective endocarditis is stagnating at a high level (between 20 to 33%) [24]. An increasingly large number of patients must undergo a heart surgery, and these remain the patients with the longest interval between onset and diagnosis of disease. Electrocardiographic and radiologic findings are not diagnostic, and cardiac catheterization is associated with a risk of embolization and infection. Therefore, echocardiography - in addition to positive blood cultures, history, and the physical examination - plays a leading role in the diagnosis [44].

Nuclear cardiologic procedures such as ^{67}GA and ^{113m}In scintigraphy and immune scintigraphy [34] complete the spectrum of diagnosis.

Cardiac catheterization, which is sometimes indicated primary to surgical intervention or at the end of medical treatment, is not the primary diagnostic technique in infective endocarditis.

The decision to perform cardiac catheterization depends on the reliability of the echocardiographic diagnosis, and on the presence of concomitant ischemic heart disease.

The principle limitation associated with echocardiographic demonstration of infective endocarditic lesions is that it is not possible to differentiate between fresh, active and healing or old, and non-active vegetations [45, 48]. Echocardiography is unable to assess the acuity of the process. Therefore, when fever, bacteremia or newly occurring murmurs are absent, echocardiography cannot differentiate between healed old endocarditis and acute infective endocarditis. It remains unclear whether textural analysis will be able to provide help in this respect.

In these cases, complementary diagnostic procedures must be used to assess the value and accuracy of cardiac ultrasound diagnosis.

| 12. | Infective Endocarditis |
| 12.5 | Follow-up and Treatment Considerations |

When there is continued, but unconfirmed, suspicion of infective endocarditis, the patient must be closely followed (usually every 2 weeks) by transthoracic and transesophageal examination. If infective endocarditis has been positively diagnosed, weekly transthoracic follow-up examinations must be performed in order to detect complications and to evaluate the results of treatment [48].

Since opinions differ as to the prognostic value of certain findings, their impact on therapy is also controversial [43]. The best predictors of a high risk are infection of a prosthetic valve, septic embolism, severe neurological complications, multi-organ failure, and evidence of highly virulent organisms (Staphlyococcus aureus and S. epidermidis, gram-negative bacteria, fungi) [26]. Very large (> 10 mm) and highly mobile vegetations are risk factors for septic embolism [10]. Large, mobile mitral valve vegetations are said to have a higher risk for septic embolism than vegetations on other valves. Should one of these constellations be present, then early, aggressive intervention would appear urgently necessary.

In patients with acute aortic insufficiency, there is an abrupt increase in diastolic and systolic wall stress. Patients with acute mitral insufficiency experience a much lesser degree of systolic wall stress, as systolic pressure compensation via the leaking valve occurs at the expense of the left atrium.

In aortic valve endocarditis with acute aortic insufficiency, the myocardial oxygen requirement continues to increase while the myocardial blood flow continues to decrease. This much more frequently develops into a situation that requires surgery than infective endocarditis of the mitral valve [11]. The abrupt hemodynamic changes resulting from an aortic valve rupture develop into severe heart failure and lead to death when emergency surgery cannot be performed [3, 33].

As compared to the mitral and aortic valves, the hemodynamic effects of right-side endocarditis with erosion and destruction of the tricuspid and/or pulmonary valve are much better tolerated; emergency surgery is hardly ever necessary. Usually, surgery is indicated due to septic pulmonary embolism.

The most common absolute indications for surgery are [15]:
- progressive heart failure due to valvular insufficiency
- intractable infection or evidence of abscess
- cerebral or recurrent peripheral septic embolism
- instability of the prosthetic valve.

Some authors also consider mycotic etiology, obstruction of the involved valve, new onset AV-block, and acute renal failure to be absolute indications for surgery. Relative indications for surgery are:
- mild heart failure due to valvular insufficiency
- non-streptococcal endocarditis
- septic embolism
- perivalvular leak
- echocardiographic evidence of vegetations
- relapse after completion of antibiotic therapy
- early-onset prosthetic valve endocarditis or negative blood cultures in prosthetic valve endocarditis with persistent fever, despite antibiotic therapy.

Although at some centers first attempts to treat bacteremia and valve infection with antibiotics before surgery, this should not be pursued until ventricular function is jeopardized. The probability of other serious complications such as severe thrombo-embolic attacks and acute renal failure also increases [14].

Doppler echocardiography is of therapeutic and prognostic significance only with regard to the detection of severe regurgitation, which often leads to rapidly progressive heart failure. Native valves with sclerotic changes often exhibit regurgitation of varying severity. However, particularly in these valves, it is difficult to identify small vegetations. Consequently, Doppler echocardiography is of only slight significance in the differentiation between non-infected sclerotic and infected sclerotic native valves.

Because homograft valves and conduits are increasingly favored for surgical management of infective endocarditis [47], preoperative echocardiographic morphometry of the native valve ring is gaining increasing significance in the preparation of homografts. Transesophageal, biplane or multiplane techniques are normally used for this purpose.

Morphometry and Ventricular Function

RVEDD   _____ mm
LAmaxD   _____ mm
LVEDD   _____ mm
LVESD   _____ mm
Fractional shortening   _____
RAEDD   _____ mm

Evidence of associated ischemic heart disease?
Wall motion analysis

Valve Morphology and Dynamics

▶ Independently moving, poorly defined, cloud-like foreign structures (vegetations) that move in the bloodstream in diastole and/or systole, that adhere to the valves or cardiac and vascular walls, that do not restrict the mobility of the valve as compared to fibrotic changes. 2-D echocardiography can determine the topographic orientation and size of the vegetations.
▶ Evidence of chordal rupture and/or leaflet perforation (cannot be reliably differentiated from vegetations).
▶ Evidence of vegetation prolapsing across the valve ring plane.
▶ Dilatation and wall separation in the region of the aortic root, *e.g.*, perivalvular echo-free spaces or an abnormal perivalvular echogenicity >10 mm, as evidence of aneurysm or abscess.
▶ Hemodynamic effects of valvular lesions (dilatated, volume-overloaded ventricles, conduction phenomenon due to irregular flows, etc.).

Valve Function and Pressure-Flow Relationships (Doppler Echocardiography)

▶ Qualitative visual proof of regurgitation
▶ Detection, velocity measurement, mapping, and follow-up of regurgitations.
▶ Graphic display of regurgitation and irregular, turbulent flow in the region of the vegetations

Transesophageal Echocardiography

▶ Superior imaging quality to that of transthoracic scans.

HISTORY / SYMPTOMATOLOGY / AUSCULTATION

Fever of unclear etiology, newly occurring heart murmur?

BLOOD CULTURES

Bacteremia, pyemia, sepsis? Determination of minimal inhibitory concentrations.

ECHOCARDIOGRAPHY

Conventional echocardiography:

Morphometry (RAEDD, RVEDD, LADmax, LVEDD, LVESD),
Ventricular function (LVFS, wall motion analysis)
and
Visualization of structural causes and complications:
Vegetations (size, mobility),
Valve morphology and dynamics

Doppler and transesophageal echocardiography:

To prove or exclude the presence of vegetations and destruction

Detection and assessment of regurgitation

Complementary procedures such as laboratory tests, nuclear medicine, and radiology.

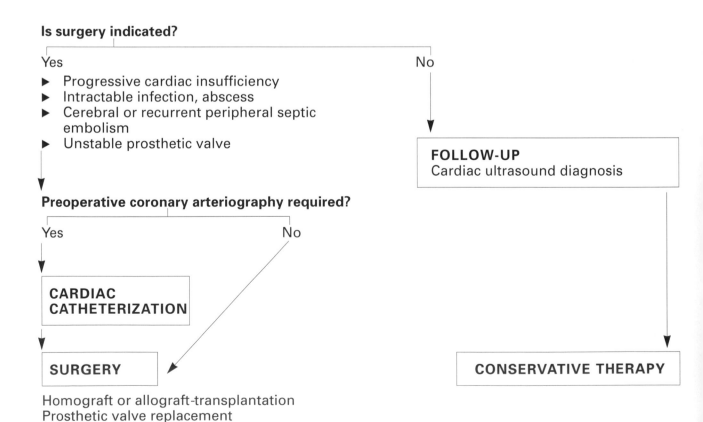

Is surgery indicated?

Yes
- ▶ Progressive cardiac insufficiency
- ▶ Intractable infection, abscess
- ▶ Cerebral or recurrent peripheral septic embolism
- ▶ Unstable prosthetic valve

No

FOLLOW-UP
Cardiac ultrasound diagnosis

Preoperative coronary arteriography required?

Yes   No

CARDIAC CATHETERIZATION

SURGERY

Homograft or allograft-transplantation
Prosthetic valve replacement

CONSERVATIVE THERAPY

1. Amsterdam EA. Value and limitations of echocardiography in endocarditis. Cardiology 1984; 71: 229-231.
2. Angrist A, Oka M, Nakao K. Vegetative endocarditis. Pathol Ann 1967; 2: 155-212.
3. Aufiero TX, Waldhausen JA. Early surgery for native left-sided endocarditis. J Am Coll Cardiol 1991; 18: 668.
4. Bansal RC, Graham BM, Jutzky KR, Shakudo M, Shah PM. Left ventricular outflow tract to left atrial communication secondary to rupture of mitral-aortic intervalvular fibrosa in infective endocarditis: Diagnosis by transesophageal echocardiography and color flow mapping. J Am Coll Cardiol 1990; 15; 499-504.
5. Bashour FA, Winchell CP. Right-sided bacterial endocarditis. Am J Med Sci 1960; 240: 411-416.
6. Biamino G, Lange L. Echokardiographie. Hoechst AG, 1983, 114.
7. Bleyl U, Döhnert G, Höpker WW, Hofmann W. Allgemeine Pathologie. Berlin, Heidelberg, New York: Springer Verlag, 1976: 179.
8. Boucher CA, Fallon JT, Myers SG, Hutter AM, Buckley MJ. The value and limitations of echocardiography in recording mitral valve vegetations. Am Heart J 1977; 94: 37-43.
9. Bryan CS. Nonbacterial thrombotic endocarditis in patients with malignant tumors. Am J Med 1969; 46: 787-793.
10. Buda AJ, Rotz RJ, LeMire MS, Bach DS. Prognostic significance of vegetations detected by two-dimensional echocardiography in infective endocarditis. Am Heart J 1986; 112: 1291-1296.
11. Ceitlin MD. The timing of surgery in mitral and aortic valve disease. Curr Probl Cardiol 1987; 12: 49-149.
12. Chan KL, Daniel L, Rakowski H, Ascah C, Baird M. Transesophageal echocardiography is crucial in the management of endocarditis. Circulation 1989; 80 (suppl II): 2656.
13. Chandraratna PAN, Langevin E. Limitations of the echocardiogram in diagnosing valvular vegetations in patients with mitral valve prolapse. Circulation 1977; 56: 436-438.
14. Cooley DA. Surgical considerations in infective endocarditis. Texas Heart J 1989; 16: 263-269.
15. Cowgill LD, Addonizio VP, Hopeman AR, Harken AH. A practical approach to prosthetic valve endocarditis. Ann Thor Surg 1987; 43: 450-457.
16. Cross AS, Steigbigel RT. Infective endocarditis and access site infections in patients of hemodialysis. Medicine 1976; 55: 453-466.
17. Dismukes WE Karchmer AW, Buckley MJ, Austen WG, Swartz MN. Prosthetic valve endocarditis. Analysis of 38 cases. Circulation 1973; 48: 365-377.
18. Edwards JE Jr, Burchell HB. Endocardial and intimal lesions (jet impact) as possible sites of origin of murmurs. Circulation 1958; 18: 946-960.
19. Erbel R, Rohmann S, Drexler M, Mohr-Kahaly S, Gerharz CD, Iversen S, Oelert H, Meyer J. Improved diagnostic value of echocardiography in patients with infective endocarditis by transesophageal approach: A prospective study. Eur Heart J 1988; 9: 43-53.
20. Estevez CM, Dillon JC, Walker PD, Feigenbaum H,Chang S. Echocardiographic manifestations of aortic cusp rupture in a myxomatous aortic valve. Chest 1976; 69: 685-687.
21. Fleck E. Frühzeitige Kunstklappenendokarditis. Münch med Wschr 1984; 124: 953-954.
22. Gentry LO, Khoshdel A. New approaches to the diagnosis and treatment of infective endocarditis. Texas Heart Inst J 1989; 16: 250-257.
23. Glazier JJ, Verwilghen J, Donaldson RM, Ross DN. Treatment of complicated prosthetic valve endocarditis with annular abscess formation by homograft aortic root replacement. J Am Coll Cardiol 1991; 17: 1177-1182.
24. Hayward D. Infective endocarditis: A changing disease. Brit Med J 1973; 273: 706-709.
25. Hubbell G, Cheitlin MD, Rapaport E. Presentation, management, and follow-up evaluation of infective endocarditis in drug addicts. Am Heart J 1981; 102: 85-94.
26. Jaffe WM, Morgan DE, Pearlman AS, Otto CM. Infective endocarditis, 1983-1988: Echocardiographic findings and factors influencing morbidity and mortality. J Am Coll Cardiol 1990; 15: 1227-1233.
27. Lee E, Schiller N. How useful is transesophageal echocardiography? Choices in Cardiology 1989; 3: 176-179.
28. Libman E, Sacks B. A hitherto undescribed form of valvular and mural endocarditis. Arch Intern Med 1924; 33: 701-737.
29. Lowry RW, Zoghbi WA, Baker WB, Wray RA, Quinones MA. Clinical impact of transesophageal echocardiography in the diagnosis and management of infective endocarditis: Siginificance of a negative finding. J Am Coll Cardiol 1992; 19 (suppl A): 237 A.
30. Lutas EM, Roberts RB, Devereux RB, Prieto LM. Relation between the presence of echocardiographic vegetations and the complication rate in infective endocarditis. Am Heart J 1986; 112: 107-113.
31. Markiewicz W, Peled B, Alroy G, Pollack S, Brook G, Rapoport J, Kerner H. Echocardiography in infective endocarditis. Lack of specifity in patients with valvular pathology. Europ J Cardiol 1979; 10: 247-257.
32. Martin RP. The diagnostic and prognostic role of cardiovascular ultrasound in endocarditis: Bigger is not better. J Am Coll Cardiol 1991; 15: 1234-1237.
33. Middlemost S, Wisenbaugh T, Meyerowitz C, Teeger S, Essop R, Skoularigis J, Cronje S, Sarelli P. A case for early surgery in native left-sided endocarditis complicated by heart failure: Results in 203 patients. J Am Coll Cardiol 1991; 18: 663-667.

34. Morguet AJ, Munz DL, Sold G, Sandrock D, Figulla HR, Emrich D, Kreuzer H. Technetium-99m labeled anti-granulocyte antibodies for immunoscintigraphy in subacute infective endocarditis. J Am Coll Cardiol 1992; 19 (suppl A): 181 A.
35. Mügge A, Daniel WG, Frank G, Lichtlen PR. Echocardiography in infective endocarditis: Reassessment of prognostic implications of vegetation size determined by the transthoracal and transesophageal approach. J Am Coll Cardiol 1989; 14: 631-638.
36. O'Brien JT, Geiser EA. Infective endocarditis and echocardiography. Am Heart J 1984; 108: 386-394.
37. Oakley CM. Letter to the editor: Antibiotic prophylaxis for bacterial endocarditis. Am J Cardiol 1980; 46: 1073.
38. Pelletier LL, Petersdorf RG. Infective endocarditis: A review of 125 cases of Washington hospitals 1963-1972. Medicine 1977; 56: 287-313.
39. Rayhaudhury T, Faichney A, Cameron EWJ, Walbaum PR. Surgical management of native valve endocarditis. Thorax 1983; 38: 168-174.
40. Rodbard S. Blood velocity and endocarditis. Circulation 1963; 27: 18-28.
41. Ross D. Allograft root replacement for prosthetic endocarditis. J Cardiac Surg 1990; 5: 5-11.
42. Rudolph W, Kraus F. Erkennung und Beurteilung der infektiösen Endokarditis. Herz 1983; 8: 241-270.
43. Sanfilippo AJ, Picard MH, Newell JB, Rosas E, Davidoff R, Thomas JD, Weyman AE. Echocardiographic assessment of patients with infectious endocarditis: predicition of risk for complications. J Am Coll Cardiol 1991; 18: 1191-1199.
44. Schmailzl KJG. Infektiöse Endocarditis. Gesichertes und Kontroverses. Antibiotika-Dialog 1988; 6: 5-6.
45. Sheikh MU, Covarrubias EA, Ali N, Lee WE, Sheikh NM, Roberts WC. M-mode echocardiographic observations during and after healing of active bacterial endocarditis limited to the mitral valve. Am Heart J 1981; 101: 37-45.
46. Shively BK, Gurule FT, Roldan CA, Leggett JH, Schiller NB. Diagnostic value of transesophageal compared with transthoracic echocardiography in infective endocarditis. J Am Coll Cardiol 1991; 18: 391-397.
47. Stelzer P, Elkins R. Homograft valves and conduits: applications in cardiac surgery. Curr Probl Surg 1989; 26: 410-413.
48. Stewart JA, Silimperi D, Harris P, Wise NW, Fraker TD, Kisslo JA. Echocardiographic documentation of vegetative lesions in infective endocarditis. Clinical implications. Circulation 1980; 61: 374-380.
49. Watanakunakoro G. Prosthetic valve endocarditis. Progr Cardiovasc Dis 1979; 22: 181-192.
50. Wise J, Bentall HH, Cleland WP, Goodwin JF, Hallidie-Smith KA, Oakley CM. Urgent aortic valve replacement for acute aortic regurgitation in infective endocarditis. Lancet 1971; 2: 115-121.

For a long time the existence of human immunodeficiency virus related cardiac disorders had not been positively established, although the Hi-virus is known to affect every other organ system, either directly or indirectly by means of opportunistic infections. In the years when no life-prolonging treatment was available, most patients either did not live long enough for life-threatening cardiac manifestations to occur, or cardiac diagnosis was neglected because other organs appeared to be affected sooner. Even back then, autopsy findings confirmed cardiac involvement due to Kaposi's sarcoma, malignant lymphoma, and opportunistic infections with systemic dissemination. We now know that transient or persistent ECG repolarization disturbances appear in the setting of wasting syndrome, but also in the AIDS-related complex (ARC) stage. It is difficult to interpret these findings correctly if one regards the heart as an innocent organ.

Descriptions of cardiac disorders affecting one or all wall layers and leading to dilated cardiomyopathy without any evidence of neoplastic or opportunistic infection posed the question of whether the Hi-virus directly interferes with heart tissue.

Hi-virus can only invade cells with T4 receptors to which it can attach its gp41 and gp120 glycoproteins. In addition to lymphocytes, cells present in heart tissue which have T4 receptors include monocytes and macrophages. It is doubtful that there are any cardiocytes that express T4 receptors. Hi-virus can destroy cells with T4 receptors by direct infection (ultimately resulting in cytolysis), or as "innocent bystander" in a manner similar to infestation of the neuroglia.

Cardiac Lesions in HIV Infection

▶ Infective and noninfective pericarditis
▶ Inflammatory and noninflammatory vascular lesions
▶ Myocarditis
▶ Dilated cardiomyopathy
▶ Opportunistic infections
▶ Infective endocarditis
▶ Cardiac neoplasms
▶ Pharmacologically induced toxic heart damage

Pericarditis occurs with neoplastic infiltration or infection. Myocardial involvement is observed in practically all cases.

Vascular lesions generally appear in the form of arteritis, or they manifest as intimal fibrosis with fragmentation of elastic connective tissue and fibrous calcification of the media, thereby obliterating the lumen [5]. Coronary artery involvement may range from stenosis and dilatation to fusiform aneurysms.

The human immunodeficiency virus itself appears to be involved in the pathogenesis of myocarditis. It was isolated from cultures taken from endomyocardial biopsies of a patient with dilated cardiomyopathy secondary to AIDS [3]. Retrospective studies show that the incidence of myocarditis is approximately 50% [1, 8], whereby no distinction is made between "primary" myocarditis associated with Hi-virus and secondary myocarditis caused by known pathogens. The diagnostic problem lies in the fact that HIV-related myocarditis appears to show inflammatory cellular infiltrates but no myocyte necrosis; thus, it fails to fulfil the classic Dallas criteria. Conversely, necrosis is observed without signs of inflammation, which would indicate a virus or an excessive level of catecholamine as the probable cause.

In addition to the obvious signs of right heart overload with right ventricular hypertrophy and dilation attributable to severe or repeated opportunistic infection of the respiratory tract, HIV infection involving the heart can also result in dilated cardiomyopathy. All these cases were shown to have myocardial lesions [1].

These lesions do not necessarily follow the pattern of an active process. This could indicate that the human immunodeficiency virus itself not only induces myocarditis, but can ultimately lead to dilated cardiomyopathy [12].

Opportunistic infections with systemic dissemination can result in cardiac involvement. Cytomegalovirus, cryptococcus, mycobacteria, and toxoplasmic infections of the heart have been described.

Among the various risk groups, the incidence of infective endocarditis involving the right heart is highest in intravenous drug abusers.

Two types of malignant neoplasms that characteristically involve the heart have been described in AIDS: Kaposi's sarcoma and malignant lymphoma.

The echomorphological appearance of HIV-related cardiac disorders varies, but there are three basic patterns:

- Noninfective and infective endocarditis,
- Neoplastic infiltration,
- Syndromes similar to myocarditis and dilated cardiomyopathy.

Compared with the features of the non-HIV-related varieties of these cardiac disorders, certain special features can be observed in the AIDS-related varieties and their precursors.

Marantic endocarditis, a special type of noninfective endocarditis, is the most common type of endocarditis reported to occur in the setting of AIDS [2, 4, 6, 7, 9]. Marantic endocarditis is characterized by vegetations composed of a crumbly, reticular network of fibrin with inclusion of inflammatory cells. It can cause systemic or cerebral embolisms, thus leading to acute and dramatic worsening episodes [11]. Classic *infective endocarditis* in the setting of AIDS generally appears amongst intravenous drug abusers, which speaks against an increased incidence as a consequence of the primary disorder. In both forms of endocarditis, vegetations, assuming they are large enough to be detected, are the primary cardiologic manifestations. Vegetations appear as indistinct cloud-like foreign structures that flutter and move independently in the bloodstream during systole and/or diastole. Vegetations adhere to the endocardial surfaces of the valves or the heart and vessel walls and show a contrasting echogenecity.

Malignant neoplasms occur in about one-third of all AIDS cases. *Kaposi's sarcoma* with cardiac involvement (usually the epicardium) was found in 28% of all autopsied cases [10]. Infiltrations can be identified on the echocardiogram as masses or as localized areas of different echo-density.

HIV-related inflammatory heart diseases resembling myocarditis and dilated cardiomyopathy exhibit echocardiographic signs ranging from those of inflammatory heart disease, *e.g.* pericardial effusion, to ventricular dilatation and impairment of systolic ventricular function. The clinical manifestations of an HIV-associated inflammatory heart disease vary according to the severity of inflammation and, if it is focal, on the localization. The clinical picture ranges from absence of cardiac symptoms to rapidly progressing heart failure. *Opportunistic infections* are well documented as one of the relevant etiological factors in HIV-associated myocarditis. The role of viruses, including Hi-virus itself, has been demonstrated in isolated cases of dilated cardiomyopathy [3]. Since viruses such as Hi-virus and cytomegalovirus can cause necrosis without provoking inflammatory responses, it is probable that they are responsible for many such autopsy findings [13]. Due to the absence of inflammatory reactions, the echomorphology of these disorder often is not spectacular, and is limited to borderline abnormality of cardiac dimensions and systolic ventricular function. Compared with the incidence of HIV-related inflammatory heart disease, the complete clinical picture of dilated cardiomyopathy is rare.

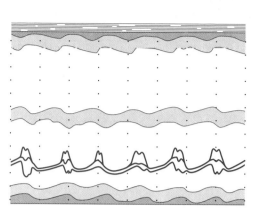

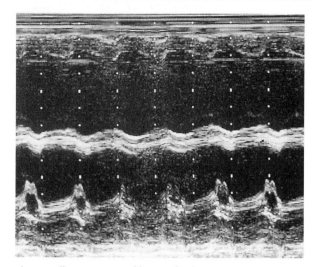

ARC in patient w/o previous history of heart disease. Incidental findings: borderline hypertrophy and severe dilatation of the right ventricle; suspected vegetation on the right mitral valve; suspected noninfective endocarditis.

M-mode recording, parasternal long-axis view.

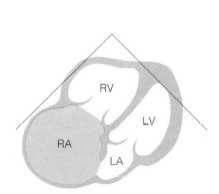

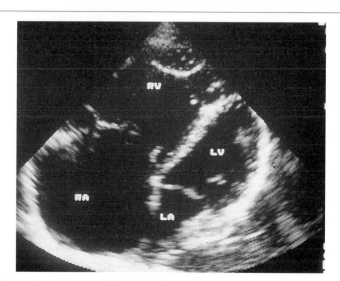

Same patient. Diastolic image. Findings: massively dilated right atrium; dimension of left cardiac cavities within reference range; structural defect in the interatrial septum.

Apical four-chamber 2-D echocardiogram.

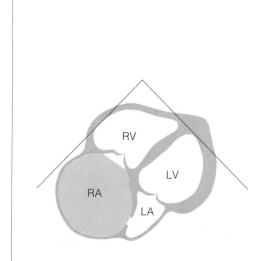

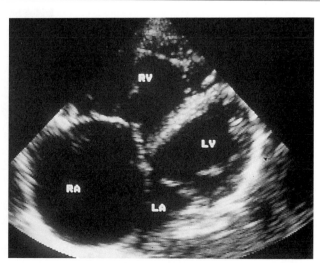

Same patient. Systolic image.

Apical four-chamber 2-D echocardiogram.

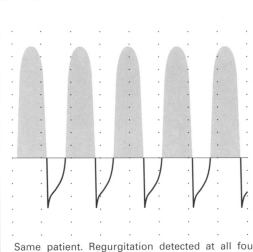

Same patient. Regurgitation detected at all four valves. Pulmonary insufficiency.

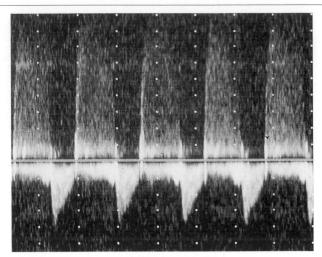

CW Doppler recording.

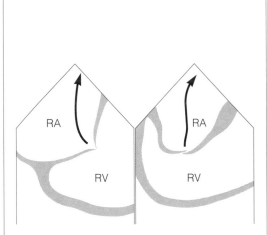

Same patient. Moderately severe tricuspid insufficiency.

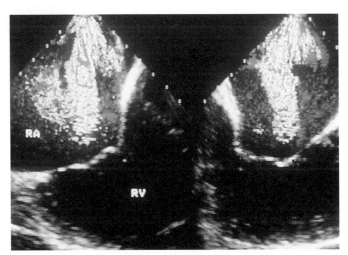

Transesophageal short and long-axis view. Color coded.

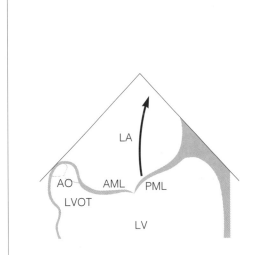

Same patient. Mild mitral insufficiency.

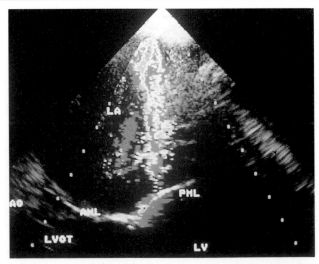

Color flow map of transesophageal short-axis 2-D echocardiogram.

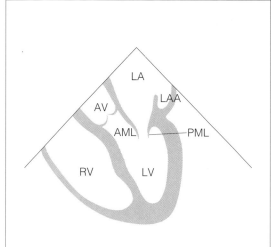

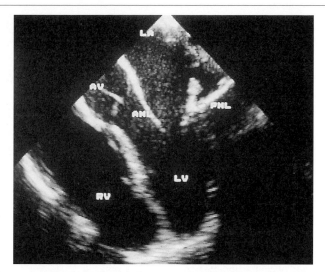

Same patient. Spontaneous contrast in the left ventricle, left ventricular outflow tract, and aorta.

Transesophageal short-axis 2-D echocardiogram.

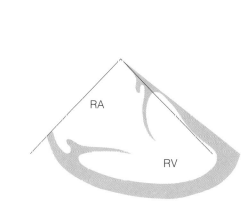

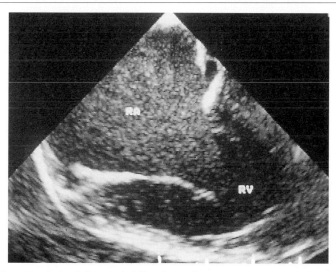

Same patient. Spontaneous contrast in the right atrium.

Transesophageal short-axis 2-D echocardiogram.

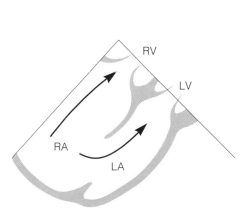

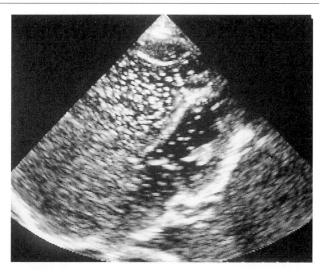

Same patient. Contrast medium visible in all four chambers of the heart. Oximetry does indicate presence of a hemodynamically significant shunt.

Contrast echocardiography, apical four-chamber 2-D scan.

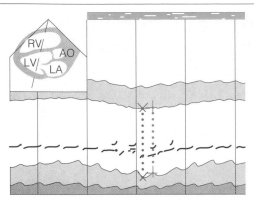

AIDS patient with shortness of breath persisting for four weeks. Pharyngoesophageal candidiasis. Possibility of cytomegalovirus, cryptococcus, mycobacteria, or toxoplasmic infection excluded. Dilation of the right and left ventricles with extremely reduced amplitude of contraction. Hemodynamically significant pericardial effusion excluded.

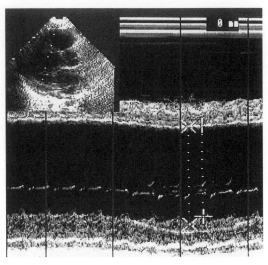

M-mode, parasternal long-axis view at the level of the ventricle.

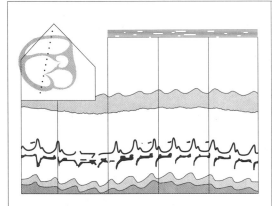

Same patient. Systemic pressure 80/55 mmHg. Sinus tachycardia 110-150/min. Tachypnea. Chest x-ray indicates pulmonary congestion. Paradoxical pulse without pericardial effusion. Respiration-related variation in right and left ventricular diameter. Reduced transmitral stroke volume.

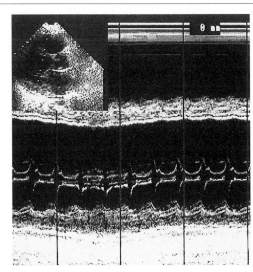

M-mode, parasternal long-axis view at mitral valve level.

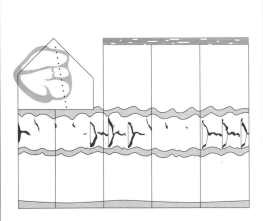

Same patient. Reduced transaortic stroke volume. Dilated left atrium.

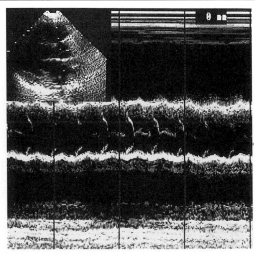

M-mode, parasternal long-axis view at the level of the aorta and left atrium.

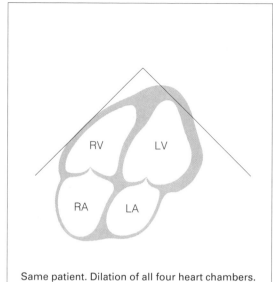

Same patient. Dilation of all four heart chambers.

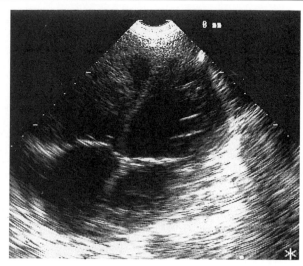

Apical four-chamber 2-D echocardiogram.

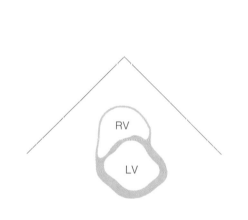

Same patient. Dilation of the right and left ventricles. Pleural effusion.

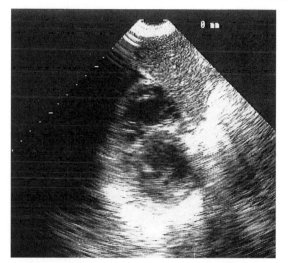

Parasternal short-axis 2-D scan at level of the ventricle.

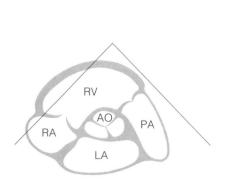

Same patient. Dilation of right heart chambers, right ventricular outflow tract, and pulmonary trunk.

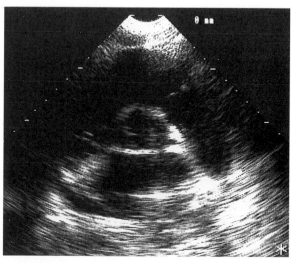

M-mode, parasternal short-axis view at the aortic valve level.

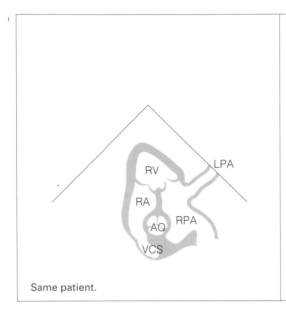

Same patient.

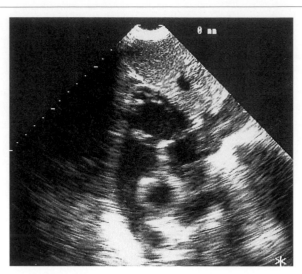

Subcostal short-axis 2-D echocardiogram.

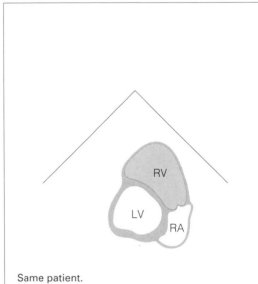

Same patient.

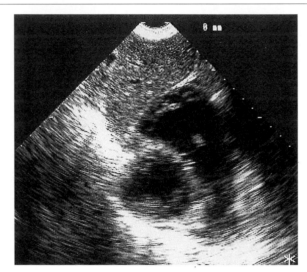

Subcostal short-axis 2-D echocardiogram.

References

1. Anderson DW, Virmani R, Reilly JM, O'Leary T, Cunnion RE, Robinowitz M, Macher AM, Punja U, Villa-flor ST, Parrillo JE, et al. Prevalent myocarditis at necropsy in the acquired immunodeficiency syndrome. J Am Coll Cardiol 1988; 11: 792-799.
2. Bryan CS. Nonbacterial thrombotic endocarditis in patients with malignant tumors. Am J Med 1969; 46: 787-793.
3. Calabrese LH, Profitt MR, Yen-Lieberman B, Hobbs RE, Ratliff NB. Congestive cardiomyopathy and illness related to the acquired immune deficiency syndrome (AIDS) associated with isolation of retrovirus from myocardium. Ann Intern Med 197; 107: 691-692.
4. Cammarasano C, Lewis W. Cardiac lesions in acquired immunodeficiency syndrome (AIDS). J Am Coll Cardiol 1985; 5: 703-706.

5. Joshi VV, Pawel B, Connor E, Sharer L, Oleske JM, Morrison S, Marin-Garcia J. Arteriopathy in children with acquired immune deficiency syndrome. Pediatr Pathol 1987; 7: 261-275.

6. Klatt EC, Meyer BR. Pathology of the heart in acquired immunodeficiency syndrome (AIDS). Arch Pathol Lab Med 1988; 112: 112-114.

7. Niedt GW, Schinella RA. Acquired immunodeficiency syndrome: clinical pathologic study of 56 autopsies. Arch Pathol Lab Med 1985; 109: 727-734.

8. Roldan EO, Moskowitz L, Hensley GT. Pathology of the heart in acquired immunodeficiency syndrome. Arch Path Lab Med 1987; 1: 1-14.

9. Rosen P, Armstrong O. Non-bacterial thrombotic endocarditis in patients with malignant neoplastic disease. Am J Med 1973; 54: 23-29.

10. Silver MA, Macher AM, Reichert CM, Levens DL, Parrillo JE, Longo DL, Roberts WC. Cardiac involvement by Kaposi's sarcoma in acquired immunodeficiency syndrome. JAMA 1984; 252: 1152-1159.

11. Snyder WD, Simpson DN, Nielsen S, Gold JWM, Metroka CE, Posner JB. Neurological complications of acquired immune deficiency syndrome: analysis of 50 patients. Ann Neurol 1983; 14: 403-418.

12. Tazelaar HD, Billingham ME. Leukocytic infiltrates in idiopathic dilated cardiomyopathy. A source of confusion with active myocarditis. Am J Pathol 1986; 10: 405-412.

13. Wink K, Schmitz H. Cytomegalovirus myocarditis. Am Heart J 1980; 100: 667-672.

Echocardiography plays an important role in the diagnosis of coronary artery disease. In the setting of myocardial ischemia, temporary or permanent contractile abnormality can occur in the affected myocardial region of the left ventricle [4, 10]. Ischemic myocardium can be detected by two-dimensional echocardiography and, in certain segments of the left ventricle, with the help of M-mode echocardiography. Ischemia-related hemodynamic changes can also be visualized with the help of Doppler echocardiography [17, 23].

| 14.1 | Detection of Ischemic Myocardium |
| 14.1.1 | Wall Motion Abnormality, Wall Thinning, Abnormal Systolic Increase in Wall Thickness |

Experimental studies have shown that, following acute coronary artery occlusion, contraction abnormalities occur with cancellation of systolic wall motion in the affected supply region and abnormal wall motion in the adjacent regions, while the rest of the myocardium exhibits a compensatory increase in contraction [1, 22]. The increased contractility of the healthy myocardium can usually maintain global left ventricular function. However, the deficits of extensive myocardial infarction can no longer be compensated for, and diastolic relaxation and compliance abnormalities and impairment of global systolic pump function therefore develop [7].

Two major features of normal wall motion are *systolic inward motion and systolic wall thickening* of the myocardium.

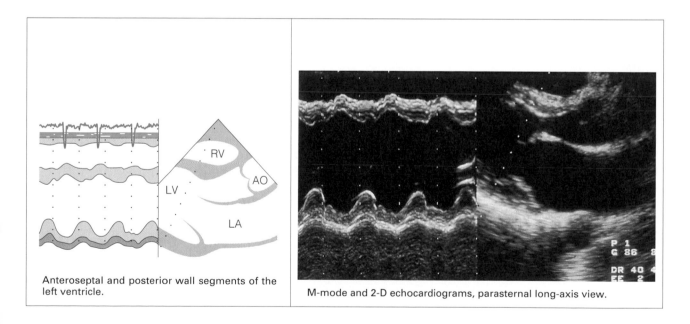

Anteroseptal and posterior wall segments of the left ventricle.

M-mode and 2-D echocardiograms, parasternal long-axis view.

Abnormalities in systolic inward motion and systolic wall thickening occur rapidly following ischemia. The magnitude of functional impairment varies in accordance with the extent of ischemia [11, 18]. Decreased systolic inward motion is defined as *hypokinesis*, and this occurs in conjunction with reduced systolic wall thickening.

The complete absence of systolic wall motion and wall thickening is defined as *akinesis*. Systolic outward motion with systolic wall thinning is defined as *dyskinesis*. The occurrence of akinesis or dyskinesis in a localized segment of the myocardium may lead to dilatation and outward bulging of the segment. This, in turn, may cause aneurysm with risk of thrombogenesis.

The described contraction abnormalities may affect all wall segments of the left ventricle, as can be visualized in different scan planes. A comparison study showed a good correlation between simultaneous echocardiographic and angiographic assessments of contractility [12].

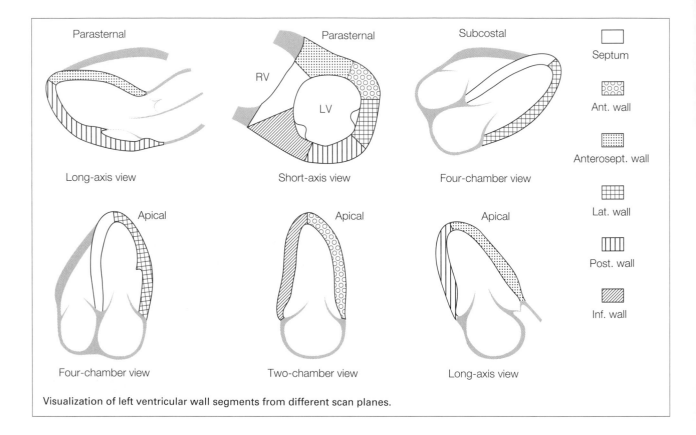

Visualization of left ventricular wall segments from different scan planes.

The basal and distal segments of the anteroseptal and posterior walls are assessed in M-mode recordings obtained from the parasternal long-axis view.

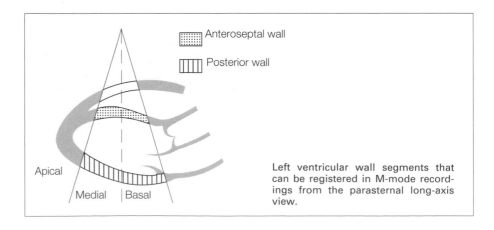

Left ventricular wall segments that can be registered in M-mode recordings from the parasternal long-axis view.

Two-dimensionally guided M-mode recordings of the anteroseptal and posterior wall can also be made from the short-axis view, however, the apical wall segments cannot always be visualized. Thus, M-mode echocardiography is limited is its capacity to visualize the left ventricle [16]. Although the M-mode beam can be positioned anywhere in the sector of the two-dimensional image, the long and short axes are the only suitable scan planes where the M-mode beam can be positioned perpendicular to the walls of the left ventricle. It is not possible to assess the inferior and lateral wall by M-mode echocardiography, and no complete assessment of the anterior wall can be made. Therefore, M-mode studies alone cannot fully exclude the possibility of wall motion abnormality.

Despite these limitations, 2-D guided M-mode echocardiography still plays an important role in the diagnosis of ischemia [5]. First of all, M-mode echocardiography permits measurement of anterior and posterior wall thickness. Therefore, in addition to detecting postinfarction wall thinning, M-mode also permits quantitation of total muscle mass. Secondly, in M-mode recordings the echo intensity of the anteroseptal and posterior walls can be assessed by direct comparison. Due to scarring, infarcted myocardium can be identified in M-mode recordings, because it is more echo-dense than normal myocardium [3]. Furthermore, M-mode echocardiography permits exact determination of left ventricular dimensions, which can be used as parameters for follow-up.

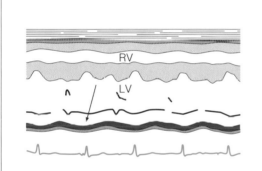

Posterior myocardial infarction. Findings: Absence of systolic inward motion and wall thickening. Normal motion in the anteroseptal wall.

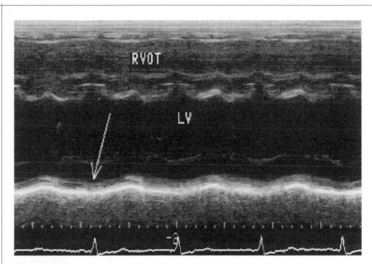

M-mode recording from the left parasternal long-axis view.

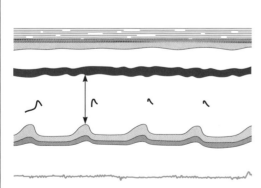

Anteroseptal infarction. Findings: Normal contractility in posterior wall. Thinned and echo-dense anteroseptal wall indicative of an old infarction.

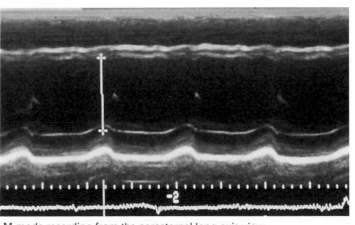

M-mode recording from the parasternal long-axis view.

14.1   Detection of Ischemic Myocardium
14.1.1   Wall Motion Abnormality, Wall Thinning,
**   Abnormal Systolic Increase in Wall Thickness**

660

All standard scan planes and additional atypical scan planes should be used when assessing left ventricular contractility. The left ventricle can then be visualized in its entirety. Because each wall segment can be visualized in more than one scan plane, abnormally contracting wall segments should be evaluated from multiple planes. Short-axis scans of the ventricle should always be made, because contractile abnormality can be assessed particularly well from the short-axis view. In short-axis scans, all left ventricular walls can be visualized in a single plane and assessed at a glance. Furthermore, when the transducer is angulated apically, the ventricular short axis can be followed up to the cardiac apex. Similarly, by angulating the transducer towards the base of the heart, the ventricle can be interrogated up to valve level. This, of course, is not possible in every case. Scanning conditions from the parasternal window are frequently restricted, especially in older patients.

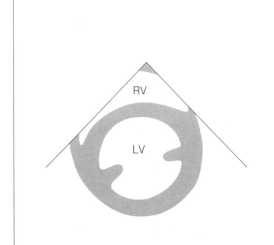

Short-axis view through the left ventricle at papillary muscle level. Diastolic image.

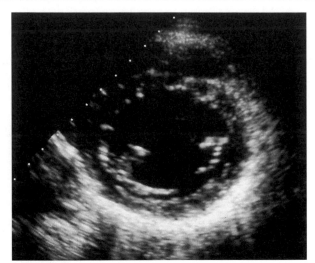

Left parasternal short-axis 2-D echocardiogram.

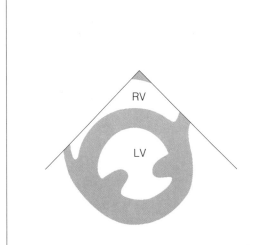

Short-axis view through the left ventricle at papillary muscle level. Systolic image.

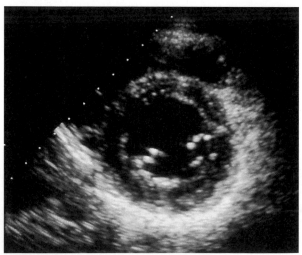

Left parasternal short-axis 2-D echocardiogram.

The papillary muscles, which are both uniformly visualized, serve as orientational structures when scanning the short axis. When contractility is normal, the left ventricular short-axis is virtually round in shape. Abnormally contractility causes systolic „unrounding" of the short axis.

14.1   **Detection of Ischemic Myocardium**   661
14.1.1   **Wall Motion Abnormality, Wall Thinning,**
          Abnormal Systolic Increase in Wall Thickness

Following myocardial infarction, contraction may be completely absent in the affected segment. Additionally, the wall may be thinner and more echo-dense (due to fibrotic changes and scarring).

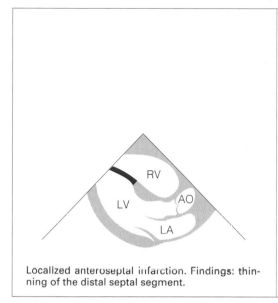

Localized anteroseptal infarction. Findings: thinning of the distal septal segment.

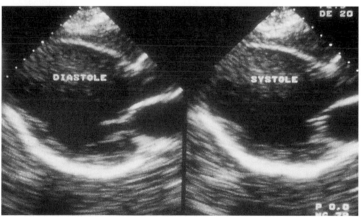

Left parasternal long-axis 2-D echocardiogram.

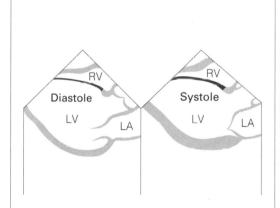

Extensive anteroseptal infarction. Findings: dilated left ventricle with thinned and echo-dense septum in absence of systolic inward motion and wall thickening. Diastolic and systolic images.

Left parasternal long-axis 2-D echocardiograms.

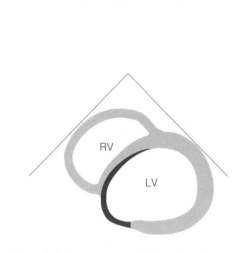

Acute inferior myocardial infarction: Findings: thinned and akinetic inferoseptal wall.

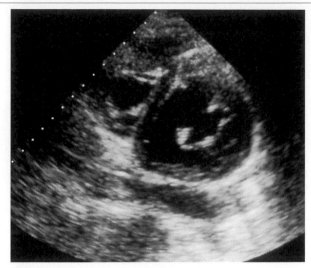

Left parasternal short-axis 2-D echocardiogram.

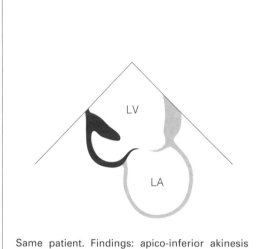

Same patient. Findings: apico-inferior akinesis with involvement of the posteromedial papillary muscle. Moderate ischemic mitral insufficiency.

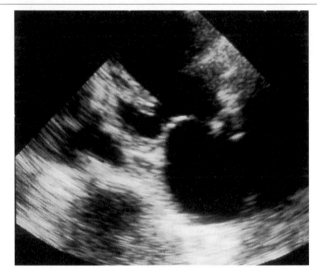

Apical two-chamber 2-D echocardiogram.

Because the basal septum is frequently involved in inferior myocardial infarctions, the basal septum should also be routinely studied. Contraction abnormalities in the posterior LV wall can be extremely localized and limited, which means they may be overlooked in standard scan planes. When there is justified suspicion of this, the left ventricle should also be investigated from atypical scan planes.

14.1   **Detection of Ischemic Myocardium**   **663**
14.1.1   **Wall Motion Abnormality, Wall Thinning,**
               Abnormal Systolic Increase in Wall Thickness

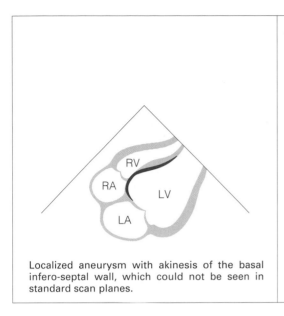

Localized aneurysm with akinesis of the basal infero-septal wall, which could not be seen in standard scan planes.

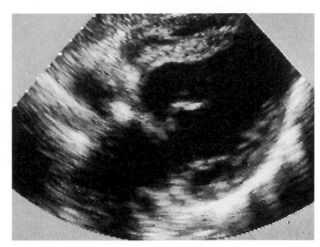

Oblique cut of the subcostal four-chamber view.

Wall motion abnormalities in the region of the lateral wall can be easily overlooked when localized and located only in distal or basal segments.

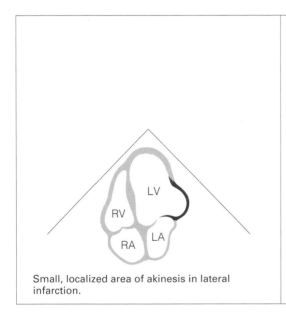

Small, localized area of akinesis in lateral infarction.

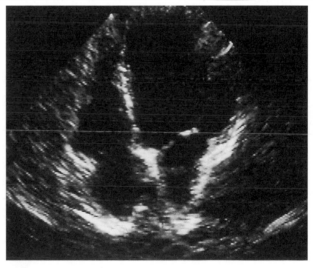

Apical four-chamber view.

Isolated lateral wall motion abnormality is rare, whereas combined anterolateral or inferolateral scarring is more common. Therefore, when lateral wall motion abnormality is found, particular attention should be paid to contractility in the anterior and inferior wall segments, which should be assessed from the apical two-chamber view. Involvement of the cardiac apex is frequently seen following anterolateral or inferolateral myocardial infarction. Therefore, these infarctions may severely affect the global left ventricular function and may eventually lead to such postinfarction complications as left ventricular dilatation.

14.1   **Detection of Ischemic Myocardium**
14.1.1   **Wall Motion Abnormality, Wall Thinning,**
               Abnormal Systolic Increase in Wall Thickness

664

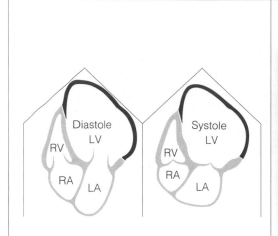

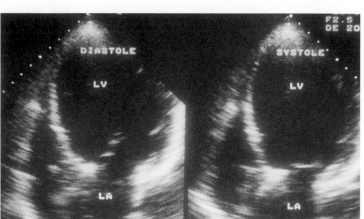

Dilated left ventricle with impaired global and regional (lateral, apical, septal) function. Diastolic and systolic images.

Apical four-chamber 2-D echocardiograms.

Frequently, contractile abnormality of posterior or posterolateral wall segments can be identified in M-mode recordings by directly comparing the contraction amplitudes of the posterior and anteroseptal walls. If the ventricular long axis cannot be visualized from the parasternal window, assessments of the posterior wall should always be made from the apical long-axis view.

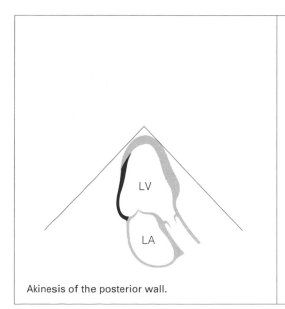

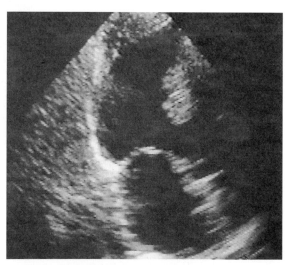

Akinesis of the posterior wall.

Apical long-axis („RAO equivalent") view.

Involvement of the cardiac apex is also common in contractile abnormality of the anterior and anteroseptal wall. Parasternal visualization of apical wall segments is limited. Therefore, apical scan planes should always be used for assessment of the cardiac apex. Thrombus must be suspected in the presence of marked contractile abnormalities and aneurysmal changes, especially in the region of the cardiac apex. These segments must then be carefully interrogated and assessed.

14.1   **Detection of Ischemic Myocardium**   **665**
14.1.1   **Wall Motion Abnormality, Wall Thinning,**
                Abnormal Systolic Increase in Wall Thickness

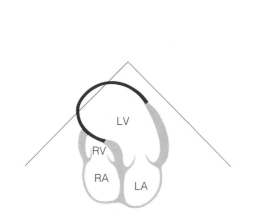

Extensive anteroseptal infarction. Findings: aneurysm of the cardiac apex; dyskinesis with systolic outward bulging of the cardiac apex and adjacent septum.

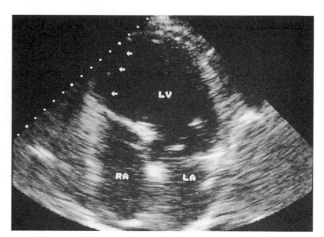

Apical four-chamber 2-D echocardiogram.

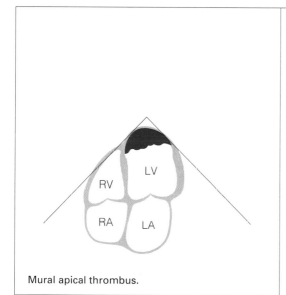

Mural apical thrombus.

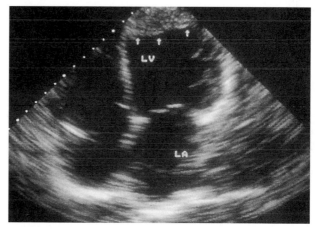

Apical four-chamber 2-D echocardiogram.

Although contractile abnormality primarily involves the left ventricle, the right ventricle cannot be disregarded. Right ventricular size and contractile function should always be assessed in scans obtained from the apical four-chamber view, especially in the presence of extensive inferior myocardial infarction. In addition to the four-chamber view, other scan planes will also be required to assess RV size and function. For example, subcostal scans are of great importance because they provide good visualization of the right ventricular free wall.

14.1   Detection of Ischemic Myocardium
14.1.1   Wall Motion Abnormality, Wall Thinning,
Abnormal Systolic Increase in Wall Thickness

666

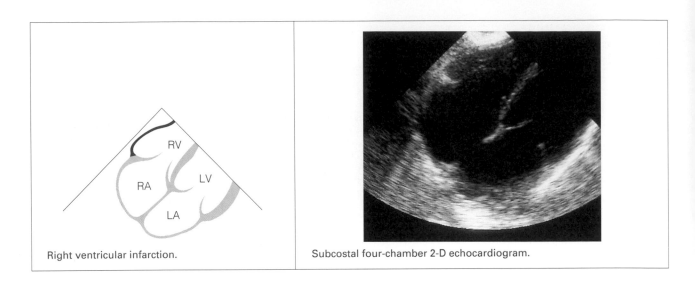

Right ventricular infarction.

Subcostal four-chamber 2-D echocardiogram.

To a limited degree, left ventricle can also be defined according to the distribution of coronary arteries supplying each segment.

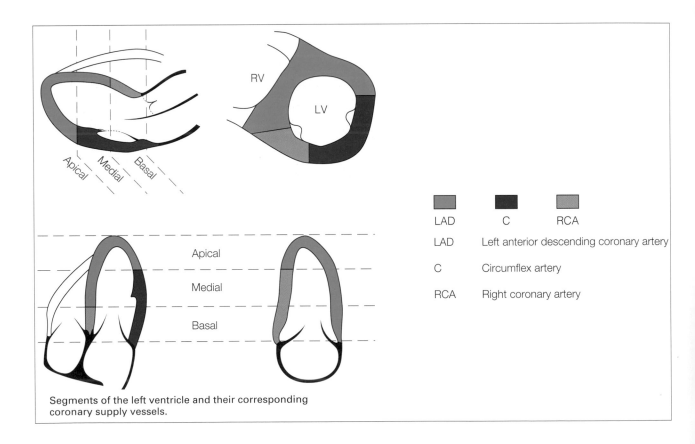

LAD   C   RCA

LAD   Left anterior descending coronary artery

C   Circumflex artery

RCA   Right coronary artery

Segments of the left ventricle and their corresponding coronary supply vessels.

Following extensive myocardial infarction with an unfavorable course, the occurrence of left ventricular dilatation with impairment of global contractile function can occur. This is defined as *ischemic cardiomyopathy*. In this case, regional wall motion abnormalities often can no longer be recognized as such. In ischemic cardiomyopathy, one usually finds a left ventricle with diastolically and systolically enlarged dimensions, with reduced contractility of all wall segments and, thus, impaired global function.

14.1   **Detection of Ischemic Myocardium**   **667**
14.1.1   **Wall Motion Abnormality, Wall Thinning,**
         Abnormal Systolic Increase in Wall Thickness

Involvement of the respective papillary muscles of the mitral valve can occur when contractile abnormality of the anteroseptal wall or posterolateral wall exists. This may result in papillary muscle dysfunction and valvular incompetence.

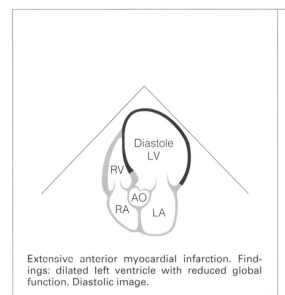

Extensive anterior myocardial infarction. Findings: dilated left ventricle with reduced global function. Diastolic image.

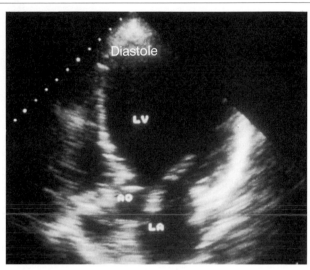

Apical four-chamber 2-D echocardiogram.

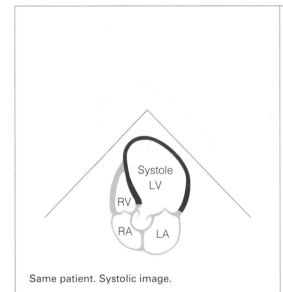

Same patient. Systolic image.

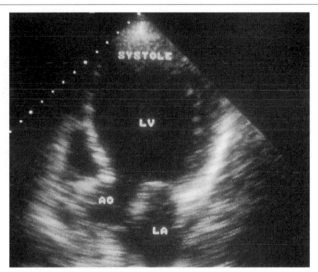

Apical four-chamber 2-D echocardiogram.

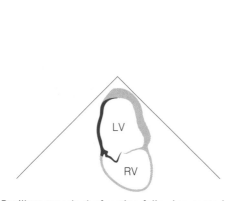

Papillary muscle dysfunction following posterior myocardial infarction. Findings: akinesis of the inferior wall following inferoposterior myocardial infarction; incompetence of the posterior mitral leaflet.

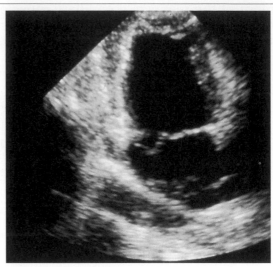

Apical two-chamber 2-D echocardiogram.

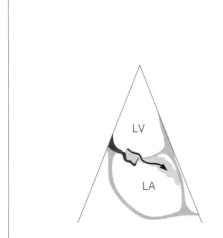

Same patient. Moderate mitral insufficiency.

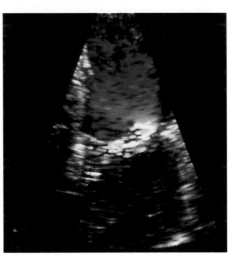

Apical four-chamber 2-D scan with color flow imaging.

Differential diagnosis: These findings must be differentiated from contractile abnormalities that occur in the setting of ventricular conduction disturbance. Left bundle-branch block can lead to uncoordinated septal contraction with decreased systolic inward motion. As compared with hypokinesis or akinesis, contractile abnormalities caused by left bundle-branch block do not affect systolic wall thickening.

Doppler echocardiographic parameters can also be used for assessment of left ventricular function. The appropriate Doppler-derived parameters are flow velocity in the left ventricular outflow tract, mitral inflow measurements, and cardiac output.

14.1   **Detection of Ischemic Myocardium**   **669**
14.1.1   **Wall Motion Abnormality, Wall Thinning,**
            Abnormal Systolic Increase in Wall Thickness

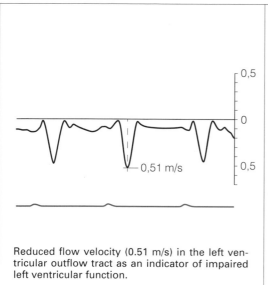

Reduced flow velocity (0.51 m/s) in the left ventricular outflow tract as an indicator of impaired left ventricular function.

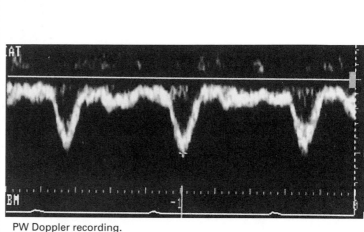

PW Doppler recording.

14.1   **Detection of Ischemic Myocardium**
14.1.2   **Quantitation of Regional and Global LV Function**

Left ventricular function plays an important role in the short and long-term prognosis in patients with acute myocardial infarction. Echocardiographic studies have shown that patients with extensive left ventricular dysfunction experience more complications and have a higher mortality rate [8, 15]. Because echocardiography is noninvasive, it can be used to perform frequent serial follow-up examinations in order to monitor left ventricular function. Thus, high-risk patients can be identified early, treated appropriately, and monitored in serial follow-ups. There are different ways to assess left ventricular function by echocardiography [9, 14].

Visual semiquantitative assessment of the left ventricle makes use of the ability of echocardiography to visualize the left ventricle from multiple scan planes; the results of visual semiquantitative assessment are good [13]. Another proven method for semiquantitation of left ventricular function is the *wall motion score index* recommended by the American Society of Echocardiography [20]. In this 16 segment model, the left ventricle is divided into 16 segments. The walls are divided into apical, medial, and basal segments, as follows:

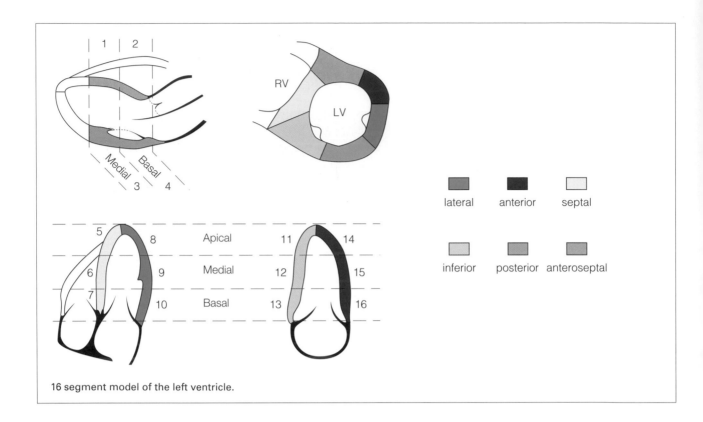

lateral   anterior   septal

inferior   posterior   anteroseptal

16 segment model of the left ventricle.

Visual semiquantitative assessment of contractility is performed, whereby the individual wall motion abnormalities are graded as follows:

1 = Normokinesis
2 = Hypokinesis
3 = Akinesis
4 = Dyskinesis
0 = Assessment not possible

The wall motion score index is calculated by summing the scores determined for all the individual wall segments and dividing this figure by the number of segments studied. Using the wall motion score index (WMSI), patients can be divided into the following four groups:

Group I   WMSI = 1
Group II   WMSI = 1.1 to 1.49
Group III   WMSI = 1.5 to 1.99
Group IV   WMSI = 2

In Group IV patients, mortality within the first year following myocardial infarction is almost 3 times higher than that of patients in Group III, and is 10 times higher than that of patients in Group II [13].

Special computer software is required for *wall motion analysis and quantitation of regional LV function*. A normal range must first be specified before the computer can distinguish between normal and abnormal contraction. Also, images utilized for these studies must be good to excellent quality 2-D echocardiograms of the left ventricular endocardium. Only then can systolic and diastolic contours be properly identified and marked.

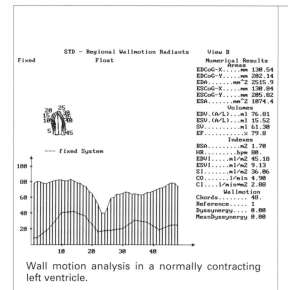

Wall motion analysis in a normally contracting left ventricle.

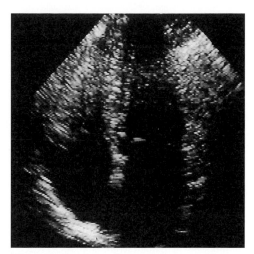

Apical four-chamber 2-D echocardiogram.

Wall motion analyses can be performed according to two different principles. *Consisting systems* are designed to compensate for rotation of the heart during the cardiac cycle. A significant drawback of the consisting system method is that contraction abnormalities that are supposed to be assessed are often „rotated out". *In fixed systems*, no corrective shift is calculated. A direct comparison of these two methods for assessment of contraction abnormality showed that the fixed system yielded superior results [2].

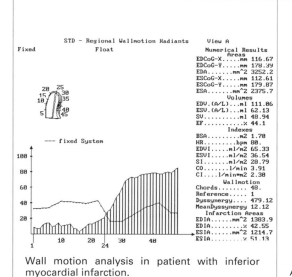

Wall motion analysis in patient with inferior myocardial infarction.

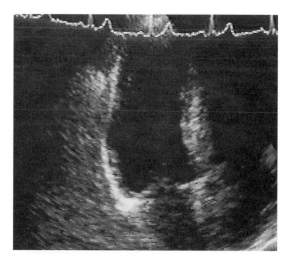

Apical four-chamber 2-D echocardiogram.

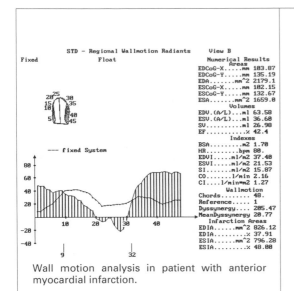

STD – Regional Wallmotion Radiants   View B
Fixed   Float

Numerical Results
Areas
EDCoG-X.....mm 103.87
EDCoG-Y.....mm 135.19
EDA.......mm^2 2179.1
ESCoG-X.....mm 102.15
ESCoG-Y.....mm 132.67
ESA.......mm^2 1659.0
Volumes
EDV.(A/L)...ml 63.58
ESV.(A/L)...ml 36.60
SV.........ml 26.98
EF.........% 42.4
Indexes
BSA........m2 1.70
HR.........bpm 80.
EDVI.....ml/m2 37.40
ESVI.....ml/m2 21.53
SI.......ml/m2 15.87
CO.......l/min 2.16
CI....l/min*m2 1.27
Wallmotion
Chords........ 48.
Reference..... 1
Dyssynergy.... 285.47
MeanDyssynergy 28.77
Infarction Areas
EDIA.....mm^2 826.12
EDIA........% 37.91
ESIA.....mm^2 796.28
ESIA........% 48.00

Wall motion analysis in patient with anterior myocardial infarction.

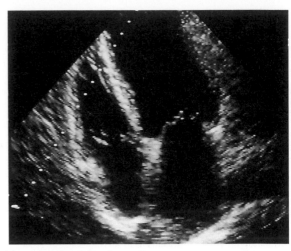

Apical four-chamber 2-D echocardiogram.

Various parameters can be used for assessment of global left ventricular function. M-mode-derived left ventricular end-diastolic and end-systolic dimensions provide an orientational assessment of left ventricular function. Using these dimensions, left ventricular fractional shortening and (with large restrictions) volumes and the ejection fraction can be calculated according to various methods (Teichholz, Gibson, Cube). The mitral leaflet to septum distance is another M-mode parameter that can be measured from the ventricular long and short axes. However, this parameter should be used with caution in patients with left bundle-branch block, concomitant lesions, extremely localized wall motion abnormalities, or right ventricular enlargement [6].

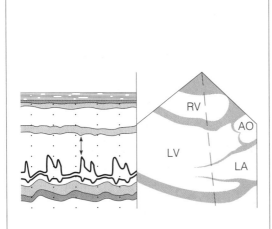

Anteroseptal infarction. Findings: echo-dense, akinetic anteroseptal wall and increased distance between the mitral leaflet and septum.

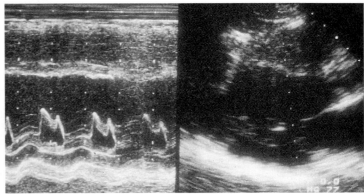

M-mode and 2-D echo, left parasternal long-axis view.

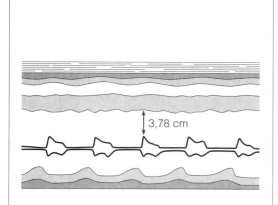

Anteroseptal infarction. Findings: echo-dense, akinetic anteroseptal wall and increased distance between the mitral leaflet and septum.

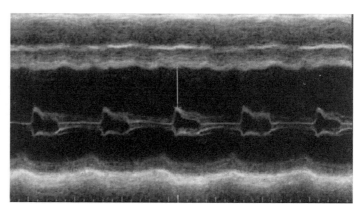

M-mode recording from the left parasternal short-axis view.

There are different ways to calculate left ventricular volume from two-dimensional images. A number of geometric formulas have been proposed, including the area-length method, which is also utilized in angiography [19, 21]. *The Simpson's rule method* appears to be the best. In this method, the systolic and diastolic left ventricular endocardial contours are first identified and marked on the image. Then, a three-dimensional ventricle is reconstructed slice for slice. The value of this method has been demonstrated in many studies for assessment of volume determination.

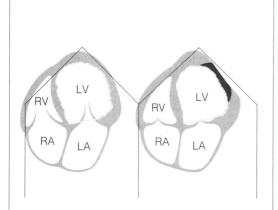

Anterolateral infarction. Diastolic and systolic still frames. In Simpson's method of volume determination, the end-diastolic and end-systolic contours of the left ventricle are marked, and the data is computed with the appropriate software.

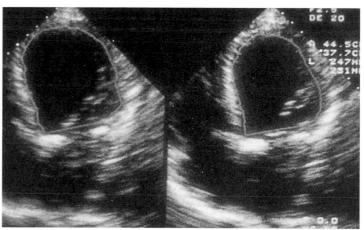

Apical four-chamber echocardiograms.

Using Doppler echocardiographic techniques, flow velocities in the left ventricular outflow tract and cardiac output can be determined. These measurements can then be used to assess left ventricular pump function. The cardiac output is measured by determining the integrals of either the aortic, mitral, tricuspid, or pulmonary flow curve and by also measuring the maximum orifice area in the region of the respective valve ring. The mitral inflow profile can also be used to assess diastolic left ventricular function. However, a discussion of the potential sources of error and limitations of each of these methods goes beyond the scope of this chapter.

1. Amano J, Thomas JX jr, Lavallee M, Mirsky I, Glover D, Manders WT, Randall WC, Vatner SF. Effects of myocardial ischemia on regional function and stiffness in conscious dogs. Am J Physiol 1987; 252: H110-H117.
2. Assmann PE, Slager CJ, van der Borden SG, Sutherland GR, Rˆlandt JR. Reference systems in echocardiographic quantitative wall motion analysis with registration of respiration. J Am Soc Echo 1991; 4 (3): 224-234.
3. Corya BC. Echocardiography in ischemic heart disease. Am J Med 1977; 63 (1): 10-20.
4. Erbel R, Schweizer P, Lambertz H, Henn G, Meyer J, Krebs W, Effert S. Echoventriculography - a simultaneous analysis of two-dimensional echocardiography and cineventriculography. Circulation 1983; 67 (1): 205-215.
5. Feigenbaum H. Coronary artery disease. In: Feigenbaum H (ed). Echocardiography. 4th ed. Lea & Febiger, Philadelphia 1987: 462-513.
6. Feigenbaum H. Echocardiographic examination of the left ventricle. Circulation 1975; 51 (1): 1-7.
7. Fisher DC, Voyles WF, Sikes W, Greene ER. Left ventricular filling patterns during ischemia: an echo-Doppler study in open-chest dogs. J Am Coll Cardiol 1985; 5: 426.
8. Gibson RS, Bishop HL, Stamm RB, Crampton RS, Beller GA, Martin RP. Value of early two-dimensional echocardiography in patients with acute myocardial infarction. Am J Cardiol 1982; 49 (5): 1110-1119.
9. Heng MK, Lang TW, Toshimitsu T, Meerbaum S, Wyatt HL, Lee SS, Davidson R, Corday E. Quantification of myocardial ischemic damage by 2-dimensional echocardiography. Circulation Suppl 1977; 56 (4): III-125.
10. Henry WL. Evaluation of ventricular function using two-dimensional echocardiography. Am J Cardiol 1982; 49: 1319-1323.
11. Kerber RE, Marcus ML, Ehrhardt J, Wilson R, Abboud FM. Correlation between echocardiographically demonstrated segmental dyskinesis and regional myocardial perfusion. Circulation 1975; 52 (6): 1097-1104.
12. Kisslo JA, Robertson D, Gilbert BW, von Ramm O, Behar VS. A comparison of real-time, two-dimensional echocardiography and cineangiography in detecting left ventricular asynergy. Circulation 1977; 55 (1): 134-141.
13. Kruck I, Biamino G. Quantitative Methoden in der M-Mode-, 2D- und Doppler-Echokardiographie. Boehringer Mannheim GmbH, 1988.
14. Meltzer RS, Woythaler JN, Buda AJ, Griffin JC, Harrison WD, Martin RP, Harrison DC, Popp RL. Two-dimensional echocardiographic quantification of infarct size alteration by pharmacologic agents. Am J Cardiol 1979; 44 (2): 257-262.
15. Nishimura RA, Tajik AJ, Shub C, Miller FA jr, Ilstrup DM, Harrison CE. Role of two-dimensional echocardiography in the prediction of in-hospital complications after acute myocardial infarction. J Am Coll Cardiol 1984; 4 (6): 1080-1087.
16. Pandian N, Wang SS, Salem D, Funai J. Ischemic myocardial disease. In: Sutton MSJ, Oldershaw P (eds). Textbook of adult and pediatric echocardiography and Doppler. Blackwell Scientific Publications, Boston 1989; 313-337.
17. Rosoff M, Funai J, Wang SS, Pandian N. Left-ventricular diastolic filling dynamics in acute myocardial-infarction: immediate effects of ischemia, time course in 1st 6 hours and relation to infarct size. J Am Coll Cardiol 1986; 7: A227.
18. Ross J jr, Gallagher KP, Matzusaki M, Lee JD, Guth B, Goldfarb R. Regional myocardial blood flow and function in experimental myocardial ischemia. Can J Cardiol 1986; 1 (suppl A): 9A-18A.
19. Schiller NB, Acquatella H, Ports TA, Drew D, Goerke J, Ringertz H, Silverman NH, Brundage B, Botvinick EH, Boswell R, Carlsson E, Parmley WW. Left ventricular volume from paired biplane two-dimensional echocardiography. Circulation 1979; 60 (3): 547-555.
20. Schiller NB, Shah PM, Crawford M, DeMaria A, Devereux R, Feigenbaum H, Gutgesell H, Reichek N, Sahn D, Silverman AH, Tajik AJ. Recommendations for quantification of the left ventricle by two-dimensional echocardiography. J Am Soc Echocardiography 1989; 2: 358-367.
21. Starling MR, Crawford MH, Sorensen SG, Levi B, Richards KL, O'Rourke RA. Comparative accuracy of apical biplane cross-sectional echocardiography and gated equilibrium radionuclide angiography for estimating left ventricular size and performance. Circulation 1981; 63 (5): 1075-1084.
22. Tennant R, Wiggers CJ. The effect of coronary occlusion on myocardial contraction. Am J Physiol 1935; 112: 351.
23. Wind BE, Dilworth LR, Buda AJ, Snider AR. Doppler evaluation of left ventricular diastolic filling in ischemic heart disease. Am Heart Assoc Monogr 1985; 0 (114): III-59.

The role of ultrasonic tissue characterization in the diagnosis of ischemic heart disease consists in identifying changes in myocardial function and structure by studying the acoustic properties of the myocardium. The goal thereby is to detect ischemia, necrosis, ischemic cardiomyopathy, and collagen deposition, and to differentiate between hibernating myocardium, stunned myocardium, and necrotic tissue.

The starting point of ultrasonic characterization of ischemic and necrotic tissue is the simple observation that calcification and fibrosis cause a uniform increase in echo amplitude [7]. Furthermore, one can study the changes in ultrasonic attenuation in myocardial tissue and attempt to relate them to increased collagen content [4] or changes in fiber architecture [1].

Echocardiographic techniques for characterization of ischemic or necrotic tissue have basically used five different acoustic parameters. They are:

1. *Acoustic impedance*, which is defined as the product of tissue density and the velocity of sound in tissue:
   $Z = qc$; $[Z] = kg\ m^{-3}\ m\ s^{-1} = kg\ m^{-2}\ s^{-1}$.

2. *Backscatter, i.e.* the amount of energy from the originally transmitted signal that returns to the transducer-receiver. Backscatter is a small portion of total scatter. Ideally, backscatter is representative of the total scatter in the target structure.

3. *Texture* – the two-dimensional spatial distribution of the reflection pattern [8].

4. *Attenuation*, which occurs due to scatter and absorption, *i.e.* conversion of some sonic energy as the wave travels through tissue.

5. *Frequency dependence* of backscatter and attenuation.

To points 1 and 4:
As compared to normal myocardium, the impedance of infarcted myocardium is lower due to increased attenuation [4]. However, in the first 24 hours after acute myocardial infarction (early postinfarction phase), attenuation decreases slightly. This may be due to proteolytic processes, increasing cell disintegration, and edema formation [6]. The increase in collagen content occurring in the course of scar tissue development can take up to three months. A continuous increase in attenuation is thereby observed, and attenuation ultimately reaches supranormal values.

To point 2: Characteristic changes in backscatter occur in the cardiac cycle, whereby an end-diastolic peak and an end-systolic trough can be observed. Areas of increased connective tissue density as well as early postischemic states lead to a dampening of this rhythm due to an increase in end-systolic scatter [2]. Upon reperfusion, the recovery of wall motion may not occur immediately (stunned myocardium) [3].

To point 5: In dilated cardiomyopathy, the frequency dependence of backscatter increases from the epicardium to the endocardium, together with a decrease in fiber diameter. In scar tissue with a simultaneous increase in fibrotic components, it decreases from the epicardium to the endocardium [9].

Details and a discussion of involved methodological problems associated with signal properties and of the dependence of the date on instrument settings can be found in Chapter 4.5.

1. Lattanzi F, Di Bello V, Picano E, Caputo MT, Talarico L, Di Muro C, Landini L, Santoro G, Giusti C, Distante A. Circulation 1992; 85: 1828-1834.
2. Lythall DA, Kushawaha SS, Norell MS, Mitchell AG, Ilsley CJD. Changes in myocardial echo amplitude during reversible ischemia in humans. Br Heart J 1992; 67: 368-376.
3. Milunski MR, Mohr GA, Waer KA, Sobel BE, Miller JG, Wickline SA. Early identification with ultrasonic integrated backscatter of viable but stunned myocardium in dogs. J Am Coll Cardiol 1989; 14: 462-471.
4. O'Donnell M, Mimbs JW, Miller JG. The relationship between collagen and ultrasonic attenuation in myocardial tissue. J Acoust Soc Am 1979; 65: 512-517.
5. O'Donnell M, Mimbs JW, Miller JG. The relationship between collagen and ultrasonic backscatter in myocardial tissue. J Acoust Soc Am 1981; 69: 580-588.
6. O'Donnell M, Mimbs JW, Sobel BE, Miller JG. Ultrasonic attenuation in normal and ischemic myocardium. In: Linzer M (ed). Ultrasonic tissue characterization II. National Bureau of Standard, Spec. Publ. No. 525, U.S. Government Printing Office, Washington D.C. 1979.
7. Rasmussen S, Corya BC, Feigenbaum H, Knoebel SB. Detection of myocardial scar tissue by M-mode echocardiography. Circulation 1978; 57: 230-237.
8. Skorton DJ, Miller JG, Wickline SA, Barzilai B, Collins SM, Perez JE. Ultrasonic characterization of cardiovascular tissue: In: Marcus ML, Schelbert HR, Skorton DJ, Wolf G (eds), Braunwald E (consulting ed). Cardiac imaging. WB Saunders, Philadelphia 1990; 538-556.
9. Wong AK, Verdonk ED, Hoffmeister BK, Miller JG, Wickline SA. Detection of unique transmural architecture of human idiopathic cardiomyopathy by ultrasonic tissue characterization. Circulation 1992; 86: 1108-1115.

14.	Ischemic Heart Disease
14.2	Stress Echocardiography
	(Ursula Wilkenshoff)

Stress echocardiography is a method that enables direct visualization of ischemic responses based on the occurrence of a new wall motion abnormality. Manifest coronary disease can usually be identified by wall motion abnormalities in the resting echocardiogram. However, this is not the case in coronary stenosis, which presents clinically as angina pectoris, but cannot at that time have caused myocardial tissue death. Even in extensive coronary artery disease, ventricular function is often completely normal at rest. With the help of different active and passive exercise testing techniques, it is possible to provoke an ischemic response, which then typically leads to wall motion abnormality in the supply area of the stenotic coronary artery.

The use of stress echocardiography for diagnosis and assessment of coronary artery disease is increasing steadily. In many cases, stress echocardiography has been able to establish the diagnosis when other methods were inconclusive or negative [2, 4].

Stress echocardiography should be performed as a supplementary diagnostic technique in patients with symptoms indicative of coronary stenosis, but negative exercise ECG results. Stress echocardiography plays a decisive diagnostic role in functional assessment of coronary stenosis and assessment of multi-vessel disease. Following myocardial infarction, stress echocardiography can also identify viable myocardium that would benefit from angioplasty [1-3, 5, 6, 8]. Stress echocardiography also has a high prognostic value [7].

A detailed description of the pathophysiology of ischemic, and of the methodology and clinical applications of stress echocardiography can be found in Chapter 5.2.

1. Crouse LJ, Harbrecht JJ, Vacek JL, Rosamond TL, Kramer PH. Exercise echocardiography as a screening test for coronary artery disease and correlation with coronary arteriography. Am J Cardiol 1991; 67: 1231-1218.
2. Feigenbaum H. Exercise echocardiography. In: Visser C, Kan G, Meltzer R (eds). Echocardiography in coronary artery disease. Kluver, Bosten 1988; 1-64.
3. McNeill AJ, Fioretti PM, El-Said EM, Salustri A, de Feyter PJ, Roelandt JR. Dobutamine stress echocardiography before and after coronary angioplasty. Am J Cardiol 1992; 69: 740-745.
4. Picano E. Stress Echocardiography, Springer, Berlin/Heidelberg/New York 1992.
5. Pierard LA, de Landsheere CM, Berthe C, Rigo P, Kulbertus HE. Identification of viable myocardium by echocardiography during dobutamine infusion in patients with myocardial infarction after thrombolytic therapy: comparison with positron emission tomography. J Am Coll Cardiol 1990; 15 (5): 1021-1031.
6. Salustri A, Fioretti PM, McNeill AJ, Pozzoli MMA, Roelandt JR. Pharmacological stress echocardiography in the diagnosis of coronary artery disease and myocardial ischemia: a comparison between dobutamine and dipyridamol. Eur Heart J 1992; 13: 1356-1362.
7. Severi S, Michelassi C, Picano E, Lattanzi F, Landi P, L'Abbate A. The prognostic value of dipyridamole-echocardiography, exercise stress electrocardiography and coronary angiography test in previous myocardial infarction. J Am Coll Cardiol 1992; 19 (suppl A): 100A.
8. Wilkenshoff U, Schr^der K, V^ller H, M͵nzberg H, Dissmann R, Spielberg C, Linderer T, Schr^der R. Detection of jeopardized myocardium after acute myocardial infarction with dipyridamole echocardiography stress test. Echocardiography; in press.

14.   **Ischemic Heart Disease**
14.3   **Follow-up and Risk Stratification**
        (Kurt J.G. Schmailzl)

The purpose of following patients with ischemic heart disease is to monitor their symptoms, to evaluate the efficacy of therapy, and to detect new exercise-induced ischemia or intercurrent myocardial infarction and progressive left ventricular dysfunction.

The role of echocardiography includes:

Echocardiographic follow-up of patients with ischemic heart disease
Diagnostic Screening
▸ Serial evaluation of various parameters of ventricular function ▸ Stress echocardiography
Techniques Addressing Special Diagnostic Questions
▸ Myocardial perfusion studies with echo contrast agents ▸ Intracoronary and intracardiac sonography ▸ Doppler catheter studies ▸ Tissue Characterization

Examinations performed in parallel to echocardiography include the patient's history, resting and exercise ECG, exercise scintigraphy, and exercise ergospirometry. Examinations that may be indicated after echocardiography are angiographic ventriculography and coronary angiography.

Additionally, electrophysiological examinations like the determination of late potentials and programmed ventricular stimulation can be performed for the purpose of risk stratification. Such nuclear medicine techniques as scintigraphic reinjection, magnetic resonance spectroscopy, and positron emission tomography can be used to determine the viability of myocardial substrate.

Serial evaluation of ventricular function is designed to assess the efficacy of reperfusion therapy and to evaluate disease progression. When any change in the therapy regimen is made, ventricular function should be reassessed and an exercise test (ECG, scintigraphy, echocardiography) should be performed. In the same vein, serial monitoring of ventricular function also plays a role in therapy planning and risk stratification in patients with ischemic cardiomyopathy.

With the improvements and quicker and wider availability of various reperfusion techniques, it is becoming increasingly important to assess the viability of localized regions of the heart that were affected by ischemia. Upon reperfusion, the recovery of wall motion may not occur immediately. The persistence of impaired contractile function may become chronic (hibernating myocardium), or may be only short-term and temporary (stunned myocardium).

Such echocardiographic techniques as low-dose dobutamine stress echocardiography are based on the concept of contractile reserve. However, no satisfactory quantitation approaches have been supplied, and these techniques suffer from the extensive interpretation of the processed data, the implied hypotheses of which could be a source of error.

In fact, this can be described as a practical problem related primarily to quantitation, clinical application, and cost-benefit relationship. Quantitation would imply exact quantification of regional contractile reserve. The transient improvement in regional contractile function may also be an unspecific response that is further complicated by passive movement that occurs as normal adjacent myocardium pulls the akinetic segment along. Cyclic triaxial heart rotation makes it even more difficult to precisely measure small changes in regional contractile function or to spatially differentiate viable myocardium from necrotic myocardium. Radio frequency signals that have not been subjected to hypothetical models to translate the signals into images of systolic inward motion and wall thickening may hold the more important data. The most clinically significant question is: How severe and how large is the irreversible damage? When the cardiologist must determine the feasibility of reperfusion therapy, analysis of the unmanipulated raw data may hold the key to precisely quantifying where and how much viable myocardium is present.

Echocardiography is an ideal method for detecting complications that occur following acute myocardial infarction. Echocardiography permits identification of high-risk patients and provides important prognostic information.

| 14.4 | Complications of Myocardial Infarction |
| 14.4.1 | Myocardial Rupture |

The development of rupture in infarcted myocardium is a dramatic complication. Myocardial rupture may occur in either the left ventricular free wall or, in rare cases, the right ventricular wall and the region of the interventricular septum; the papillary muscles may also be involved [43]. Approximately 15% of all deaths following myocardial infarction can be attributed to myocardial rupture [46]. When rupture is suspected, the quick establishment of a definitive diagnosis and quick surgical intervention are two factors that play a critical role in the prognosis [29]. In most cases, a bedside diagnosis of myocardial rupture can be made with the help of two-dimensional and Doppler echocardiography.

| 14.4.1 | Myocardial Rupture |
| 14.4.1.1 | Rupture of the left ventricular Free Wall and Pseudoaneurysm |

Rupture of the left ventricular free wall usually runs an acute course with hemopericardium and subsequent pericardial tamponade. When the course is subacute with incomplete rupture and slow leakage of blood into the pericardium, hemopericardium may not develop due to local thrombosis. In this case, a pseudoaneurysm that communicates with the left ventricular cavity develops instead [5, 60]. In most cases, echocardiography can identify the pseudoaneurysm as aneurysmal dilation with a characteristically narrow neck [18, 22]. When considering surgical intervention, it is essential to determine whether the aneurysm is a true aneurysm or false aneurysm; however, this may prove difficult [13, 31].

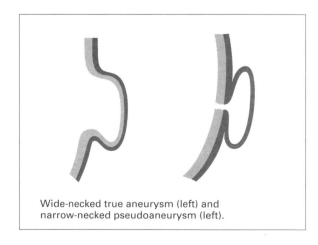

Wide-necked true aneurysm (left) and narrow-necked pseudoaneurysm (left).

Doppler echocardiography can be helpful in this regard [4, 56]. Pseudoaneurysms usually have either low or non-detectable flow velocities due to their narrow portal of entry into the ventricle. True aneurysms, on the other hand, usually have detectable blood flow, which can be demonstrated with conventional Doppler and Doppler color flow imaging. However, flow may be restricted in extensive aneurysms.

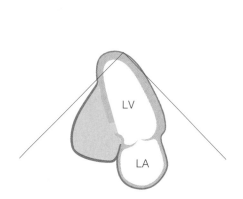

Large pseudoaneurysm that is almost as large as the left ventricle itself is located on the posterolateral wall.

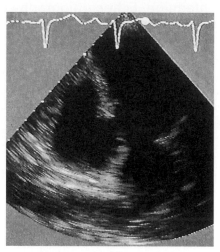

Apical two-chamber 2-D echocardiogram.

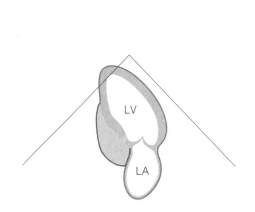

Pseudoaneurysm with typical sickle-shaped configuration due to its narrow neck; extent is restricted by the pericardium.

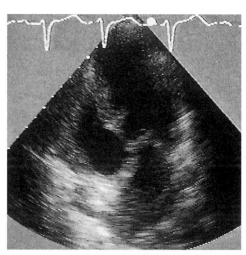

Apical two-chamber 2-D echocardiogram.

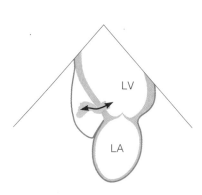

Same patient. Visualization of flow between the left ventricle and pseudoaneurysm. Flow velocity in the pseudoaneurysm is low, and can hardly be visualized on the color Doppler flow map.

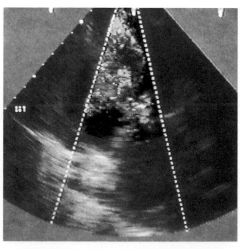

Color flow map of apical two-chamber 2-D echocardiogram.

Ventricular septal rupture is another serious complication of myocardial infarction. In anterior myocardial infarction, the rupture is usually located in the apical septum, whereas the basal septum is more commonly involved in inferior myocardial infarction. As compared to apical septal ruptures, basal septal ruptures have a poorer prognosis [39]. The prognosis is also affected by the size of the defect, the degree of left-to-right shunt, and involvement of the right ventricle [47]. Two-dimensional echocardiography is often able to establish the diagnosis in cases where ventricular septal rupture is suspected due to the new occurrence of a sharp, loud systolic murmur in the left or right parasternal region, or increasing signs of biventricular heart failure within hours to a few days after acute myocardial infarction. Often, the first noted sign of basal septal rupture following inferior myocardial infarction is an aneurysm in the basal septum or in the region of the inferoposterior wall; the muscle is thinned and echo-dense [55]. The findings in apical septal rupture are similar. Since ruptures typically occur at the junction between infarcted necrotic tissue and noninfarcted tissue following infarction expansion [50], one should carefully interrogate the transition zone for defects. Gross, readily visible defects can be visualized on 2-D echocardiograms without any great difficulty [16, 37, 48]; thus, the location and size of the defect can be defined. In some cases, it is helpful to scan from atypical planes when attempting to locate the defect.

Still, many defects cannot be visualized on 2-D echocardiograms, even when images are obtained from atypical scan planes [53]. In this case, intravenous administration of an echo contrast agent may be helpful. However, the presence of a septal defect cannot be excluded by the absence of contrast agent leakage or by the absence of „wash-out" phenomena [19, 64]. When the morphological features of postinfarction ventricular septal rupture cannot be identified by 2-D echocardiography, and when scans performed after the administration of echo contrast agent still are not conclusive, Doppler echocardiography is usually helpful in establishing the diagnosis [8, 12, 38, 42]. Parasternal long and short-axis views and apical two and four-chamber views can be used to measure transseptal flow. The full extent of the septum can be visualized in the four-chamber view, but a large angle is formed between the Doppler beam and the direction of shunt flow; this has negative effects on jet detection and velocity measurements. Scanning from the short-axis view seems to be more advantageous; however, high-seated septal defects are sometimes overlooked from this position [28]. Generally speaking, one should obtain images from all the above-mentioned scan planes, because shunts occurring after ventricular septal rupture often flow in an atypical direction. Color Doppler techniques provide direct visualization of transseptal flow across the septal defect. As compared to other Doppler techniques, this technique is faster and clearer, and should therefore be performed at the beginning of the Doppler examination. Using Doppler color flow imaging, one should interrogate the interventricular septum from the parasternal long and short axes, section by section. In order to detect apical ruptures, the septum must be thoroughly interrogated from the apical two and four-chamber views. The possibility of quantitating the shunt size by measuring the color jet area on a 2-D echocardiogram has been described [52]; however, this technique appears to be limited in the case of ventricular septal ruptures. It is very difficult to measure the color jet in its entirety: following ventricular septal rupture, the course of the jet may be atypical or, in the presence of multiple small defects, the jet may extend diffusely along the septum.

When the blood flow velocity is low, color encoding of shunt flow may need enhancement. In this case, an echo contrast agent can be administered to enhance the signal and to improve visualization of shunt flow [64].

One advantage of using pulsed-wave Doppler is that flow velocities can be measured at a defined site. PW Doppler permits point by point interrogation of the interventricular septum in its entirety for detection of accelerated flow. When the defect is localized, and when the flow velocity exceeds the Nyquist limit, continuous-wave Doppler should then be used. CW Doppler is able to measure high-velocity flow. The Doppler-determined peak flow velocity can be used to estimate the interventricular pressure difference. The extent of left-to-right shunts can be determined by evaluating the aortic to pulmonary flow velocity ratio.

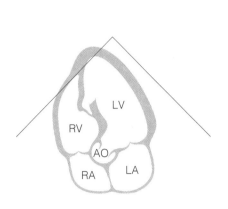

Rupture in the medial septum. A nearly 2 cm long defect was found at the junction of infarcted to intact tissue two days after acute inferior myocardial infarction.

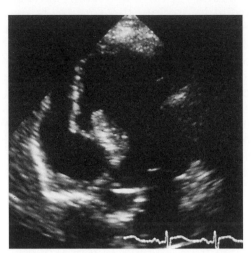

Apical four-chamber 2-D echocardiogram.

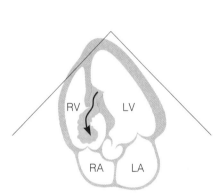

Findings: turbulent transseptal shunt jet from the left to the right ventricle; postinfarction septal rupture with a hemodynamically significant ventricular septal defect.

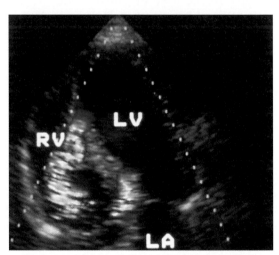

Color flow map of apical four-chamber 2-D echocardiogram.

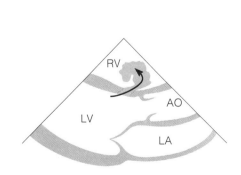

Ventricular septal defect. After administration of echo contrast agent, signal intensity and color-encoding of the shunt are enhanced.

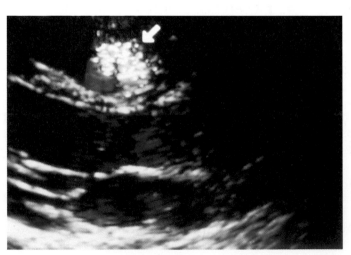

Color flow map of left parasternal long-axis 2-D scan.

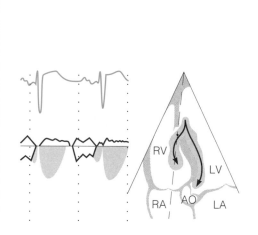

Same patient. Predominantly systolic transseptal, high-velocity flow. Slight amount of flow in diastole.

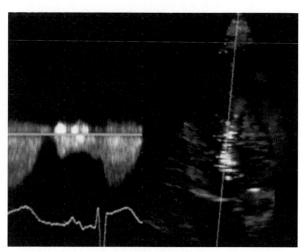

CFMs of CW Doppler recording and apical four-chamber 2-D scan.

14.4   Complications of Myocardial Infarction
14.4.2   Lesions of the Mitral Valve Apparatus

Partial or complete rupture of the papillary muscles or chordae tendineae can occur secondary to acute transmural myocardial infarction. This complication is relatively rare, but is an acute risk for the patient [40]. Complete papillary muscle rupture with sudden massive mitral insufficiency is incompatible with life. Particularly from the transesophageal access, partial papillary muscle ruptures can be identified as structural changes in the mitral valve apparatus; these ruptures cause severe mitral insufficiency, which can be detected using Doppler echocardiography [7, 44]. Different papillary muscles are involved, corresponding to the site of infarction. Involvement of the anterior papillary muscle may be seen in anterolateral myocardial infarction [6, 10]. Rupture of the right papillary muscles, which can lead to massive tricuspid insufficiency, and combined papillary muscle and ventricular septal ruptures, and ruptures of the left ventricular free wall have been described; these ruptures should be taken into consideration when severe complications occur secondary to myocardial infarction [30]. When papillary muscle rupture is suspected due to hemodynamic complications or due to the occurrence of a new systolic murmur, echocardiography can quickly provide an assessment of the morphological and functional status of the valve and valvular apparatus.

In partial papillary muscle rupture or chordal rupture, two freely moving structures are commonly seen; oscillating, prolapsing leaflet motion can also be seen. The M-mode indicator of this situation is „chaotic" motion of the leaflet and valvular apparatus, which can be seen fluttering in the bloodstream. Transesophageal multiplane echocardiography makes it possible to reliably differentiate between papillary muscle and chordal ruptures, and also makes it possible to visualize small lesions.

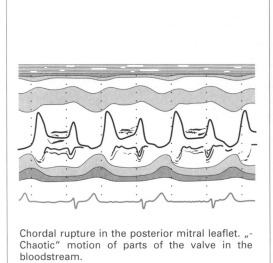

Chordal rupture in the posterior mitral leaflet. „-Chaotic" motion of parts of the valve in the bloodstream.

M-mode recording from the left parasternal long axis view.

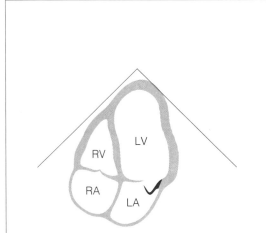

Chordal rupture in the posterior mitral leaflet. Findings: pseudoprolapse with valve echoes in the left atrium in systole.

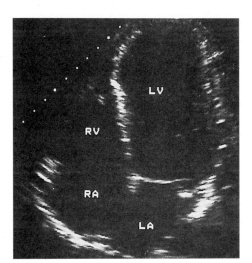

Apical four-chamber 2-D echocardiogram.

Partial rupture of the mitral valve apparatus gives rise to mitral valve incompetence. Commonly, mitral incompetence is so severe that surgical intervention is needed. Frequently, marked contractile abnormality of the involved infarcted wall segment is suggestive of mitral valve involvement. Regional akinesis to dyskinesis with papillary muscle involvement and left ventricular dilatation may result in incomplete mitral valve closure and regurgitation. In most cases, infarction or partial infarction of the papillary muscle does not cause such severe insufficiency as is seen in papillary muscle rupture or in ruptures involving the subvalvular apparatus.

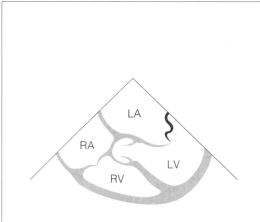

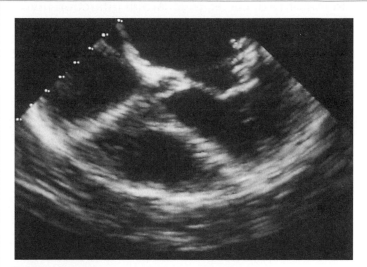

Chordal rupture in posterior mitral valve. Pseudo-prolapse with evidence of valve echoes in the left atrium in systole.

Transesophageal short-axis 2-D echocardiogram.

Mitral insufficiency secondary to papillary muscle dysfunction following myocardial infarction cannot always be clearly differentiated from ventricular septal defect on the basis of the auscultatory findings. However, conventional and color Doppler techniques are highly reliable methods for detecting mitral insufficiency and for differentiating this lesion from ventricular septal defects. Sometimes, especially in septal ruptures proximal to the valve, both lesions may exist and result in complications over the course of disease [15]. Mitral insufficiency can be visualized by both color and CW Doppler and graded according to its severity. Transesophageal echocardiography with color flow mapping of the regurgitant jet provides additional information that is helpful when quantifying mitral insufficiency.

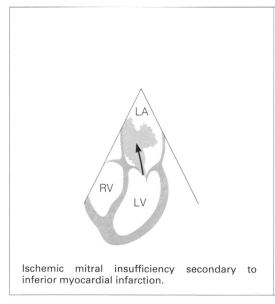

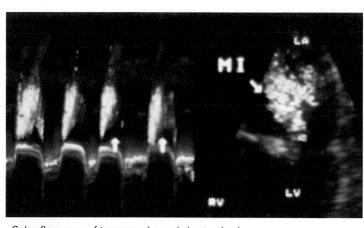

Ischemic mitral insufficiency secondary to inferior myocardial infarction.

Color flow map of transesophageal short-axis view.

In the majority of cases, myocardial infarction involves the left ventricle or the interventricular septum. However, involvement of the right ventricle is found in around one-third of all inferior myocardial infarctions [23, 51]. Because of its low oxygen consumption, isolated right ventricular myocardial infarction is very rare, and is found in only 3 to 5 % of all autopsy-confirmed myocardial infarctions. These cases usually involve patients with chronic bronchopulmonary disease and right ventricular hypertrophy [27], who have an increased right ventricular oxygen demand [20]. Left ventricular infarction can seldom be detected in M-mode recordings obtained from the parasternal long-axis view. This is because the free inferior and lateral walls, which cannot be visualized from this scan plane, are usually involved. Sometimes, the only clue will be enlargement of the right ventricle.

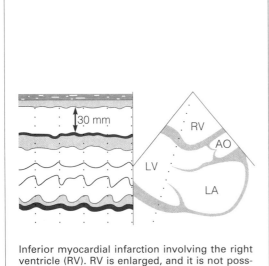

Inferior myocardial infarction involving the right ventricle (RV). RV is enlarged, and it is not possible to define the exact site of infarction.

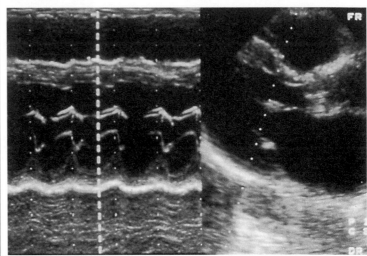

M-mode and 2-D scans, left parasternal long-axis view.

Visualization from the short-axis view, which readily demonstrates the right ventricular free wall, is somewhat better. As a rule, however, scan must be obtained from the apical and subcostal four-chamber views in order to fully establish the diagnosis.

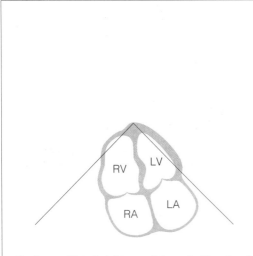

Findings: dilated right ventricle and akinesis of the right ventricular free wall.

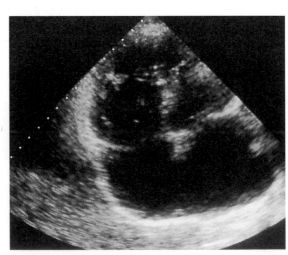

Apical four-chamber 2-D echocardiogram.

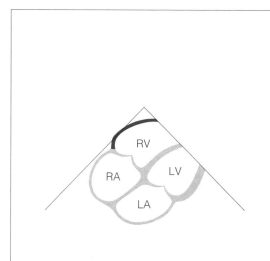

Same patient. In this scan, akinesis of the RV free wall is seen more clearly.

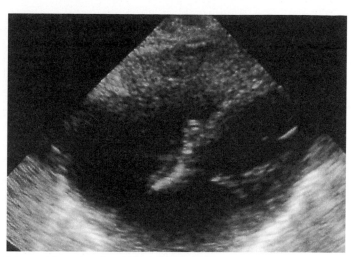

Subcostal four-chamber 2-D echocardiogram.

The diagnosis of right ventricular infarction is of decisive clinical importance and prognostic relevance [62, 65]. When hemodynamic changes suggestive of right ventricular infarction are found (increased right ventricular filling index, normal to slightly elevated end-diastolic left ventricular pressure, diminished heart index) are found [11], echocardiography can be used to establish the diagnosis [35]. Because the right ventricle is affected primarily when inferior myocardial infarction occurs, akinesis of the inferior and sometimes interoposterolateral wall of the left ventricle can be seen in two or four-chamber scans obtained in systole. Dilatation and impaired contractility of the right ventricle are typical findings in subcostal four-chamber echocardiograms [25]. In some cases, segmental contractile abnormality (hypokinesis or akinesis) of the right ventricular free wall is found in addition to global right ventricular dysfunction [2]. Paradoxical motion of the interatrial septum and premature closure of the pulmonary valve can also be observed in some cases [14, 34].

14.4   **Complications of Myocardial Infarction**
14.4.4   **Ventricular Aneurysm**

Left ventricular aneurysm is a complication that commonly occurs secondary to acute myocardial infarction. In ca. 8 to 15 % of all myocardial infarction survivors, an aneurysm develops as a localized, noncontractile, thin-walled dilatation in the region of the infarcted tissue [17]. Whereas the walls of pseudoaneurysms are composed of pericardium and thrombotic material, the aneurysmal wall contains myocardial components that are mainly necrotic and scarred [49]. The aneurysm only passively moves with each contraction. Ventricular aneurysms can become as large as 8 cm in size [1]. Depending on the extent of the aneurysm, a certain portion of the stroke volume travels in and out of the aneurysm [43]. Apical aneurysms and aneurysms of the anterior wall are much more common than aneurysms of the inferoposterior wall [1].

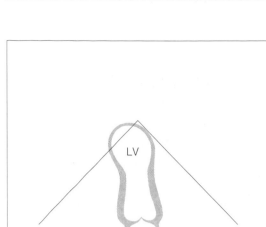

Anteroseptal infarction with small, localized apical aneurysm.

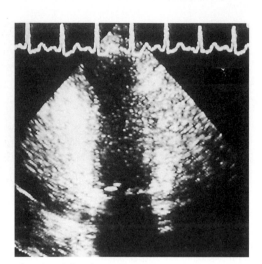

Apical two-chamber 2-D echocardiogram.

Two-dimensional echocardiography is the method of choice for detecting left ventricular aneurysms [63]. The typical changes are found in most cases [35, 59]. The echocardiographic appearance of ventricular aneurysm is that of localized, outward bulging of the ventricular contour, which can usually be clearly delineated from the rest of the intact myocardium.

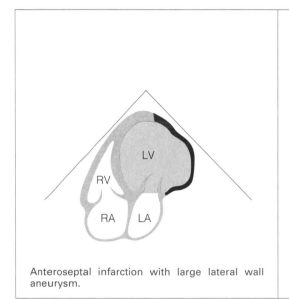

Anteroseptal infarction with large lateral wall aneurysm.

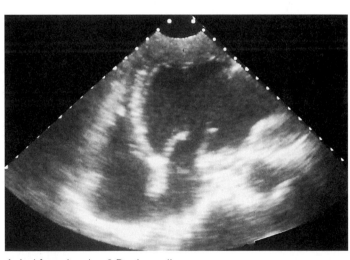

Apical four-chamber 2-D echocardiogram.

The septal walls are relatively thin, and they do not become any thicker during systole. Because of scarring, the wall of the aneurysm is much more echo-dense than the rest of the myocardium.

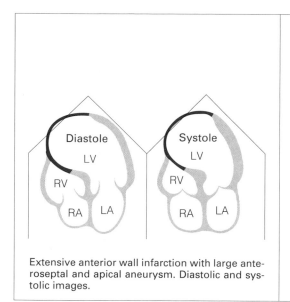

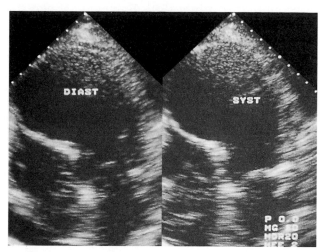

Extensive anterior wall infarction with large anteroseptal and apical aneurysm. Diastolic and systolic images.

Apical four-chamber 2-D echocardiograms.

It is not always easy to differentiate between true and false aneurysms [31], because true aneurysms may also have the narrow neck that is characteristic of pseudoaneurysms. Pseudoaneurysms can become very extensive and, in many case, they may be as large as the left ventricle. True aneurysms, on the other hand, hardly ever become this large. The best planes for assessment are the apical two and four-chamber views and the parasternal long-axis view.

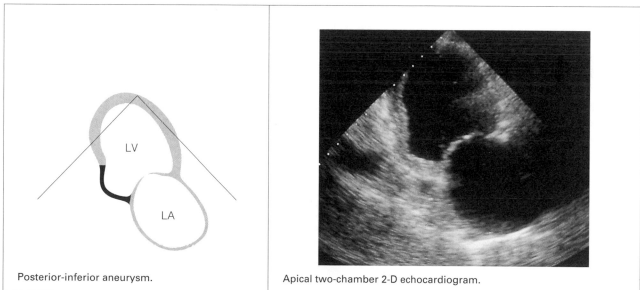

Posterior-inferior aneurysm.

Apical two-chamber 2-D echocardiogram.

A slight amount of turbulence can be visualized in true aneurysms using Doppler color flow imaging. The flow velocity is usually reduced, which makes these lesions predestined for clot formation. In some cases, a mural thrombus may completely line the wall of the aneurysm, which creates the impression that the wall is thicker than it really is. Then, the aneurysmal wall may be mistaken for myocardium. Right ventricular aneurysm, which is very rare, may occur secondary to right ventricular infarction [41].

One of the most common complications of acute myocardial infarction is the development of left ventricular thrombus [58]. Basically, these thrombi can occur in any myocardial infarction, but are more common in patients with extensive infarctions. In accordance with the site of infarction, mural thrombi can be located at various sites in the left ventricle; the most common location is the cardiac apex. Aneurysms or pseudoaneurysms secondary to myocardial infarction are sites of predilection, especially when they affect the anterior septal wall or apex. The incidence of left ventricular thrombus, as confirmed by echocardiography, is reported to be 20 to 40 % [21, 24]. Intraventricular thrombi can usually be visualized well with the help of two-dimensional echocardiography [3]. The texture and shape of thrombi may vary.

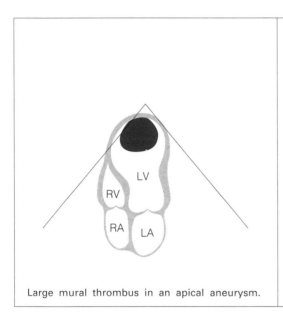

Large mural thrombus in an apical aneurysm.

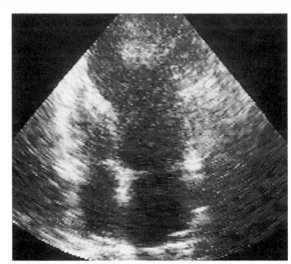

Apical four-chamber 2-D echocardiogram.

The echo texture of clots varies according to their age. New thrombi are more inhomogeneous and faint, and are of low echo intensity. As a clot becomes more organized, its echo density increases, and the clot appears brighter, more compact and more homogeneous on 2-D echocardiograms.

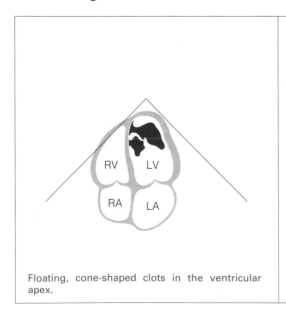

Floating, cone-shaped clots in the ventricular apex.

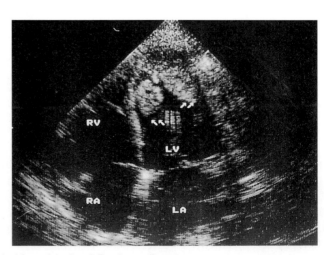

Apical four-chamber 2-D echocardiogram.

Clots come in different shapes and sizes; those that are smaller than 0.5 cm cannot be detected by echocardiography. Mural thrombi line the endocardium like „wallpaper", and are usually more firmly adherent to the wall than free mobile thrombi that extend into the lumen. These thrombi are associated with a risk of systemic embolization [26, 61].

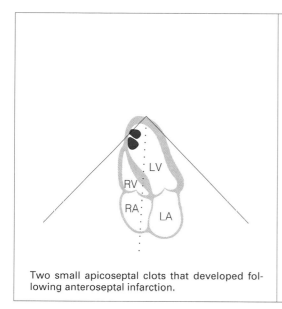

Two small apicoseptal clots that developed following anteroseptal infarction.

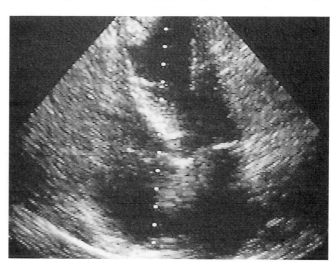

Apical four-chamber 2-D echocardiogram.

Parasternal scan planes are not suitable for visualization of thrombus, and M-mode echocardiography also is not helpful. This is because these techniques do not provide visualization of the decisive segments of the ventricle. Apical scan planes are much better suited for this. However, when scanning conditions are suboptimal, the ventricular apex sometimes cannot be fully visualized, and hypoechogenic apical thrombi may be overlooked. A false-positive diagnosis is often made due to acoustic shadowing and artifacts from the ribs. Extensive trabeculation and prominent papillary muscles occasionally simulate thrombus. A decisive criterion for establishing the diagnosis of thrombus is that the clot must be visualized in two different, preferably perpendicular, scan planes.

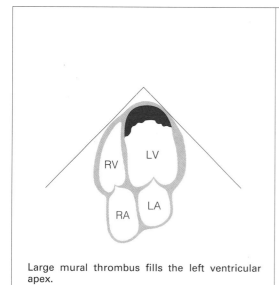

Large mural thrombus fills the left ventricular apex.

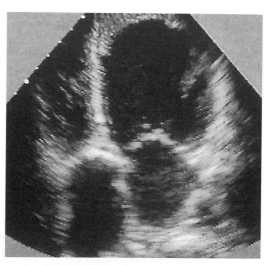

Apical four-chamber 2-D echocardiogram.

When the results are equivocal, multiplane transesophageal echocardiograpy can provide clarity. Anticoagulation therapy should always be considered when the diagnosis of left ventricular thrombus has been established.

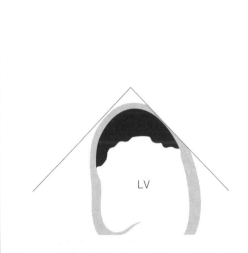

Same patient. In this enlarged image, it is easier to differentiate the thrombus from the heart wall.

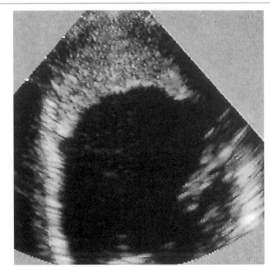

Apical four-chamber 2-D echocardiogram.

14.4   Complications of Myocardial Infarction
14.4.6   Postinfarction Pericarditis

The development of pericardial effusion following acute myocardial infarction is not uncommon. Actually, pericardial effusion is not considered to be a complication, because it usually does not lead to clinically significant problems. Postinfarction pericardial effusions occur in around 17 to 25% of all patients [9, 45], without clinical signs of pericarditis [54]. However, pericarditis with pericardial friction, typical pain symptoms, and typical ECG changes can occur two to four days after the onset of acute myocardial infarction [57]. In these cases, most pericardial effusions are small and are seldom hemodynamically significant. In the setting of Dressler's syndrome, clinically relevant fibrinous pericarditis that may cause complications can develop two to ten weeks after the onset of myocardial infarction [32, 33].

Pericardial effusion is easy to identify by echocardiography. All scan planes can be used for this purpose. In any case, subcostal scans should be used, because even small-sized pericardial effusions anterior to the right ventricle can be visualized from the subcostal view.

A *swinging heart*, characterized by swinging motion of the entire heart, can occur in extensive pericardial effusion. However, because swinging heart is a rare complication of myocardial infarction, the possibility of hemopericardium should also be considered. The width of the effusion should always be measured at end diastole, and should always be measured at the same site in the course of serial follow-up.

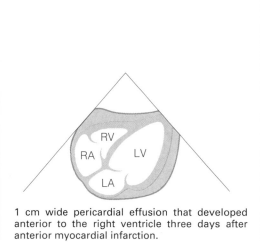

1 cm wide pericardial effusion that developed anterior to the right ventricle three days after anterior myocardial infarction.

Subcostal four-chamber 2-D echocardiogram.

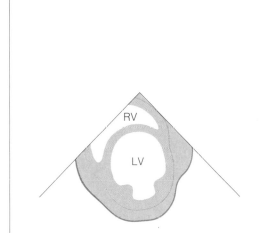

Circular pericardial effusion (1.5 cm wide).

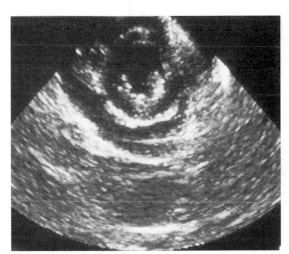

Left parasternal short-axis 2-D echocardiogram.

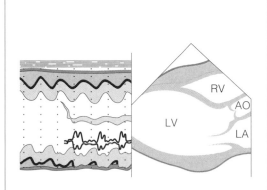

Circular pericardial effusion is found after extensive anterior wall infarction.

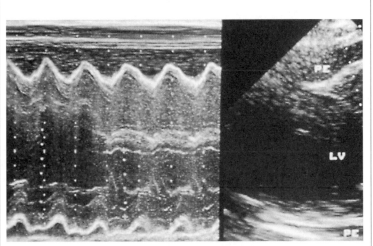

M-mode and 2-D echocardiograms, left parasternal long-axis view.

1. Abrams DL, Edelist A, Luria MH, Miller AJ. Ventricular aneurysm: A reappraisal based on a study of 65 consecutive autopsied cases. Circulation 1963; 27: 164.
2. Arditti A, Lewin RF, Hellman C, Sclarovsky S, Strasberg B, Agmon J. Right ventricular dysfunction in acute inferoposterior myocardial infarction. An echocardiographic and isotopic study. Chest 1985; 87: 307-314.
3. Asinger RW, Mikell FL, Elsperger J, Hodges M. Incidence of left-ventricular thrombosis after acute transmural myocardial infarction. Serial evaluation by two-dimensional echocardiography. N Engl J Med 1981; 305: 297-302.
4. Bach M, Berger M, Hecht SR, Strain JE. Diagnosis of left ventricular pseudoaneurysm using contrast and Doppler echocardiography. Am Heart J 1989; 118: 854-856.
5. Balakumaran K, Verbaan CJ, Essed CE, Nauta J, Bos E, Haalebos MM, Penn O, Simoons ML, Hugenholtz PG. Ventricular free wall rupture: sudden, subacute, slow, sealed and stabilized varieties. Eur Heart J 1984; 5: 282-288.
6. Barbour DJ, Roberts WC. Rupture of a left ventricular papillary muscle during acute myocardial infarction: analysis of 22 necropsy patients. J Am Coll Cardiol 1986; 8: 588-565.
7. Barzilai B, Gessler C jr, Perez JE, Schaab C, Jaffe AS. Significance of Doppler detected mitral regurgitation in acute myocardial infarction. Am J Cardiol 1988; 61: 220-223.
8. Bhatia SJ, Plappert T, Theard MA, Sutton MS. Transseptal Doppler flow velocity profile in aquired ventricular septal defect in acute myocardial infarction. Am J Cardiol 1987; 60: 372-373.
9. Charlap S, Greenberg S, Greengart A, Budzilowicz L, Gelbfish J, Hollander G, Shani J, Lichstein E. Pericardial effusion early in acute myocardial infarction. Clin Cardiol 1989; 12: 252-254.
10. Coma-Canella I, Gamallo C, Onsurbe PM, Jadraque LM. Anatomic findings in acute papillary muscle necrosis. Am Heart J 1989; 118: 1188-1192.
11. Coma-Canella I, Lopez-Sendon J, Gamallo C. Low output syndrome in right ventricular infarction. Am Heart J 1979; 98: 613-620.
12. Come PC. Doppler detection of aquired ventricular septal defect. Am J Cardiol 1985; 55: 586-588.
13. Davies MJ. Ischemic ventricular aneurysms: True or false? Br Heart J 1988; 60: 95-97.
14. Doyle T, Troup PJ, Wann LS. Mid-diastolic opening of the pulmonary valve after right ventricular infarction. J Am Coll Cardiol 1985; 5: 366-368.
15. Eisenberg PR, Barzilai B, Perez JE. Noninvasive detection by Doppler echocardiography of combined ventricular septal rupture and mitral regurgitation in acute myocardial infarction. J Am Coll Cardiol 1984; 4: 617-620.
16. Farcot JC, Boisante L, Rigaud M, Bardet J, Bourdarias JP. Two-dimensional echocardiographic visualization of ventricular anterior rupture after acute septal myocardial infarction. Am J Cardiol 1980; 45: 370-377.
17. Faxon DP, Ryan TJ, Davis KB, McCabe CH, Myers W, Lesperance J, Shaw R, Tong TG. Prognostic significance of angiographically documented left ventricular aneurysm from the Coronary Artery Sugery Study (CASS). Am J Cardiol 1982; 50 (1): 157-164.
18. Feigenbaum H. Echocardiography. In: Braunwald E (ed). Heart Disease. A textbook of cardiovascular medicine. Saunders 1992; 64-115.
19. Foale R. Contrast Echocardiography. In: Sutton MSJ, Oldershaw P (eds). Textbook of adult and pediatric echocardiography and Doppler. Blackwell Scientific Publications, Bosten 1989; 507-520.
20. Forman MB, Wilson BH, Sheller JR, Kopelman HA, Vaughn WK, Virmani R, Friesinger GC. Right ventricular hypertrophy is an important determinat of right ventricular infarction complicating acute inferior left ventricular infarction. J Am Coll Cardiol 1987; 10: 1180-1187.
21. Funke-K̦pper AJ, Verheugt F WA, Peels CH, Galema TW, Roos JP. Left ventricular thrombus incidence and behavior studied by serial two-dimensional echocardiography in acute anterior myocardial infarction: left ventricular wall motion, systemic wall motion, systemic embolism and oral anticoagulation. J Am Coll Cardiol 1989; 13: 1514-1520.
22. Hamilton K, Ellenbogen K, Lowe JE, Kisslo J. Ultrasound diagnosis of pseudoaneurysm and contiguous ventricular septal defect complicating inferior myocardial infarction. J Am Coll Cardiol 1985; 6: 1160-1163.
23. Haupt HM, Hutchins GM, Moore GW. Right ventricular infarction: role of the moderator band artery in determining infarct size. Circulation 1983; 67: 1268-1272.
24. Jugdutt BI, Sivaram CA, Wortman C. Prospective two-dimensional echocardiographic evaluation of left ventricular thrombus and embolism after acute myocardial infarction. J Am Coll Cardiol 1989; 13: 554-564.
25. Jugdutt BI, Sussex BA, Sivaram CA, Rossall RE. Right ventricular infarction: two dimensional echocardiographic evaluation. Am Heart J 1984; 107: 505-518.
26. Keren A, Goldberg S, Gottlieb S, Klein J, Schuger C, Medina A, Tzivoni D, Stern S. Natural history of left ventricular thrombi: their appearance and resolution in the posthospitalization period of acute myocardial infarction. J Am Coll Cardiol 1990; 15: 790-800.

27. Kopelman HA, Forman MB, Wilson BH, Kolodgie FD, Smith RF, Friesinger GC, Virmani R. Right ventricular myocardial infarction in patients with chronic lung disease: possible role of right ventricular hypertrophy. J Am Coll Cardiol 1985; 5: 1302-1307.

28. Kruck I, Biamino G (eds). Quantitative Methoden in der M-mode-, 2D- und Doppler-Echokardiographie. Mannheim 1988; 122.

29. Labovitz AJ et al. Mechanical complications of acute myocardial infarction. Cardiovasc Rev Rep 1984; 5: 948.

30. Lader E, Colvin S, Tunick P. Myocardial infarction complicated by rupture of both ventricular septum and right ventricular papillary muscle. Am J Cardiol 1983; 52: 423-424.

31. Lascault G, Reeves F, Drobinski G. Evidence of the inaccurancy of standard echocardiographic and angiographic criteria used for the recognition of true and „false" left ventricular inferior aneurysms. Br Heart J 1988; 60: 125-127.

32. Lichstein E, Arsura E, Hollander G, Greengart A, Sanders M. Current incidence of postmyocardial infarction (Dressler's) syndrome. Am J Cardiol 1982; 50: 1269-1271.

33. Lichstein E, Liu HM, Gupta P. Pericarditis complicating acute myocardial infarction: incidence of complications and significance of electocardiogram on admission. Am Heart J 1974; 87: 246-252.

34. Lopez-Sendon J, Lopez de Sa E, Roldan I, Fernandez de Soria R, Ramos F, Martin Jadraquel. Inversion of the normal interatrial septum convexity in acute myocardial infarction: Incidence, clinical relevance and prognostic significance. J Am Coll Cardiol 1990; 15: 801-805.

35. Lopez-Sendon J, Garcia-Fernandez MA, Coma-Canella I, Yangueela MM; Banuelos F. Segmental right ventricular function after acute myocardial infarction: two-dimensional echocardiographic study in 63 patients. Am J Cardiol 1983; 51: 390-396.

36. Matsumoto M, Watanabe F, Goto A, Hamano Y, Yasui K, Minamino T, Abe H, Kamada T. Left ventricular aneurysm and the prediction of left ventricular enlargement studied by two-dimensional echocardiography: quantitative assessment of aneurysm size in relation to clinical course. Circulation 1985; 72: 280-286.

37. Mintz GS, Victor MF, Kotler MN, Parry WR, Segal BL. Two-dimensional echocardiographic identification of surgically correctable complications of acute myocardial infarction. Circulation 1981; 64): 91-96.

38. Miyatake K, Okamoto M, Kinoshita N, Park YD, Nagata S, Izumi S, Fusejima K, Sakakibara H, Nimura Y. Doppler echocardiographic features of ventricular septal rupture in myocardial infarction. J Am Coll Cardiol 1985; 5: 182-187.

39. Moore CA, Nygaard TW, Kaiser DL, Cooper AA, Gibson RS. Postinfarction ventricular septal rupture: the importance of location of infarction and right ventricular function in determining survival. Circulation 1986; 74: 45 55.

40. Nishimura RA, Schaff HV, Shub C, Gersh BJ, Edwards WD, Tajik AJ. Papillary muscle rupture complicating acute myocardial infarction: analysis of 17 patients. Am J Cardiol 1983; 51: 373-377.

41. Pandian N, Wang SS, Salem D, Funai J. Ischemic myocardial disease. In: Sutton MSJ, Oldershaw P (eds). Textbook of Adult and Pediatric Echocardiography and Doppler. Blackwell Scientific Publications, Boston 1989; 313-337.

42. Panidis IP, Mintz GS, Goel I, McAllister M, Ross J. Acquired ventricular septal defect after myocardial infarction: detection by combined two-dimensional and Doppler echocardiography. Am Heart J 1986; 111: 427-429.

43. Pasternak RC, Braunwald E, Sobel BE. Acute myocardial infarction. In: Braunwald E (ed). Heart Disease. A textbook of cardiovascular medicine. Saunders, 1992; 1200-1291.

44. Patel AM, Miller FA jr, Khandheria BK, Mullany CJ, Seward JB, Oh JK. Role of transesophageal echocardiography in the diagnosis of papillary muscle rupture secondary to myocardial infarction. Am Heart J 1989; 118: 1330-1333.

45. Pierard LA, Albert A, Henrard L, Lempereur P, Sprynger M, Carlier J, Kulbertus HE. Incidence and significance of pericardial effusion in acute myocardial infarction as determined by two-dimensional echocardiography. J Am Coll Cardiol 1986; 8: 517-520.

46. Pohjola-Sintonen S, Muller JE, Stone PH, Willich SN, Antman EM, Davis VG, Parker CB, Braunwald E. Ventricular septal and free wall rupture complicating acute myocardial infarction: experience in the Multicenter Investigation of Limitation of Infarct Size. Am Heart J 1989; 117: 809-818.

47. Radford MJ, Johnson RA, Daggett WM jr, Fallon JT, Buckley MJ, Gold HK, Leinbach RC. Ventricular septal rupture: a review of clinical and physiologic features and an analysis of survival. Circulation 1981; 64: 545-553.

48. Scanlan JG, Seward JB, Tajik AJ. Visualization of ventricular septal rupture utilizing wide angle two-dimensional echocardiography. Mayo Clin Proc 1979; 54: 381-384.

49. Schlichter J, Hellerstein HK, Katz LN. Aneurysm of the heart: a correlative study of 102 proved cases. Medicine 1954; 33: 43.

50. Schuster EH, Bulkley BH. Expansion of transmural myocardial infarction: a pathophysiologic factor in cardiac rupture. Circulation 1979; 60: 1532-1538.

51. Shah PK, Maddahi J, Berman DS, Pichler M, Swan HJ. Scintigraphically detected predominant right ventricular dysfunction in acute myocardial infarction: clinical and hemodynamic correlates and implications for therapy and prognosis. J Am Coll Cardiol 1985; 6: 1264-1272.

52. Sherman FS, Sahn DJ, Valdez-Cruz LM, Chung KJ, Elias W. Two-dimensional Doppler color flow mapping for detecting atrial and ventricular septal defects. Studies in an animal model and in the clinical setting. Herz 1987; 12: 212-216.

53. Smith G, Endresen K, Sivertssen E, Semb G. Ventricular septal rupture diagnosed by simultaneous cross-sectional echocardiography and Doppler ultrasound. Eur Hear J 1985; 6: 631-636.

54. Somolinos M, Violan S, Sanz R, Marrero P. Early pericarditis after acute myocardial infarction: a clinical echocardiographic study. Crit Care Med 1987; 15: 648-651.

55. Stephens JD, Giles MR, Banim SO. Ruptured postinfarction ventricular septal aneurysm causing chronic congestive cardiac failure. Detection by two-dimensional echocardiography. Br Heart J 1981; 46: 216-219.

56. Sutherland GR, Smyllie JH, Roelandt JR TC. Advantages of colour flow imaging in the diagnosis of left ventricular pseudoaneurysm. Br Heart J 1989; 61: 59-64.

57. Tofler GH, Muller JE, Stone PH, Willich SN, Davis VG, Poole WK, Robertson T, Braunwald E. Pericarditis in acute myocardial infarction: characterization and clinical significance. Am Heart J 1989; 117: 86-92.

58. Visser CA, Kan G, Lie KI, Durrer D. Incidence and one year follow-up of left ventricular thrombus following acute myocardial infarction: an echocardiographic study of 96 patients. J Am Coll Cardiol 1983; 1: 648.

59. Visser CA, Kan G, Meltzer RS, Moulijn AC, David GK, Dunning AJ. Assessment of left ventricular aneurysm resectability by two-dimensional echocardiography. Am J Cardiol 1985; 56: 857-860.

60. Vlodaver Z, Coe JI, Edwards JE. True and false left ventricular aneurysms. Propensity for the altter to rupture. Circulation 1975; 51: 567-572.

61. Weintraub WS, Ba'albaki HA. Decision analysis concerning the application of echocardiography to the diagnosis and treatment of mural thrombi after anterior wall acute myocardial infarction. Am J Cardiol 1989; 64: 708-716.

62. Wellens HJ. Right ventricular infarction. N Engl J Med 1993; 328: 1036-1038.

63. Weyman AE, Peskoe SM, Williams ES, Dillon JC, Feigenbaum H. Detection of left ventricular aneurysms by cross-sectional echocardiography. Circulation 1976; 54: 936-944.

64. Wilkenshoff U, Gast D, Kruck I, Schlief R, Schrˆder R. Contrast-Echo: a comparison of color Doppler, contrast echo and enhanced color Doppler in the detection of cardiac shunts in adults. J Am Coll Cardiol 1990; 15 (suppl A): 195A.

65. Zehender M, Kasper W, Kauder E, Schoenthaler M, Geibel A, Olschewski M, Just H. Right ventricular infarction as an independent predictor of prognosis after acute inferior myocardial infarction. N Engl J Med 1993; 328: 981-988

14.4	**Complications of Myocardial Infarction**
14.4.7	**Remodeling**

Acute myocardial infarction first causes more or less extensive death of functional tissue. Immediately following the acute episode, a number of structural changes occur in the left ventricle. This change or adaptation process in the left ventricle following acute myocardial infarction is defined as *remodeling* [8]. The underlying concept of this is that the left ventricle attempts to compensate for the loss of contractile myocardial tissue by means of various mechanisms.

The extent of remodeling is determined primarily by *infarct expansion* [11]. It was demonstrated that five basic risk factors are associated with infarct expansion. Infarct expansion is more common in first-time infarctions, large infarctions, and transmural infarctions. It occurs almost exclusively following anterior infarction, and occurs when the infarcted vessel remains obstructed [6, 7, 10, 14].

Remodeling occurs in three stages:

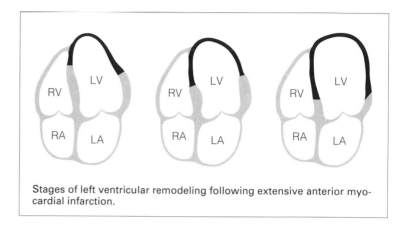

Stages of left ventricular remodeling following extensive anterior myocardial infarction.

In Stage 1, which lasts for hours to a few days after the acute episode, a loss of contractility with thinning and stretching of the infarcted muscle occurs shortly after vessel occlusion. Dilatation of the infarcted area increases steadily. The typical silhouette of the heart is lost. At the beginning of Stage 2, the heart is already globular in shape [17]. Additional, slight infarct expansion occurs in Stage 2, which lasts approximately three weeks, but the primary development is hypertrophy of the remaining contractile muscle. Stage 3 begins three to four weeks after acute myocardial infarction, and is defined as the chronic stage. This stage is characterized by scar tissue formation in the infarcted region and global dilatation of the left ventricle.

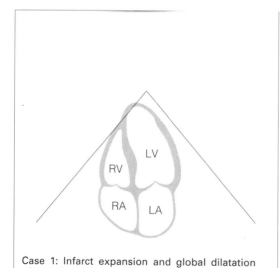

Case 1: Infarct expansion and global dilatation of the left ventricle following anterolateral infarction.

Apical four-chamber 2-D echocardiogram.

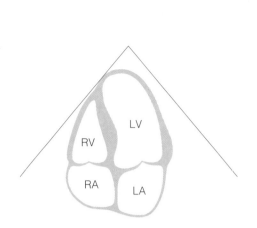

Case 2: Infarct expansion and global dilatation of the left ventricle following anterolateral infarction.

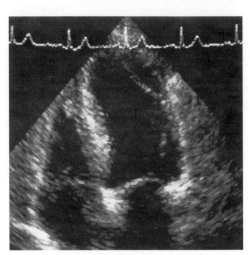

Apical four-chamber 2-D echocardiogram.

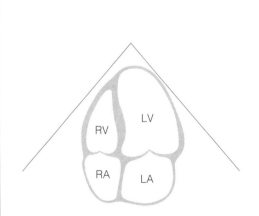

Case 3: Infarct expansion and global dilatation of the left ventricle following anterolateral infarction.

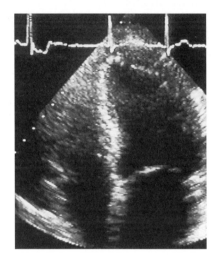

Apical four-chamber 2-D echocardiogram.

In the past few years, the efforts of many work groups have been centered around the avoidance of infarct expansion. The site of infarction is a risk factor that cannot be influenced. However, other risk factors can be influenced to some degree. For example, it has been shown that the infarction expands less often in patients with patent infarcted vessels or well developed collateral circulation. Furthermore, these patients have a lower incidence of left ventricular dilatation and infarction complications, and their overall prognosis is better [1-3]. Large studies have demonstrated the value of early reperfusion (in up to six hours) in the form of systemic thrombolysis [5, 15, 16].

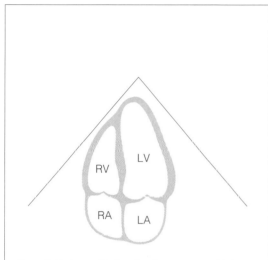

Case 1: Patient with localized anteroseptal infarction: no remodeling.

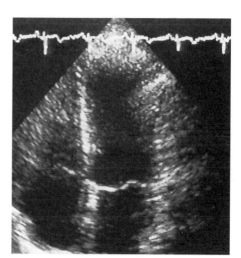

Apical four-chamber 2-D echocardiogram.

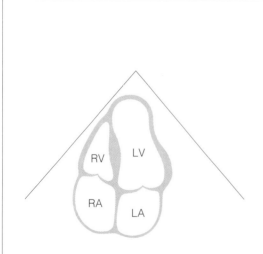

Case 2: Patient with localized anteroseptal infarction: no remodeling.

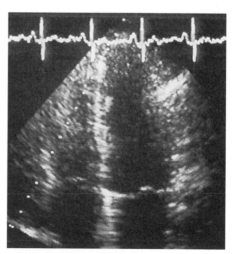

Apical four-chamber 2-D echocardiogram.

Later reperfusion is also reported to be of value [13].

Another fundamental approach is medical therapy to prevent progressive ventricular dilatation. The course of myocardial infarction was favorably influenced by ACE inhibitors [9, 12]. Similar results were obtained with intravenous nitroglycerin [4].

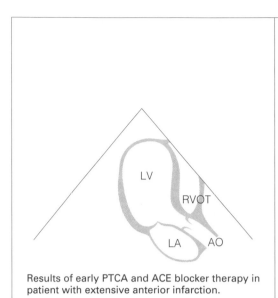

Results of early PTCA and ACE blocker therapy in patient with extensive anterior infarction.

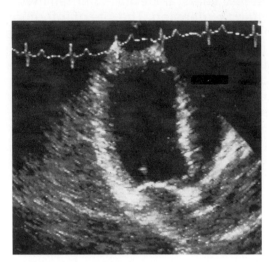

Apical two-chamber 2-D echocardiogram.

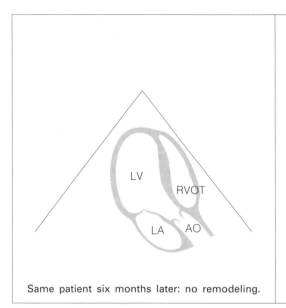

Same patient six months later: no remodeling.

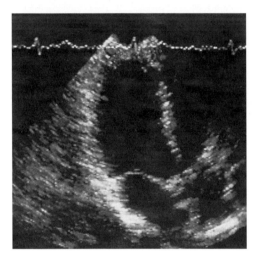

Apical two-chamber 2-D echocardiogram.

References

1. Braunwald E. Myocardial reperfusion, limitation of infarct size, reduction of left ventricular dysfunction, and improved survival. Should the paradigm be expanded? Circulation 1989; 79: 441-444.
2. Hirai T, Fujita M, Nakajima H, Asanoi H, Yamanishi K, Ohno A, Sasayama S. Importance of collateral circulation for prevention of left ventricular aneurysm formation in acute myocardial infarction. Circulation 1989; 79: 791-796.
3. Jeremy RW, Hackworthy RA, Bautovich G, Hutton BF, Harris PJ. Infarct artery perfusion and changes in left ventricular volume in the month after acute myocardial infarction. J Am Coll Cardiol 1987; 9: 989-995.
4. Jugdutt BI, Warnica JW. Intravenous nitroglycerin therapy to limit myocardial infarct size, expansion, and complications. Effect of timing, dosage, and infarct location. Circulation 1988; 78: 906-919.

5. Marino P, Zanolla L, Zardini P. Effect of streptokinase on left ventricular modeling and function after myocardial infarction: The GISSI (Gruppo Italiano per lo Studio della Streptochinasi nell'Infarto Miocardico) Trial. J Am Coll Cardiol 1989; 14: 1149-1158.

6. Meizlish JL, Berger HJ, Plankey M, Errico D, Levy W, Zaret BL. Functional left ventricular aneurysm formation after acute anterior transmural myocardial infarction: Incidence, natural history, and prognostic implications. N Engl J Med 1984; 311: 1001-1006.

7. Mitchell GF, Lamas GA, Vaughan DE, Pfeffer MA. Left ventricular remodeling in the year following first anterior myocardial infarction: a quantitative analysis of contractile segment lengths and ventricular shape. J Am Coll Cardiol 1992; 19: 1136-1144.

8. Mitchell GF, Pfeffer MA. Left ventricular remodeling after myocardial infarction: Progression toward heart failure. Heart Failure 1992; 4: 55-69.

9. Pfeffer JM, Pfeffer MA, Braunwald E. Influence of chronic captopril therapy on the infarcted left ventricle of the rat. Circ Res 1985; 57: 84-95.

10. Picard MH, Wilkins GT, Gillam LD, Thomas JD, Weymann AE. Immediate regional endocardial surface expansion following coronary occlusion in the canine left ventricle: disproportionate effects of anterior versus inferior ischemia. Am Heart J 1991; 121: 753-762.

11. Pirolo JS, Hutchins GM, Moore GW. Infarct expansion: pathologic analysis of 204 patients with a single myocardial infarct. J Am Coll Cardiol 1986; 7: 349-354.

12. Raya TE, Gay RG, Aguirre M, Goldman S. Importance of venodilatation in prevention of left ventricular dilatation after chronic large myocardial infarction in rats: a comparison of captopril and hydralazine. Circ Res 1989; 64: 330-337.

13. Schröder R, Neuhaus KL, Linderer T, Brueggemann T, Tebbe U, Wegscheider K. Impact of late coronary artery reperfusion on left ventricular function one month after acute myocardial infarction: results from the ISAM study. Am J Cardiol 1989; 64: 878-884.

14. Schuster EH, Bulkley BH. Expansion of transmural myocardial infarction: a pathophysiologic factor in cardiac rupture. Circulation 1979; 60: 1532-1538.

15. Sheehan FH, Braunwald E, Canner P, Dodge HT, Gore J, van Natta P, Passamani ER, Williams DO, Zaret B. The effect of intravenous thrombolytic therapy on left ventricular function: a report on tissue-type plasminogen activator and streptokinase from the Thrombolysis in Myocardial Infarction (TIMI Phase I) Trial. Circulation 1987; 75: 817-829.

16. Touchstone DA, Beller GA, Nygaard TW, Tedesco C, Kaul S. Effects of successful intravenous reperfusion therapy on regional myocardial function and geometry in humans: a tomographic assessment using two-dimensional echocardiography. J Am Coll Cardiol 1989; 13: 1506-1513.

17. Weisman HF, Bush DE, Mannisi JA, Bulkley BH. Global cardiac remodeling after acute myocardial infarction: a study in a rat model. J Am Coll Cardiol 1985; 5: 1355-1362

14.5 **Echocardiography of Coronary Arteries**
14.5.1 **Transesophageal Assessment of Coronary Arteries and of Coronary Artery Perfusion**
(C. Memmola, V.F. Napoli, M. Ayuso, K. Valsamis, S. Iliceto, P. Rizzon)

Our knowledge of the anatomy and hemodynamics of coronary circulation is owed primarily to the performance of invasive diagnostic examinations like cardiac catheterization and digitalized angiography [3]. However, the feasibility and repeatability of these techniques have obvious limitations. Therefore, the interest in non-invasive methods such as those involving radioisotopes and echocardiography is increasing.

Over the past 20 years, echocardiography has proved to be useful, particularly in identifying and evaluating the proximal tract of the left coronary [8, 9], even though potential applications are limited by the fact that the quality of obtainable images is frequently insufficient. The favorable transducer position used in transesophageal echocardiography makes it possible to achieve high- resolution images of cardiac structures; the Doppler signal can be recorded from the heart cavities and from the large vessels. Hence, this technique has prospects of becoming a useful approach for studying the hemodynamic characteristics of coronary circulation.

Visualization of the coronary arteries and identification of coronary stenosis

During a transesophageal echocardiography examination, the coronary arteries can be visualized through both horizontal and longitudinal scans. The appropriate views are obtained by positioning the transducer immediately above the aortic valvular plane. The left coronary originates from the left coronary sinus, and the left main coronary artery (LM) is perpendicular to the aorta, which bifurcates after a few millimeters into the circumflex artery (C) and into the left anterior descending artery (LAD). The C continues from the LM and runs for a few centimeters below the left atrial appendage; on the other hand, the LAD runs downwards and becomes medially parallel to the ultrasound beam.

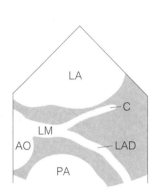

Scan showing the distal left main coronary artery (LM) and its bifurcation. The circumflex artery (C) is located below the left atrial appendage and appears continuously with the LM.

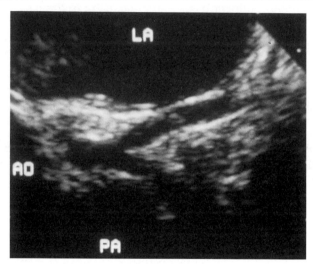

Transesophageal short-axis 2-D echocardiogram.

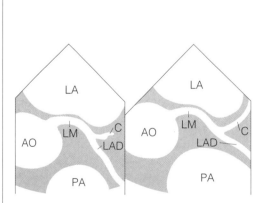

View of proximal left coronary arteries visualizing, on different tomographic levels, the left anterior descending artery (left panels) and the circumflex artery (right panels).

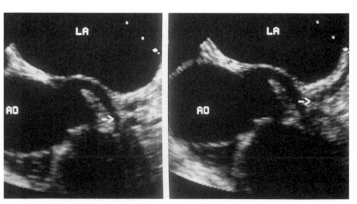

Transesophageal short-axis 2-D echocardiograms.

14.5   Echocardiography of Coronary Arteries
**14.5.1 Transesophageal Assessment of Coronary Arteries and of
         Coronary Artery Perfusion**

703

The right coronary artery and its ostium can be visualized in the same projection by rotating the transducer slightly to the right at a slightly different tomographic level from that of the left coronary artery.

A longitudinal view through the origin of the left coronary artery can be obtained with a biplane transducer by scanning in a projection that images the long axis of the outflow tract of the right ventricle, where the artery appears as a vessel running parallel to the pulmonary artery.

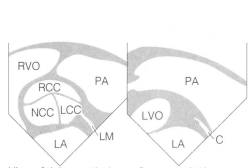
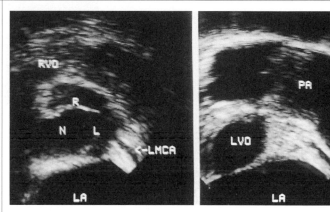

View of right ventricular outflow tract (RVO) showing the origin of the left main coronary artery (LM) (left panels). The circumflex artery (C), which lies parallel to the pulmonary artery (PA), is seen in the right panels. LVO = left ventricular outflow.

Transesophageal long-axis 2-D echocardiograms.

In a recent study [6], we evaluated the capability of this technique to identify proximal stenoses of the left coronary artery by subjecting 160 consecutive patients to transesophageal echocardiography before performing diagnostic angiography. The coronary segments under examination (LM, proximal LAD, proximal C) were assessed as follows:

- *patent* if hyper-reflecting calcific plaques were absent or non-stenosing;
- *stenotic* if hyper-reflecting plaques were present, and/or when non-calcific narrowing of the lumen reduced vessel caliber by at least 50%.

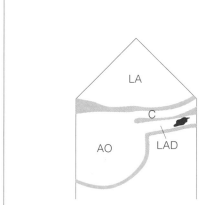
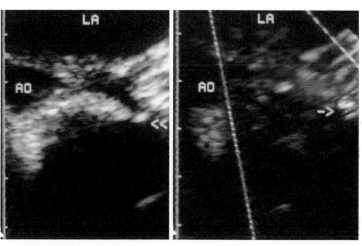

View of plaque and proximal stenosis of the LAD. A calcific plaque narrowing the lumen is seen in the left panel. Doppler color flow imaging detected a small „variance area" indicating turbulent prestenotic flow (arrow).

Transesophageal short-axis view. Color-encoded.

14.5   **Echocardiography of Coronary Arteries**
14.5.1   **Transesophageal Assessment of Coronary Arteries and of Coronary Artery Perfusion**

704

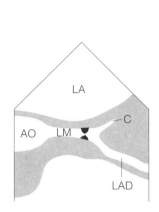

Identification of proximal LAD stenosis. Hyper-reflecting plaque severely narrows the vessel (left panel). Turbulent flow in the proximity of the stenosis is detected via Doppler color flow mapping.

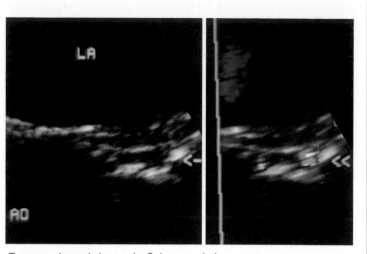

Transesophageal short-axis. Color-encoded.

The results of echocardiography and angiocardiography were compared using analogous diagnostic criteria.

Accuracy of transesophageal echocardiography in detecting proximal coronary stenosis.

	Transesophageal echocardiography					
	LM		LAD		C	
	pat	*sten*	*pat*	*sten*	*pat*	*sten*
ANGIOGRAPHY						
Patent	103	2	43	5	73	14
Stenotic	0	6	13	50	11	13
Sensitivity	100 %		79 %		54 %	
Specificity	98 %		89 %		84 %	

LM	Left main coronary artery
LAD	Left anterior descending artery
C	Circumflex artery
pat	Patent
sten	Stenotic

14.5   **Echocardiography of Coronary Arteries**   **705**
14.5.1   **Transesophageal Assessment of Coronary Arteries and of**
                Coronary Artery Perfusion

The percentage of segments that could be visualized was higher in the LM (94%) and C (82%) than in the LAD (78%). In 111 out of 160 patients (70%), all of the explored segments were visible during transesophageal echocardiography. The sensitivity and specificity of transesophageal echocardiography in this group of patients was 100% and 98% for the LM, 79% and 89% for the LAD, and 54% and 84% for the C, respectively.

The greatest feasibility problems are related to the nonuniform tomographic position of different vessels with respect to the ultrasound beam, which gives better resolution of the walls to the LM and C and poor lateral resolution to the LAD. With regard to accuracy, it is often difficult to identify eccentric or non-calcific stenoses of the vessel and false reduction of the lumen due to non-stenosing calcific plaques. Both factors can lead to false negative findings. Despite these limitations, transesophageal echocardiography makes it possible to non-invasively explore the LM of the left coronary artery and its proximal branches in the majority of patients.

In a subsequent study [7], we attempted to improve the diagnostic accuracy of transesophageal echocardiography in identifying proximal stenoses of the LAD by means of Doppler color flow mapping. Turbulent flow through a stenotic portion of the vessel that caused disorganization of surrounding laminar flow was thereby adopted as an additional diagnostic criterion.

Combined use of the two diagnostic criteria (positive two-dimensional transesophageal echocardiography and/or positive Doppler color flow mapping) significantly increased the sensitivity of the technique (94%) without causing any significant reduction in specificity (88%). In the study, color Doppler mapping of coronary flow was consistently performed in the LAD only. Only infrequently were the LM or C mapped, due to the wide angle formed between these vessels and the exploring ultrasound beam.

Characteristics of Coronary Flow and Coronary Reserve

The diagnostic and pathophysiological potentials of transesophageal echocardiography in evaluating the coronary circulation seem to be especially dependent on the possibility of correctly measuring by Doppler the coronary flow velocity in 80% of all cases. Using Doppler color flow mapping as an optical guide, it is possible to position the sample volume in the proximal tract of the LAD. Because of its favorable position parallel to the direction of the ultrasound beam, the LAD can easily be explored via this technique. The recorded velocity pattern is biphasic and is made up of two anterograde components: a greater diastolic one and a smaller systolic one.

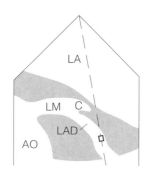

Coronary blood flow velocity. The sample volume was placed in the proximal LAD with the help of color flow mapping (left panel). A biphasic pattern with a small systolic component and a larger diastolic component was observed in normal subjects (right panel).

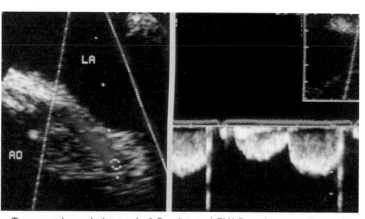

Transesophageal short-axis 2-D echo and PW Doppler recording, with color flow mapping.

14.5   Echocardiography of Coronary Arteries
**14.5.1   Transesophageal Assessment of Coronary Arteries and of
           Coronary Artery Perfusion**

706

The ratio of the diastolic and systolic components as well as their morphology and direction can be modified by different pathological conditions, which thereby create a characteristic velocity pattern. In agreement with our pathological knowledge, coronary flow was more markedly altered in patients with conditions that obstruct the left ventricular outflow tract (*e.g.*, aortic stenosis and hypertrophic obstructive cardiomyopathy).

We compared the coronary flow velocity pattern in 10 patients with hypertrophic obstructive cardiomyopathy with that of 10 normal subjects [4]. The coronary flow pattern revealed in transesophageal echocardiography was characterized by a reduced systolic component that was sometimes retrograde and a larger than normal diastolic component. Consequently, the diastolic/systolic flow ratio was wider than that of the control group, even in baseline conditions. Moreover, the diastolic component, which showed a tendency to decelerate, was significantly slower than normal. This was presumably due to the increased diastolic stiffness of the hypertrophic ventricle.

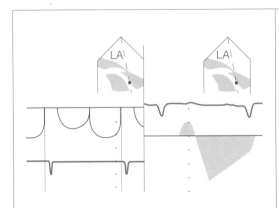

Coronary blood flow velocity characteristics in hypertrophic obstructive cardiomyopathy. The systolic component is small and often shows flow reversal. The diastolic component is larger than normal (left panel) and shows a low deceleration rate due to reduced diastolic compliance of the left ventricle (right panel).

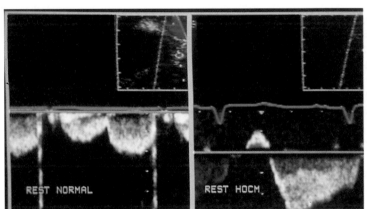

PW Doppler recordings from TEE short-axis 2-D scans.

These observations show the strict dependency of coronary flow on its diastolic value in patients with obstructive hypertrophic heart disease. Furthermore, it demonstrates the potentials of transesophageal echocardiography in studying the characteristics of coronary flow.

Transesophageal echocardiography can also be applied to measure rapid variations in coronary flow velocity. Such variations can be induced by administering coronary drugs such as nitrate and dipyridamole. Particularly during infusion of dipyridamole (D), both components of the velocity pattern increase considerably in normal subjects without significantly modifying the caliber of epicardial vessels. Such velocity variation in absence of epicardial vessel size change can be considered an expression of a real increase in coronary flow within a wide range of variations of the same, as recent studies have demonstrated [10]. The technique therefore can be used to evaluate the coronary reserve, which is obtained as a ratio of hyperemic diastolic velocity (after administration of dipyridamole) to the baseline diastolic velocity of coronary flow, analogous to the procedure applied in the intracoronary Doppler catheterizat-ion [10].

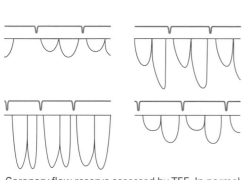

Coronary flow reserve assessed by TEE. In normal subjects (upper left), both the systolic and diastolic components of coronary flow velocity increase significantly 2 min after dipyridamole (D) infusion (upper right). The increases amount to at least three times the baseline values 4 min. after D (lower left). Velocity returns to rest values after administration of aminophylline (lower right).

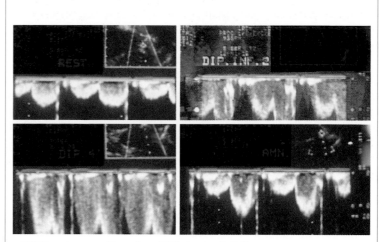

PW Doppler recordings from TEE short-axis 2-D scans.

A validation study of the method was performed on six patients with isolated, severe stenosis of the left anterior descending artery ($\geq$ 75% narrowing) [2]. The coronary flow reserve measured in these patients was significantly lower than that obtained in nine normal subjects.

Transesophageal Doppler measurement of coronary flow reserve

	B-MDV	B-MSV	D-MDV	D-MSV	CFR
N	35 ± 11	104 ± 21*	24 ± 7	48 ± 7*	3,2 ± 0,9
ST	54 ± 14	76 ± 20°	29 ± 10	40 ± 19	1,4 ± 0,4°

*   p < 0.01 (B vs. D)
°   p < 0.01 (N vs. ST)

B-MDV, D-MDV	Maximal diastolic velocity in baseline conditions (B) and after dipyridamole (D)
B-MSV, D-MSV	Maximum systolic velocity in baseline conditions (B) and after dipyridamole
CFR	Coronary flow reserve
N	Normal subjects
ST	Patients with proximal stenosis of the LAD coronary artery

This new method has the undoubted advantage of being only slightly invasive and therefore can easily be repeated in the same patient. However, due to scanning geometry, this evaluation can be made virtually only by Doppler mapping of the left anterior descending artery and is therefore limited in the evaluation of regional pathologies such as the one under consideration. The study of coronary flow reserve was therefore extended to those forms of myocardial ischemia that occur in the presence normal epicardial arteries (*e.g.*, small vessel disease).

A study with an analogous protocol was performed in 5 patients with Syndrome X, 8 patients with hypertrophic obstructive cardiomyopathy, and 9 patients with dilated cardiomyopathy. Our study [5] has pin-pointed a similarly significant reduction in the coronary flow reserve in these groups of patients, which somehow seems to be connected with different pathophysiological mechanisms.

Coronary flow reserve assessment in microvascular angina				
	N	XS	DC	HOCM
B-MDV	35 ± 11	44 ± 9	46 ± 17	51 ± 7*
D-MDV	104 ± 21	67 ± 4*	75 ± 24*	114 ± 2
CFR	3.2 ± 0,9	1.6 ± 0.3*	1,7 ± 0.5*	2.2 ± 0.5*
* p < 0.01 (vs. N)				

B-MDV, D-MDV   maximum diastolic velocity in baseline conditions (B) and after dipyridamole (D)
CFR   coronary flow reserve
N   normals
XS   syndrome X
DC   dilated cardiomyopathy
HOCM   hypertrophic obstructive cardiomyopathy

- In XS and DC, the coronary flow reserve appears to be reduced because of the presence of low hyperemic velocity. These subjects show normal baseline flow, indicating that there is impaired vasodilation in the microcirculatory bed (increased vasomotor tone of pre-arteriolar vessels).

- In hypertrophic obstructive cardiomyopathy, on the other hand, the higher velocity of baseline flow is responsible for a reduced increased in velocity after vasodilation, which occurs in the presence of normal hyperemic values.

On the whole, it is evident that this technique can be useful in the diagnosis and follow-up microvascular insufficiency and in the study of its pathophysiological mechanisms.

Limitations and Technological Prospects

This non-invasive technique undoubtedly has interesting prospects, but is limited by the fact that only a reduced extent of the coronary area can be explored by means of 2-dimensional scanning. Complete Doppler flow mapping of these vessels is therefore limited. However, recent technological advances promise to overcome some of these intrinsic limitations, thereby giving the technique more extensive and useful applications. In particular, utilization of the new multiplane transducer may make it possible to scan a greater number of tomographic planes in cardiac structures.

Moreover, the use of new echocontrastography agents capable of traversing the pulmonary circulation may be able to strengthen of the Doppler signal in sections of the left heart and in systemic vessels. We therefore tested the efficiency of one echocontrastography substance (SHU-508-A, Schering AG).

After injecting it into a peripheral vein, we verified its effectiveness in improving Doppler cardiac signals [1]. Furthermore, SHU-508-A made it possible to highlight and study longer sections of the LAD, and it provided virtually constant visualization of the C and LM. This, in turn, enabled us to visualize areas of turbulent flow located in more distal positions.

Conclusions

Despite its above-mentioned limitations, transesophageal echocardiographic assessment is of interest in diagnostic and pathophysiological studies of the coronary arteries.

- Transesophageal echocardiography can detect proximal narrowing of coronary sections;
- It can verify the hemodynamic efficiency of coronary active drugs;
- It is useful in the diagnosis and follow-up of various forms of microvascular angina and in the verification of the pathogenetic mechanisms of this condition; and
- It is useful in the study of different pathophysiological aspects of coronary hemodynamics.

References

1. Caiati C, Schlief R, Aragona P, Memmola C, Sublimi Saponetti L, Iliceto S, Rizzon P. Enhanced PW and color doppler signal intensity in the left coronary artery after intravenous SHU-508-A injection. A transesophageal echo doppler study. Eur Heart J 1991; 12: (suppl) 161.
2. Iliceto S, Marangelli V, Memmola C, Rizzon P. Transesophageal Doppler echocardiography evaluation of coronary blood flow velocity in baseline conditions and during dipyridamole-induced vasodilation. Circulation 1991; 83: 61-69.
3. Marcus ML, Wilson RF, White CW. Methods of measurement of myocardial blood flow in patients: a critical review. Circulation 1987; 76: 245-253.
4. Memmola C, Iliceto S, Carella L, Napoli VF, de Martino G, Marangelli V, Rizzon P. Transesophageal doppler evaluation of coronary blood flow. Velocity in hypertrophic obstructive cardiomyopathy. J Am Coll Cardiol 1992; 19 (suppl A): 323A.
5. Memmola C, Iliceto S, Marangelli V, Carella L, de Martino G, Biasco G, Rizzon P. Mechanisms of coronary flow reserve. Impairment assessed by transeophageal echo doppler in patients with microvascular angina. Circulation 1992; 86: 726.
6. Memmola C, Iliceto S, Sublimi L, Pellegrini C, Rizzon P. Detection of proximal stenosis of left coronary artery by digital cine loop transesophageal-2D echo. Feasibility, sensitivity and specificity. Circulation 1990; 82: 245.
7. Memmola C, Iliceto S, Valsamis K, D'Ambrosio G, Carella L, Rizzon P. Combined use of transesophageal 2D-echo and color doppler in detecting proximal coronary artery stenosis. Circulation 1991; 84 (suppl): II708.
8. Presti CF, Feigenbaum H, Armstrong WF, Ryan T, Dillon JC. Digital two-dimensional echocardiographic imaging of the proximal left anterior descending coronary artery. Am J Cardiol 1987; 60: 1254-1259.
9. Weyman AE, Feigenbaum H, Dillon JC, Johnston KW, Eggleton RC. Noninvasive visualization of the left main coronary artery by cross-sectional echocardiography. Circulation 1976; 54: 169-174.
10. Wilson RF, Laughlin DE, Ackell PH, Chilian WM, Holida MD, Hartley CJ, Armstrong ML, Marcus ML, White CW. Transluminal, subselective measurement of coronary blood flow velocity and vasodilator reserve in man. Circulation 1985; 72: 82-92.

14.5   **Echocardiography of the Coronary Arteries**   710
14.5.2   **Multiplane Scanning of the Coronary Arteries**
(Kirsten van Kooten, Kurt J.G. Schmailzl)

Multiplane transesophageal echocardiography systems make it possible to obtain tomographic sections over a range of 0° to 180°. By also angulating the tip of the echoscope and rotating the shaft of the echoscope, it is possible to view the heart in an almost infinite number of planes.

Multiplane transesophageal echocardiography permits visualization of the left anterior descending coronary artery and distal segments of the main coronary arteries in a larger percentage of patients. Of at least equal importance is the fact that, in multiplane transesophageal echocardiography, one can better position the Doppler beam with respect to the direction of blood flow. Thus, multiplane transesophageal echocardiography velocity measurements and the functional assessments derived from these measurements are more reliable.

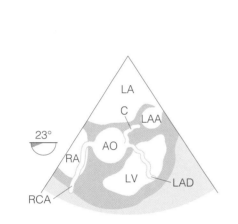

Simultaneous visualization of the left anterior descending (LAD), circumflex (C), and right (RCA) coronary arteries.

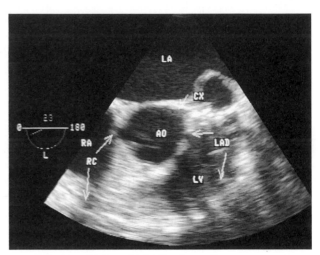

Transesophageal multiplane (23°) 2-D echocardiogram .

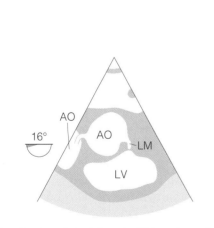

Visualization of the left main (LM) and proximal LAD coronaries.

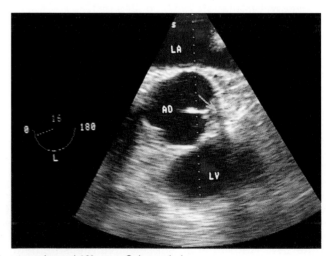

Transesophageal 16°-scan. Color coded.

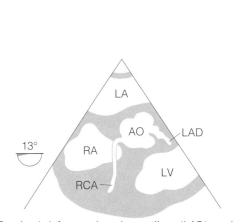

Proximal left anterior descending (LAD) and medial right (RCA) coronary arteries.

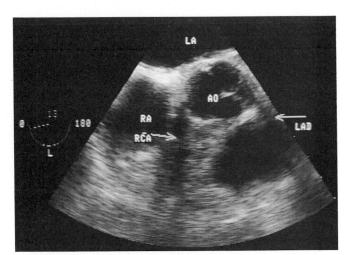

Transesophageal multiplane (13°) 2-D echocardiogram.

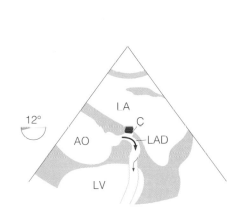

Left main (LM) and proximal LAD. Plaque and turbulence in the proximal LAD.

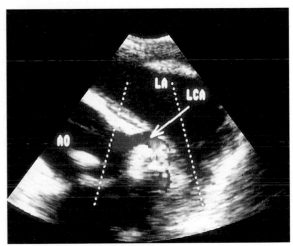

Transesophageal 12°-scan. Color coded.

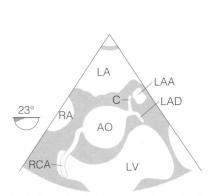

Proximal circumflex (C) artery, and proximal and medial right coronary artery (RCA).

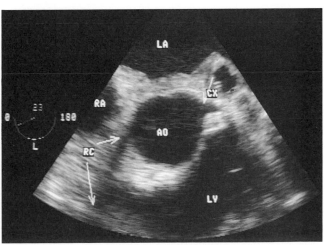

Transesophageal multiplane (23°) 2-D echocardiogram.

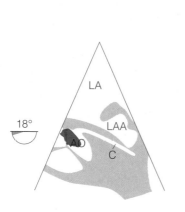

Proximal and medial circumflex (C) coronary artery. Findings indicate aortic stenosis.

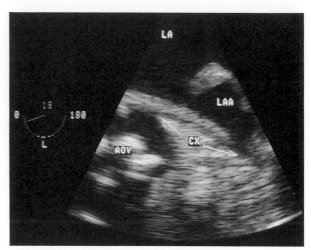

Transesophageal multiplane (18°) 2-D echocardiogram.

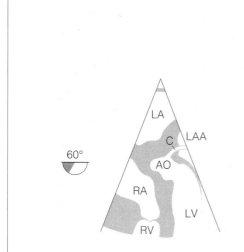

Proximal circumflex (C) coronary artery.

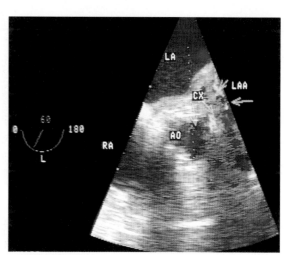

Transesophageal 60°-scan. Color coded.

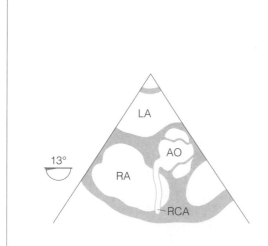

Proximal and medial right coronary artery (RCA).

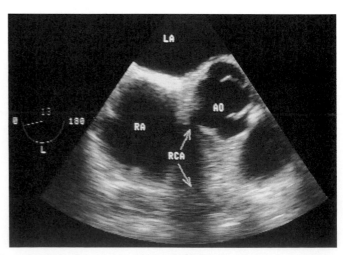

Transesophageal multiplane (13°) 2-D echocardiogram.

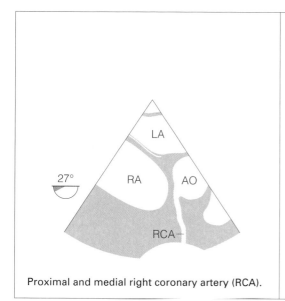

Proximal and medial right coronary artery (RCA).

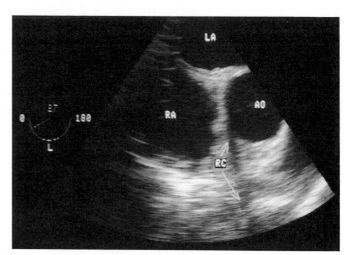

Transesophageal multiplane (27°) 2-D echocardiogram.

Intracardiac masses that impinge upon or invade the heart can be caused by neoplastic diseases of the heart, adjacent structures, or other organs, by thrombus, vegetations, and morphological anomalies.

Intracardiac Masses

- ▸ Vegetations
- ▸ Thrombus
- ▸ Tumors and cysts
- ▸ Foreign objects

With the advent of transesophageal echocardiography, not only the diagnostic potentials, but also the possibility of false-positive diagnoses, has increased. The best insurance against false-positive diagnosis is a thorough knowledge of morphology and topography and familiarity with the most common artifacts.

Cardiac masses can be simulated by large eustachian valves (Valvula v. cavae inferioris), tissue folds that extend to the valve level, and by the triangle created by the apex of the right atrium and the superior vena cava, which can cause strong echo reflection. In the apical third of the right ventricle, the moderator band and the thebesian valve (Valvula v. cavae superioris) can also lead to confusion. In all cases, following the course of the structure is helpful for clarification. False-positive diagnosis of thrombus in the left atrial appendage (which is not uncommon) is usually attributable to the pectinate muscles, the narrow edges of which can usually be identified well and delineated. The echogenicity of the pectinate muscles is constant and is identical with that of the wall of the left atrial appendage. The pectinate muscles move with the left atrial appendage, they are not calcified, their spatial orientation appears relatively regular, and they never completely occupy the left atrial appendage. A tissue duplicature is located near the origin of the left superior pulmonary vein in the left ventricle. When this duplicature produces highly reflective echoes, it can be mistaken for a mass.

The most common predisposing factors for left atrial thrombi are left atrial dilation and mitral stenosis, whereby akinesis or dyskinesis of wall segments after acute myocardial infarction (with or without aneurysm) and large hypokinetic ventricles are the most common predisposing factors for left ventricular thrombi.

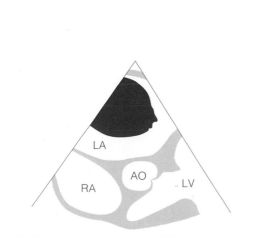

Findings: Large, organized old thrombus in the left atrial appendage (LAA) in patient with mitral stenosis.

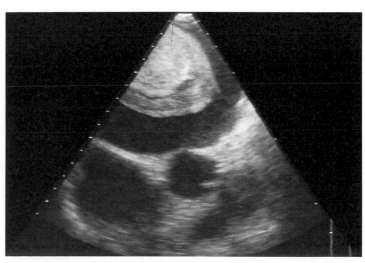

Transesophageal short-axis 2-D echocardiogram.

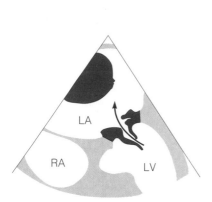

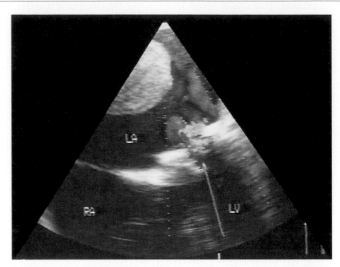

Same patient. Findings: Large, organized old thrombus in the left atrial appendage (LAA) in patient with mitral stenosis. Calcified mitral valve with turbulent stenotic flow jet. Visualization of flow in pulmonary vein and left atrial appendage.

Color flow map of transesophageal short-axis 2-D echocardiogram.

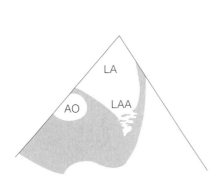

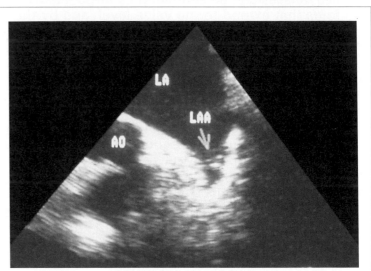

Left atrial appendage (LAA). Findings normal; no evidence of thrombus. The echo-dense structures in LAA correspond to the pectinate muscles.

Transesophageal short-axis 2-D echocardiogram.

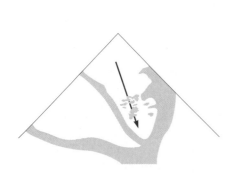

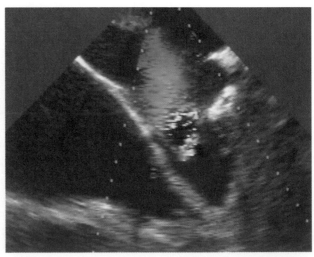

Left atrial appendage (LAA). Findings normal; no evidence of thrombus. Flow in LAA normal.

Color flow map of transesophageal short-axis 2-D echocardiogram.

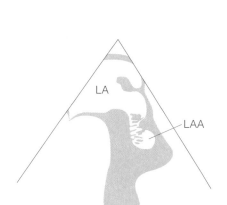

Left atrial appendage (LAA). Findings questionable. Echo-dense, difficult to delineate structures were found in the LAA. Clinical examination and MR found no evidence of thrombus.

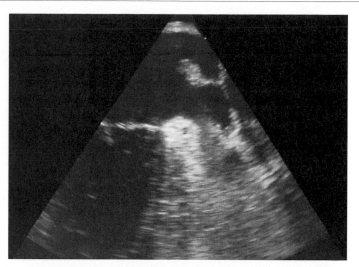

Transesophageal long-axis 2-D echocardiogram.

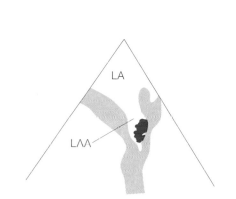

Left atrial appendage (LAA). Echo-dense structure in the LAA has irregular borders which, however, can be delineated.

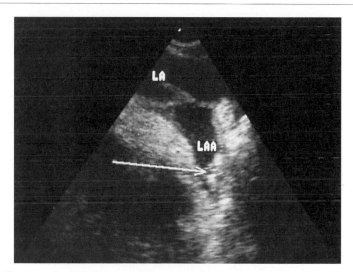

Transesophageal short-axis 2-D echocardiogram.

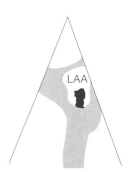

Left atrial appendage (LAA). Echo-dense structure, the borders of which can be delineated, is seen floating in the LAA. Diagnosis: thrombus.

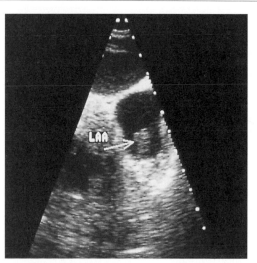

Transesophageal short-axis 2-D echocardiogram.

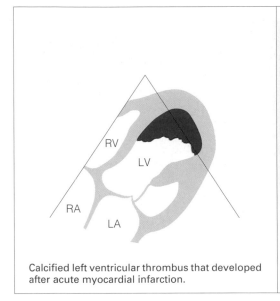

Calcified left ventricular thrombus that developed after acute myocardial infarction.

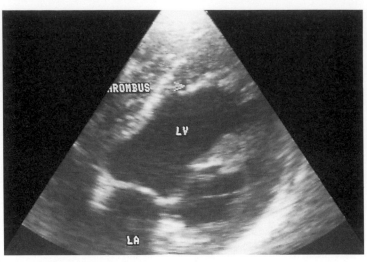

Apical four-chamber 2-D echocardiogram.

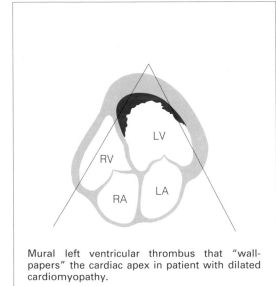

Mural left ventricular thrombus that "wall-papers" the cardiac apex in patient with dilated cardiomyopathy.

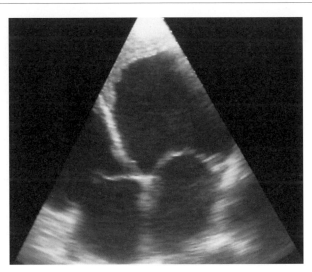

Apical four-chamber 2-D echocardiogram.

Generally, atrial fibrillation is considered to be an additional risk factor. Sites of predilection are the left atrial appendage and the apex of the left ventricle.

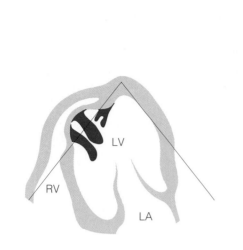

Floating thrombus in apical anterior wall aneurysm.

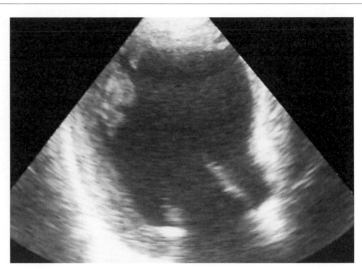

Apical four-chamber 2-D echocardiogram.

This is the reason for the superiority of 2-D over M-mode echocardiography, and for the superiority of transesophageal over transthoracic techniques. Transesophageal studies of suspected thrombus should be performed as the routine cardiac ultrasound examination whenever atrial fibrillation occurs in addition to the above-mentioned predisposing factors.

At many hospitals, suspected cardiac embolism is the most common indication for transesophageal echocardiography. This is because transesophageal echocardiography can detect a large number of the etiologic causes of ischemic cerebral attacks [9], on the one hand, and is due to the disappointing results of transthoracic echocardiography, on the other hand [8].

The examination should specifically search for the following primary diseases commonly associated with cardiac thrombo-embolism.

Possible and probable causes of embolism (modified from [3])
▸ General predisposing factors for cardiogenic thrombo-embolism 　　Valvular heart disease 　　Wall motion abnormalities
▸ Possible cause of cardiac embolism 　　Patent foramen ovale 　　Atrial septal defect 　　Atrial septal aneurysm 　　Spontaneous echocardiographic contrast as an indicator of increased risk
▸ Probable cause of cardiac embolism 　　Left atrial thrombus 　　Left ventricular thrombus 　　Prominent mobile plaques in the aorta 　　Vegetations 　　Neoplastic heart disease

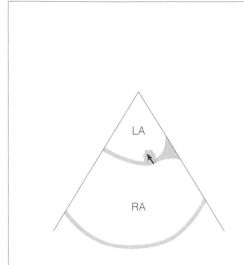

Patent foramen ovale.

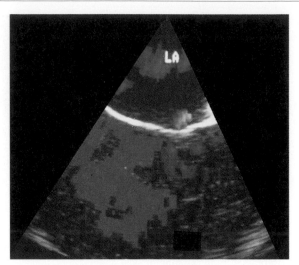

Transesophageal short-axis view. Color coded.

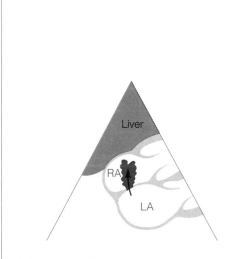

Atrial septal defect.

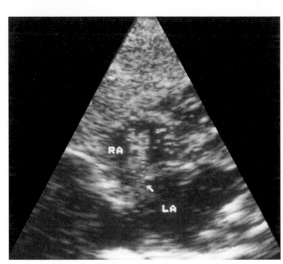

Subcostal four-chamber view. Color coded.

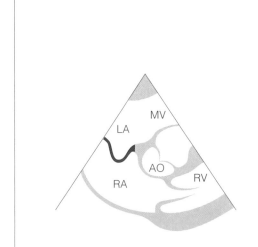

Atrial septal aneurysm.

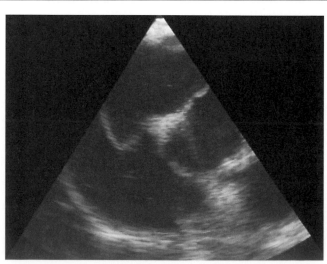

Transesophageal short-axis 2-D echocardiogram.

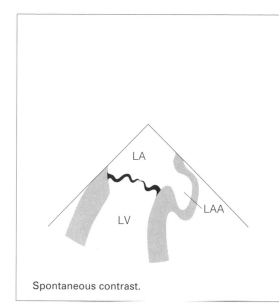

Spontaneous contrast.

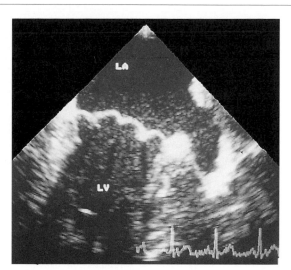

Transesophageal long-axis 2-D echocardiogram.

The problem in searching for the source of cardiac embolism is that predominantly fresh thrombi embolize. Therefore, after thrombo-embolism has occurred, signs of thrombus can no longer be found. Conversely, it is hard to judge the clinical significance of an organized and partially calcified old thrombus in absence of an acute thrombo-embolic attack.

In serial studies, thrombotic material was found in the left atrium of approximately 5% of patients examined by transesophageal echocardiography after an ischemic cerebral attack [8, 10]. None of the available studies permit any reliable conclusion about the clinical and therapeutic consequences of such findings. Therefore, the clinician must decide from case to case whether to initiate thrombolysis, heparinization, or anticoagulative therapy with serial follow-up examinations.

As in the case of left ventricular thrombi, the lack of transesophageal echocardiographic proof of left atrial thrombus cannot be taken as exclusion of the presence of thrombus, because the sensitivity of the method is not 100%. When in doubt, and when justified clinical suspicion persists, supplementary techniques such as cardangiography, MRI, and ultra-fast CT are indicated.

The prognostic implications of spontaneous echocardiographic contrast in absence of a concomitant primary heart disease predisposing to thrombo-embolism are unknown. The same is true of alternative therapeutic strategies in patients with spontaneous contrast [4].

Prominent, mobile, usually pedicled atheromatous plaques in the aorta are associated with an increased risk of cerebral embolism. In patients with a history of ischemic cerebral attacks, endarterectomy therefore seems to be a justifiable consideration [13].

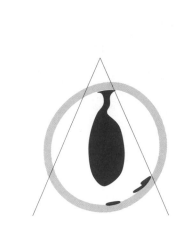

Hypertrophy of the media. Pedicled thrombus and atheromatous plaques in the aorta.

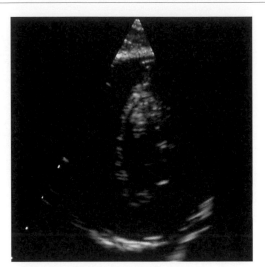

Transesophageal short-axis 2-D echocardiogram.

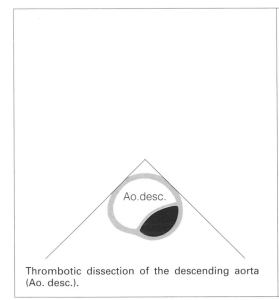

Thrombotic dissection of the descending aorta (Ao. desc.).

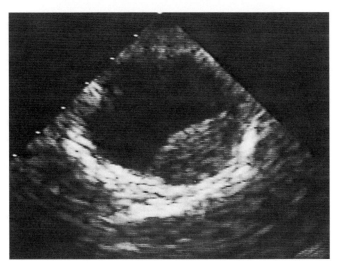

Transesophageal short-axis 2-D echocardiogram.

---

15.   **Intra- and Extracardiac Masses**
15.2   **Cardiac Tumors**

The first *ante mortem* diagnosis of a cardiac tumor (by angiography) was made in 1951, and was followed by an unsuccessful attempt to remove the myxoma [11]. The advances in imaging technology in cardiology have revolutionized the diagnosis of intracardiac masses. Echocardiographic visualization of cardiac tumors is a demonstrative example of this type of sensational, *prima vista* diagnosis that can be made within seconds, and which has become the gold standard [5].

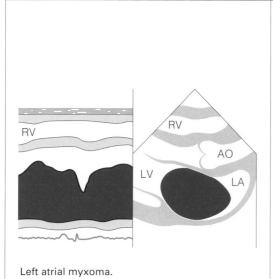

Left atrial myxoma.

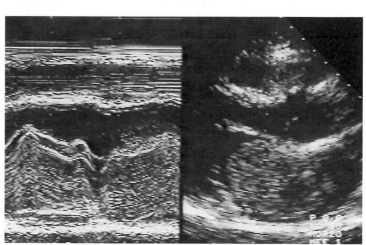

Parasternal long-axis M-mode and 2-D echocardiograms.

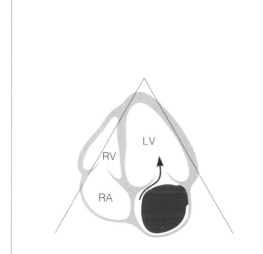

Left atrial myxoma.

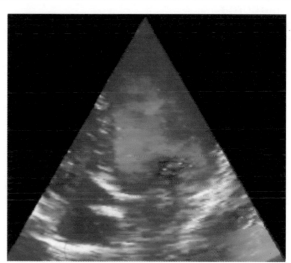

Color flow map of apical four-chamber 2-D echocardiogram.

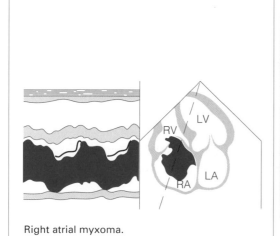

Right atrial myxoma.

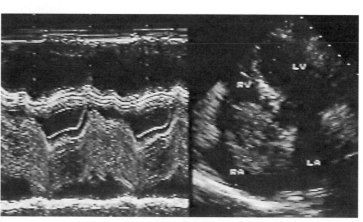

Apical four-chamber M-mode and 2-D echocardiograms.

This is underscored by frustrating clinical efforts [2] based on obstructive, embolic and systemic manifestations, which arrive at the correct diagnosis in only 5 to 10% of all cases [12].

Relatively common intra- and extracardiac neoplasms (> 3%) (modified from [1])	
Benign	**Percentage Frequency**
Myxoma	24.4
Pericardial cysts	15.4
Lipoma	8.4
Papillary fibroelastoma	7.9
Rhabdomyoma	6.8
Fibroma	3.2
Subtotal	66.1
Malignant	
Angiosarcoma	7.3
Rhabdomyosarcoma	4.9
Mesothelioma	3.6
Subtotal	15.8
Other	18.1
Total	100.0

Efforts to differentiate between tumor and thrombus focus on such indications as the site of attachment, the presence of echolucent areas, echo-free areas, and calcification, the shape and contours of the observed mass, and (when applicable) the involvement of adjacent structures. Techniques of tissue characterization may one day provide a reliable means of differentiation.

Such radiologic techniques as computed tomography and magnetic resonance imaging have taken the leading role in the diagnosis of extracardiac tumors.

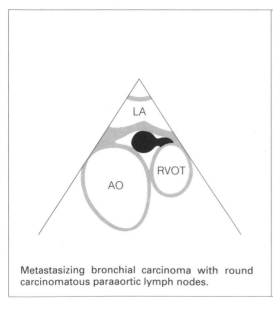

Metastasizing bronchial carcinoma with round carcinomatous paraaortic lymph nodes.

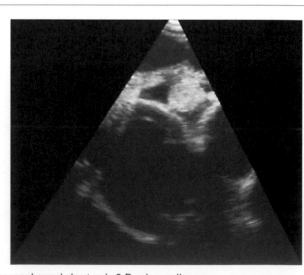

Transesophageal short-axis 2-D echocardiogram.

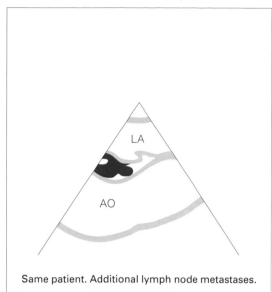

Same patient. Additional lymph node metastases.

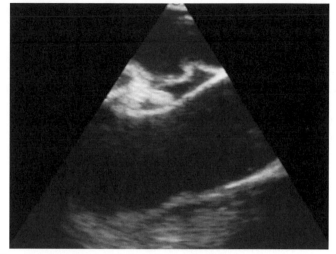

Transesophageal long-axis 2-D echocardiogram.

15.2   Cardiac Tumors
15.2.1   Intracardiac Tumors

Etiology and location of intracardiac tumors (modified from [7])

▶ Right atrium
     Myxoma
     Rhabdomyosarcoma
     Renal cell carcinoma

▶ Right ventricle
     Ectopic thyroid tissue

▶ Left atrium
     Myxoma
     Rhabdomyosarcoma

▶ Left ventricle
     Rhabdomyosarcoma

▶ Aorta
     Malignant histiocytoma

Etiology and location of intracardiac tumors (modified from [7])

▶ Right paracardial
     Pericardial cyst
     Malignant lymphoma
     Bronchial carcinoma
     Other

▶ Left paracardial
     Pericardial cyst
     Malignant lymphoma
     Bronchogenic and embryonal cysts
     Other

▶ Paraaortic
     Malignant lymphoma

15.2   **Cardiac Tumors**
15.2.3   **Foreign Objects**

This group includes valve prostheses, pace-makers, and circulatory support systems. All of these devices are associated with increased thrombogenicity and may cause sterile or infectious thrombus or embolism.

References

1. Beppu S, Park Y, Sakakibara H, Nagata S, Nimura Y. Clinical features of intracardiac thrombosis based on echocardiographic observation. Jpn Circul J 1984; 48: 75-82.
2. Bloor CM, O'Rourke RA. Cardiac tumors: clinical presentations and pathologic correlations. Curr Probl Cardiol 1984; 9: 1-415.
3. Camp A, Labovitz AJ. Evaluation of cardiac sources of emboli. In: Dittrich HC (ed). Clinical transesophageal echocardiography. Mosby, St. Louis 1992: 54 (tbl. 4-2).
4. Camp A, Labovitz AJ. Evaluation of cardiac sources of emboli. In: Dittrich HC (ed). Clinical transesophageal echocardiography. Mosby, St. Louis 1992: 62.
5. Dunnigan A, Oldham HN, Serwer GA, Benson DW. Left atrial myxoma: is cardiac catheterization essential? Am J Dis Child 1981; 135: 420-421.
6. McAllister HA jr, Fenoglio JJ jr. Tumors of the cardiovascular system. Armed Forces Institute of Pathology, Washington D.C. 19715.
7. Mügge A, Stottmeister Chr, Bargheer K, Daniel WG. Detection of cardiac and paracardiac masses. In: Dittrich HC (ed). Clinical transesophageal echocardiography. Mosby, St. Louis 1992: 92 (tbl. 6-3).
8. Pearson AC, Labovitz AJ, Tatineni S, Gomez CR. Superiority of transesophageal echocardiography in detecting cardiac source of embolism in patients with cerebral ischemia of uncertain etiology. J Am Coll Cardiol 1991; 17: 66-72.
9. Pearson AC, Nagelhout D, Camp A, Gomez CR, Labovitz AJ. Atrial septal aneurysm and stroke: A transesophageal echocardiographic study. J Am Coll Cardiol 1991; 18: 1223-1229.
10. Pop G, Sutherland GR, Koudstaal PJ et al. Transesophageal echocardiography in the detection of intracardiac embolic sources in patients with transient ischemic attacks. Stroke 1990; 21: 560-565.
11. Pritchard RW. Tumors of the heart. Review of the subject and report of one hundred and fifty cases. Arch Pathol 1951; 51: 98-1215.
12. Silverman NA. Primary cardiac tumors. Ann Surg 1980; 191: 127-1315.
13. Tunick PA, Culliford AT, Lamparello PJ et al. Atheromatosis of the aortic arch as an occult source of multiple systemic emboli. Ann Intern Med 1991; 114: 391-392.

The pericardium consists of two portions: a *serous-visceral* (epicardial) layer that forms part of the epicardium, and a multilayered *parietal* (fibrous) layer that is firmly adherent to the diaphragm, the aorta up to the aortic arch, and the pulmonary trunk up to its bifurcation, and is loosely adherent to venae cavae up to their atrial origins, the esophagus, and the pleural cavities. Along the pulmonary veins and the venae cavae, the two pericardial layers form reflections which are firmly attached to anterior wall of the left atrium, thereby forming the oblique sinus.

Echocardiography permits assessment of the diastolic communication between the two ventricles and provides optical guidance in pericardiocentesis. Echocardiographic findings are of central importance in the diagnosis of intra- and extrapericardial masses.

Pericardial diseases (adapted from [2])
1. Malformations (agenesis, partial defect, congenital cysts and diverticula)
2. Pathological contents of the pericardial sac ▸ Hydropericardium (due to transudate in congestive heart failure or hypalbuminemia) ▸ Hematopericardium (in transmural myocardial infarction, dissecting aneurysm of the aorta, pericardial carcinosis, and hemorrhagic diathesis) ▸ Chylopericardium (in thoracic duct injuries) ▸ Pneumopericardium (in injuries to the respiratory tract or esophagus)
3. Inflammatory pericardial disease (pericarditis, epicarditis, perimyocarditis)
4. Malignant pericarditis
5. Metabolic disease with pericardial involvement (uremic pericardial effusion, myxedema)

This list contains overlapping groups: malformations can simulate pericardial effusion, and inflammatory pericardial diseases are associated with serous, serofibrinous, fibrinous, and hemorrhagic pericardial effusions. The most common pericardial diseases are cryptogenic (-usually postviral) pericardial effusion and pericardial effusion in the setting of viral pericarditis, postpericardiotomy syndrome and Dressler's postinfarction syndrome, tuberculous pericarditis, pericarditis secondary to autoimmune disease, collagenosis-associated pericarditis (systemic lupus erythematosus, scleroderma), and uremic pericardial effusion.

Conventional echocardiography is the method of choice for diagnosis and assessment of pericardial effusion. Echocardiographic studies provide the definitive indication for further testing (pericardial biopsy, pericardioscopy) and treatment (pericardiocentesis, pericardiotomy, pericardial fenestration, pericardiectomy).

The echocardiographic diagnosis of pericardial effusion is based on detection of an echo-free space either posterior to the left ventricle or anterior to the right ventricle. The amplitude of motion of the parietal pericardium is also diminished in the presence of effusion fluid. An additional sign of pericardial effusion is the disappearance of the observed echo-free space at the reflection of the pericardium onto the pulmonary veins (at the atrioventricular groove).

Echocardiographic quantitation of pericardial effusion is performed primarily by M-mode. This method infers the volume of effusion fluid from the degree of diastolic separation of the pericardial layers. Admittedly, the validity of this method has great limitations, because a uniform distribution of effusion fluid cannot be assumed.

Semiquantitation of pericardial fluid		
Very small	< 50 ml	Only systolic separation of the pericardial layers on the left ventricular posterior wall
Small	50 to 100 ml	Only flat systolic anterior motion of the parietal pericardium
Moderate	100 to 300 ml	Separation of the pericardial layers persists through the entire cardiac cycle
Large	> 300 ml	Separation of the pericardial layers along the entire left ventricular posterior wall is > 10 mm

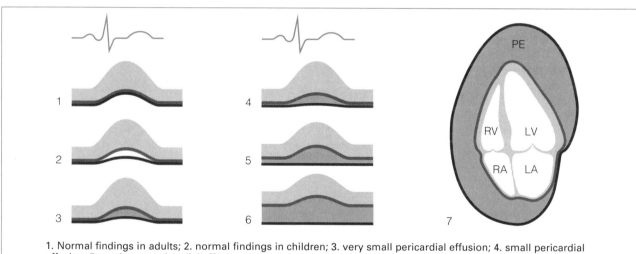

1. Normal findings in adults; 2. normal findings in children; 3. very small pericardial effusion; 4. small pericardial effusion; 5. moderate pericardial effusion; 6. large pericardial effusion; 7. swinging heart.

The size of pericardial effusion is best appreciated by two-dimensional echocardiography, which permits assessment of the spatial distribution of pericardial effusion. Only in 2-D echocardiograms can circular effusions and large local effusions suitable for pericardiocentesis be visualized. The standard echocardiographic planes are the subcostal and apical four-chamber views and the parasternal short and long-axis views. Very small and small pericardial effusions are located mostly posterobasal and inferobasal. Moderate effusions extend in the apical and lateral directions, and large effusions circumscribe the heart. "Swinging heart" is characterized by counter-clockwise rotational movement that occurs in addition to the triangular rotation of the heart in the chest cavity; this produces dance-like motion. Two-dimensional echocardiography can readily demonstrate fibrous tissue strands that extend through the pericardial cavity and pericardial effusion in uremic effusion, many chronic effusions, radiation pericarditis, and tumorous pericarditis.

The significance of the size of pericardial effusions usually boils down to the following questions:

- Is the pericardial effusion hemodynamically significant; does it require treatment? Does cardiac tamponade exist?
- Has the volume of effusion changed over the course of disease?
- Does constriction exist?

Hemodynamically significant effusion must be assumed when swinging heart is observed.

The development of cardiac tamponade is dependent on the speed of development of pericardial effusion. Thus, a swinging heart does not necessarily indicate the development of tamponade. On the other hand, even slight amounts of pericardial fluid can give rise to cardiac tamponade and increased intrapericardial pressure, which can become higher than the right ventricular end-diastolic pressure. Echocardiographic indications of cardiac tamponade are paradoxical volume changes of the ventricle in dependence with the respiration cycle, similar to the clinical phenomenon of pulsus paradoxus. Cardiac tamponade is probable when the right ventricular volume increases while the left ventricular volume decreases during deep inspiration, and the right ventricular volume decreases (<< 10 mm) and the left ventricular volume increases on expiration.

Findings associated with cardiac tamponade

- Increase in right ventricular size on inspiration and reduction on expiration (RVEDD << 10 mm)
- Decrease in left ventricular size on inspiration and increase on expiration, similar to findings in pulsus paradoxus (diminished inspiratory pulse)
- Diastolic collapse of the right ventricle and, in some cases, left ventricle
- Right atrial compression or collapse; left atrial compression
- Abnormal respiratory variations in transtricuspid and transmitral flow velocities
- Diminished EF slope
- Pseudoprolapse of the mitral valve
- Dilated inferior vena cava without inspiratory collapse
- Swinging heart

In constrictive pericarditis, the echocardiographic diagnosis is based primarily on the detection of thickened and echo-dense pericardial layers that move parallel to the posterior wall of the left ventricle, from which they are frequently separated by a narrow echo-free margin corresponding to an old, organized effusion. This finding alone does not permit diagnosis of hemodynamically significant constriction. A more specific but unsensitive finding, similar to the finding in angiography, is the square root phenomenon, in which the diastolic posterior motion of the posterior wall appears to stop prematurely and abruptly during the rapid filling phase, then proceeds horizontally in the further course of diastole. In constrictive pericarditis, the posterior endocardial line of the interventricular septum exhibits very little or abnormal motion in systole. In diastole the anterior relaxation motion during atrial systole may reverse, creating an arch-shaped motion pattern when atrial blood is ejected into the stiff left ventricle.

Although echocardiography is highly sensitive for detection of pericardial effusion, it lacks significance in clarification of etiopathogenetic questions. Echocardiography still cannot reliably differentiate between clear and protein-rich or blood-containing effusions.

Specificity problems and misinterpretations ensure from the following sources of error [1]:

- Epicardial fat can usually be detected in front of the anterior right ventricular wall, but does not compress it. Also, no alterations in the motion of the interventricular septum nor of the left ventricular posterior wall can be detected.
- A localized echo-free space corresponding to the coronary sinus is frequently seen at the junction of the left atrium and left ventricle, and may also be mistaken for pericardial effusion.
- A circular echo-free space corresponding to the descending aorta is located posterior to the proximal left atrium may also lead to misinterpretation.
- Pleural effusion extends beyond the pleuro-pericardial duplicature near the ventricular-atrial border posterior to the atrium. In concomitant pericardial effusion, pleural effusion is localized posterior and lateral to it.

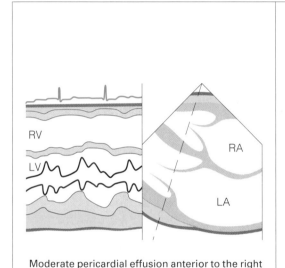

Moderate pericardial effusion anterior to the right ventricle and posterior to the left ventricle.

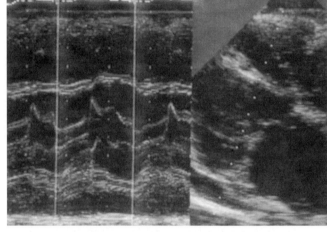

Parasternal long-axis M-mode and 2-D echocardiograms.

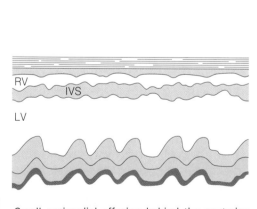

Small pericardial effusion behind the posterior wall of the left ventricle.

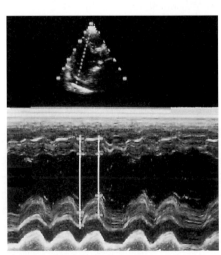

Parasternal long-axis M-mode recording.

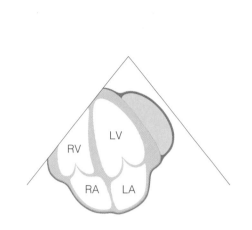

Large pericardial effusion extending along the lateral wall of the left ventricle.

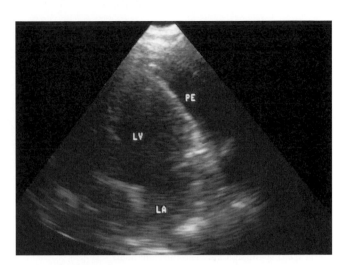

Apical four-chamber 2-D echocardiogram.

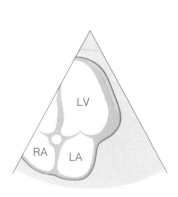

Small pericardial effusion and small pleural effusion. Both are separated by the thin parietal pericardium.

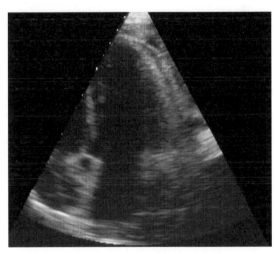

Apical four-chamber 2-D echocardiogram.

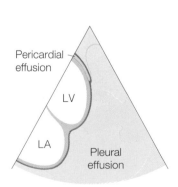

Small pericardial effusion and large pleural with large protein-rich inclusions that float to and flow

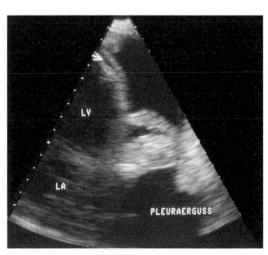

Apical four-chamber 2-D echocardiogram.

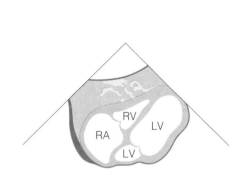

Large pericardial effusion between the right heart cavities and the diaphragm.

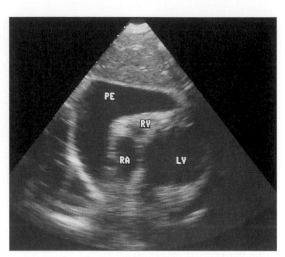

Subcostal four-chamber 2-D echocardiogram.

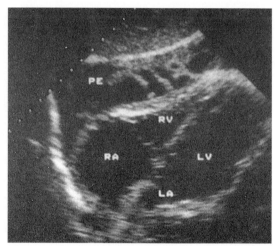

Large uremic pericardial effusion with fibrinous inclusions, located anterior to the right ventricle.

Subcostal four-chamber 2-D echocardiogram.

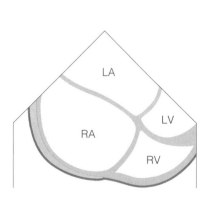

Narrow seam of pericardial effusion anterior to the right atrium.

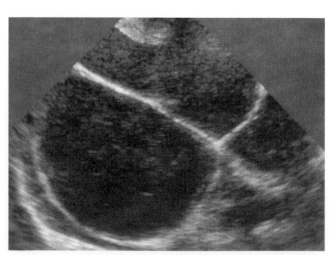

Transesophageal short-axis 2-D echocardiogram.

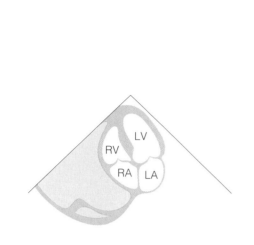

Large loculated pericardial cyst (PZ) adjacent to the right atrium.

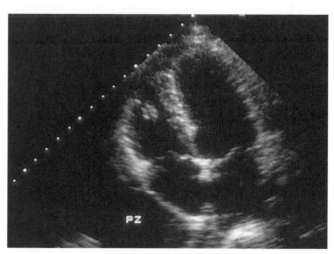

Apical four-chamber 2-D echocardiogram.

References

1. Horowitz MS, Schultz CS, Stinson EB. Sensitivity and specifity of echocardiographic diagnosis of pericardial effusion. Circulation 1974; 50: 239.
2. Maisch B. Myocarditis and pericarditis - old questions and new answers. Herz 1992; 17: 65-70.

Since Christiaan Barnard performed the first cardiac transplantation in Cape Town on December 3rd, 1967, cardiac transplantation has become an established surgical procedure [2, 19]. A world-wide total of more than 22,600 cardiac transplantations had been reported to the International Society for Heart and Lung Transplantation as of April 1993 [15]. A total of approximately 3000 cardiac transplantations are performed around the world each year [14].

The most common indications for cardiac transplantation are final-stage dilated and ischemic cardiomyopathies. In rare cases, cardiac transplantation may also be indicated in traumatic and congenital heart diseases.

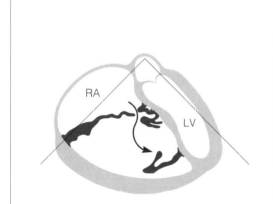

Ebstein's malformation in a female heart transplant candidate. Findings: ventricularized tricuspid valve with posterior leaflet displaced into the right ventricle; adhesive septal leaflet; small, residual right ventricle; hypoplastic left ventricle.

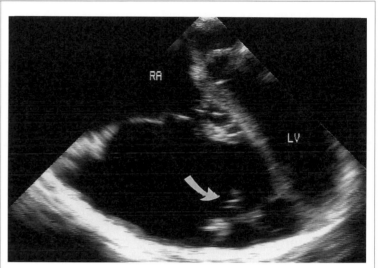

Transoesophageal short axis 2 D echocardiogram.

By standardizing the surgical technique and by modifying the immunosuppressive treatment strategies (combination treatment with cyclosporine A, azathioprine, and low-dose corticosteroids), perioperative mortality has been reduced to 10%. Currently, the world-wide one-year and five-year survival rates are 84% and 69%, respectively.

Although immunosuppressive treatment has significantly improved in the last few years, still almost every heart transplant patient experiences rejection episodes, despite the introduction of cyclosporine A. In fact, the reported frequency of rejection has remained basically unchanged [12]. Next to infections, rejection is the most common complication [11, 16, 21], and is the most frequent cause of death in the postoperative phase after cardiac transplantation [13]. Therefore, the early diagnosis of acute rejection, before irreversible damage has occurred, is of utmost importance.

Currently, the endomyocardial biopsy technique described by Caves and Billingham [4, 5] is still the gold standard for early and reliable diagnosis of transplant rejection. After applying local anesthesia, a venous sheath is placed in the right internal jugular vein. Then a bioptome is advanced under fluoroscopic control to the right ventricular apex. Multiple (3 to 6) biopsy specimens are obtained from different sites. Histologic alterations should be assessed according to the recommendations of the International Society for Heart and Lung Transplantation [3].

Although the above-described endomyocardial biopsy technique is a low-risk procedure, it is invasive and causes the patient some discomfort. Therefore, comparable noninvasive techniques have been developed. Noninvasive techniques, which can be performed daily, provide an early diagnosis of acute rejection reaction with less discomfort to the patient.

Over the past few years, our hospital has adopted various noninvasive techniques for diagnosis of heart transplant rejection. The techniques that we use to monitor transplant patients in the early postoperative phase are: cytoimmunologic monitoring (CIM), which was developed by the Institute of Surgical Research at the University of Munich in 1984 [9, 18]; Fast Fourier Transform ECG (FFT-ECG) [8]; and echocardiography [1]. These techniques are also suitable for long-term follow-up. The chest x-ray findings and clinical diagnostic parameters provide further information for diagnosis of rejection after heart transplantation.

A study comparing the results of transmural biopsy with those of the above-described noninvasive techniques confirmed that the sensitivity and specificity of these techniques is good [20]. FFT-ECG properly identified incipient rejection episodes in 89% of all cases. CIM also detected the onset of rejection reactions in the majority of cases. The sensitivity and specificity of CIM were 85% and 80%, respectively. These parameters are suitable for diagnosis of rejection, but not for follow-up monitoring.

Echocardiography is a simple and reliable technique that can be repeated at any time. It is a meaningful addition to the other noninvasive examination techniques.

Echocardiography permits assessment of transplant function and early diagnosis of transplant rejection. Associated complications such as acute transplant failure and hemodynamically significant pericardial effusion can also be diagnosed by echocardiography.

M-mode echocardiographic indices for assessment of transplant function are left and right ventricular end-diastolic dimensions and wall thicknesses of the interventricular septum and left ventricular wall, as described by the American Society of Echocardiography. The parasternal long-axis view is the standard plane for measuring ventricular dimensions and wall thicknesses. Measurements are made at the level of the chordae tendineae at end-diastole, cutting the structures perpendicularly. The percent systolic diameter shortening, *i.e.* left ventricular fractional shortening, is calculated using the following formula:

LVFS = (LVEDD - LVESD) / (LVEDD)

LVEDD   Left ventricular end-diastolic diameter
LVESD   Left ventricular end-systolic diameter

Two-dimensional echocardiographic visualization and assessment of left and right ventricular wall motion has also been proven effective. Scans are made from the standard imaging planes.

The primary goal of the echocardiographic examination is early detection and diagnosis of heart transplant rejection. Changes in the ventricular myocardium and in cardiac pump function of great significance. In order to make accurately compare different echocardiographic findings, the examination technique must be extensively standardized, *i.e.* fairly reproducible. Immediate postoperative recording of baseline echocardiographic findings is imperative. This permits comparison of the baseline data with the findings of later echocardiographic studies and reproduction of the corresponding imaging planes. In cardiac transplant patients, echocardiographic postoperative monitoring should be performed daily.

Qualitative echocardiographic markers of acute rejection are:

- Increased thickening of the interventricular septal wall and the left ventricular posterior wall. Such thickening is caused mainly by rejection-related myocardial edema and cellular infiltration. Differential diagnosis: Developing hypertrophy secondary to hypertension, which can occur as a side-effect of cyclosporine A, can also produce a similar encrease in wall thickness and change in left ventricular diastolic function.

It is important that one distinguish this from the changes due to transplant rejection. When in doubt, myocardial biopsy should be performed to provide the definitive diagnosis.

- Increased right ventricular wall thickness. This can be an isolated, sole sign of heart rejection, as animal experiments have shown [10].
- Reduction in left ventricular fractional shortening as an expression of impaired systolic pump function. Reduction in left ventricular fractional shortening, *i.e.* outside the limits of normal, is not an absolute measure. Studies at our hospital have shown that, in patients with bioptically confirmed heart rejection, the left ventricular fractional shortening was normal in the majority of patients, despite worsening of systolic and diastolic function. Therefore, precise follow-up studies and comparison with the initial baseline findings is absolutely essential for identifying acute rejection episodes.
- Reduction in isovolumic relaxation time as an expression of impaired diastolic function and increased ventricular stiffness [6, 7].
- Global enlargement of the left ventricle.
- New occurrence of paradoxical septal motion.
- Increased amount of pericardial effusion.
- Overall structural "loosening" in 2-D echocardiograms.

Studies at our hospital have shown that, by using all of the available echocardiographic markers, acute cardiac rejection can be diagnosed noninvasively [1]. Suspicion of acute rejection is based on changes identified by comparing later findings with those of the initial baseline findings.

References

1. Angermann CE, Spes C, Hart RJ, Kemkes BM, Gokel M, Theisen K. Echokardiografische Diagnose akuter Abstoßungsreaktionen bei herztransplantierten Patienten unter Cyclosporintherapie. Z Kardiol 1989; 78: 243-252.
2. Barnard CN. The operation. A human cardiac transplantation: an interim report of the successful operation performed at the Groote Schuur Hospital, Cape Town. South African Med J 1967; 41: 1271-1274.
3. Billingham ME, Cary NR, Hammond ME, Kemnitz J, Marboe C, McCallister HA, Snovar DC, Winters GL, Zerbe A. A working formulation for the standardization of nomenclature in the diagnosis of heart and lung rejection: Heart Rejection Study Group. J Heart Transplant 1990; 9: 587-593.
4. Caves PK, Stinson EB, Billingham ME, Shumway NE. Serial transvenous biopsy of the transplanted human heart - improved management of the acute rejection episodes. Lancet 1974; 862: 821-826.
5. Caves PK, Stinson EB, Billingham ME, Rider AK, Shumway NE. Diagnosis of human cardiac allograft rejection by serial cardiac biopsy. J Thorac Cardiovasc Surg 1973; 66: 461-466.
6. Dawkins KD, Jamieson SW, Oldershaw PJ et al. Changes in diastoic function as a noninvasive marker of cardiac allograft rejection. Heart Transplant 1984; 3: 286-294.
7. Furniss SS, Murray A, Hunter S, Dougenis V, McGregor CGA. Value of Echocardiographic Determination of Isovolumic Relxation Time in the Detection of Heart Transplant Rejection. J Heart Lung Transplant 1991; 10: 557-561.
8. Haberl R, Weber M, Reichenspurner H, Kemkes BM, Osterholzer G, Anthuber M, Steinbeck G. Frequency analysis of the surface electrocardiogram for recognition of acute rejection after orthotopic cardiac transplantation in man. Circulation 1987; 76: 101-108.
9. Hammer C, Reichenspurner H, Ertel W, Lersch C, Plahl M, Prendel W, Reichart B, Überfuhr P, Welz A, Kemkes BM, Reble B, Funccius W, Gokel M. Cytological and immunological monitoring of cyclosporin - treated human heart recipients. J Heart Transplant 1984; 3: 228-231.
10. Havernich A, Scott WC, Dawkins KD, Billingham ME, Jamieson SW. Asymmetric pattern of rejection following orthotopic cardiac transplantation in primates. J Heart Transplant 1984; 3: 280-285.
11. Hetzer R, Warnecke H, Schüler S, Süthoff U, Borst HG. Heart transplantation - a two year experience. Z Kardiol 1985; 74: 51-58.
12. Hunt SA. Complications of heart transplantation. J Heart Transplant 1983; 3: 70-74.

13. Jamieson SW, Oyer PE, Reitz BA, Baumgartner WA, Bieber CP, Stinson EB, Shumway NE. Cardiac transplatation at Stanford. Heart Transplant 1981; 1: 86-91.
14. Kaye MP, Kriett JM. Heart Registry Report 1991. 11th Annual Meeting of the International Society for Heart Transplantation. Paris, France, April 7-9, 1991.
15. Kaye MP. The Registry of the International Society for Heart and Lung Transplantation: Tenth Official Report - 1993. Meeting of the International Society for Heart and Lung Transplantation, Boca Raton, USA, March 31 - April 3, 1993.
16. Kemkes BM, Reichenspurner H, Osterholzer G, Erdmann E, Lersch C, Schad N, Gokel JM, Klinner W. Herztransplantation. Internist 1986; 27: 322-330.
17. Reichart B, Überfuhr P, Welz A, Kemkes BM, Klinner W, Reble B, Funccius W, Hammer C, Ertel W, Reichenspurner H, Peters D, Gokel JM, Franke N, Land W: Heart transplantation at the University of Munich - the first one and a half years. J Heart Transplant 1983; 2: 266-269.
18. Reichenspurner H, Kemkes BM, Haberl R, Angermann CH, Lersch CH, Osterholzer G, Anthuber M, Weber M, Gokel JM. Patientenüberwachung nach Herztransplantation an der Universitätsklinik München, Großhadern. Z Herz-, Thorax-, Gefäßchir 1987; 1: 79.
19. Schütz A, Kemkes BM, Kugler C, Angermann C, Schad N, Rienmüller R, Fritsch S, Anthuber M, Neumaier P, Gokel M. The influence of rejection episodes on the development of coronary artery diseases after heart transplantation. Eur J Cardio-thorac Surg 1990; 4: 300-308.
20. Schütz A. Die Kinetik und Dynamik der akuten Abstoßungsreaktion nach Herztransplantation im täglichen invasiven und nichtinvasiven Monitoring. Wolfgang Papst Verlag, Lengerich 1992.
21. Yacoub MH, Reid CJ, Al-Khadimi RH, Radley-Smith R. Cardiac transplantation - the London experience. Z Kardiol 1985; 74: 45-50.

Left ventricular hypertrophy is defined as an increase in left ventricular muscle mass due to left ventricular pressure or volume overload. Histologically, this corresponds to enlargement of muscle cells, while the number of cells remains constant [19]. The left ventricular volume is normal in concentric left ventricular hypertrophy, and is increased in *eccentric* left ventricular hypertrophy. *Hypertensive heart disease* is the cardiac consequence of hypertension, expressed as hypertrophy and impaired ventricular function. In the early stages, it is characterized by concentric left ventricular hypertrophy with reduced left ventricular diastolic function and diminished coronary flow reserve. In the advanced stage, there is eccentric hypertrophy and impaired systolic left ventricular function.

Echocardiographic Diagnosis

Echocardiography is the most sensitive technique for diagnosis of left ventricular hypertrophy [21, 22].

M-Mode Echocardiography

In M-mode echocardiography, left ventricular wall thicknesses are measured in recordings obtained from parasternal long or short-axis views. Using the standard technique recommended by the American Society of Echocardiography, measurements are made below mitral valve level and are ECG-triggered to occur with the Q wave; leading edge methodology is used [2, 23, 24].

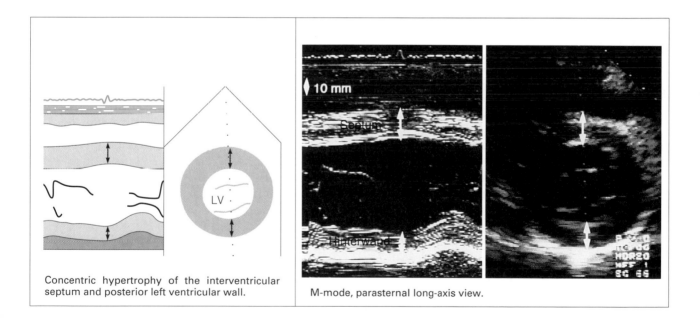

Concentric hypertrophy of the interventricular septum and posterior left ventricular wall.

M-mode, parasternal long-axis view.

Using leading edge methodology, measurements are made from the leading edge (facing the transducer) of the first echo boundary to the leading edge of the second echo boundary.

The maximum diastolic interventricular septal and left ventricular posterior wall thickness is 11 mm. The left ventricular (muscle) mass is calculated assuming that the shape of the left ventricle is ellipsoid. The standard left ventricular mass calculation formula is as follows:

LVM = (1.04)[(IVS-EDD + LVEDD + LVPW-EDD)³ - (LVEDD)³]

LVM	Left ventricular mass
IVS-EDD	End-diastolic diameter of the interventricular septum
LVEDD	Left ventricular end-diastolic dimension
LVPW-EDD	Left ventricular posterior wall end-diastolic dimension

---

The maximum normal values (sum of the mean and two times the standard deviation) for left ventricular mass, the left ventricular mass index, and the left ventricular mass corrected for body size are 294 g, 150 g/m² and 163 g/m, respectively in men, and 198 g, 120 g/m², and 121 g/m, resp. in women [17].

Validation studies have demonstrated the superiority of left ventricular mass calculations using the *Penn convention* [10, 14], which requires exclusion of the thickness of endocardial interfaces. The Penn convention formula for left ventricular mass calculation is:

LVM = (1.04)[(IVS-EDD + LVEDD + LVPW-EDD)³ - (LVEDD)³] - 13.6 g

LVM	Left ventricular mass
IVS-EDD	End-diastolic diameter of the interventricular septum
LVEDD	Left ventricular end-diastolic dimension
LVPW-EDD	Left ventricular posterior wall end-diastolic dimension

---

Using the Penn formula, the maximum normal values for left ventricular mass, the left ventricular mass index, and the left ventricular mass corrected for body size are 260 g, 132 g/m², and 144 g/m, respectively in men, and 190 g, 109 g/m², and 114.8 g/m, resp. in women [10, 13].

Sources of Error

Error will arise if the left ventricular shape does not correspond to the assumed geometry, *i.e.* prolate ellipsoid. This is the case when the left ventricle has become globular or small and elongated in shape, or when regional wall motion abnormalities have developed. Furthermore, measurement error can occur when the scan plane is not perpendicular to the ventricular long axis. Error may also arise when the chordae tendineae of the mitral or tricuspid valves are mistaken for endocardial boundaries. The reproducibility of M-mode measurements of wall thicknesses, and of measurements made using leading edge methodology, is good [20, 28].

Two-Dimensional Echocardiography

In two-dimensional echocardiography, left ventricular mass is determined by visualization of the left ventricle in apical four-chamber and parasternal short-axis views at the level of the papillary muscles [28]. Calculations are based on the assumption that the left ventricular geometry corresponds to that of a cylindrical hemi-ellipse. The following formula is used:

V = 5/6 A L/2

V	Volume of the left ventricle
A	Area of the left ventricle
L	Length of the left ventricle

The left ventricular long axis is measured from the apical four-chamber view, from mitral valve level to the apical endocardium or epicardium. The left ventricular cross-sectional area is measured by planimetering the total left ventricular volume enclosed by the endo- and epicardial surfaces. Measurements are made in the parasternal short axis at the level of the papillary muscles (midlevel). However, the papillary muscles are not included in measurements of wall thickness. The left ventricular mass is calculated by subtracting the left ventricular volume enclosed by the endocardial surface (cavitary volume) from the volume enclosed by the epicardial surface (total volume). The specific weight of the myocardium is also taken into account.

LVM = (1.055)[(total volume) - (cavitary volume)]

Sources of Error and Problems

In the apical four-chamber view, the measured left ventricular long axis will be underestimated if the beam is angulated, *i.e.* not perpendicular to the target structures. If imaging conditions are suboptimal, and if lateral resolution is poor, error in identification of septal surfaces and lateral left ventricular segments can occur; this will falsify left ventricular area calculations. The left ventricular mass will be overestimated if the papillary muscles in the left ventricular cavity are not accounted for. In the advanced stage of hypertensive heart disease, which is characterized by eccentric hypertrophy and impaired systolic function, the echocardiographic findings will resemble those of dilated cardiomyopathy, especially when left ventricular walls are no longer thickened.

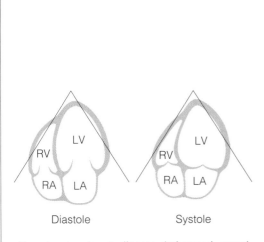

Hypertensive heart disease (advanced stage). Only slightly enlarged wall thickness, dilated left ventricle with impaired function.

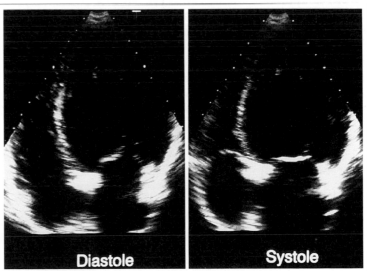

Apical four-chamber view. End-diastole and end-systole.

Relative mitral insufficiency also is commonly found in the advanced stages of hypertensive heart disease.

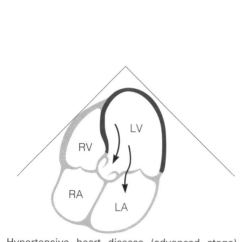

Hypertensive heart disease (advanced stage). Findings: "relative mitral insufficiency" and dilatation of the left ventricle.

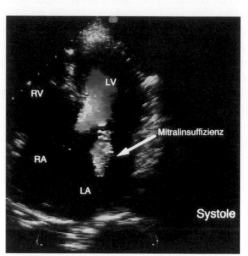

Color flow map of apical four-chamber 2-D echocardiogram. Systole.

Doppler Echocardiography

Hypertension leads to impairment of both left ventricular contractility and vascular compliance [3, 11]. Left ventricular hypertrophy is associated with changes in diastolic left ventricular function. Early diastolic relaxation and the passive late diastolic pressure-volume relationship are thereby altered; increased relaxation and reduced chamber compliance are characteristic findings. This produces changes in both the diastolic flow velocity at mitral valve level and the isovolumic relaxation time. PW Doppler can be used to measure the diastolic flow velocity across the mitral valve. The sample volume is thereby positioned in the left ventricle, at the level of the tips of the leaflets of the opened mitral valve. Using the Doppler spectral display, the peak early diastolic (V_E) and late diastolic (V_A) velocities can be determined. In Doppler echocardiography, the isovolumic relaxation time is calculated as the time difference between the end of systolic flow in the left ventricular outflow tract and the beginning of diastolic flow across the mitral valve. In normal individuals, the early diastolic peak flow velocity (V_E) is greater than the late diastolic peak flow velocity (V_A): $V_E > V_A$.

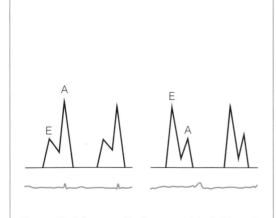

Transmitral flow profile in concentric (left) and eccentric (right) hypertrophy. Findings: reduced ($V_E < V_A$) early diastolic peak flow velocity (left); increased ($V_E < V_A$) early diastolic peak flow velocity (right), and impaired systolic function.

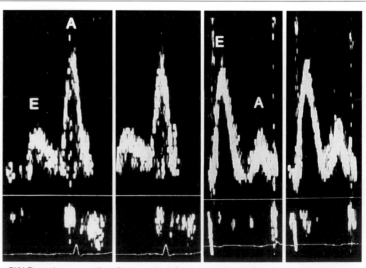

CW Doppler recording from apical four-chamber 2-D echocardiograms.

When left ventricular relaxation is impaired, the isovolumic relaxation time increases and the early diastolic peak flow velocity decreases ($V_E < V_A$). In reduced chamber compliance, the early diastolic flow velocity is decreased ($V_E > V_A$). In the early stages of hypertensive heart disease, which is characterized by concentric left ventricular hypertrophy and normal systolic function, the typical flow velocity pattern of impaired relaxation is usually observed. In the advanced stage of the disease, which is characterized by eccentric hypertrophy and impaired left ventricular function, the typical flow pattern of impaired compliance is found [6].

Increased stiffness of the left ventricle leads to an increase in filling time. Mitral valve closure is thus slow, and the EF slope is diminished. This should not be misinterpreted as an expression of mitral stenosis. In contrast to mitral stenosis, hypertensive heart disease can be identified by the delicate leaflet structure, normal initial opening motion, and normal motion pattern of the posterior leaflet. A further consequence of increased left ventricular stiffness is a compensatory increase in filling pressure, which can lead to dilatation of the left atrium.

Sources of Error and Problems

Doppler-derived flow velocities and their relationships (V_E:V_A) are not constant; they vary with heart rate, blood pressure, preload, and the inotropic state, and can also be influenced by vasodilators. Therefore, one can find smooth transitions and apparent normalization of the flow patterns characteristic of relaxation and compliance abnormalities. Therefore, Doppler echocardiography is often unable to provide a reliable diagnosis of diastolic function [9].

Regression of Left Ventricular Hypertrophy

Left ventricular hypertrophy is associated with an increased risk of cardiac failure [15], increased occurrence of arrhythmias [25], and a worse prognosis [8, 16]. Medical treatment of hypertension can bring about regression of left ventricular hypertrophy. This effect has been confirmed in angiotensin conversion enzyme blockers, calcium antagonists, and sympatholytic agents. No regression has been observed under therapy with vasodilators that increase the heart rate. An ongoing controversy exists on the value of diuretics in causing regression of left ventricular hypertrophy. Echocardiography is the method of choice for performing follow-up studies and for monitoring the results of treatment in patients with left ventricular hypertrophy.

References

1. Angermann CE, Spes CH, Willems S, Dominiak P, Kemkes B, Theisen K. Regression of left ventricular hypertrophy in hypertensive heart transplant recipients treated with enalapril, furosemide, and verapamil. Circulation 1991; 84: 583-593.
2. Blasini R. Neue Entwicklungen auf dem Gebiet der Echokardiografie und Doppler-Kardiografie. Bildgebung/Imaging 1988; 56: 5-18.
3. Blasini R, Schad H, Heimisch W, Denkinger K, Mendler N, Blömer H. Einfluß von Angiotensin-induziertem Hochdruck auf die vaskuläre Compliance großer Arterien: Experimentelle Untersuchungen mit simultaner intravaskulärer Ultraschallbildgebung und Druckmessung Z Kardiol 1992; 81: 39.
4. Blasini R, Lutilsky L, Unger-Gräber B, Blömer H. Different onset of action of Isosorbide Dinitrate and Isosorbide-5-Moninitrate. Europ Heart J 1989; 10: 154.

5. Blasini R, Tiessen V, Töpfer M, Lutilsky L, Blömer H. Streßechokardiografie: Stellenwert zusätzlicher Doppler-echokardiografischer Messungen Z Kardiol 1992; 81: 187.
6. Blasini R, Tiessen V, Schömig A. Functional alterations in left ventricular hypertropy: Diagnosis of impaired diastolic function in patients with hypertension. Clin Invest 1993 (*in press*).
7. Brilla CG, Janicki JS, Weber KT. Cardioreparative effects of lisinopril in rats with genetic hypertension and left ventricular hypertrophy. Circulation 1991; 83: 1771-1779.
8. Cooper RS, Simmons BE, Castaner A, Santhanam V, Ghali J, Mar M. Left ventricular hypertrophy is associated with worse survival independent of ventricular function and number of coronary arteries severely narrowed. Am J Cardiol 1990; 65: 441-445.
9. DeMaria AN, Wisenbaugh TW, Smith MD, Harrison MR, Berk MR. Doppler echocardiographic evaluation of diastolic dysfunction. Circulation 1991; 84: I-228 - I-295.
10. Devereux RB, Lutas EM, Casale PN, Kligfield P, Eisenberg RR, Hammond IW, Miller DH, Reis G, Alderman MH, Larcher JH. Standardization of M-mode echocardiographic left ventricular anatomic measurements. J Am Coll Cardiol 1984; 4: 1222-1230.
11. Fouad FM. Left ventricular diastolic function in hypertensive patients. Circulation 1987; 75: I-48.
12. Frenzel H. Morphologische Befunde bei Rückbildung einer Herzhypertrophie. Z Kardiol 1985; 74: 107-118.
13. Hammond IW, Devereux RB, Alderman MH, Lutas EM, Spitzer MC, Crowley JS, Laragh JH. The prevalence and correlates of echocardiographic left ventricular hypertrophy among employed patients with uncomplicated hypertension. J Am Coll Cardiol 1986; 7: 639-650.
14. Helak JW, Reichek N. Quantitation of human left ventricular mass and volume by two-dimensional echocardiography: in vitro anatomic validation. Circulation 1981; 63: 1398-1407.
15. Kannel WB, Levy D, Cupples LA. Left ventricular hypertrophy and risk of cardiac failure: insights from the Framingham Study. J Cardiovasc Pharmacol 1987; 10: 135-140.
16. Koren MJ, Devereux RB, Casale PN, Savage DD, Laragh JH. Relation of left ventricular mass and geometry to morbidity and mortality in uncomplicated essential hypertension. Ann Intern Med 1991; 114: 345-352.
17. Levy D, Savage DD, Garrison RJ, Anderson KM, Kannel WB, Castelli WP. Echocardiographic criteria for left ventricular hypertrophy: the Framingham Heart Study. Am J Cardiol 1987; 59: 956-960.
18. Motz W, Strauer BE. Rückbildung der hypertensiven Herzhypertrophie durch chronische Angiotensin-Konversionsenzymhemmung. Z Kardiol 1988; 77: 53-60.
19. Panidis IP, Kotler MN, Ren JF, Mintz GS, Ross J, Kalman P. Development and regression of left ventricular hypertrophy. J Am Coll Cardiol 1984; 3: 1309-1320.
20. Pietro DA, Voelkel AG, Ray BJ, Parisi AF. Reproducibility of echocardiography. A study evaluating the variability of serial echocardiographic measurements. Chest 1981; 79: 29-32.
21. Reichek N, Devereux RB. Left ventricular hypertrophy: relationship of anatomic, echocardiographic and electrocardiographic findings. Circulation 1981; 63: 1391-1398.
22. Reichek N, Helak J, Plappert T, Sutton M, Weber KT. Anatomic validation of left ventricular mass estimates from clinical two-dimensional echocardiography: initial results. Circulation 1983; 67: 348-352.
23. Sahn DJ, DeMaria A, Kisslo J, Weyman A. Recommendations regarding quantitation in M-mode echocardiography: results of a survey of echocardiographic measurements. Circulation 1978; 58: 1072-1082.
24. Schiller NB. Two-dimensional echocardiographic determination of left ventricular volume, systolic function and mass. Circulation 1991; 84: I-280-I-287.
25. Siegel D, Cheitlin MD, Black DM, Seeley D, Hearst N, Hulley SB. Risk of ventricular arrhythmias in hypertensive men with left ventricular hypertrophy. Am J Cardiol 1990; 65: 742-747.
26. Strauer BE, Mahmoud MA, Bayer F, Bohn I, Motz U. Reversal of left ventricular hypertrophy and improvement of cardiac function in man by nifedipine. Eur Heart J 1984 5: 53-60.
27. Sugishita Y, Iida K, Yukisada K, Itto I. Cardiac determinants of regression of left ventricular hypertrophy in essential hypertension with antihypertensive treatment. J Am Coll Cardiol 1990; 15: 665-671.
28. Wyatt HL, Haendchen R V, Meerbaum S, Corday E. Assessment of quantitative methods for 2-dimensional echocardiography. Am J Cardiol 1983; 52: 396-401.

In transthoracic echocardiography, the heart must be scanned from multiple transducer positions to diagnose and assess diseases of the aorta. Left parasternal scans are used to visualize the proximal ascending aorta and the middle segment of the descending thoracic aorta; suprasternal scans are used to visualize the aortic arch and the proximal descending thoracic aorta; subcostal scans are used to visualize the distal descending thoracic aorta.

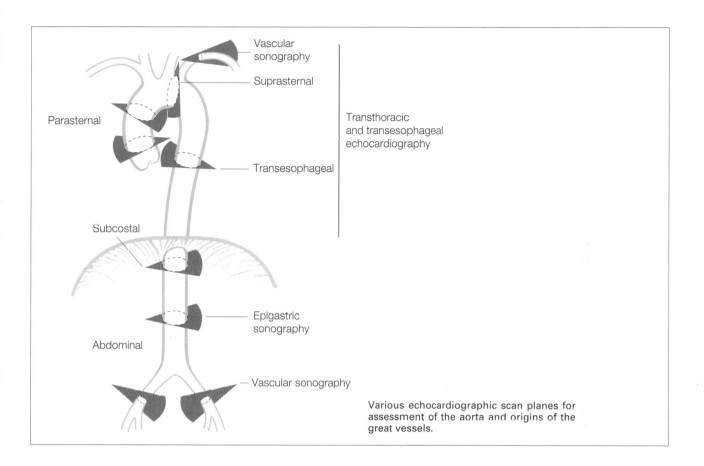

Various echocardiographic scan planes for assessment of the aorta and origins of the great vessels.

Still, in only around 70% of all cases did transthoracic echocardiography correctly diagnose distal aortic dissection - the most significant pathological change in the descending aorta [3, 10]. Furthermore, sonographic studies of the cerebral supply vessels, the abdominal aorta, and the iliac vessels must also be made in order to define the total extent of dissection.

Transesophageal echocardiography has significantly improved the diagnosis of aortic disease. It provides the following advantages:

1. Better morphological resolution because the aorta is closer to the esophageal echoscope.
2. High-frequency transducers (5 MHz) can be used.

Transesophageal color Doppler registration of blood flow in the aorta is also possible. However, scans of the ascending and descending aorta usually cannot be utilized for quantitative assessments, because the Doppler beam is situated approximately 90° to the direction of flow. The different segments of the aorta can be visualized is short-axis (transverse), long-axis (longitudinal), and multiplane views. Cross-sectional images of the aorta are obtained from the short-axis plane. Usually, the beam cuts the aortic valve tangentially, due to the curved course of the aorta.

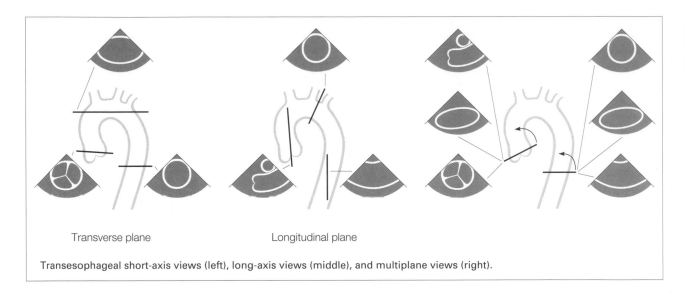

Transverse plane   Longitudinal plane

Transesophageal short-axis views (left), long-axis views (middle), and multiplane views (right).

The ascending aorta can be viewed in cross section around 3 to 4 cm above the valve, at the bifurcation of the pulmonary artery. The more cranial segments of the ascending aorta cannot be visualized, because the interposed left main bronchus and trachea obscure them from view.

Between 6 to 8 cm of the ascending aorta can be continuously visualized in long-axis views, or in planes tangential to the long axis. With multiplane transesophageal echocardiography systems, short and long-axis views can be individually optimized, and a multitude of tangential planes between the two extreme positions can be scanned. Multiplane transesophageal echocardiography also allows better differentiation of artifacts that frequently occur when imaging ectatic vessels in the short-axis plane.

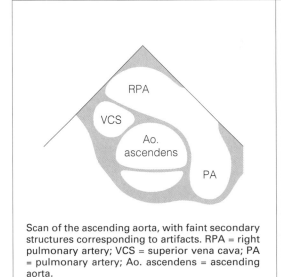

Scan of the ascending aorta, with faint secondary structures corresponding to artifacts. RPA = right pulmonary artery; VCS = superior vena cava; PA = pulmonary artery; Ao. ascendens = ascending aorta.

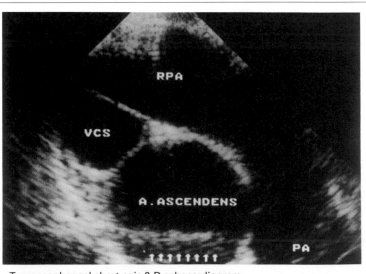

Transesophageal short-axis 2-D echocardiogram.

In transesophageal echocardiography the descending aorta can be visualized in a number of different short-axis planes, similar to computed tomography.

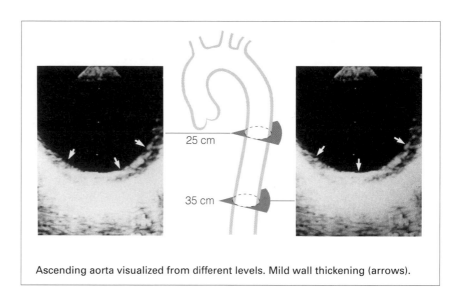

Ascending aorta visualized from different levels. Mild wall thickening (arrows).

The echoscope is advanced into the stomach, then the descending aorta is followed from the subdiaphragmatic region up to the aortic arch, *i.e.*, from ca. 42 cm below the incisors to 25 cm below the incisors. It is important to remember that the relationship between the descending aorta and esophagus changes.

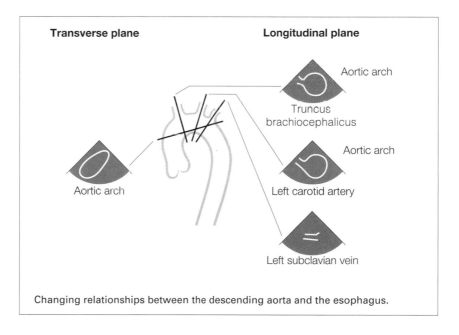

Changing relationships between the descending aorta and the esophagus.

The aorta lies in front of the esophagus at the level of the aortic arch, whereas the esophagus lies in front of the aorta at the level of the diaphragm. Therefore, progressive rotation of the transducer is essential when retracting the transducer [22].

Between 5 to 6 cm of the descending aorta can be continuously visualized in long-axis scans. However, only ca. 1 cm of the aortic wall proximal to the transducer is seen, whereas 5 to 6 cm of the distal wall can be seen.

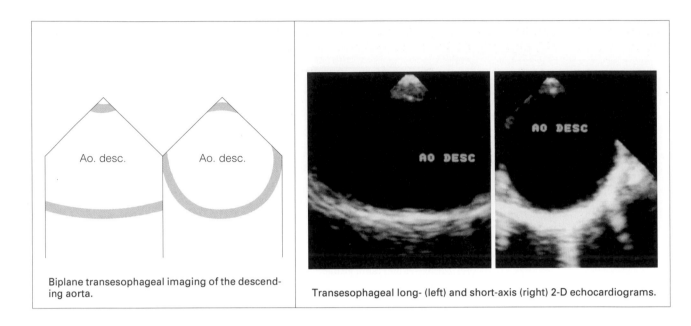

Biplane transesophageal imaging of the descending aorta.

Transesophageal long- (left) and short-axis (right) 2-D echocardiograms.

In addition to permitting individual optimization of the above-mentioned planes, multiplane transesophageal echocardiography also permits imaging of oblique and tangential planes (see above figure). Short-axis scans tangentially visualize the long axis of the aortic arch, whereas long-axis scans provide cross-sectional images of the aortic arch. Long-axis scans also permit visualization of the origins of the cerebral supply vessels [1, 19].

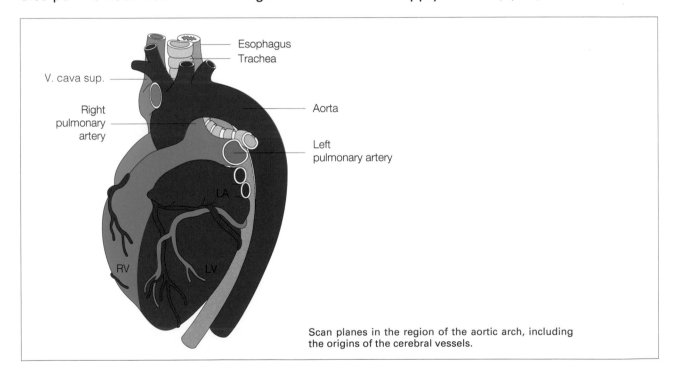

Scan planes in the region of the aortic arch, including the origins of the cerebral vessels.

The primary feature of multiplane transesophageal echocardiography is individual optimization of the above-mentioned scan planes.

In a collective of adults, the diameter of the aorta was shown to increase linearly with increasing age by ca. 35%, and the cross-sectional area increased by ca. 90% [15].

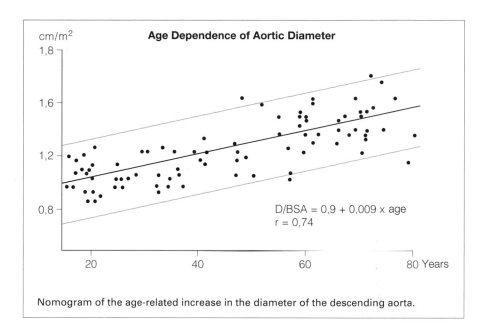

Nomogram of the age-related increase in the diameter of the descending aorta.

The wall thickness also increased with increasing age by up to 40%.

Aortic diameter / BSA	=	$0.9 + 0.009 \times age$ (cm/m²)
Aortic wall thickness	=	$0.3 + 0.0025 \times age$ (cm)

In these measurements, the maximum width of the aorta was 3.6 cm.

Ectasia of the aorta (diameter > 3.6 cm) and localized fusiform aneurysms can be diagnosed by biplane transesophageal echocardiography, and can be viewed and measured in the short and long-axis planes.

Thrombus may be included in saccular aneurysms.

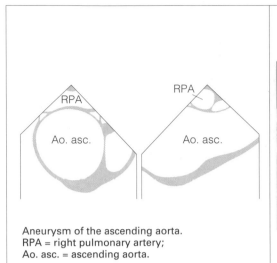

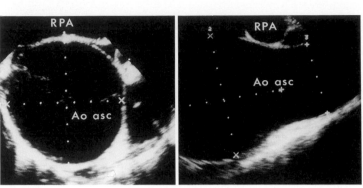

Aneurysm of the ascending aorta.
RPA = right pulmonary artery;
Ao. asc. = ascending aorta.

Transesophageal short-axis (left) and long-axis (right) 2-D echocardiograms.

| 19. | Diseases of the Aorta |
| 19.3 | Atherosclerosis |

Atherosclerotic wall changes are frequently found in the descending aorta and in the aortic arch. They can be divided into three grades of severity [12, 25]:

Grade I	Echo-intense areas in the region of the vessel inner wall with absence of changes in the inner wall contours
Grade II	Extensive plaques that protrude into the lumen
Grade III	Complicated plaques that extend throughout the entire thickness of the aortic wall, associated with wall thickening and thrombus

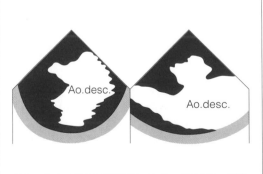

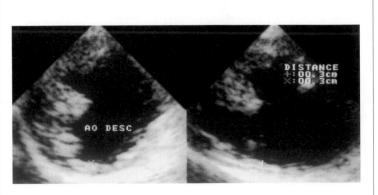

Extensive atherosclerotic wall changes with thrombotic masses that protrude into the lumen.

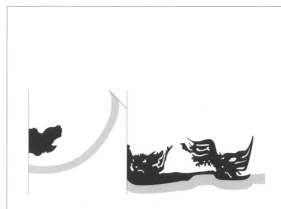

Thrombus in the descending aorta. Floating motion detected in M-mode recording (right).

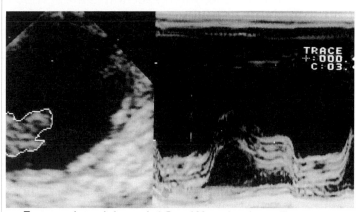

Transesophageal short-axis 2-D and M-mode echocardiograms.

| 19. | Diseases of the Aorta |
| 19.4 | Aortic Dissection |

Aortic dissections are classified as proximal (DeBakey types I and II, Stanford type A) or distal (DeBakey type III, Stanford type B). Because the mortality rate in acute proximal dissection is particularly high, a definitive diagnosis should be established as quickly as possible. Dissections should be further classified as communicating or noncommunicating, as the prognosis in these dissections varies [7].

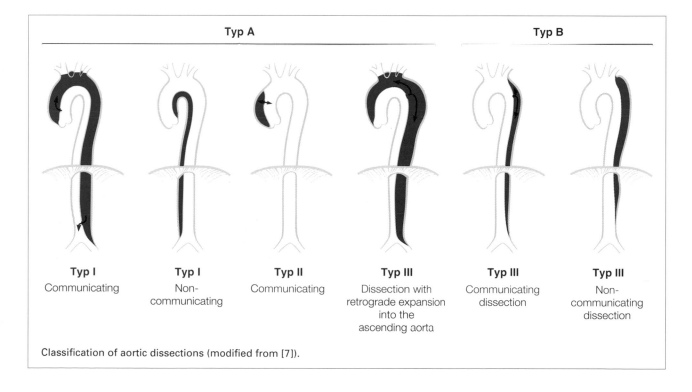

Classification of aortic dissections (modified from [7]).

Also, knowing whether the dissection is antegrade or retrograde is of importance when planning surgical therapy. Proximal dissections require immediate surgery, whereas patients with distal dissections can usually be managed with conservative medical therapy. Patients with imminent rupture or with hemorrhagic pleural effusion or a mediastinal hematoma are exceptions. Mortality is particularly high in these patients.

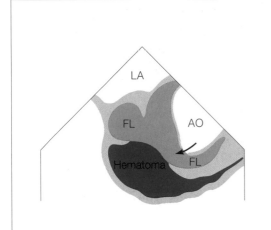

Acute dissection of the ascending aorta with anterior mediastinal hematoma.
TL = true lumen; FL = false lumen;
LA = left atrium.

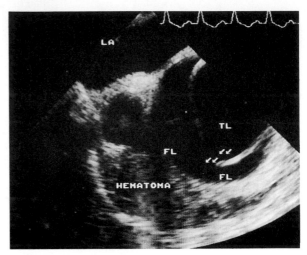

Transesophageal short-axis 2-D echocardiogram.

The primary goal of the diagnostic examination in patients with suspected aortic dissection is to confirm or to safely exclude the presence of dissection by identifying the dissection membrane. When aortic dissection is found, determination of the extent of dissection is important for treatment planning. The lumen is thereby divided into two parts - the true lumen and the false lumen.

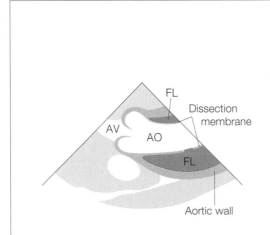

Dissection membrane in the ascending aorta.
AV = aortic valve; TL = true lumen;
FL = false lumen.

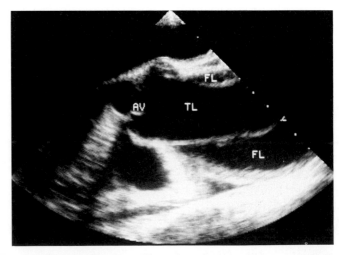

Transesophageal 2-D echocardiography using a multiplane transducer.

Echocardiography also facilitates the detection of complications such as pericardial effusion, pleural effusion, aortic insufficiency, and mediastinal hematoma.

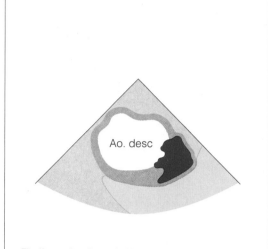

Findings: Aortic wall thickening and mural hematoma. Pleural effusion.

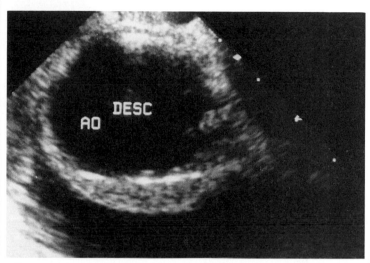

Transesophageal short-axis 2-D echocardiogram.

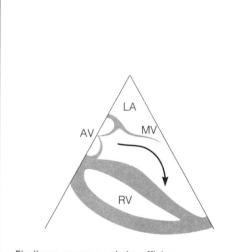

Findings: severe aortic insufficiency.

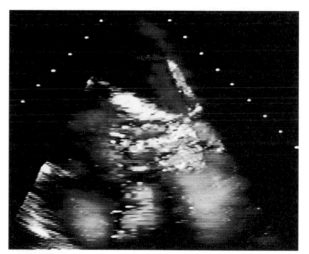

Transesophageal short-axis 2-D echocardiogram with color flow imaging.

Bedside echocardiographic examinations in the intensive care unit with utilization of the transesophageal access were shown to be more sensitive and specific for detection of acute aortic dissection than angiography and computed tomography [6]. Therefore, a transesophageal echocardiographic diagnosis of acute proximal dissection obviate the need for further diagnostic screening before initiating surgical treatment. In subacute or chronic cases, magnetic resonance imaging is recommended as a complementary diagnostic technique. Magnetic resonance imaging permits visualization and assessment of the entire aorta and the origins of the great vessel origins [11, 18].

In acute communicating dissections, the dissection membrane often exhibits marked motion amplitude. In some cases, the dissection membrane is virtually circumferential.

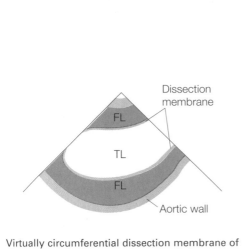

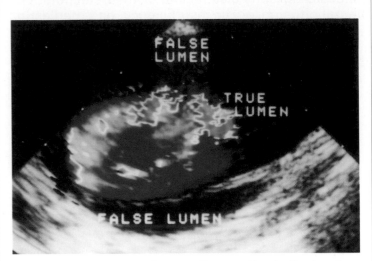

Virtually circumferential dissection membrane of the aortic arch. Flow is registered only in the true lumen.

Transesophageal long-axis 2-D echocardiogram with color flow imaging.

One note of caution: indistinctly contoured, faint secondary echoes in the region of the aortic root, seen primarily in ectatic vessels, correspond to echoes, and should not be misinterpreted. One special type of incipient noncommunicating dissection is characterized by hemorrhage into the wall that leads to wall thickening of > 7 cm without evidence of a dissection membrane. This is called intramural hemorrhage or intramural hematoma. Close follow-up monitoring is necessary in these cases, ca. 30% of these cases lead to typical aortic dissection, and another 30% lead to rupture of the aorta [17, 26].

In the majority of cases, the dissection membrane divides the true lumen from the false lumen. Characteristic findings are increased expansion of the true lumen in systole, and compression in diastole. The true lumen is usually narrower than the false lumen. Aneurysmal dilatation of the false lumen can occur in chronic dissections [14]. In the false lumen, particularly in chronic aortic dissection, spontaneous echocardiographic contrast and partial thrombosis is frequently found.

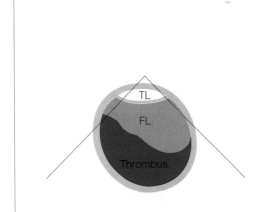

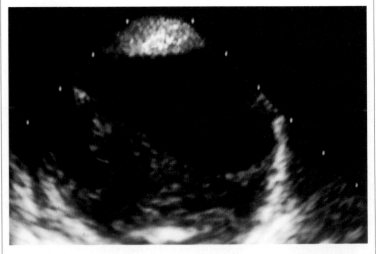

Chronic dissection of the descending aorta with detection of fluid in the compromised true lumen and the aneurysmally dilated false lumen. Partial thrombosis can be seen within the false lumen.

Transesophageal short-axis 2-D echocardiogram with color flow imaging.

Communication between the true lumen and the false lumen can be demonstrated by Doppler color flow imaging in approximately 80% of all cases, as compared to only ca. 20% using two-dimensional echocardiography. Multiple communications are common. It has been shown that flow across these communications in multiphasic in 80% of all cases. In other words, blood flows from the true lumen to the false lumen in systole, and one or more flow reversals occur in diastole, depending on the instantaneous pressure difference between the true lumen and the false lumen.

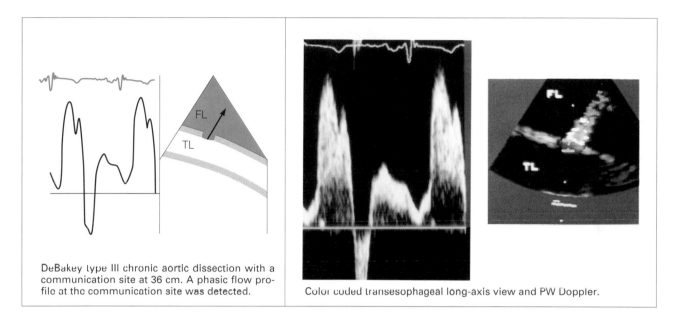

DeBakey type III chronic aortic dissection with a communication site at 36 cm. A phasic flow profile at the communication site was detected.

Color coded transesophageal long-axis view and PW Doppler.

In patients with a postoperatively persistent, large proximal communications in the aortic arch or in the proximal descending aorta, the development of thrombus in the false lumen is usually mild or even absent. These patients have a higher rate of complications. Spontaneous healing of chronic distal dissections under general medical therapy is possible [7, 14].

Using biplane or multiplane transesophageal echocardiography, it now is possible to detect the exact pathomechanism of aortic insufficiency (which occurs in 80 to 100% of all proximal dissections) and to make a semiquantitative assessment of severity in vivo [20].

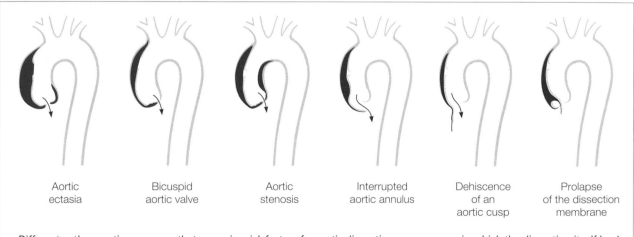

| Aortic ectasia | Bicuspid aortic valve | Aortic stenosis | Interrupted aortic annulus | Dehiscence of an aortic cusp | Prolapse of the dissection membrane |

Different pathogenetic processes that comprise risk factors for aortic dissection, or processes in which the dissection itself leads to aortic insufficiency.

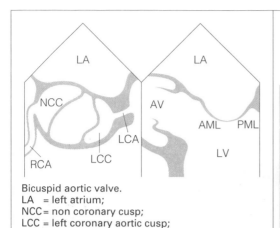

Bicuspid aortic valve.
LA = left atrium;
NCC= non coronary cusp;
LCC = left coronary aortic cusp;
AML= anterior mitral leaflet;
PML= posterior mitral leaflet;
LV = left ventricle;
LCA = left coronary artery;
AV = aortic valve.

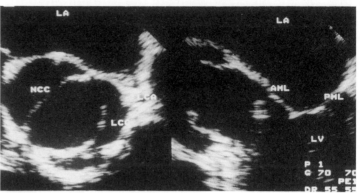

Transesophageal long- and short-axis (right) 2-D echocardiograms.

A bicuspid aortic valve is found in ca. 10% of all cases of aortic dissection. Other predisposing conditions are annuloectasia of the ascending aorta, as in Marfan's syndrome, and aortic stenosis with poststenotic dilatation. The dissection process can cause dehiscence of the aortic annulus, malcoaptation of the valve cusps, or prolapse of the dissection membrane into the left ventricular outflow tract. Identification of the pathomechanism is important for planning surgical therapy, because valve preservation by surgically resuspending the aortic valve has lead to better long-term results. In particular, this is due to the avoidance of anticoagulation-related bleeding complications associated with mechanical valve prostheses. Valve replacement is still necessary in annuloectasia and associated aortic valve disease. Transesophageal echocardiography is also useful for serial follow-up of patients with aortic dissection, *i.e.*, for monitoring vessel grafts and anastomoses and to assess the competence of the aortic valve.

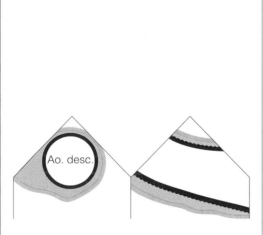

Graft replacement of the descending aorta due to DeBakey type III aortic dissection. Follow-up scan.

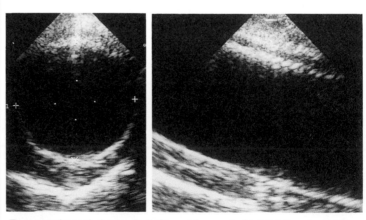

Transesophageal short-axis (left) and long-axis (right) 2-D echocardiograms.

Initially, follow-up examinations are performed every six months. After one year, they can be performed annually. A particular purpose of the follow-up examination is to assess the width of the false lumen, where aneurysms develop in approximately 30% of all cases.

In echocardiograms of the descending aorta obtained from the suprasternal notch, coarctation of the aorta (stenosis of the aortic isthmus) can be detected in 90% of all cases. In ca. 80% of all children and in 50% of all adults, the gradient across the aortic stenosis can calculated according to the Bernoulli equation using CW Doppler-derived measurements obtained from the suprasternal position [9, 13]. Forward flow into the descending aorta that persists into diastole is a conspicuous finding.

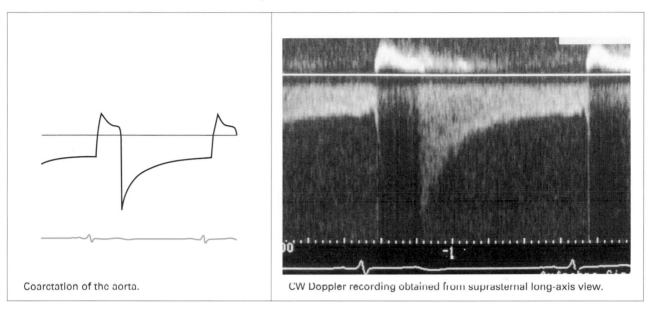

Coarctation of the aorta. | CW Doppler recording obtained from suprasternal long-axis view.

However, the Bernoulli equation can be used only in short stenoses. Furthermore, the prestenotic velocity must also be taken into consideration:

$$p_1 - p_2 = 4 \, (v_1^2 - v_2^2).$$

The exact location and morphological features of the stenosis can only rarely be assessed from the suprasternal notch, due to the curved course of the aorta. Using short-axis scans, and particularly with multiplane transesophageal echocardiography, assessment of the stenotic vessel segment and diameter and area measurements are possible [23].

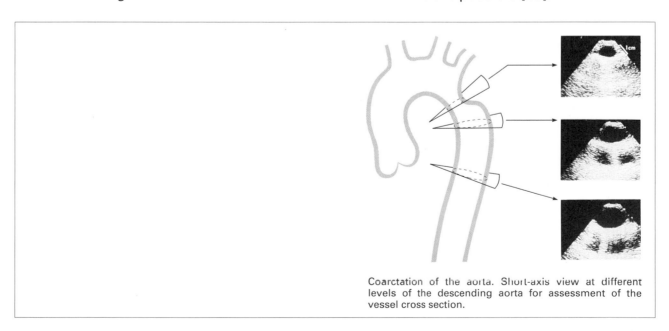

Coarctation of the aorta. Short-axis view at different levels of the descending aorta for assessment of the vessel cross section.

Interventional angioplasty of the aorta should also be monitored using transesophageal echocardiography, because angioplasty causes temporarily raised intimal areas or dissections in up to 50% of all cases [4]. Such surgical interventions as aortic graft, anastomosis, or bypass surgery can also be monitored by means of transesophageal echocardiography.

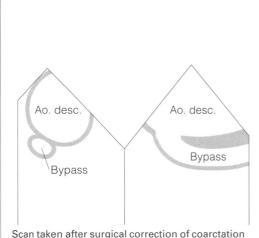

Scan taken after surgical correction of coarctation of the aorta, demonstrating the para-aortic bypass.

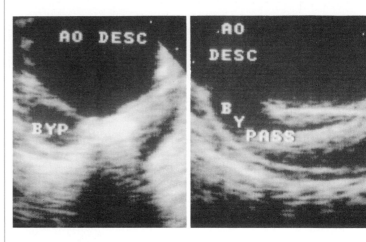

Transesophageal short- (left) and long-axis (right) 2-D echocardiograms.

References

1. Bansal RC, Shakudo M, Shah PM. Biplane transesophageal echocardiography: technique, image orientation, and preliminary experience in 131 patients. J Am Soc Echo 1990; 3: 348-366.
2. Börner N, Erbel R, Braun B, Henkel B, Meyer J, Rumpelt J. Diagnosis of aortic dissection by transesophageal echocardiography. Am J Cardiol 1984; 54: 1157-1158.
3. Bubenheimer P, Schmuzinger M, Roskamp H. Ein- und zweidimensionale Echokardiographie bei Aneurysmen und Dissektionen der Aorta. Herz 1980; 5: 226-240.
4. Erbel R, Bednarczyk I, Pop T, Todt M, Henrichs KJ, Brunier A, Thelen M, Meyer J. Detection of dissection of the aortic intima and media after angioplasty of coarctation of the aorta. Circulation 1990; 81: 805-814.
5. Erbel R, Börner N, Steller D, Brunier J, Thelen M, Pfeiffer C, Mohr-Kahaly S, Oelert H, Meyer J. Detection of aortic dissection by transesophageal echocardiography. Br Heart J 1987; 58: 45-51.
6. Erbel R, Engberding R, Daniel W, Roelandt J, Visser C, Rennollet H, the European Cooperative Study Group for Echocardiography. Echocardiography in diagnosis of aortic dissection. Lancet 1989; 1: 457-461.
7. Erbel R, Oelert H, Meyer J, Puth M, Mohr-Kahaly S, Hausmann D, Daniel W, Maffei S, Caruso A, Covino FE et al. Effect of medical and surgical therapy on aortic dissection evaluated by transesophageal echocardiography. Implications for prognosis and therapy. The European Cooperative Study Group for Echocardiography. Circulation 1993; 87: 1604-1615.
8. Gore I, Seiwert VJ. Dissecting aneurysms of the aorta: pathologic aspects: an analysis of eighty-five fatal cases. Arch Pathol 1952; 53: 121-141.
9. Huhta JC, Gutgesell HP, Latson LA, Huffines FD. Two-dimensional echocardiographic assessment of the aorta in infants and children with congenital heart disease. Circulation 1984; 70: 417-424.
10. Iliceto S, Ettorre G, Francioso G, Antonelli G, Biaco G, Rizzon P. Diagnosis of aneurysm of the thoracic aorta. Comparison between two non-invasive techniques: two-dimensional echocardiography and computed tomography. Eur Heart J 1984; 5: 545-555.

11. Just M, Mohr-Kahaly S, Kreitner KF, Grebe P, Erbel R, Meyer J, Thelen M. Magnetresonanztomographie bei chronischer Aortendissektion. Fortschr Röntgenstr 1993; 158: 109-114.
12. Karalis DG, Chandrasekaran K, Victor MF, Ross JJ jr, Mintz GS. Recognition and embolic potential of intraaortic atherosclerotic debris. J Am Coll Cardiol 1991; 17: 73-78.
13. Marx GR, Allen HD, Accuracy and pitfalls of Doppler evaluation of the pressuregradient in aortic coarctation. J Am Coll Cardiol 1986; 7: 1379-1385.
14. Mohr-Kahaly S, Erbel R, Rennollet H, Wittlich N, Drexler M, Oelert H, Meyer J. Ambulatory follow-up of aortic dissection by transesophageal two-dimensional and color-coded Doppler echocardiography. Circulation 1989; 80: 24-33.
15. Mohr-Kahaly S, Erbel R, Scharf N, Meyer J. Age related normal values for the descending thoracic aorta analyzed by biplane transesophageal echocardiography. J Am Coll Cardiol 1992; 19 (suppl A): 280A.
16. Mohr-Kahaly S, Erbel R, Steller D, Börner N, Drexler M, Meyer J. Aortic dissection detected by transesophageal echocardiography. Int J Cardiac Imag 1986; 2: 31-35.
17. Mohr-Kahaly S, Puth M, Erbel R, Meyer J. Intramural hematoma visualized by transesophageal echocardiography - an early sign of aortic dissection. J Am Coll Cardiol 1991; 17 (suppl A): 20A.
18. Nienaber C, Spielmann RP, von Kodolitsch Y, Siglow V, Piepho A, Jaup T, Nicolas V, Weber P, Triebel HJ, Bleifeld W. Diagnosis of thoracic aortic dissection: magnetic resonance imaging versus transesophageal echocardiography. Circulation 1992; 85: 434-447.
19. Omoto R, Kyo S, Matsumura M, Shah PM, Adachi H, Matsunaka T. Biplane color Doppler transesophageal echocardiography: its impact on cardiovascular surgery and further technological process in the probe, a matrix phased-array biplane probe. Echocardiography 1989; 6: 423-430.
20. Perry GJ, Helmcke F, Nanda NC, Byard C, Soto B. Evaluation of aortic insufficiency by Doppler flow mapping. J Am Coll Cardiol 1987; 9: 952-959.
21. Roberts CS, Roberts WC. Dissection of the aorta associated with congenital malformation of the aortic valve. J Am Coll Cardiol 1991; 17: 712-716.
22. Seward JB, Khandheria BK, Oh JK, Abel MD, Hughes RW jr, Edwards WD, Nichols BA, Freeman WK, Tajik AJ. Transesophageal echocardiography: technique, anatomic correlations, implementation, and clinical applications. Mayo Clinic Proc 1988; 63: 649-680.
23. Stern H, Erbel R, Schreiner G, Henkel B, Meyer J. Coarctation of the aorta: quantitative analysis by transesophageal echocardiography. Echocardiography 1987; 4: 387-395.
24. Taams MA, Gussenhoven WJ, Schippers LA, Roelandt J, van Herwerden LA, Bos E, de Jong N, Bom N. The value of transesophageal echocardiography for diagnosis of thoracic aorta pathology. Eur Heart J 1988; 9: 1308-1316.
25. Tunick PA, Kronzon I. Protruding atherosclerotic plaque in the aortic arch of patients with systemic embolization: a new finding seen by transesophageal echocardiography. Am Heart J 1990; 120: 658-660.
26. Zotz RJ, Erbel R, Meyer J. Noncommunicating intramural hematoma: an indication of developing aortic dissection? J Am Soc Echocardiogr 1991; 4: 636-638.

Pulmonary hypertension has many features that distinguish it from systemic hypertension. It is much more difficult to diagnose, and can usually be quantitated only by invasive methods (right heart catheterization). Therefore, serial follow-up at close intervals is hardly possible. With the help of echocardiography, new methods have been developed that permit not only semiquantitative assessment, but also quantitative assessment of pulmonary artery pressure. Echocardiographic techniques can be performed as bedside procedures, and they expand the realm of conventional diagnostics.

The differential diagnosis of pulmonary hypertension is multiple. Acute pulmonary hypertension in the form of pulmonary embolism is numerically significant. In Germany, between 10,000 to 20,000 individuals still die of this disease each year [12, 23].

Secondary pulmonary hypertension (*e.g.* obstructive or restrictive respiratory disorders), coronary artery disease, and systemic hypertension are among the most common heart diseases in patients over 60 years of age. The development of pulmonary hypertension determines the prognosis of chronic obstructive respiratory tract disease [3]. Pulmonary hypertension is reported to reduce the two-year survival rate to 40% [29].

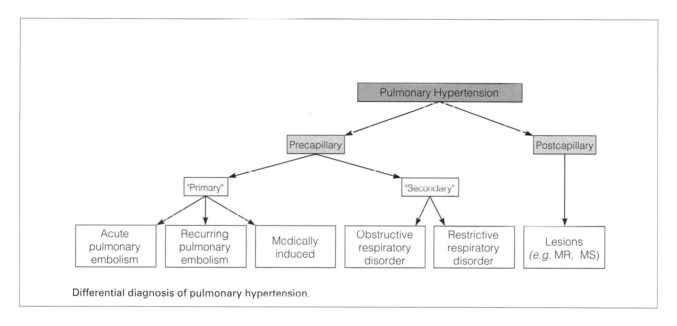

Differential diagnosis of pulmonary hypertension.

Generally, pulmonary artery pressure is said to be elevated when the mean pressure exceeds 20 mmHg at rest, and when the systolic pulmonary artery pressure exceeds 30 mmHg at rest [16, 20]. Echocardiographic techniques, regardless of whether semiquantitative or quantitative, are indirect diagnostic techniques. Therefore, they provide only an estimate of pulmonary artery pressure.

20. **Cor Pulmonale and Pulmonary Embolism**
20.1 **Right Ventricle**

An increase in pulmonary artery pressure affects the motion pattern of the pulmonary valve. In M-mode echocardiography, the reduced atrial systolic motion is expressed as reduced A wave amplitude. A second M-mode marker is mesosystolic closure of the pulmonary valve.

Increased diameter of the pulmonary trunk may be the first indication of pulmonary hypertension. These structures can only seldom be visualized satisfactorily in patients where scanning conditions are poor.

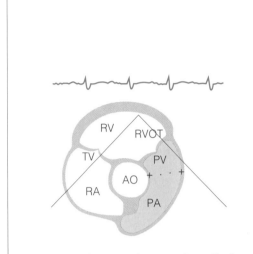

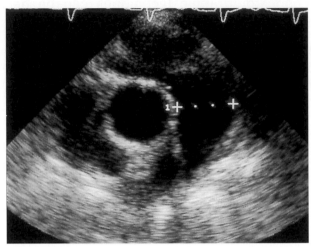

Extensive pulmonary hypertension. Findings: dilatation of the pulmonary trunk.

Parasternal short-axis view showing the right ventricular outflow tract and the pulmonary trunk.

The complex geometry of the right ventricle poses a major problem in assessment and measurement of the right chamber of the heart. The right ventricle can be broken down into separate inflow and outflow parts. The main part is crescent-shaped in cross section. Additional complicating factors are its retrosternal location and anterior position with respect to the left ventricle. The position of the right ventricle also varies with the axis of the heart. In light of these factors, echocardiographic assessment of the right ventricle has seen little standardization and is only rarely part of the routine echocardiographic examination. Possibilities for using echocardiography for assessment of the right ventricle will be described below. Those with further interest may refer to the literature [2, 8, 21, 23, 27].

Right Ventricular Inflow Tract

The right ventricular inflow tract (RVIT) is situated between the tricuspid valve ring and the proximal part of the right ventricle. The long (RVIT1) and the short (RVIT3) axes of the right ventricular inflow tract (RVIT, one-third the distance from the annulus to the right ventricular apex) can be determined in parasternal long-axis scans and in four-chamber scans.

Reference ranges for the right ventricular inflow tract				
	Mean		Standard Deviation (cm)	Range (cm)
RVIT1	4.5	±	0.5	3.7 - 5.4
RVIT3	2.4	±	0.4	1.5 - 3.0

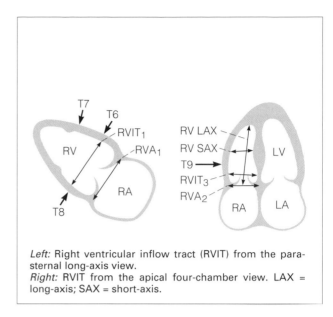

Left: Right ventricular inflow tract (RVIT) from the parasternal long-axis view.

Right: RVIT from the apical four-chamber view. LAX = long-axis; SAX = short-axis.

Right Ventricular Outflow Tract

The dimensions of the right ventricular outflow tract (RVOT) can be assessed well in parasternal long (RVOT1) and short-axis (RVOT3) echocardiograms recorded directly below the pulmonary valve.

Reference ranges for the right ventricular outflow tract

	Mean		Standard Deviation (cm)	Range (cm)
RVOT1	2.2	±	0.3	1.8 - 3.0
RVOT3	2.0	±	0.3	1.5 - 2.6

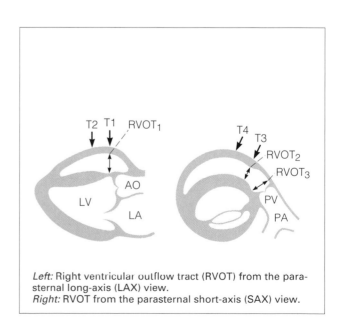

Left: Right ventricular outflow tract (RVOT) from the parasternal long-axis (LAX) view.

Right: RVOT from the parasternal short-axis (SAX) view.

Dimensions of the Main Body of the Right Ventricle

The main body of the right ventricle is measured in the apical four-chamber view (long axis = RV LAX, short axis = RV SAX):

Reference ranges for the main body of the right ventricle				
	Mean		Standard Deviation (cm)	Range (cm)
RV LAX	4.4	±	0.4	3.6 - 5.4
RV SAX	1.8	±	0.2	1.4 - 2.2

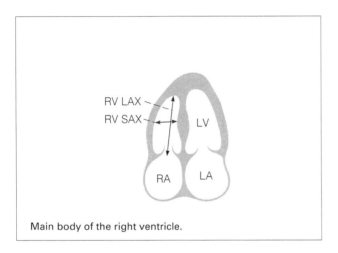

Main body of the right ventricle.

Right Ventricular Wall Thicknesses

The figures show different sampling sites for determination of the thickness of the fight ventricular free wall. T1 - T5 are measurements from the region of the right ventricular outflow tract; T6 - T10 are measurements from the region of the right ventricular inflow tract and from the main body of the right ventricle.

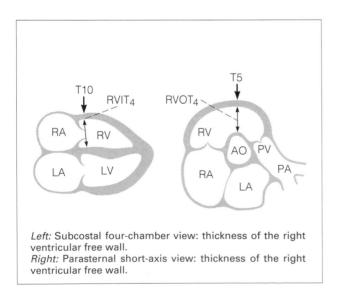

Left: Subcostal four-chamber view: thickness of the right ventricular free wall.
Right: Parasternal short-axis view: thickness of the right ventricular free wall.

Naturally, not all of these sampling points are investigated in a routine examination. T1, T2, and T9 are commonly used sampling points. The right ventricular wall thickness in the middle segment usually does not exceed 4 mm in normals, but can be as much as 7 mm in isolated cases. Right ventricular wall thicknesses of more than 7 mm can reliably be interpreted as pathological. Right ventricular enlargement or hypertrophy may indicate an increase in pulmonary artery pressure, which should be investigated in consecutive examinations.

| 20. | Cor Pulmonale and Pulmonary Embolism |
| 20.2 | Pulmonary Embolism |

Intra-atrial or intraventricular thrombus may occur secondary to deep leg vein thrombosis, and usually requires immediate therapeutic intervention. Thrombi in the pulmonary vascular bed can be directly visualized from the suprasternal notch. This provides a reliable noninvasive diagnosis of embolism.

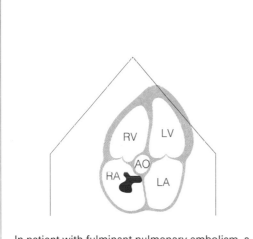

In patient with fulminant pulmonary embolism, a large thrombus is found in the right atrium, close to the interatrial septum.

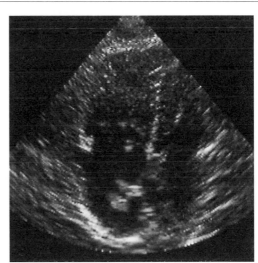

Apical four-chamber view.

Hypokinetic to akinetic right ventricular wall motion as an expression of diminished left ventricular filling is another echocardiographic sign of pulmonary embolism. Additionally, paradoxical septal motion can be detected in many cases [1, 4, 6, 12].

20.	Cor Pulmonale and Pulmonary Embolism
20.3	Semiquantitation of
	Pulmonary Hypertension

Pulmonary valve acceleration time is defined as the time from opening of the pulmonary valve until the time of peak transvalvular flow velocity. The acceleration time is significantly reduced (< 90 ms) in patient with pulmonary hypertension.

20.   **Cor Pulmonale and Pulmonary Embolism**   766
20.3   **Semiquantitation of**
        Pulmonary Hypertension

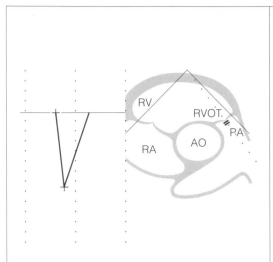

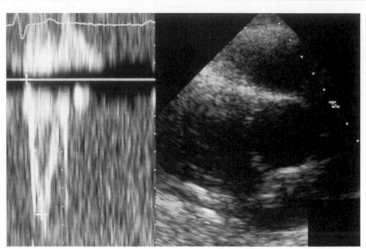

Significantly reduced acceleration time; dome-like flow profile.

PW Doppler and parasternal short-axis 2-D echocardiogram of the RV outflow tract. Systole.

This reduction in acceleration time is due to increased stiffness and impaired capacity of the pulmonary vascular tree. The flow profile reveals a dome-like pattern, as compared to the triangular flow profile seen in patients with normal pulmonary artery pressure [16].

Other semiquantitative techniques, *i.e.* for determination of right ventricular isovolumic relaxation time or of right ventricular pre-ejection time, are less specific and are hard to reproduce [7, 17, 27].

Additional techniques are centered around the flow profiles in the peripheral veins, *i.e.* the inferior vena cava and the hepatic veins. Flow relationships in the inferior vena cava or in the large hepatic veins provide indirect information about the hemodynamics of the right ventricle. The presence of tricuspid insufficiency can be determined by indirect echocardiographic evidence. It is even possible to differentiate between mild and severe tricuspid insufficiency.

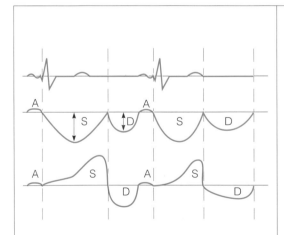

Flow relationships in the hepatic veins and inferior vena cava in mild to severe tricuspid insufficiency. Hepatic veins exhibit systolic-diastolic pendular flow.

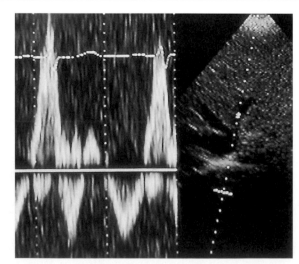

PW Doppler recording and 2-D echocardiogram of the liver.

Evaluation of tricuspid regurgitation by pulsed-wave (PW) Doppler blood flow patterns in the hepatic veins is helpful in patients with poor parasternal and apical imaging windows (*e.g.* patients with pulmonary emphysema), where the subcostal position provides the only suitable portal. The disadvantage of this method is that it can provide only qualitative, not quantitative, information [13, 19, 21].

Normal flow in the inferior vena cava is directed away from the transducer and, thus, produces a negative wave. Flow in the vena cava has three components (A, S, D):

- Positive flow in late diastole due to atrial contraction (A wave),
- Negative systolic wave as an expression of atrial relaxation and shifting of the valve plane (S wave), and
- Negative diastolic wave as an expression of passive right ventricular filling (D wave).

In the presence of mild tricuspid insufficiency, the amplitude of the antegrade systolic flow velocity is diminished. In severe tricuspid insufficiency, the negative systolic wave is replaced by a retrograde positive systolic wave (positive S wave, type 3).

When right ventricular compliance is impaired, the normally negative diastolic wave is replaced by a retrograde positive diastolic wave. The magnitude of the Doppler shift (S, D) sufficiently correlated with right atrial and right ventricular diastolic pressure. A quantitative assessment of pulmonary artery pressure cannot be derived from this.

The flow profile in the hepatic vein corresponds largely with that of the inferior vena cava.

| 20. | Cor Pulmonale and Pulmonary Embolism |
| 20.4 | Quantitation of Pulmonary Hypertension |

Continuous-wave (CW) Doppler enables quantitative assessment of pulmonary artery pressure. Right ventricular to right atrial pressure gradients or pulmonary artery to right ventricular pressure gradients can be detected based on the presence of a regurgitant jet across the tricuspid valve or pulmonary valve. A regurgitant jet across the tricuspid valve can be found in 50 to 70% of the normal population, and across the tricuspid valve in 30 to 50% [30]. The incidence of regurgitant jets is increased in patients with pulmonary hypertension [10, 11, 18, 25, 26, 30].

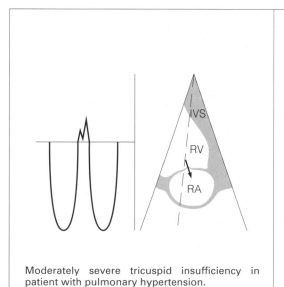

Moderately severe tricuspid insufficiency in patient with pulmonary hypertension.

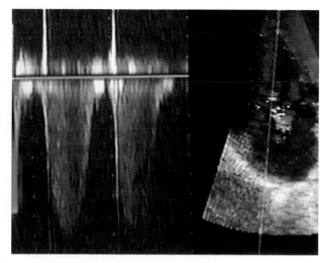

Color coded apical four-chamber view. CW Doppler

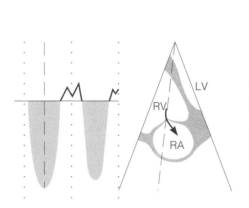

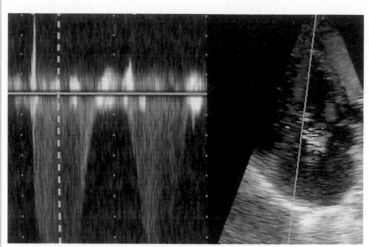

Tricuspid insufficiency in pulmonary hypertension, with a regurgitant jet
(peak velocity = 4.02 m/s).

Color coded apical four-chamber view. CW Doppler

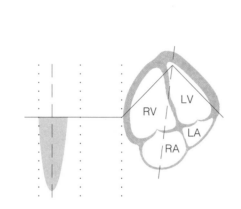

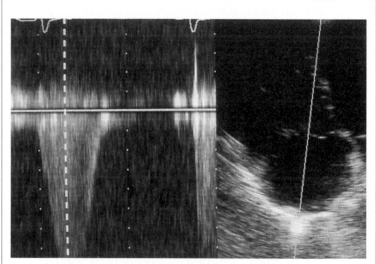

Tricuspid insufficiency in pulmonary hypertension, with regurgitant jet (peak velocity = 3.93 m/s).

CW Doppler recording from apical four-chamber view.

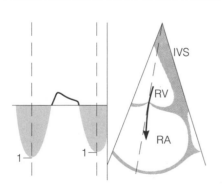

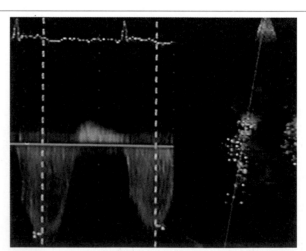

Calculation of right ventricular systolic pressure for two different intervals, based on the peak instantaneous velocity of the tricuspid regurgitant jet. The pressure fluctuates from 70 to 90 mmHg with basic rhythm of atrial fibrillation. The estimated right atrial pressure must also be added.

CW Doppler recording and apical four-chamber 2-D echocardiogram, with color flow imaging. Calculation of pulmonary artery pressure for two different systolic intervals in patient with atrial fibrillation.

Calculation of Systolic Right Ventricular Pressure

Color flow mapping of transtricuspid flow to confirm or exclude the presence of a regurgitant jet can be performed from either the apical four-chamber or the parasternal short-axis view. The peak flow velocity of the regurgitant jet is used to calculate the right ventricular systolic pressure with the modified Bernoulli equation of Hatle and Anderson:

$$RVSP = 4\ v^2$$

After the right atrial pressure has been estimated with the help of the jugular vein pulse or according to inspiratory collapse of the inferior vena cava, the systolic pulmonary artery pressure can be determined as follows:

$$PASP = RVSP = DP\ (4v^2) + RAP_e$$

PASP	Pulmonary artery systolic pressure
RVSP	Right ventricular systolic pressure
DP	Maximum pressure gradient across the tricuspid valve
RAP_e	Estimated atrial pressure

Calculation of Diastolic Right Ventricular Pressure

First the right ventricular outflow tract is visualized in the parasternal short-axis view. The flow velocity of the regurgitant jet measured across the pulmonary valve is converted to the end-diastolic transvalvular pressure gradient using the modified Bernoulli equation.

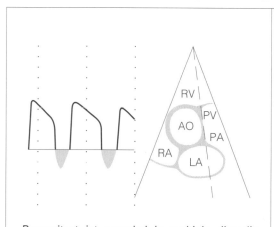

Regurgitant jet recorded in multiple diastolic intervals in patient with pulmonary insufficiency.

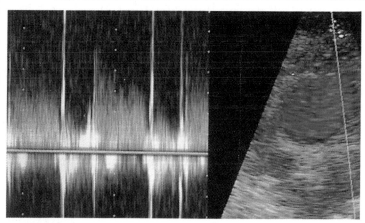

Color coded parasternal short-axis view. CW Doppler.

The pressure gradients calculated according to this method correlated very well with the diastolic right ventricular pressure and diastolic pulmonary artery pressure. The peak regurgitant jet velocity at the onset of diastole correlated well with the mean pulmonary artery pressure. The pulmonary artery pressure can thereby be estimated [15]. One problem with this method of CW Doppler detection of pulmonary regurgitation is positioning the Doppler beam parallel to the regurgitant jet. Also, in patients with severely increased end-diastolic right ventricular pressure, this method tends to underestimate the diastolic pulmonary artery pressure [15].

$$PA\text{-}EDP = 4\ v^2_{ed}$$

PA-EDP	Pulmonary artery end-diastolic pressure
V_{ed}	End-diastolic velocity of the pulmonary regurgitant jet

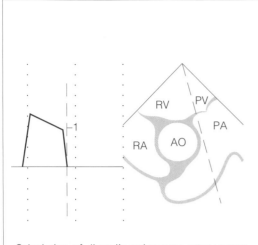

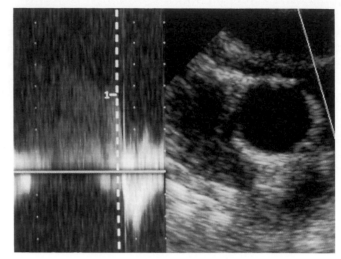

Calculation of diastolic pulmonary artery pressure using the end-diastolic velocity of the regurgitant jet across the pulmonary valve.

CW Doppler recording from parasternal SAX scan.

Estimation of Right Atrial Pressure

Flow in the inferior vena cava is dependent on right atrial pressure and respiration. In order to estimate the right atrial pressure, the inferior vena cava is scanned 2 cm proximal to its site of entry in the atrium. The diameter of the inferior vena cava is measured at resting respiration and at maximum inspiration. When the inferior vena cava collapses by more than 40% at maximum inspiration, the right atrial pressure is estimated to be 5 mmHg. It is estimated to be 10 mmHg when it collapses by less than 40%.

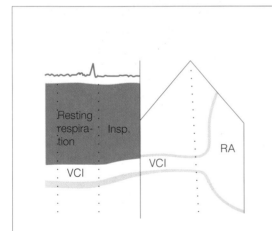

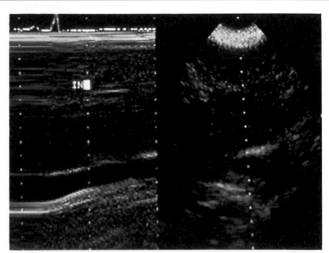

Entry of the inferior vena cava (VCI) in the right atrium (RA). The diameter of the VCI is measured 2 cm before its site of entry in the RA at resting respiration and at maximum inspiration.

M-mode and 2-D echo. Diameter of the VCI at resting respiration and maximum inspiration.

Improved Sensitivity with Echo Contrast Agents

Echo contrast agents significantly enhance the CW Doppler signal and improve visualization of the regurgitant jet across the tricuspid valve. The sensitivity of the technique is thereby increased to 80 to 90 %. In patients with chronic obstructive respiratory tract disease who exhibit normal pressure relationships at rest, contrast-enhanced Doppler exercise echocardiography is able to reveal "latent" pulmonary hypertension [9, 11].

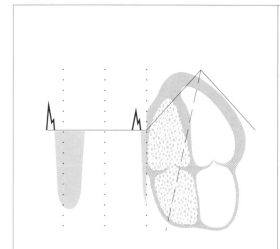

Enhancement of the CW Doppler recording of the tricuspid regurgitant jet by use of echo contrast agent.

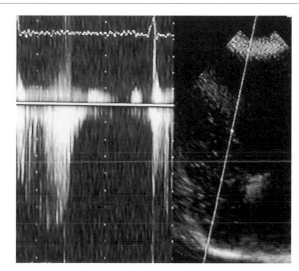

CW Doppler recording from apical four-chamber scan in systole.

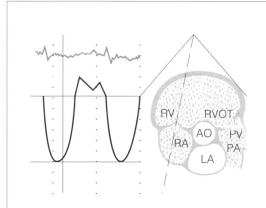

Calculation of RV systolic pressure using the peak instantaneous tricuspid regurgitant jet velocity after administration of echo contrast agent. The estimated right atrial pressure must also be added.

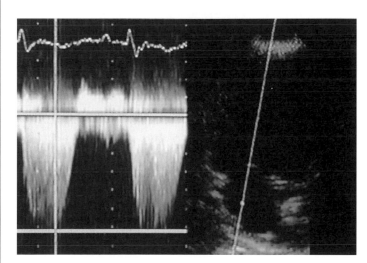

Parasternal short-axis view. CW Doppler.

Three-dimensional reconstruction may one day facilitate the detection of regurgitant jets. Intravascular ultrasound techniques and Doppler catheters can also be expected to improve the diagnosis of pulmonary hypertension. The former method may permit direct echocardiographic visualization of the proximal pulmonary circulation, and the latter may permit quantitative assessment via flow measurements in the proximal pulmonary vascular tree.

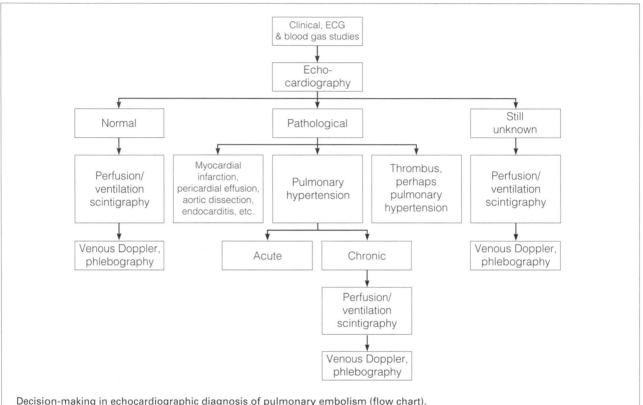

Decision-making in echocardiographic diagnosis of pulmonary embolism (flow chart).
Reprinted with permission from: H. Hoffmann, T. Meinertz, W. Kaper, A. Geibel, H Just: Echokardiographie in der Diagnostik der Lungenembolie. Dtsch Med Wochenschr, 1992; 117: 21f.

Echocardiographic Criteria		
Pulmonary Hypertension		Right Ventricular Myocardial Infarction
Acute	Chronic	
RVEDD* > 30 mm or > 16 mm/m^2 or RV > LV** IVS paradoxical motion Δ IVC$_{insp}$ < 40 % v$_{max\text{-}TR}$ > 2.8 m/s AT$_{PA}$ < 90 ms RPA < 12 mm/m^2 RV wall motion abnormality	RVAW-EDD* > 5 mm or > 16 mm/m^2 v$_{max\text{-}TR}$ > 3.8 m/s RV normo- or hyperkinesis v$_{max, PR}$ > 1.6 m/s	RV wall motion abnormality RVEDD* > 30 mm or > 16 mm/m^2 or RV > LV** RPA < 12 mm/m^2 v$_{max\text{-}TR}$ > 2.8 m/s
M-mode, parasternal long-axis view, left lateral position at end expiration **2-D echocardiography, apical four-chamber view		

Echocardiographic differential diagnosis.
Reprinted with permission from: H. Hoffmann, T. Meinertz, W. Kaper, A. Geibel, H Just: Echokardiographie in der Diagnostik der Lungenembolie. Dtsch Med Wochenschr, 1992; 117: 21f.

1. Aglio VD, Nicolosi GL, Zanuttini D: Transthoracic and transoesophageal echocardiography documentation of disappearance of massive right atrial and pulmonary artery thrombemboli after fibrinolytic therapy and normalization of left ventricular dimensions and function. Eur Heart J 1990; 11: 863-865.
2. Bommer W, Weinert L, Newmann A, Neef J, Mason DT, DeMaria A: Determination of right atrial and right ventricular size by two dimensional echocardiography. Circulation 1979; 60: 91-100.
3. Brockmann M, Müller KM: Morphologie des Cor pulmonale und der pulmonalen Hypertension: Atemw-Lungenkrkh 1990; 11: 523-529.
4. Come PC, Kim D, Parker A, Goldhaber S, Braunwald E, Markis J: Early reversal of right ventricular dysfunction in patients with acute pulmonary embolism after treatment with intravenous tissue plasminogen activator. J Am Coll Cardiol 1987; 10: 971-978.
5. Dabestani A, Mahan G, Gardin J M, Takenaka K, Burn C, Allfie A, Henry WL: Evaluation of pulmonary artery pressure and resistance by pulsed Doppler echocardiography. Am J Cardiol 1987; 59: 662-668.
6. Dittrich HC, Chow LC, Nikod PH: Early improvement in left ventricular diastolic function after relief of chronic right ventricular pressure overload. Circulation 1989; 80: 823-830.
7. Ferrazza A, Marino B, Giusti V, Affiniy V, Ragnose P: Usefulness of left and right oblique subcostal view in the echo-Doppler investigation of pulmonary arterial blood flow in patients with chronic obstructive pulmonary disease. Chest 1990; 98: 286-289.
8. Foale R, Nihoyannonpoulus P, McKenna W, Klienebenne A, Nadazdin A, Rowland E, Smith G: Echocardiographic measurement of the normal adult right ventricle. Br Heart J 1986; 56: 33-44.
9. Himelman RB, Abott JA, Lee E, Schiller NB,Dean NC, Stulbarg MS: Doppler echocardiography and ultrafast cine computed tomography during dynamic exercise in chronic parenchymal pulmonary disease: Am J Cardiol 1989; 64: 528-533.
10. Himelman RB, Struve SN, Brown JK, Nammum P Schiller NB: Improved recognition of cor pulmonale in patients with severe chronic pulmonary disease. Am J Med; 84: 891-898.
11. Himelman RB, Stulbarg M, Kircher, Lee E, Kee L, Ean NC, Golden J, Christopher LW, Schiller NB: Noninvasive evaluation of pulmonary artery pressure during exercise by saline-enhanced Doppler echocardiography in chronic pulmonary disease. Circulation 1988; 79: 863-871.
12. Hofmann H, Meinertz T, Kaper W, Geibel A, Just H: Echokardiografie in der Diagnostik der Lungenarterienembolie. Dtsch Med Wschr 1992; 117: 21-26.
13. Laaban JP, Dibold B, Zelinski R, Lafay M, Raffoul H, Rochemoure J: Noninvasive estimation of systolic pulmonary artery pressure using Doppler echocardiography in patients with chronic obstructive pulmonary disease. Chest 1989, 6: 1258 1262.
14. Marchandise B, Bruyne B, Delanois L, Kremer R: Noninvasive prediction of pulmonary hypertension in chronic obstructive pulmonary disease by Doppler echocardiography. Chest 1987; 3: 361-365.
15. Masuyama T, Kodama K, Kitabatake A, Sato H, Nanto S, Inque M: Continuous wave echocardiographic detection of pulmonary regurgitation and its appplication to noninvasive estimation of pulmonary artery pressure. Circulation 1986; 74: 484-492.
16. Matsuda M, Sekiguchi T, Sugishita Y, Kuwako K, Ilda K, Ito I: Reliability of noninvasive estimates of pulmonary hypertension by pulsed Doppler echocardiography. Br Heart J 1986; 56:158-64.
17. Migueres M, Escamilla R, Cocu F, Didier A, Krempf M: Pulsed Doppler echocardiography in the diagnosis of pulmonary Hypertension in chronic obstructive pulmonary disease. Chest 1990; 98: 280-285.
18. Mopurgo M, Denolin H, Jezek V: Noninvasive assessment of pulmonary arterial hypertension in chronic lung disease: Why and how? Eur Heart J 1987; 8: 564-568.
19. Pennestri F, Loperfido F Salvatori MP: Assessment of tricuspid regurgitation by pulsed Doppler ultrasonography of the hepatic veins. Am J Cardiol 1984; 54: 363-368.
20. Riedel M, Rudolph W: Hämodynamik und Gasaustausch bei akuter Lungenarterienembolie. Herz 1989; 14: 109-114.
21. Sakai K, Nakamura K, Satomi G, Kondo M, Hirosawa K: Evaluation of tricuspid regurgitation by blood flow pattern in the hepatic vein using pulsed Doppler technique. Am Heart J 1984; 108: 516-523.
22. Schnittger I, Gordon EP, Fitzgerald PJ, Popp RL: Standardized intracardiac measurements of two dimensional echocardiography. J Am Coll Cardiol 1983; 2: 934-938.
23. Schulte HD: Lungearterienembolie. Chirurgische Aspekte. Dtsch Ärztebl 1979; 76: 85.
24. Starling MR, Crawford MN, Sorensen SG, Rourke RA. A new two dimensional echocardiographic technique for evalution of right ventricular size and performance in patients with obstructive lung disease. Circulation 1982; 66: 612-620.
25. Torbicki a, Skwarski K, Hawrylkiewicz I, Pasierski T, Miskiewicz Z, Zielinski J: Attempts at measuring pulmonary arterial pressure by means of Doppler echocardiography in patients with chronic lung disease. Eur Respir J 1989; 2: 856-860.
26. Tramarin R, Torbicki A, Marchandise B, Laaban JP, Morpurgo M: Doppler echocardiographic evaluation of pulmonary artery pressure in chronic obstructive pulmonoary disease: A European Heart Journal multicentre study. Eur Heart J 1991; 12: 103-111.
27. Vogel M, Weil J, Stern H, Bühlmeyer K: Responsiveness of raised pulmonary vascular resistance to oxygen by pulsed Doppler echocardiography. Br Heart J 1991; 66: 277-280.

28. Watanabe T, Katsume H, Matsukobo H, furukawa K, Ijichi H. Estimation of right ventricular volume with two dimensional echocardiography. Am J Cardiol 1982; 50: 1360-1375.

29. Weitzenblum E, Hirt C, Ducolone A, Mirhom R, Rasaholinjanahary J, Ehrhart M: Prognostic value of pulmonary artery pressure in chronic obstructive pulmonary disease. Thorax 1981; 36: 752-758.

30. Yagi H, Yamada H, Kobayashi T, Sekiguchi M: Doppler assessment of pulmonary hypertension induced by breathing in subjects susceptible to high altitude pulmonary edema. Am Rev Respir Dis 1990, 142: 796-801.

31. Yock PG, Naasz C, Schnittger I, Popp RL: Doppler tricuspid and pulmonic regurgitation in normals: is it real? Circulation 1984, 70: 40.

Echocardiography is an invaluable tool for helping surgeons and anesthesiologists make appropriate clinical decisions in the day-to-day management of patients with forms of cardiovascular disease. Transthoracic and transesophageal echocardiography are rapidly advancing diagnostic imaging techniques the provide clinicians with exact anatomic and hemodynamic information. Transthoracic echocardiography remains the procedure of choice in the assessment of valvular, pericardial and myocardial disease. Guidelines have been established for the timing of surgery in valvular heart disease and prosthetic valve dysfunction. Transesophageal echocardiography has been extremely valuable in evaluating the mitral valve, prosthetic valves, complications of endocarditis, and aortic dissection. Doppler echocardiography is useful to delineate constrictive and tamponade physiology and all of the complications of myocardial infarction. In this chapter, we will discuss how both transesophageal and transthoracic echocardiographic procedures contribute to definitive surgical treatment of various forms of cardiovascular disease.

21.1	**Native Valves**
21.1.1	**Mitral Stenosis**

Critical mitral stenosis is defined as a valve area of less than 1.0 cm². The correlation of echocardiography and catheterization findings with mean mitral valve gradients (r=0.97) and mitral valve area (r=0.92) is extremely reliable for assessing the degree of stenosis [47]. Echocardiography is particularly useful in determining a patient's suitability for commissurotomy. Those patients with extensive calcification of the valvular or subvalvular apparatus and/or significant mitral regurgitation, for example, are not good candidates for valve repair.

Echocardiography is also helpful in diagnosing associated and coexistent conditions such as atrial septal defect and aortic and tricuspid valve pathology [6]. It has been suggested that, in young patients with pure mitral stenosis, preoperative cardiac catheterization may not be necessary [47]. Transesophageal echocardiography is accurate for assessing the presence of left atrial and left atrial appendage thrombi [5], which may prompt further surgical intervention such as appendage clipping or thrombectomy. These procedures are not routinely performed at our institution.

21.1	**Native Valves**
21.1.2	**Mitral Regurgitation**

Transthoracic echocardiography has been shown to be useful in the semiquantitation of mitral regurgitation.

The timing of surgery in asymptomatic patients with severe mitral regurgitation is when the ejection fraction is greater than 50%, the end-systolic diameter is less than 2.6 cm/m², and the end-diastolic diameter is greater than 75 mm [6, 60].

A recently published report [17] on the determinants of survival and left ventricular performance after mitral valve replacement listed the following factors as poor predictors of operative outcome: ejection fraction $\leq$ 50%, mean pulmonary artery pressure > 20 mmHg, and end-systolic volume > 50 ml/m^2.

Transesophageal echocardiography is routinely used at our institution during mitral valve repair to assess both the adequacy of repair and left ventricular function.

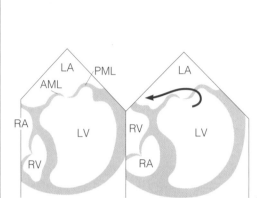

Preoperative transesophageal short-axis scans with color flow mapping. Prolapse of both mitral leaflets (left). The posterior leaflet (PML) is prolapsing more than the anterior leaflet (AML). Eccentric mitral regurgitation (MR) (right). LA = left atrium; LV = left ventricle.

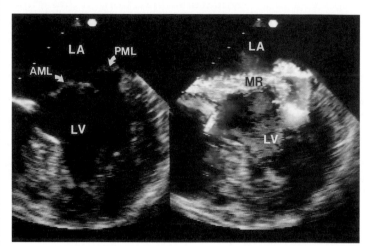

Preoperative transesophageal short-axis 2-D echocardiograms.

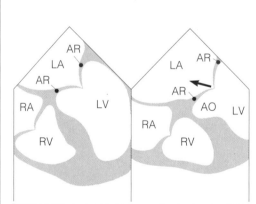

Postoperative transesophageal short-axis 2-D echocardiograms with color flow mapping. Annuloplasty (left). Right panel shows trivial residual mitral regurgitation (MR). LA = left atrium; LV = left ventricle; AR = annuloplasty ring.

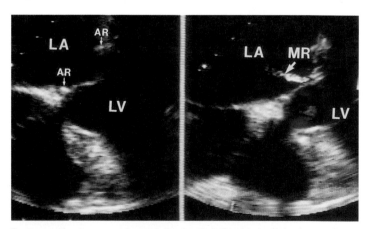

Postoperative transesophageal short-axis 2-D echocardiograms.

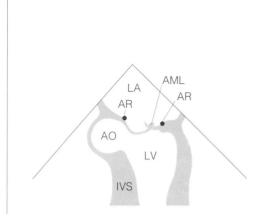

The patient was readmitted with profound hemolysis two months after mitral valve repair. Note buckling of the mitral leaflet against the annuloplasty ring. See p. 776 for abbreviations.

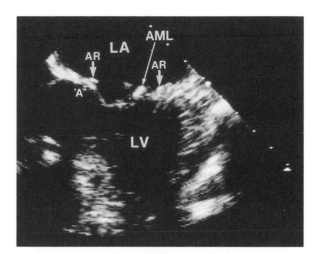

Transesophageal short-axis 2-D echocardiogram.

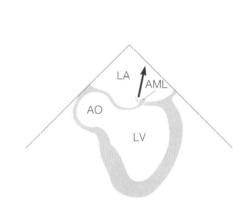

Same patient. The echocardiogram illustrates 2+ mitral regurgitation originating from the site of abnormal anterior leaflet motion. See p. 776 for abbreviations.

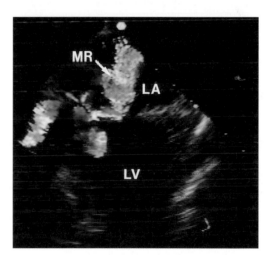

Color flow map of transesophageal short-axis 2-D echocardiogram.

Indications for reoperation include residual mitral regurgitation (> 2+) and left ventricular outflow tract obstruction. In patients with significant ischemic mitral regurgitation, moderately depressed left ventricular ejection fraction, and coronary artery disease, the aim of surgery is to improve left ventricular function with revascularization [6]. Transesophageal has been particularly helpful in assessing for the need for annuloplasty at the time of bypass surgery. In patients with acute mitral regurgitation, transesophageal echocardiography can reliably establish the etiology (ruptured chordae tendineae, ruptured papillary muscle, vegetation) and allows for preoperative surgical planning.

Critical aortic stenosis is defined as an orifice area of less than 0.75 cm^2. Cardiac catheterization traditionally measures the peak-to-peak gradient, whereas echocardiography measures the instantaneous peak gradient, which is often 10 to 15 mmHg higher [8, 76]. Calculation of the aortic valve area by the continuity equation, however, yields extremely accurate results [3, 69]. The agreement between the two methods in determining critical versus noncritical aortic stenosis is 98% [76]. Heavily calcified aortic valves are often challenging, and sometimes impossible, to cross during catheterization. Furthermore, in an unstable patient with critical aortic stenosis, it may be prudent to simply perform coronary angiography and utilize the echographic data with respect to the severity of the stenosis and assessment of left ventricular function.

Finally, asymptomatic patients with moderate or severe aortic stenosis may be followed clinically and echocardiographically to determine the appropriate timing for surgery.

| 21.1 | Native Valves |
| 21.1.4 | Aortic Insufficiency |

Surgery is indicated in patients with severe, symptomatic aortic insufficiency. Because echocardiography combines all the modalities of conventional and Doppler ultrasound-assisted procedures [28, 43, 44, 54, 58, 73, 74], it is a sensitive tool not only in assessing the severity of aortic insufficiency, but also in documenting other associated lesions (*i.e.* bicuspid aortic valve, aortic root disease, coarctation of the aorta, endocarditis, ventricular septal defect) [6]. The management of asymptomatic patients with severe aortic insufficiency, on the other hand, is less straightforward. Echocardiographic indices have proven useful in following patients with this condition for appropriate timing of surgery. The likelihood of developing complications (symptoms, left ventricular dysfunction, death) can be predicted by following left ventricular end-systolic and diastolic dimensions. The ejection fraction, fractional shortening, or both, have also been used as a guideline for timing of surgery. Predictors of good postoperative outcome include end-systolic diameter ≤ 55 mm, end-diastolic diameter ≤ 70 mm, ejection fraction > 50%, and short duration of symptoms [6, 9, 26, 32, 33].

| 21.1 | Native Valves |
| 21.1.5 | Tricuspid Valve Disease |

Echocardiography is the most useful diagnostic procedure for determining the presence and severity of tricuspid regurgitation.

Angiography is less useful because of the problems caused by catheter-induced regurgitation. Tricuspid regurgitation is frequently associated with other cardiac lesions (especially mitral stenosis). Tricuspid annuloplasty should probably be undertaken when a patient has mitral stenosis with pulmonary hypertension and significant tricuspid regurgitation. In this situation, preoperative echocardiography is helpful in planning surgery.

Doppler echocardiography is an excellent procedure for assessing prosthetic valve dysfunction. Since gradients and valve areas have been established for most biological and mechanical valves, the diagnosis of valvular obstruction can be made by echocardiography alone [1, 10, 12, 21, 23, 59, 61, 72, 75]. Sudden, severe regurgitation may be induced by crossing most mechanical valves with a catheter. Thus, in older prostheses, coronary angiography may be all that it is necessary to do in the catheterization laboratory. When obstruction is present in a relatively recently implanted valve, cardiac catheterization may not be necessary at all. Transesophageal echocardiography has also aided in identifying thrombus as a mechanism of acute obstruction [22].

Regurgitant prosthetic valves resulting in hemolysis or significant hemodynamic compromise can be demonstrated with good accuracy by transesophageal echocardiography, particularly in the mitral position [2, 39, 50]. Transthoracic echocardiography is helpful in the quantification of prosthetic valve aortic insufficiency and in the delineation of the mechanism of the regurgitation in biologic mitral valves (*i.e.*, torn or flail cusps) [13, 37].

| 21. | State of the Art: The Heart Surgeon's Point of View |
| 21.3 | Hypertrophic Obstructive Cardiomyopathy |

Before the advent of echocardiography, hypertrophic obstructive cardiomyopathy was diagnosed on the basis of typical clinical primary symptoms and angiographic findings. Echocardiography and Doppler presently provide precise assessment of the extent of hypertrophy and the coexistence of unrelated mitral valve anomalies, with the exception of typical systolic anterior motion (SAM) phenomena. The accuracy of echocardiography in documenting intraventricular gradient is also excellent.

Therefore, patients now must not necessarily undergo complicated hemodynamic testing in the catheterization laboratory that was necessary in the past. Coronary angiography and right ventricular pressure alone may provide adequate preoperative information.

| 21. | State of the Art: The Heart Surgeon's Point of View |
| 21.4 | Infective Endocarditis |

The indications for surgery in patients with acute or subacute endocarditis include hemodynamic instability, recurrent embolization, refractory bacteremia, infection with fungal organisms, and possibly prosthetic valve infection and the presence of abscess [36, 45]. Although the diagnosis of endocarditis is based on clinical and bacteriological findings, both transesophageal and transthoracic echocardiography can clearly define the size, extent, and mobility of vegetations, the presence of abscess (aortic root and mitral annular), and the severity of hemodynamic complications [18, 23, 25, 48, 68, 71]. The young ill patient with acute endocarditis requiring surgery can undergo the procedure based on the echocardiographic data alone. In the older patient with several risk factors, coronary angiography is indicated prior to surgery.

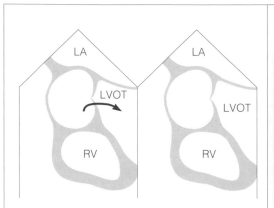

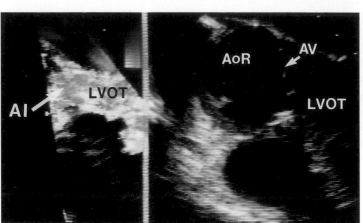

Short-axis view at the level of the aortic valve (AV) and left ventricular outflow tract (LVOT) in a patient with infective endocarditis (right panel). Severe aortic insufficiency (AI) can be seen in the left panel. AoR = aortic root.

Color flow map of transesophageal short-axis 2-D echocardiogram.

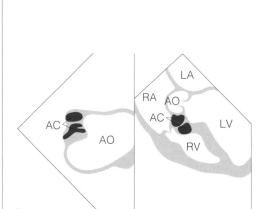

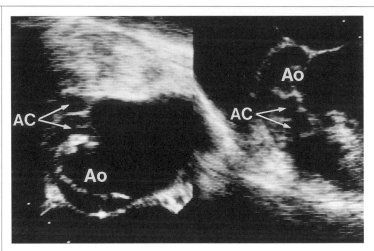

Same patient. Transesophageal short-axis view (right) illustrates an abscess cavity (AC) in the region of the right coronary sinus. Transesophageal long-axis view (left) illustrates the same abscess cavity. Ao = aorta.

Split-screen display of transesophageal 2-D echocardiograms.

21.   **State of the Art: The Heart Surgeon's Point of View**
21.5   **Ischemic Heart Disease**

In the setting of acute myocardial infarction, echocardiography is not only helpful in assessing the extent of myocardial damage, but also allows for prognostication and may guide the clinician to more aggressive intervention [7, 19, 35, 53, 56].

Surgical complications of acute myocardial infarction are detected with excellent accuracy. These include left ventricular aneurysm and pseudoaneurysm [62, 63], acute mitral regurgitation secondary to torn chordae tendineae or papillary muscle rupture [16, 52, 57, 70], and ventricular septal defect [20, 29, 46, 66, 67]. Most of these conditions require emergency surgery and, in such cases, echocardiography provides rapid, safe anatomic and hemodynamic information for preoperative planning. For all of these conditions coronary angiography may be the only diagnostic procedure necessary prior to surgery.

Pericardial effusion is common following open heart surgery. Most cases of pericardial effusion do not result in hemodynamic compromise.

Two-dimensional and Doppler echocardiography facilitate the assessment of pericardial tamponade and will guide the cardiologist to perform pericardiocentesis or the surgeon to perform pericardial windowing, depending upon the clinical scenario [64].

Doppler echocardiography additionally helps to differentiate pericardial constriction from restriction [3, 11, 15, 24, 27, 31, 34, 41, 55]. The Doppler signs of constrictive physiology disappear following successful pericardiectomy and, in fact, may be a predictor of which patients will benefit from the procedure.

21.   State of the Art: The Heart Surgeon's Point of View
21.7   Aortic Dissection

A high mortality is associated with ascending aortic dissection early after patients present with the condition. Therefore, rapid diagnosis of this condition is essential [40]. In the acute phase of dissection, the surgeon needs to differentiate between the common sites of origin and extent of the lesion.

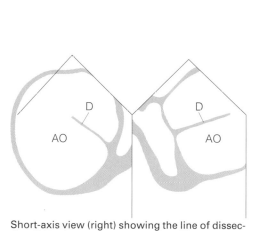

Short-axis view (right) showing the line of dissection (D) in the proximal aortic root. The long-axis view (left) shows the origin of the dissection in the proximal aorta just beyond the aortic valve. AO = aorta.

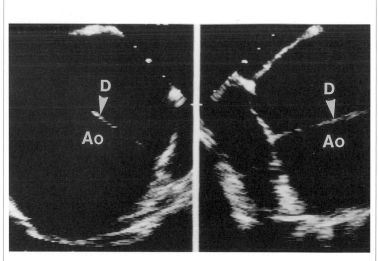

Transesophageal long and short-axis 2-D echocardiograms.

In Type A dissection, which begins just above the coronary orifices, involvement of the aortic valve is common, and the probability of rupture with fatal hemopericardium is high. Type A dissections are therefore an indication for emergency or immediate surgery. Type B dissection, which begins at the aortic isthmus and involves the descending thoracic aorta, may not require operation and often can be managed conservatively.

Transesophageal echocardiography is recognized as a sensitive, rapid and safe screening test for the diagnosis of aortic dissection and provides most of the information the surgeon needs to know preoperatively [4, 14, 42]. Transesophageal echocardiography provides the most practical means of defining the anatomic location of acute aortic dissection. The sensitivity of this technique for assessment of the ascending aorta compared with other segments of the aorta, however, is reportedly lower [51].

| 21. | State of the Art: The Heart Surgeon's Point of View |
| 21.8 | Cardiac Masses |

Two-dimensional echocardiography has been very useful in detecting cardiac masses. Left atrial myxoma, the most common cardiac tumor, is a pedunculated mobile mass attached to the interarterial septum, often prolapsing across the mitral valve.

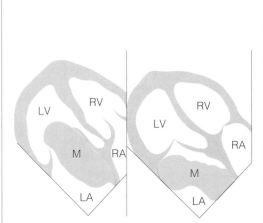

The left panel demonstrates a left atrial myxoma (M) prolapsing across the mitral valve during diastole. The right panel shows the myxoma in the left atrium (LA) during systole. LV = left ventricle.

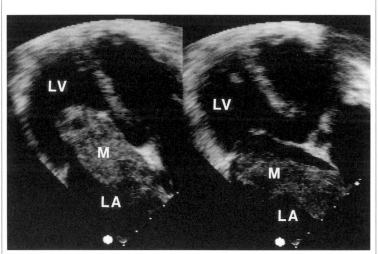

Transesophageal short-axis 2-D echocardiograms; diastole and systole.

Less common sites of tumor involvement that are also easily detected by echocardiography are the right atrium, mitral valve, and left ventricle. Two-dimensional echocardiography allows effective follow-up of patients with recurrent disease, especially those with familial-type tumors.

Transesophageal echocardiography may help to delineate the extent of tumor involvement, particularly in the cases of malignant or metastatic masses [49]. Transesophageal echocardiography has also been used successfully at our institution for intraoperative assessment of the adequacy of tumor debridement.

Transesophageal echocardiography has become a very useful adjunct in the operating room. In a large study by Scheik et al. [65], transesophageal echocardiography modified surgery in 19% of cases, 10% of which were of major significance.

After bypass surgery, the primary utility of transesophageal echocardiography is to assess the adequacy of mitral valve repair and left ventricular function. With respect to valve repair, a repeat operation was performed in 10% of all patients for residual mitral regurgitation, left ventricular outflow tract obstruction, or residual stenosis following commissurotomy [65]. Postoperative left ventricular dysfunction occurred in 9 to 30% of patients and was a predictor of poor outcome (postoperative congestive heart failure and death) [65]. Transesophageal echocardiography is also effective in perioperative hemodynamic management of patients. In a study by Ballal et al. [4], 3.1% of patients undergoing valve surgery required repeat cardiopulmonary bypass to correct problems detected by transesophageal echocardiography, including suture dehiscence, residual regurgitation, aortic dissection, thrombus, and iatrogenic ventricular septal defect.

References

1. Alam M, Rosman HS, Lakier JB, Kemp S, Khaja F, Hautamaki K, Magilligan DJ Jr, Stein PD. Doppler and echocardiographic features of normal and dysfunctioning bioprosthetic valves. J Am Coll Cardiol 1987; 10: 851-858.
2. Alam M, Rosman HS, McBroom D, Graham L, Magilligan DJ Jr, Khaja F, Stein PD. Color flow Doppler evaluation of St. Jude Medical prosthetic valves. Am J Cardiol 1989; 64: 1387-1389.
3. Appleton CP, Hatle LK, Popp RL. Cardiac tamponade and pericardial effusion: respiratory variation in transvalvular flow velocities studied by Doppler echocardiography. J Am Coll Cardiol 1988; 11: 1020-1030.
4. Ballal RS, Nanda NC, Jain H, Sanyal RS, Helmcke F, Samdarshi TE, Pizzano N. Second run bypass based on intraoperative transesophageal echocardiography: avoidance of unfavorable outcome. Circulation 1991; 84 (suppl II): II-130.
5. Bansal RC, Shah PM. Transesophageal echocardiography. Curr Probl Cardiol 1990; 15: 641-720.
6. Bansal RC, Shah PM. Usefulness of echo-Doppler in management of patients with valvular heart disease. Curr Probl Cardiol 1989; 14: 281-350.
7. Barzilai B, Gessler C Jr., Perez JE, Schaab C, Jaffe AS. Significance of Doppler-detected mitral regurgitation in acute myocardial infarction. Am J Cardio 1988; 61: 220-223.
8. Berger M, Berdoff R, Gallerstein P, Goldberg E. Evaluation of aortic stenosis by continuous wave Doppler ultrasound. J Am Coll Cardiol 1984; 3: 150-156.
9. Bonow RO, Rosing DR, Maron BJ, McIntosh CL, Jones M, Bacharach SL, Green MV, Clark RE, Epstein SE. Reversal of left ventricular dysfunction after aortic valve replacement for chronic aortic regurgitation: influence of duration on preoperative left ventricular dysfunction. Circulation 1984; 70: 570-579.
10. Burstow DJ, Nishimura RA, Bailey KR, Reeder GS, Holmes DR Jr, Seward JB, Tajik AJ. Continuous wave Doppler echocardiographic measurement of prosthetic valve gradients: a simultaneous Doppler-catheter correlative study. Circulation 1989; 80: 504-514.
11. Burstow DJ, Oh JK, Bailey KR, Seward JB, Tajik AJ. Cardiac tamponade: characteristic Doppler observations. Mayo Clin Proc 1989; 64: 312-324.
12. Chafizadeh ER, Zoghbi WA. Doppler echocardiographic assessment of the St. Jude Medical prosthetic valve in the aortic position using the continuity equation. Circulation 1991; 83: 213-223.
13. Chambers JB, Monaghan MJ, Jackson G, Jewitt DE. Doppler echocardiographic appearance of cusp tears in tissue valve prostheses. J Am Coll Cardiol 1987; 10: 462-466.
14. Chandrasekaran K, Currie PJ. Transesophageal echocardiography in aortic dissection. Journal of Invasive Cardiology 1989; 1: 6.
15. Chuttani K, Pandian NG, Mohanty PK, Rosenfield K, Schwartz SL, Udelson JE, Simonetti J, Kusay BS, Caldeira ME. Left ventricular diastolic collapse: an echocardiographic sign of regional cardiac tamponade. Circulation 1991; 83: 1999-2006.
16. Come PC, Riley MF, Weintraub R, Morgan JP, Nakao S. Echocardiography detection of complete and partial papillary muscle rupture during acute myocardial infarction. Am J Cardiol 1985; 56: 787-789.
17. Crawford MH, Soucheck J, Oprian CA, Miller DC, Rahimtoola S, Giacomini JC, Sethi G, Hammermeister KE. Determinants of survival and left ventricular performance after mitral valve replacement. Department of Veterans' Affairs Cooperative Study on Valvular Heart Disease. Circulation 1990; 81: 1173-1181.

18. Daniel WG, Muegge A, Martin RP, Lindert O, Hausmann D, Nonnast-Daniel B, Laas J, Lichtlen PR. Improvement in the diagnosis of abscesses associated with endocarditis by transesophageal echocardiography. N Engl J Med 1991; 324: 795-800.

19. De Servi S, Vaccari L, Assandri J. Clinical significance of mitral regurgitation in patients with recent myocardial infarction. Europ Heart J 1988; 9 (suppl F): 5-9.

20. Drobac M, Gilbert B, Howard R, Baigrie R, Rakowski H. Ventricular septal defect after myocardial infarction: diagnosis by two-dimensional contrast echocardiography. Circulation 1983; 67: 335-341.

21. Dumesnil JG, Honos GN, Lemieux M, Beauchemin J. Validation and applications of indexed aortic prosthetic valve areas calculated by Doppler echocardiography. J Am Coll Cardiol 1990; 16; 637-643.

22. Dzavik V, Cohen G, Chan KL. Role of transesophageal echocardiography in the diagnosis and management of prosthetic valve thrombosis. J Am Coll Cardiol 1991; 18: 1829-1833.

23. Effron MK, Popp RL. Two-dimensional echocardiographic assessment of bioprosthetic valve dysfunction and infective endocarditis. J Am Coll Cardiol 1983; 2: 597-606.

24. Eisenberg MJ, Schiller NB. Bayes' theorem and the echocardiographic diagnosis of cardiac tamponade. Am J Cardiol 1991; 68: 1242-1244.

25. Erbel R, Rohmann S, Drexler M, Mohr-Kahaly S, Gerharz CD, Iversen S, Oelert H, Meyer J. Improved diagnostic value of echocardiography in patients with infective endocarditis by transesophageal approach. A prospective study. Europ Heart J 1988; 9: 43-53.

26. Fioretti P, Roelandt J, Bos RJ, Meltzer RS, Van Hoogenhuijze D, Serruys PW, Nauta J, Hugenholtz PG. Echocardiography in chronic aortic insufficiency: Is valve replacement too late when left ventricular end-systolic dimension reaches 55 mm? Circulation 1983; 67: 216-221.

27. Gillam LD, Guyer DE, Gibson TC, King ME, Marshall JE, Weyman AE. Hydrodynamic compression of the right atrium: a new echocardiographic sign of cardiac tamponade. Circulation 1983; 68: 294-301.

28. Griffin BP, Flachskampf FA, Siu S, Weyman AE, Thomas JD. The effects of regurgitant orifice size, chamber compliance, and systemic vascular resistance on aortic regurgitant velocity slope and pressure half-time. Am Heart J 1991; 122: 1049-1056.

29. Harrison MR, MacPhail B, Gurley JC, Harlamert EA, Steinmetz JE, Smith MD, Demaria AN. Usefulness of color Doppler flow imaging to distinguish ventricular septal defect from acute mitral regurgitation complicating acute myocardial infarction. Am J Cardiol 1989; 64: 697-701.

30. Hatle L, Angelsen BA, Tromsdal A. Non-invasive assessment of aortic stenosis by Doppler ultrasound. Brit Heart J 1980; 43: 284-292.

31. Hatle LK, Appleton CP, Popp RL. Differentiation of constrictive pericarditis and restrictive cardiomyopathy by Doppler echocardiography. Circulation 1989; 79: 357-370.

32. Henry WL, Bonow RO, Boder JS, Ware JH, Kent KM, Redwood DR, McIntosh CL, Morrow AG, Epstein SE. Observations on the optimum time for operative intervention for aortic regurgitation. I. Evaluation of the results of aortic valve replacement in symptomatic patients. Circulation 1980; 61: 471-483.

33. Henry WL, Bonow RO, Rosing DR, Epstein SE. Observations on the optimum time for operative intervention for aortic regurgitation. II. Serial echocardiographic evaluation of asymptomatic patients. Circulation 1980; 61: 484-492.

34. Himelman RB, Kircher B, Rockey DC, Schiller NB. Inferior vena cava plethora with blunted respiratory response: a sensitive echocardiographic sign of cardiac tamponade. J Am Coll Cardiol 1988; 12: 1470-1477.

35. Jaarsma W, Visser CA, Kupper AJ. Usefulness of two-dimensional exercise echocardiography shortly after myocardial infarction. Am J Cardiol 1986; 57: 86-90.

36. Jaffe WM, Morgan DE, Pearlman AS, Otto CM. Infective endocarditis, 1983-1988: echocardiographic findings and factors influencing morbidity and mortality. J Am Coll Cardiol 1990; 15: 1227-1233.

37. Kapur KK, Fan P, Nanda NC, Yoganathan AP, Goyal RG. Doppler color flow mapping in the evaluation of prosthetic mitral and aortic valve function. J Am Coll Cardiol 1989; 13: 1561-1571.

38. Kelly TA, Rothbart RM, Cooper CM, Kaiser DL, Smucker ML, Gibson RS. Comparison of outcome of asymptomatic to symptomatic patients older than 20 years of age with valvular aortic stenosis. Am J Cardiol 1988; 61: 123-130.

39. Khandheria BK, Seward JB, Oh JK, Freeman WK, Nichols BA, Sinak LJ, Miller FA Jr, Tajik AJ. Value and limitations of transesophageal echocardiography in assessment of mitral valve prostheses. Circulation 1991; 83: 1956-1968.

40. Khandheria BK, Tajik AJ, Taylor CL, Safford RE, Miller FA Jr, Stanson AW, Sinak LJ, Oh JK, Seward JB. Aortic dissection: review of value and limitations of two-dimensional echocardiography in a six-year experience. J Am Soc Echocardiogr 1989; 2: 17-24.

41. King SW, Pandian NG, Gardin JM. Doppler echocardiographic findings in pericardial tamponade and constriction. Echocardiography 1988; 5: 361-372.

42. Krozon I, Demopoulos L, Schrem SS, Pasternack P. McCauley D, Freedberg RS. Pitfalls in the diagnosis of thoracic aortic aneurysm by transesophageal echocardiography. J Am Soc Echocardiogr 1990; 3: 145-148.

43. Labovitz AJ, Ferrara RP, Kern MJ, Bryg RJ, Mrosek DG, Williams GA. Quantitative evaluation of aortic insufficiency by continuous wave Doppler echocardiography. J Am Coll Cardiol 1986; 8: 1341-1347.

44. Masuyama T, Kodama K, Kitabatake A, Nanto S, Sato H, Uematsu M, Inoue M, Kamada T. Noninvasive evaluation of aortic regurgitation by continuous wave Doppler echocardiography. Circulation 1986; 73: 460-466.

45. Middlemost S, Wisenbaugh T, Meyerowitz C, Teeger S, Essop R, Skoularigis J, Cronje S, Sareli P. A case for early surgery in native left-sided endocarditis complicated by heart failure: results in 203 patients. J Am Coll Cardiol 1991; 18: 663-667.

46. Miyatake K, Okamoto M, Kinoshita N, Park YD, Nagata S, Izumi S, Fusejima K, Sakakibara H, Nimura Y. Doppler echocardiographic features of ventricular septal rupture in myocardial infarction. J Am Coll Cardiol 1985; 5: 182-187.

47. Motro M, Neufeld H. Should patients with pure mitral stenosis undergo cardiac catheterization? Am J Cardiol 1980; 46: 515-516.

48. Mügge A, Daniel WG, Frank G, Lichtlen PR. Echocardiography in infective endocarditis: reassessment of prognostic implications of vegetation size determined by the transthoracic and the transesophageal approach. J Am Coll Cardiol 1989; 14: 631-638.

49. Mügge A, Daniel WG, Haverich A, Lichtlen PR. Diagnosis of noninfective cardiac mass lesions by two-dimensional echocardiography: comparison of the transthoracic and transesophageal approaches. Circulation 1991; 83: 70-78.

50. Nellessen U, Schnittger I, Appleton CP, Masuyama T, Bolger A, Fischell TA, Tye T, Popp RL. Transesophageal two-dimensional echocardiography and color Doppler flow velocity mapping in the evaluation of cardiac valve prostheses. Circulation 1988; 78: 848-855.

51. Nienaber CA, Spielmann RP, von Kodolitsch Y, Siglow V, Piepho A, Jaup T, Nicolas V, Weber P, Triebel HJ, Bleifeld W. Diagnosis of thoracic aortic dissection: magnetic resonance imaging versus transesophageal echocardiography. Circulation 1992; 85: 434-447.

52. Nishimura RA, Schaff HV, Shub C, Gersh BJ, Edwards WD, Tajik AJ. Papillary muscle rupture complicating acute myocardial infarction: analysis of 17 patients. Am J Cardiol 1983; 51: 373-377.

53. Nishimura RA, Tajik AJ, Shub C, Miller FA, Ilstrup DM, Harrison CE. Role of two-dimensional echocardiography in the prediction of in-hospital complications after acute myocardial infarction. J Am Coll Cardiol 1984; 4: 1080-1087.

54. Oh JK, Hatle LK, Sinak LJ, Seward JB, Tajik AJ. Characteristic Doppler echocardiographic pattern of mitral inflow velocity in severe aortic regurgitation. J Am Coll Cardiol 1989; 14: 1712-1717.

55. Pandian NG, Skorton DJ, Kieso RA, Kerber RE. Diagnosis of constrictive pericarditis by two-dimensional echocardiography: studies in a new experimental model and in patients. J Am Coll Cardiol 1984; 4: 114-173.

56. Parisi AF, Moynihan PR, Folland ED, Strauss WE, Sharma GVRK, Sasahara AA. Echocardiography in acute and remote myocardial infarction. Am J Cardiol 1980; 46: 1205-1214.

57. Patel AM, Miller FA, Khandheria BK, Mullany CJ, Seward JB, Oh JK. Role of transesophageal echocardiography in the diagnosis of papillary muscle rupture secondary to myocardial infarction. Am Heart J 1989; 118: 1330-1333.

58. Perry GJ, Helmcke F, Nanda NC, Byard C, Soto B. Evaluation of aortic insufficiency by Doppler color flow mapping. J Am Coll Cardiol 1987; 9: 952-959.

59. Reisner SA, Meltzer RS, Rochester NT. Normal values of prosthetic valve Doppler echocardiographic parameters: a review. J Am Soc Echocardiogr 1988; 1: 201-210.

60. Ross J. Afterload mismatch in aortic and mitral valve disease: implications for surgical therapy. J Am Coll Cardiol 1985; 5: 811-826.

61. Rothbart RM, Castriz JL, Harding LV, Russo CD, Teague SM. Determination of aortic valve area by two-dimensional and Doppler echocardiography in patients with normal and stenotic bioprosthetic valves. J Am Coll Cardiol 1990; 15: 817-824.

62. Rueda B, Panidis IP, Gonzales R, McDonough M. Left ventricular pseudoaneurysm: detection and postoperative follow-up by color Doppler echocardiography. Am Heart J 1990; 120: 990-992.

63. Saner HE, Asinger RW, Daniel JA, Olson J. Two-dimensional echocardiographic identification of left ventricular pseudoaneurysm. Am Heart J 1986; 112: 977.

64. Schiller NB, Botvinick EH. Right ventricular compression as a sign of cardiac tamponade (an analysis of echocardiographic ventricular dimensions and their clinical implications). Circulation 1977; 56: 774.

65. Sheikh KH, de Bruijn NP, Rankin JS, Clements FM, Stanley T, Wolfe WG, Kisslo J. The utility of transesophageal echocardiography and Doppler color flow imaging in patients undergoing cardiac valve surgery. J Am Coll Cardiol 1990; 15: 363-372.

66. Smyllie J, Dawkins K, Conway N, Sutherland GR. Diagnosis of ventricular septal rupture after myocardial infarction: value of color flow mapping. Brit Heart J 1989; 62: 260-267.

67. Smyllie JH, Sutherland GR, Geuskens R, Dawkins K, Conway N, Roelandt JR. Doppler color flow mapping in the diagnosis of ventricular septal rupture and acute mitral regurgitation after myocardial infarction. J Am Coll Cardiol 1990; 15: 1449-1455.

68. Stafford WJ, Petch J, Radford DJ. Vegetations in infective endocarditis (clinical relevance and diagnosis by cross-sectional echocardiography). Brit Heart J 1985; 53: 310-313.

69. Stamm RB, Martin RP. Quantification of pressure gradients across stenotic valves by Doppler ultrasound. J Am Coll Cardiol 1983; 2: 707-718.

70. Stoddard MF, Keedy DL, Kupersmith J. Transesophageal echocardiographic diagnosis of papillary muscle rupture complicating acute myocardial infarction. Am Heart J 1990; 120: 690-692.

71. Taams MA, Gussenhoven EJ, Bos E, de Jaegere P, Roelandt JR, Sutherland GR, Bom N. Enhanced morphological diagnosis in infective endocarditis by transesophageal echocardiography. Brit Heart J 1990; 63: 109-113.

72. Taams MA, Gussenhoven EJ, Cahalan MK, Roelandt JR, van Herwerden LA, The HK, Bom N, de Jong N. Transesophageal Doppler color flow imaging in the detection of native and Bjork-Shiley mitral valve regurgitation. J Am Coll Cardiol 1989; 13: 95-99.

73. Teague SM, Heinsimer JA, Andersen JL, Sublett K, Olson EG, Voyles WF, Thadani U. Quantification of aortic regurgitation utilizing continuous wave Doppler ultrasound. J Am Coll Cardiol 1986; 8: 592-599.

74. Tribouilloy C, Avinee P, Shen WF, Rey JL, Slama M, Lesbre JP. End diastolic flow velocity just beneath the aortic isthmus assessed by pulsed Doppler echocardiography: a new predictor of the aortic regurgitant fraction. Brit Heart J 1991; 65: 37-40.

75. Wilkins GT, Gillam LD, Kritzer GL, Levine RA, Palacios IG, Weyman AE. Validation of continuous wave Doppler echocardiographic measurements of mitral and tricuspid prosthetic valve gradients: a simultaneous Doppler-catheter study. Circulation 1986; 74: 786-795.

76. Zoghbi WA. Echocardiographic and Doppler ultrasonic evaluation of valvular aortic stenosis. Echocardiography 1988; 5: 23-38.

The continuous development and increasingly widespread use of cardiac ultrasound diagnostic techniques has altered the approach to clinical cardiologic problems. Conventional radiology for cardiac diagnosis has been pushed into the background, and the indication spectrum for nuclear cardiology has shifted from the determination of ejection fraction and perfusion relationships to the study of cardiac metabolism. Cardiac ultrasound diagnosis in conjunction with computer-assisted and interventional techniques has become the fifth pillar of standard cardiac diagnosis, next to patient history evaluation and physical examination, electrocardiographic techniques, electrophysiologic techniques, and catheter-assisted invasive techniques.

On the one hand, cardiac ultrasound diagnosis differs from rival or complementary imaging techniques by providing highly precise measurement data. On the other hand, many echocardiographic findings are worthless or misleading due to limitations of the acoustic windows, lack of skill and experience, and uncritical or incorrect interpretation of images. This is the simple reason why the value of cardiac ultrasound diagnosis is ranked very differently from one department to another. Any cardiosurgery department that has received many correct echocardiographic findings as well as many incorrect ones or findings that deviate significantly from cardiac catheterization data will have a skeptical opinion of echocardiography.

Furthermore, cardiosurgery and anesthesiology residency programs play an anti-progressive role that should not be underestimated. As long as these residencies do not cover even the basics of cardiac ultrasound imaging, heart surgeons will be unable to utilize echocardiographic images with the same skill as cardiac catheterization films. They will be unable to apply the same strict standards to echo findings as to coronary angiograms. In the latter case, the heart surgeon might discover that a particular vessel segment is missing in a particular projection angiogram, or he or she would be able to evaluate collateralization to plan a revascularization strategy, etc.

User training raises the issues of training procedure and quality control. In order to obtain certification in a particular specialty, the resident is usually required to receive supervised training in one department, to complete a specified program of courses, and to protocol and evaluate a specific number of cases. This system has not been able to prevent extreme quality differences in hospitals as well as in private practices. As in all branches of medicine, receiving specialized training in a specific department such as the echocardiography laboratory implies dependence on superiors. They decide on the resident's time of rotation, the timing of his or her examination for certification in the specialty and, thus, the speed of one's career advancement. The established system of courses has largely become a business in which the practice of self-expression and didactic teaching by training physicians closely associated with equipment manufacturers outranks the much more useful practice of practical training in small groups with individualized instruction.

This situation is mirrored by uncertainty with regard to quantitation attempts. However, if we unnecessarily confine ourselves to qualitative assessments, the chance to develop a non-invasive method of quantitative cardiology will be lost.

In order to keep measurement error within a tolerable and calculable range, an established method of quality control is of inestimable value for both novice and experienced laboratory echocardiographers. If a patient's standard measurement values change by more than 20 percent within six months, there must be a good explanation. If a disease-related explanation is not found, the findings should be rejected.

To maintain these standards, examination conditions should be standardized. Furthermore, inter- and intra-observer measurement variability for all members of any echocardiography laboratory should be assessed at the end of the training period and in regular intervals thereafter. This conforms with the established procedures for laboratory quality control.

This means that equipment manufacturers still have to close a large gap between user demands and the reality of resolution. Creating a means for adequate echocardiographic diagnosis and assessment of the notorious emphysema patient or a means of performing orthogonal imaging in unusually located hearts in order to reliably measure end-diastolic and end-systolic left ventricular dimensions would be a far more revolutionary step than making slight improvements in two-dimensional imaging from nonproblematic acoustic windows, developing new ergonometric analytical software, or developing new user philosophies.